Hospital-Associated Infections: Epidemiology, Prevention and Control

Hospital-Associated Infections: Epidemiology, Prevention and Control

SECOND EDITION

Neeta Patwardhan
MD (Microbiology)
Consultant Microbiologist
Department of Microbiology
Kamalnayan Bajaj Hospital and Marathwada Research Institute
Aurangabad, Maharashtra, India

Co-author
Satish Patwardhan
DCP MD (Microbiology)
Consulting Microbiologist
Department of Microbiology
Kamalnayan Bajaj Hospital and Marathwada Reasearch Institute
Aurangabad, Maharashtra, India

Foreword
Mrudula A Phadke

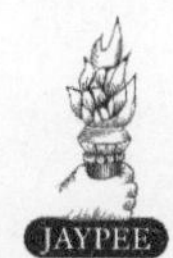

JAYPEE BROTHERS MEDICAL PUBLISHERS
The Health Sciences Publisher
New Delhi | London

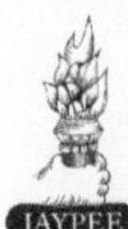

JAYPEE **Jaypee Brothers Medical Publishers (P) Ltd**

Headquarters
EMCA House
23/23-B, Ansari Road, Daryaganj
New Delhi 110 002, India
Landline: +91-11-23272143, +91-11-23272703
+91-11-23282021, +91-11-23245672
E-mail: jaypee@jaypeebrothers.com

Corporate Office
4838/24, Ansari Road, Daryaganj
New Delhi 110 002, India
Phone: +91-11-43574357
Fax: +91-11-43574314
E-mail: jaypee@jaypeebrothers.com

Overseas Office
J.P. Medical Ltd
83 Victoria Street, London
SW1H 0HW (UK)
Phone: +44 20 3170 8910
E-mail: info@jpmedpub.com

EU GPSR Authorised Representative
Logos Europe, 9 rue Nicolas Poussin
17000, La Rochelle, France
Phone: +33 (0) 6 67 93 73 78
E-mail: contact@logoseurope.eu

Website: www.jaypeebrothers.com
Website: www.jaypeedigital.com

Hospital-Associated Infections: Epidemiology, Prevention and Control

First Edition: 2006

Second Edition: 2017

Reprint: **2025**

ISBN 978-93-5270-018-9

Printed in India

Dedicated to

My beloved parents
Late Dr Ramesh Gupte
and
Late Dr (Mrs) Nalini Gupte

And

My beloved in-laws
Late Mr Shripad Patwardhan
and
Late Mrs Sunanda Patwardhan

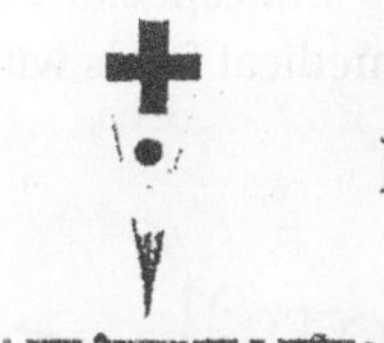

महाराष्ट्र आरोग्य विज्ञान विद्यापीठ, नाशिक
Maharashtra University of Health Sciences, Nashik
म्हसरुळ, दिंडोरी रोड, नाशिक – 422 004 Mhasrul, Dindori Road, Nashik-422 004
Tel (0253) 2531835, Fax: (0253) 2531836 Mumbai (off) Telefax (022) 22653543
Website: www.muhsnashik.com, email: vc@muhsnashik.com / muhsvc@hotmail.com

डॉ. मृदुला अ. फडके
कुलगुरु

Dr. Mrs. Mrudula A. Phadke
MD, DCH, FIAP, MRCP(UK), FRCPCH(U
Vice Chancellor

Foreword

The extent of morbidity and mortality caused by hospital-associated infections (HAIs) has reached an appalling level the world over and the awfully more in the developing countries. Of late, quite a few books have come out emphasizing the urgency of extending the focus of teaching of microbiology from the conventional study of biology of microorganisms to the applicability of clinical microbiology and study of infectious diseases. With a sweeping pace, the medical sciences continue to take strides inventing new methods, newer antibiotics, and newer modes of investigations involving a major role of technology bringing amazing accuracy in diagnosis. The medical science can proudly boast of increasing the average life-span of human beings. This has naturally increased the frequency of being hospitalized and getting discharged in good health. However, this very frequency of being hospitalized has also made us vulnerable to become victims of hospital-associated infections.

While the medical science has acquired a formidable might in battling against most of the dreaded diseases, it seems to have been caught unaware by the fatal emergence of new pathogens through their adaptation and genetic mutations. This is a dreadful threat the treating physicians are confronted with today. An alarm has already been raised by to WHO in this regard. Global haste in resorting to taking preventive means has successfully brought down mortality caused by HAI, especially in the developed countries. However, the underdeveloped and developing countries have to face the burden of dense population and overcrowded public hospitals along with some ignorance about the mortality caused by HAI.

In Indian context, except some sophisticated hospitals in a few big cities, most of the hospitals throughout the country are under the ominous shadow of this threat. Dr Neeta Patwardhan's book is one of the few, which has been written at the right time with right perspective. It is one of those few books that assure us that we are not too late.

I must appreciate Dr Neeta Patwardhan's zeal and passion with which she has laboriously gathered the scattered information from remote sources. This book reflects her rich critical insight and concern with which extensive, in-depth analyses as well as intensive preventive measures are offered to contain HAI and the resultant morbidity and mortality.

I am sure this will prove to be of immense use to the students, teachers and especially to hospitals. This is an essential handbook that should efficiently equip the medical fields with formidable weaponry in its war against the HAI.

Mrudula A Phadke
MD DCH FIAP MRCP (UK) FRCPCH (UK)
Vice-Chancellor
Maharashtra University of Health Sciences
Nashik, Maharashtra, India

Preface to the Second Edition

The first edition of this book had been written about eleven years back as a response to a call that has gone unheeded since unpardonably long. It was a call invoking help as, stalking amidst us, there is a menacingly mighty spectre to ignore which any longer will be suicidal. This spectre that is looming large is the mortality and morbidity caused by hospital-associated infections (HAIs). The prevalence of HAI according to a survey by WHO ranges from 3% to 21%, it is much higher in countries like India that is about 30–50%. Surveillance data is not adequately available from Indian hospitals, besides, lack of awareness and inertia of the hospital staff in cooperation makes surveillance difficult to carry out. Whatever information is available on HAI is not compiled systematically in one book, scattered bits of information can be had from different books most of which are written by authors from different countries and are published from different nooks of the world.

This precisely is the predicament, which triggered in my mind the necessity of writing this book that would collectively offer the scattered information, its analysis and possible remedies for the evil of HAI. And hence this book comes into being with a hope that it would prove itself to be of immense use to everyone in the medical field. Lately, strict rules have been formulated and enforced to ensure monitoring of hospitals, regarding disinfection of operation theaters, testing the efficiency of autoclaves, monitoring device-associated infection rates, monitoring outbreaks of infection in the hospital and so many other aspects related to HAIs. With this, more and more books on HAI are coming into the market. The Center for Disease Control (CDC) also has been updating guidelines related to these topics. So the necessity for updating the book and bringing out the second edition came to my mind, with a hope that this book would then be of immense use to everyone in the medical field. I hope this book will be of wide help to hospitals run by government institutions as well as to private hospitals.

I have taken efforts to ensure that this book encompasses all theoretical and practical aspects of HAI. It includes practical aspects of surgical site infections, hospital-acquired urinary tract infections, intravascular catheter-associated infections, ventilator-associated pneumonia, etc. Also, it deals with postexposure prophylaxis for hepatitis B vaccine (HBV) and human immunodeficiency virus (HIV) infections, and monitoring of HBV infections in the dialysis units. In addition, it attempts to deal in details with waste disposal, use of prophylactic antibiotics in hospitals, infections in intensive care units (ICUs), hospital infections associated with every department including kitchen, laundry and monitoring of operation theaters (OT). Collecting OT swabs for testing OT surfaces is deemed outdated today for routine purposes. However, except in extremely sophisticated operation theaters of hospitals in big cities, these conventional methods continue to be in practice; and, therefore, they have been given a deserving inclusion in this book. New chapters like 'Central Sterile Supply Department (CSSD)', 'Antibiotic Policy' and 'Infection Control in Cardiac Catheterization Units' have been introduced in the second edition. So also almost all chapters have been updated according to the latest guidelines.

In nutshell, I have tried to make all information, analysis and remedies related to hospital-associated infections, available in one single book so as to facilitate a possible organized countering of evils caused by HAIs. This book is based on all information heeded by me during my tenure as 'Hospital Infection Control In-Charge' in the Government Medical College and then as a Consultant Microbiologist and 'Hospital Infection Control In-Charge' in a tertiary care multispecialty hospital and on my painstakingly assembled information collected from far flung and scattered sources.

The arch impulse behind writing this book is to facilitate an effective management that will tame down the beast of hospital-associated infections and minimize the resultant mortality and morbidity mainly in the Indian context.

May I earnestly mention that this book suffers from no complacency of any proud sense of achievement. Any suggestion is welcome, as it will certainly strengthen the possibilities of my efforts and concern coming to fruiting.

Neeta Patwardhan

Preface to the First Edition

This book is written as a response to a call that has gone unheeded since unpardonably long. It is a call invoking help as, stalking amidst us, there is a menacingly mighty spectre to ignore which any longer will be suicidal. This spectre that is looming large is the mortality and morbidity caused by hospital-associated infections (HAIs). While the incidence of HAI in most part of the world ranges from 3% to 21%, it is much higher in India that is 35%. Surveillance data is not adequately available from Indian hospitals, besides, lack of awareness and inertia of the hospital staff in cooperation makes surveillance difficult to carry out. Whatever information is available is not compiled systematically in one book, scattered bits of information can be had from different books most of which are written by authors from different countries and are published from different nooks of the world.

This precisely is the predicament, which triggered in my mind the necessity of writing this book that would collectively offer the scattered information, its analysis and possible remedies for the evil of HAI. And hence this book comes into being with a hope that it would prove itself to be of immense use to everyone in the medical field. Lately, strict rules have been formulated and enforced to ensure monitoring of hospitals, regarding fumigation of operation theaters (OT), testing the efficiency of autoclaves, etc. The rules also ask the hospital staff to maintain registers which are checked by concerned authorities. I hope this book will be of wide help to hospitals run by government institutions as well as to private hospitals.

I have taken efforts to ensure that this book encompasses all theoretical and practical aspects of HAI. It includes practical aspects of surgical site infections, hospital-acquired urinary tract infections, intravascular catheter-associated infections, etc. Also, it deals with postexposure prophylaxis for hepatitis B virus (HBV) and human immunodeficiency virus (HIV) infections, and monitoring of HBV infections in the dialysis units. In addition, it attempts to deal in details with waste disposal, use of prophylactic antibiotics in hospitals, infections in ICUs, hospital infections associated with every department including kitchen, laundry and monitoring of operation theaters (OT). Collecting OT swabs for testing OT surfaces is deemed outdated today for routine purposes. However, except in extremely sophisticated operation theaters of hospitals in big cities, these conventional methods continue to be in practice; and, therefore, they have been given a deserving inclusion in this book.

In nutshell, I have tried to make all information, analysis and remedies related to hospital-associated infections, available in one single book so as to facilitate a possible organized countering of evils caused by HAIs. This book is based on all information heeded by me during my tenure as 'Hospital Infection Control In-Charge' and on my painstakingly assembled information collected from far flung and scattered sources.

The arch impulse behind writing this book is to facilitate an effective management that will tame down the beast of hospital-associated infections and minimize the resultant mortality and morbidity mainly in the Indian context.

May I earnestly mention that this book suffers from no complacency of any proud sense of achievement. Any suggestion is welcome, as it will certainly strengthen the possibilities of my efforts and concern coming to fruiting.

Neeta Patwardhan

Acknowledgments

I am deeply indebted to my husband Dr Satish Patwardhan, for his intense involvement in this painstaking task. In spite of his busy schedule as a Consultant Microbiologist, he assiduously helped me all day all night during the past two years in every bit of this book, and instilled cheer and spirit into it. Due to his deep involvement and concern, this tremendous work could never be affected by monotony. I cannot imagine the completion of this work without his dedicated and invaluable help.

I also express my sincere gratitude to Dr (Mrs) Mrudula A Phadke, Vice-Chancellor, Maharashtra University of Health Sciences (MUHS), Nashik, Maharashtra, India, for the keen interest she took in this book, and I was really delighted when she happily accepted to write a foreword for this book.

I must also express my gratitude to Mr Shrotre, whose meticulous and keen guidance in this book, right from typing the manuscript to all the aspects, transformed this work into a book. Certainly, without his help this book might not have seen the light of the day. I am also very thankful to a close friend of mine Mrs Rohini Karandikar, who has added picturesque dimension to my book with diagrams for which she has taken efforts. I am also very thankful to our family friend Mr Pradeep Deshpande, for his immense help in every possible way. I would also like to thank Mr Vinod Kalam, our technician at Kamalnayan Bajaj Hospital, for his help in computer work.

I would also like to thank Mr Gawde CS of M/s Jaypee Brothers Medical Publishers (Mumbai branch) who, in fact, has motivated me to write this book. His ceaseless persuasion kept alive my interest in writing. Together with him I owe my profuse thanks to Mrs Jyoti Bardapurkar, the Chief Librarian of our college and a close friend of mine, for her constant encouragement and furnishing me with all necessary material from the library from time to time.

I feel it necessary to express my gratitude to my in-laws Mr SG Patwardhan and Mrs SS Patwardhan and my daughters Shweta and Prajakta, who never made me feel that they were being neglected during these years consumed by this work. These loving ones showed exemplary considerateness and encouragement that was vital in keeping me inspired. Thanks are due to my dear sister Dulari Qureshi, my dear brother Sachin Gupte, for their affection and concern that gave me a constant source of encouragement.

I am also grateful to the past and present Dean, Government Medical College as their help was conducive to the completion of this work. I would like to thank all my colleagues in the Department of Microbiology, Government Medical College and the Pathology Laboratory of Kamalnayan Bajaj Hospital, who have been a constant source of inspiration and help to me.

Lastly, I owe my heartfelt thanks to Shri Jitendar P Vij (Group Chairman), Mr Ankit Vij (Group President) and their staff of M/s Jaypee Brothers Medical Publishers (P) Ltd, New Delhi, India, for their cooperation and keen interest in publishing this book.

Contents

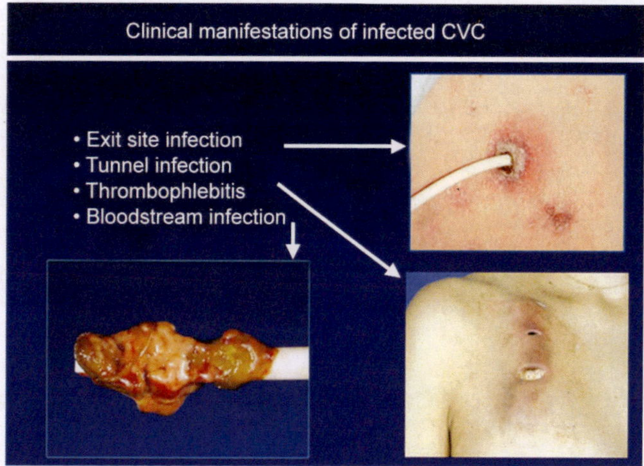

Fig. 15.2: Clinical manifestations of central venous catheter-associated infections

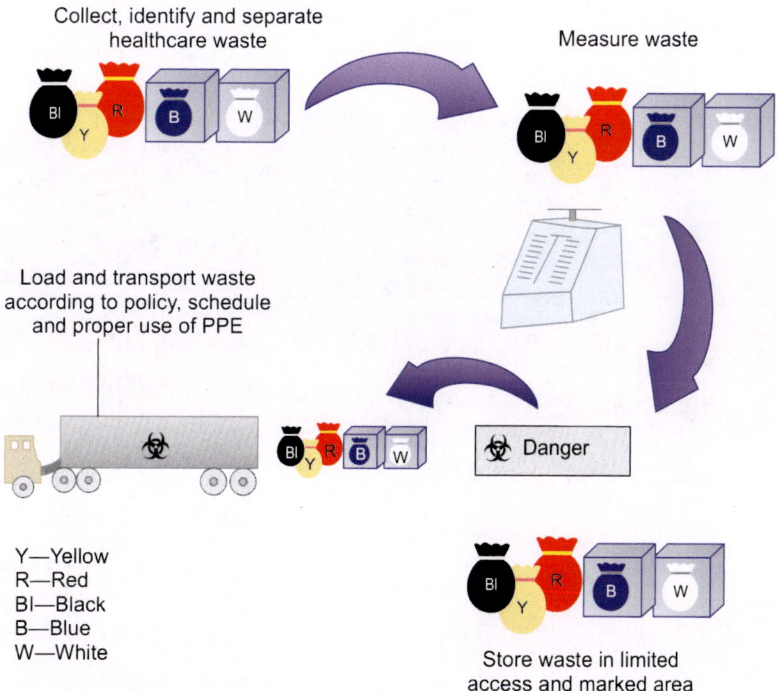

Fig. 24.1: Waste management process

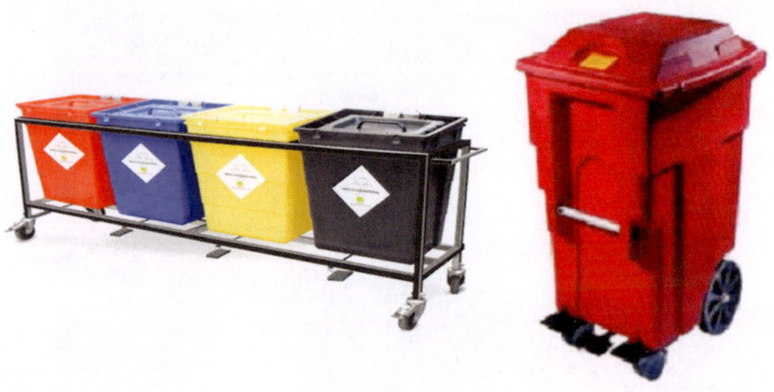

Fig. 24.2: Internal transport

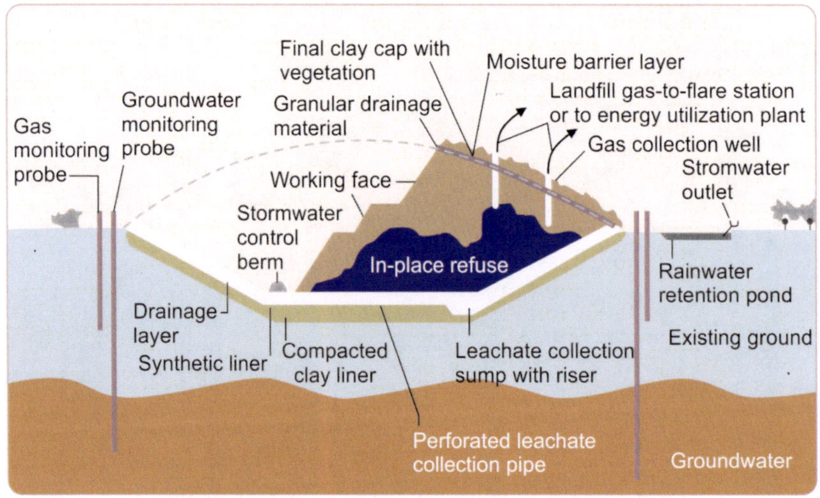

Fig. 24.13: Modern sanitary landfill cross-section

Plate 3

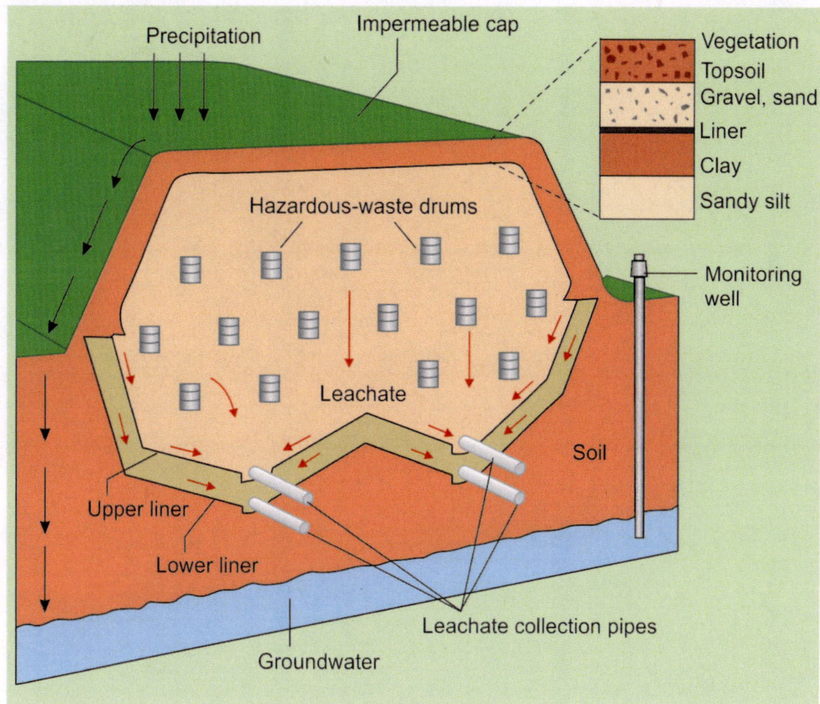

Fig. 24.14: Secure landfill

Source: www.britannica.com/technology/hazardous-waste-management#ref593344.

Chapter 1

Hospital-acquired Infection

Chapter Outline

- Selected CDC Surveillance Definitions of Nosocomial Infection
- Simplified Criteria for Surveillance of Nosocomial Infections

INTRODUCTION

Hospital-acquired infection (HAI) or nosocomial infection or healthcare-associated infection can be defined as 'An infection acquired in the hospital by a patient who was admitted for some other infection, other than that infection' or It is an infection occurring in a patient in a hospital or other healthcare facility in whom the infection was not present or incubating at the time of admission. This includes infection acquired in the hospital but appearing after discharge and also occupational infections among staff of the facility.[1] Considering time period, infections occurring more than 48 hours after admission are usually considered as nosocomial.[2]

Hospital-acquired infections are widespread. They contribute to the increased morbidity and mortality in hospitals. With an increasing population, increased number of people with impaired immunity (age, illness, treatment), emergence of new organisms like human immunodeficiency virus (HIV) and increased bacterial drug resistance to antibiotics, this problem is going to increase. hospital-acquired infections (HAIs) thereby increase the economic burden of the hospital by increasing the bed occupancy due to prolonged hospital stay. Infection control measures are suboptimal in most hospitals in underdeveloped and developing countries and therefore pose a risk of increase in accidental infections with HIV, Epstein-Barr virus (EBV), hepatitis C virus (HCV) and other blood-borne pathogens.

History of Hospital-acquired Infections

The history of HAIs started with Hippocrates who said, if you wish to become a physician follow the maxim, "first do no harm to the patient." Then it was Florence Nightingale who was also of the opinion as Hippocrates and thought that the very first requirement in a hospital is that it should do the sick no harm. At almost the same time it was Ignaz Semmelweis from Europe who realized that it was the hospital staff who were largely responsible for the dreadful death toll of puerperal fever in the maternity units. By a series of exclusion experiments, he was able to discover that by getting the hospital staff to wash their hands between seeing the patients, he could reduce the death rate by almost 96%.[2]

HAIs in the 20th–21st Century[2]

The present era of healthcare-associated infections (HAI) started with the Center for Disease Control and Prevention (CDC) in the USA. It started the national nosocomial infection surveillance system (NNIS) in 1950s and the SENIC (study of efficacy of nosocomial infection control) project in 1974. It was observed that one-third of healthcare-associated infections were preventable through effective infection control. Many guidelines were produced by Healthcare Infection Control Practices Advisory Committee (HICPAC). In 2005, hospitals started contributing data to National Healthcare Safety Network (NHSN).

"Bundle" measures are the most recent initiative to improve healthcare. Since 2005, various member countries of the world have signed the pledge of WHO's First Global Patient Safety Challenge.

Introducing low-cost measures, such as hand hygiene, staff education and inclusion of basic principles of infection control in medical and paramedical curricula can reduce healthcare associated infections. The human and economic toll of healthcare-associated infections is high and controlling it is possible.

Burden of Healthcare-associated Infection[2]

HAI Fact Sheet (WHO)

HAI are the most frequent form of adverse event in healthcare delivery worldwide

- Hundreds of millions of patients are affected by HAI worldwide each year, leading to significant mortality and financial losses for health systems.
- Of every 100 hospitalized patients at any given time, 7 in developed and 10 in developing countries will acquire at least one HAI.
- The endemic burden of HAI is also significantly higher in low- and middle-income than in high-income countries, in particular in-patients admitted to intensive care units and in neonates.

HAI in high-income countries: At any given time, the prevalence of HAI in these countries varies between 3.5% and 12%. The estimated rate in USA was 4.5% in 2002, corresponding to 9.3 infections per 1,000 patient-days and 1.7 million affected patients, with 99,000 deaths annually. The direct medical cost of HAI ranged from $28-45 billion.

The European Centre for Disease Prevention and Control reports an average prevalence of 7.1% in European countries. The cumulative incidence of infection in adult high-risk patients is 17.0 episodes per 1,000 patient-days.

HAI in low- and middle-income countries: Limited data, often of low quality, are available from this group of countries. At any given time, the prevalence of HAI varies between 5.7% and 19.1%. Average prevalence is significantly higher in high quality than in low-quality studies (15.5% vs 8.5%, respectively).

HAI data from India: HAI surveillance is a highly demanding and challenging task and settings with limited resources experience many constraints to evaluate the burden. In low- and middle-income countries, regular monitoring of data may not be feasible at national level thus, Ministry of Health and Family Welfare (MOHFW) is unable to report the burden. In addition, the limited number of studies in these settings has been published in the scientific literature.

A review of studies performed revealed an extremely fragmented picture of the endemic burden of HAI in India. The limited number of studies with broad scope, together with a lack of national surveillance systems, significantly hamper any attempts to estimate the burden of HAI in the country at regional/ national level. Studies from single hospitals cannot be considered representative of the endemic epidemiology of HAI in the country. In particular most of these studies were conducted in private hospitals, which represent a specific type of context and not the broad range of healthcare settings in India.

Challenges in India[2]

- The disparate health systems, wherein the public hospitals are free, too few and overloaded, the majority of healthcare (80%) lies in private hands in the form of large corporate hospitals, smaller nursing homes and day care clinics
- The overwhelming number of sick people with a huge dearth of trained, skilled healthcare professionals (nurse to patient ratio being 1:100 and doctor: patient = 1: 900)
- Care is individualized and concentrates on curative medicine
- Lack of systems approach and poor underdeveloped public health facilities
- The arrogant hierarchy which pushes the clinical practice to perception based rather than evidence-based medicine
- Cost of healthcare is largely borne by the patient themselves, and therefore, there is no accountability of healthcare providers on cost-effective care
- No regulatory body to oversee or monitor quality of care
- Lack of transparency of healthcare organizations whether public or private.

The Main Solutions and Perspectives for Improvement Identified by Who

Clean Care is Safer Care

- Identifying local determinants of the HAI burden
- Improving reporting and surveillance systems at the national level
- Ensuring minimum requirements in terms of facilities and dedicated resources available for HAI surveillance at the institutional level, including microbiology laboratories' capacity
- Ensuring that core components for infection control are in place at the national and healthcare setting levels
- Implementing standard precautions, particularly best hand hygiene practices at the bedside
- Improving staff education and accountability
- Conducting research to adapt and validate surveillance protocols based on the reality of developing countries
- Conducting research on the potential involvement of patients and their families in HAI reporting and control.

The way forward: If we are as serious and far-sighted, we should:

At the organization level

i. Set up the infection control program with a multidisciplinary committee to guide the processes and monitor the outcome.
ii. Surveillance of healthcare-associated infections and antimicrobial resistant pattern (using standardized international methods), to measure the burden of the disease.
iii. Implement practical evidence based, low cost and simple preventive strategies first.
iv. Antimicrobial stewardship programs and other interventions to reduce the development of multiple drug-resistant organisms (MDROs).
v. Do studies that include analysis of economic, behavioral, communication and organizational strategies that optimize the implementation of and adherence to the best practices.

At state/national level

i. Promote funded research projects through Indian Council of Medical Research (ICMR), Department of Biotechnology (DBT) and state agencies.
ii. Produce more trained infection control professionals: nurses, hospital epidemiologists and public health personnel.

iii. Promote growth of microbiology laboratories and involve the clinical microbiologists in decision making.
iv. Regulatory bodies to monitor the quality of drugs, and over the counter sale of antibiotics.
v. Develop state laws for compulsory HAI reporting.
vi. Physicians should be made responsible for HAI and condition of their patients.
vii. Empowerment of Hospital Infection Control Committees.

Strengthening of the infection control measures will result in reassuring the health care workers and patients attending the hospitals. Reduction in incidence of HAI will also save the finances, which would have been spent on treatment of HAI, and reduce the bed occupancy, make more beds available for other patients. It is an established fact that HAI can be effectively reduced by rigid implementation of aseptic and antiseptic policies.

Nosocomial infection occurs in about 5 to 10% of hospital admissions and most commonly involves the urinary tract, the respiratory tract and the blood stream. *Escherichia coli, Staphylococcus aureus, Enterococci, Pseudomonas aeruginosa* and coagulase-negative staphylococci are the most frequently isolated organisms.[3] The importance of nosocomial pathogen obviously varies according to the site of infection. Moreover, there are also wide variations from hospital to hospital, from one unit to another within a single hospital and within the same unit over a period of time. Operation theaters, ICUs and waste disposal methods are termed as the most sensitive areas for infection control followed by laundry, kitchen, wards, etc. The source of most infection cases reported in the recent past has been the operation theater (OT)/operation room (OR). Experts say that proper design and ventilation of the OT is necessary to prevent air-borne infections. Besides there should be a proper record of fumigation/fogging and disinfection measures.[4]

The perioperative use of antibiotics has prevented infections from limiting the progress of surgery. The third generation cephalosporin antibiotics have played an important role in the treatment of nosocomial infections. These agents are often used alone or in combination with aminoglycosides for initial empiric therapy of nosocomial infections. Sometimes, it is necessary to supplement or substitute this therapy with definitive therapy for specific infections. Such agents include isoxazolyl penicillin such as cloxacillin for penicillinase producing staphylococci, vancomycin for multidrug-resistant staphylococci and enterococci and nitroimidazoles to cover anaerobes after gut surgery.

There is a tendency to disregard microbiology when a patient is responding adequately to empiric therapy, so also not many efforts are taken for microbiologic documentation of nosocomial infections. This is very unfortunate, since even if making a precise bacteriologic diagnosis in the individual patient is considered to be limited, the microbiological information in each case of nosocomial infection in the hospital is vital to the interpretative value of conclusions drawn from the summary of statistics provided by the hospital microbiology unit.

The prevalence of hospital-acquired infection has been reported in a survey conducted by WHO (1992) as 3–21% with a mean of 8.4%.[5] In India, the prevalence of nosocomial infections has been said to be up to 30–50% (2002).[4,6] Even if there is no obvious infection in patients admitted in hospitals, it causes a change in the microbial flora of some patients in whom the normal flora becomes gradually replaced by drug resistant micro-organisms.[7] The increasing problems of drug resistance limit the use of many antibiotics, both for prophylaxis and treatment.[8]

The global data suggests that the nosocomial infections, the SSI incidence rate varies from 1.5% to 20%.[9,10] Recently CDC has found a prevalence rate for SSI to be 31%.[11] In India six studies reported an overall incidence of 9–23% for all surgical procedures.[12]

Of the nosocomial infections approximately 36–40% involve the urinary tract, 80% of which are catheter-associated urinary tract infections.[13-15] While according to CDC, urinary tract infections account for more than 12% of healthcare-associated infections, all of which are virtually caused by instrumentation of the urinary tract.[16]

Incidence of bloodstream infections (BSIs) is reported to be between 1% (in intensive care patients) and 36% (in bone marrow transplant patients).[17-20] Hospital-associated pneumonias (HAP) constitute about 15% of HAIs.[21,22]

WHO and other studies have shown that the highest prevalence of nosocomial infections occurs in intensive care units and in emergency surgical and orthopedic wards.

In a number of studies from India from 2006 to 2014, the prevalence of nosocomial infections was found to vary between 8% and 29%. Most of the studies found a prevalence between 26% and 29%. Risk factors like use of antibiotics, invasive devices, surgery and time of hospitalization were associated with patients with healthcare-associated infections.[23-26]

The most common HAI category was urinary tract infection followed by respiratory tract infections, and surgical site infection. Most common organisms isolated were *Pseudomonas aeruginosa, Acinetobacter baumannii, E. coli, Klebsiella* and *Staphylococcus aureus.*[5]

Technologic advances in medical care, surgery, transfusion therapy and blood banking, mechanical ventilation, intravascular therapy, urinary catheter drainage has contributed, directly or indirectly, to an increase in certain nosocomial infections. The prolonged survival in hospital of susceptible persons including premature newborns and persons with extensive burns, neutropenia or suppressed immunity also increase both the likelihood and severity of nosocomial infections.

Surveillance of nosocomial infections has identified many previously unappreciated nosocomial infections. A desire to control the direct costs of nosocomial infections has contributed to the development of infection control programs. The most ambitious attempt to measure the impact of hospital epidemiology, the study of the efficacy of nosocomial infection control (SENIC), estimated that hospitals with surveillance and control programs experienced 32% fewer nosocomial infections than hospitals that did not.[27]

The range of surveillance methods is broad, extending from self-reporting by patients and physicians, to the surveillance by trained personnel. Additional surveillance methods include review of microbiology laboratory results and chest radiography reports, review of nurses, records, interviews with the nursing staff, and interviews and examinations of patients. In general, the more intensive the surveillance, the larger the number of infections identified.[27]

To sum up, the advancing age of the patients admitted to the health care settings, greater prevalence of chronic diseases among admitted patients and the increased use of diagnostic and therapeutic procedures which effect the host defenses will provide continuing pressure on nosocomial infections in future.[1]

HAIs may be caused by infectious agents from endogenous or exogenous sources:

- Endogenous sources are body sites, such as the skin, nose, mouth, gastrointestinal (GI) tract, or vagina that are normally inhabited by microorganisms.
- Exogenous sources are those external to the patient, such as patient care personnel, visitors, patient care equipment, medical devices, or the healthcare environment.

Other important considerations include the following:

- Clinical evidence may be derived from direct observation of the infection site (e.g. a wound) or review of information in the patient chart or other clinical records
- For certain types of infection, a physician or surgeon diagnosis of infection derived from direct observation during an invasive

procedure, endoscopic examination, or other diagnostic studies or from clinical judgment may be an acceptable criterion for an HAI, unless there is compelling evidence to the contrary. For example, one of the criteria for SSI is "surgeon or attending physician diagnosis." Unless stated explicitly, physician diagnosis alone is not an acceptable criterion for any specific type of HAI.

- Infections occurring in infants that result from passage through the birth canal are considered HAIs if they meet the definition of HAI.

The following infections are not considered healthcare associated:

- Infections associated with complications or extensions of infections already present on admission, unless a change in pathogen or symptoms strongly suggests the acquisition of a new infection
- Infections in infants that have been acquired transplacentally (e.g. herpes simplex, toxoplasmosis, rubella, cytomegalovirus, or syphilis) and become evident on the day of birth or the next day
- Reactivation of a latent infection [e.g. herpes zoster (shingles), herpes simplex, syphilis, or tuberculosis].

The following conditions are not infections:

- Colonization, which means the presence of microorganisms on skin, on mucous membranes, in open wounds, or in excretions or secretions but are not causing adverse clinical signs or symptoms.
- Inflammation that results from tissue response to injury or stimulation by noninfectious agents, such as chemicals.

SELECTED CDC SURVEILLANCE DEFINITIONS OF NOSOCOMIAL INFECTION[28]

Surgical Site Infection

A. Incisional infection must occur at the incision site within 30 days after surgery and involve skin, the subcutaneous tissue, or muscle located above the fascial layer and any of the following:
   1. Purulent drainage from the incision or drain located above the fascial layer.
   2. Organism isolated from culture of fluid from wound closed primarily.
   3. Surgeon deliberately opens wound, unless wound is culture negative.
   4. Surgeon's or attending physician's diagnosis of infection.

B. Deep surgical wound infection—must occur at the operative site within 30 days after surgery, if no implant is left in place, or within one year if implant is in place and infection involves tissues or spaces and any of the following:
   1. Purulent discharge from the drain placed beneath the fascial layer.
   2. Wound spontaneously dehisces or is deliberately opened by surgeon, when patient has fever (>38°C) and/or localized pain or tenderness, unless wound culture is negative.
   3. An abscess or any other evidence of infection seen on direct examination, during surgery or by histopathologic examination.
   4. Surgeon's diagnosis of infection.

Urinary Tract Infection (UTI)[29,30]

Asymptomatic Bacteremic Urinary Tract Infection (ABUTI) Criterion

Patient with* or without an indwelling urinary catheter **has no signs or symptoms** (i.e., for any age patient, no fever (>38°C); urgency; frequency; dysuria; suprapubic tenderness; costovertebral angle pain or tenderness OR for a patient ≤1 year of age; no fever (>38°C core); hypothermia (<36°C core); apnea; bradycardia; dysuria; lethargy; or vomiting)

and

a positive urine culture of $\geq 10^5$CFU/mL with no more than 2 species of uropathogen microorganisms

and

a positive blood culture with at least 1 matching uropathogen microorganism to the urine culture, or at least 2 matching blood cultures drawn on separate occasions if the matching pathogen is a common skin commensal.

Note: For surveillance of UTIs count symptomatic UTI (SUTI) only, not asymptomatic bacteriuria (ASB)

- Exception is "ABUTI" (asymptomatic bacteremic UTI)—
  (**Ref:** Surveillance definitions for UTI recently modified in NHSN (as of Jan 2009)
- Please refer to NHSN Patient Safety Manual http://www.cdc.gov/nhsn/library.html

Symptomatic Urinary Tract Infection (SUTI)

Must meet at least *one* of the following criteria:

1a

Patient had an indwelling urinary catheter in place for >2 calendar days, with day of device placement being day 1, and catheter was in place on the date of event

and

at least 1 of the following signs or symptoms: fever (>38°C); suprapubic tenderness**; costovertebral angle pain or tenderness**

and

a positive urine culture of $\geq 10^5$ colony-forming units (CFU)/mL with no more than 2 species of microorganisms.

-----OR-----

Patient had an indwelling urinary catheter in place for >2 calendar days and had it removed the day of or the day before the date of event

and

at least 1 of the following signs or symptoms: fever (>38°C); urgency**; frequency**; dysuria**; suprapubic tenderness**; costovertebral angle pain or tenderness**

and

a positive urine culture of $\geq 10^5$ colony-forming units (CFU)/mL with no more than 2 species of microorganisms.

1b

Patient did not have an indwelling urinary catheter that had been in place for >2 calendar days and in place at the time of or the day before the date of event

and

has at least 1 of the following signs or symptoms: fever (>38°C) in a patient that is ≤65 years of age; urgency**; frequency**; dysuria**; suprapubic tenderness**; costovertebral angle pain or tenderness**

and

a positive urine culture of $\geq 10^5$ CFU/mL with no more than 2 species of microorganisms.

2a

Patient had an indwelling urinary catheter in place for >2 calendar days, with day of day of device placement being with day of device placement being day 1, and catheter was in place on the day of event

and

at least 1 of the following signs or symptoms: fever (>38°C); suprapubic tenderness*; costovertebral angle pain or tenderness*

and

at least 1 of the following findings:

a. positive dipstick for leukocyte esterase and/or nitrite

*Patient had an indwelling urinary catheter in place for >2 calendar days, with day of device placement being day 1, and catheter was in place on the date of event.

**With no other recognized cause.

b. pyuria [urine specimen with ≥10 white blood cells (WBC)/mm^3 of unspun urine or >5 WBC/high power field of spun urine]
c. microorganisms seen on Gram's stain of unspun urine

and

a positive urine culture of ≥10^3 and <10^5 CFU/mL with no more than 2 species of microorganisms. Elements of the criterion must occur within a timeframe that does not exceed a gap of 1 calendar day between two adjacent elements.

------OR------------------------------------

Patient with an indwelling urinary catheter in place for >2 calendar days and had it removed the day of or the day before the date of event

and

at least 1 of the following signs or symptoms: fever (>38°C); urgency*; frequency*; dysuria*; suprapubic tenderness*; costovertebral angle pain or tenderness*

and

at least 1 of the following findings:

a. positive dipstick for leukocyte esterase and/or nitrite
b. pyuria (urine specimen with ≥10 WBC/mm3 of unspun urine or >5 WBC/high power field of spun urine
c. microorganisms seen on Gram's stain of unspun urine

and

a positive urine culture of ≥10^3 and <10^5 CFU/mL with no more than 2 species of microorganisms. Elements of the criterion must occur within a timeframe that does not exceed a gap of 1 calendar day between two adjacent elements.

2b

Patient did not have an indwelling urinary catheter, that had been in place for >2 calendar days and in place at the time of, or the day before the date of event

and

has at least 1 of the following signs or symptoms: fever (>38°C) in a patient that is ≤65 years of age; urgency*; frequency*; dysuria*; suprapubic tenderness*; costovertebral angle pain or tenderness*

and

at least 1 of the following findings:

a. positive dipstick for leukocyte esterase and/or nitrite
b. pyuria (urine specimen with ≥10 WBC/mm^3 of unspun urine or >5 WBC/high power field of spun urine
c. microorganisms seen on Gram's stain of unspun urine

and

a positive urine culture of ≥10^3 and <10^5 CFU/mL with no more than 2 species of microorganisms. Elements of the criterion must occur within a timeframe that does not exceed a gap of 1 calendar day between two adjacent elements.

3

Patient ≤1 year of age with** or without an indwelling urinary catheter has at least 1 of the following signs or symptoms: fever (>38°C core); hypothermia (<36°C core); apnea*; bradycardia*; dysuria*; lethargy*; vomiting*

and

a positive urine culture of ≥10^5 CFU/mL with no more than 2 species of microorganisms.

4

Patient ≤1 year of age with** or without an indwelling urinary catheter has at least 1 of the following signs or symptoms: fever (>38°C core); hypothermia (<36°C core); apnea*; bradycardia*; dysuria*; lethargy*; vomiting*

---

*With no other recognized cause

and

at least 1 of the following findings:

a. positive dipstick for leukocyte esterase and/or nitrite
b. pyuria (urine specimen with ≥10 WBC/mm^3 of unspun urine or >5 WBC/high power field of spun urine
c. microorganisms seen on Gram's stain of unspun urine

and

a positive urine culture of between ≥10^3 and <10^5 CFU/mL with no more than two species of microorganisms.

Comments

- Laboratory cultures reported as "mixed flora" represent at least 2 species of organisms. Therefore, an additional organism recovered from the same culture, would represent >2 species of microorganisms. Such a specimen cannot be used to meet the UTI criteria
- Urinary catheter tips should not be cultured and are not acceptable for the diagnosis of a urinary tract infection
- Urine cultures must be obtained using appropriate technique, such as clean catch collection or catheterization. Specimens from indwelling catheters should be aspirated through the disinfected sampling ports
- In infants, urine cultures should be obtained by bladder catheterization or suprapubic aspiration; positive urine cultures from bag specimens are unreliable and should be confirmed by specimens aseptically obtained by catheterization or suprapubic aspiration
- Urine specimens for culture should be processed as soon as possible, preferably within 1 to 2 hours. If urine specimens cannot be processed within 30 minutes of collection, they should be refrigerated, or inoculated into primary isolation medium before transport, or transported in an appropriate urine preservative. Refrigerated specimens should be cultured within 24 hours
- Urine specimen labels should indicate whether or not the patient is symptomatic
- Report only pathogens in both blood and urine specimens for ABUTI
- Report *Corynebacterium* (urease positive) as either *Corynebacterium* species.

Short Summary of Definition of Symptomatic UTI

Symptoms you have to look for
In adults

- At least 1 of the following signs or symptoms: fever (>38°C); suprapubic tenderness; costovertebral angle pain or tenderness

(if catheter is in place)

and

- at least 1 of the following signs or symptoms: fever (>38°C); urgency; frequency; dysuria; suprapubic tenderness; costovertebral angle pain or tenderness.

(if catheter is removed)

In children <1 year of age: with or without an indwelling catheter

- Has at least one of the following symptoms: Fever (>38°C), hypothermia (<36°C); apnea, bradycardia, dysuria, lethargy, vomiting.

Culture Report

- A positive urine culture of ≥10^5 colony-forming units (CFU)/mL with no more than 2 species of microorganisms

*With no other recognized cause.

** Patient had an indwelling urinary catheter in place for >2 calendar days, with day of device placement being day 1, and catheter was in place on the date of event.

or

at least 1 of the following findings:

a. positive dipstick for leukocyte esterase and/or nitrite
b. pyuria [urine specimen with ≥10 white blood cells (WBC)/mm^3 of unspun urine or >5 WBC/high power field of spun urine]
c. microorganisms seen on Gram's stain of unspun urine

and

a positive urine culture of ≥10^3 and <10^5 CFU/mL with no more than 2 species of microorganisms. Elements of the criterion must occur within a timeframe.

Pneumonia

Possible Ventilator-associated Pneumonia (Possible VAP)

On or after calendar day 3 of mechanical ventilation and within 2 calendar days before or after the onset of worsening oxygenation, one of the following criteria is met:

a. purulent respiratory secretions (from one or more specimen collections)
   - Defined as secretions from the lungs, bronchi, or trachea that contains >25 neutrophils and <10 squamous epithelial cells per low power field.

OR

b. positive culture (qualitative, semi-quantitative or quantitative) of sputum*, endotracheal aspirate*, bronchoalveolar lavage*, lung tissue, or protected specimen brushing*.

Probable Ventilator-associated Pneumonia (Probable VAP)

On or after calendar day 3 of mechanical ventilation and within 2 calendar days before or after the onset of worsening oxygenation, one of the following criteria is met:

a. purulent respiratory secretions from one or more specimen collections (as defined for possible VAP)

and

one of the following:

a. positive culture of endotracheal aspirate*, ≥10^5 CFU/mL or equivalent semi-quantitative result
b. positive culture of bronchoalveolar lavage*, ≥10^4 CFU/mL or equivalent semi-quantitative result
c. positive culture of lung tissue, ≥10^4 CFU/g or equivalent semi-quantitative result
d. positive culture of protected specimen brush*, ≥10^3 CFU/mL or equivalent semi-quantitative result.

Bloodstream Infection (BSI)

Laboratory-confirmed Bloodstream Infection (LCBI)

Must meet one of the following criteria:

LCBI 1

Patient has a recognized pathogen cultured from one or more blood cultures

and

organism cultured from blood is not related to an infection at another site.

LCBI 2

Patient has at least one of the following signs or symptoms: fever (>38°C), chills, or hypotension

and

positive laboratory results are not related to an infection at another site

and

the same common commensal (i.e. diphtheroids [*Corynebacterium* species

**Excludes the following:*

- Normal respiratory/oral flora, mixed respiratory/oral flora or equivalent
- *Candida* species or yeast not otherwise specified
- Coagulase-negative *Staphylococcus* species
- *Enterococcus* species

not *C. diphtheriae*], *Bacillus* species [not *B. anthracis*], *Propionibacterium* species coagulase-negative staphylococci [including *S. epidermidis*], viridans group streptococci, *Aerococcus* species, and *Micrococcus* species) is cultured from two or more blood cultures drawn on separate occasions.

LCBI 3

Patient ≤1 year of age has at least one of the following signs or symptoms: fever (>38°C core), hypothermia (<36°C core), apnea, or bradycardia

and

positive laboratory results are not related to an infection at another site

and

the same common commensal (i.e. diphtheroids [*Corynebacterium* species not *C. diphtheriae*], *Bacillus* species [not *B. anthracis*], *Propionibacterium* species, coagulase-negative staphylococci [including *S. epidermidis*], viridans group streptococci, *Aerococcus* species, *Micrococcus* species) is cultured from two or more blood cultures drawn on the same or consecutive days and separate occasions.

SIMPLIFIED CRITERIA FOR SURVEILLANCE OF NOSOCOMIAL INFECTIONS

Types of nosocomial infections	Simplified criteria
1. Surgical site infection	Any purulent discharge, abscess or spreading cellulitis at the surgical site within a month after the operation or one year if implant is present
2. Urinary tract infection	Positive urine culture with (1 or 2 species) with at least 10^5 bacteria/mL with or without clinical symptoms

Contd...

Contd...

Types of nosocomial infections	Simplified criteria
3. Respiratory tract infection	Respiratory symptoms with at least two of the following signs appearing during • Hospitalization • Cough • Purulent sputum • New infiltrate on chest radiography consistent with infection
4. Vascular catheter infection	Inflammatory lymphangitis or purulent discharge at the site of insertion of the catheter
5. Septicemia	Fever or rigors and at least one positive blood culture

REFERENCES

1. Ducel G, Fabry J, Nicolle L. Prevention of hospital-acquired infections. A practical guide. In: WHO Manual, 2nd edition; 2002.p.1.
2. Chugh TD. Hospital Infection Control—Are we serious? Accessed from www.apiindia.org/pdf/medicine-update-2012/infectious-disease-14.pdf.)
3. Mukherjee S*, Nanivadekar AS. Nosocomial infections. An epidemiologic and microbiologic perspective. Guidelines for antibiotic policy: In Issue special from Net Address. Accessed on Jan, 2004.
4. Holla U. Lack of training and awareness hamper control measures. In India's No. 1 Newspaper for Health Care Business. Issue 16–31 July 2001 (From Net) available at Address htp://www.expresshealthcaremgmt.com/20010731/cover2.htm.
5. Shriniwas. Hospital-acquired infections. Guidelines for control. Govt of India. Ministry of Health and Family Welfare, Nirman Bhavan, New Delhi; 1992.p.1.
6. Combat nosocomial infections in India. In India's No. 1 Newspaper for Health Care Business. Issue 1–15 June 2001 (From Net) available at www.expresshealthcaremgmt.com/20010615/editorial1-htm.

**Same organism exclusions as noted for Possible VAP.*

7. Chakraborty P. Textbook of Microbiology, 2nd edition. New Central Book Agency (P) Ltd, Kolkata; 2003.p.690.
8. Shriniwas. Emmergence of drug resistance amongst common hospital pathogens. Indian J Med Microbiol. 1987;5:71-84.
9. Leaper DJ, Van Goor H, Reilly J, Petrosillo N, Geiss HK, Torres AJ, et al. Surgical site infection—a European perspective of incidence and economic burden. Int Wound J. 2004;1(4):247-73. Accessed on 8th June 2016.
10. Hospital acquired infection. From Wikipedia. Available at www.en.wikipedia.org/wiki/hospital-acquired-infection. Accessed on 9th July, 2016.
11. In surgical site infection (SSI) event—Centers for disease Control. Available at www.cdc.gov/nhsn/pdfs/pscmanual/9pscssicurrent.pdf.Jan 2016 (9-29). Accessed on 8th June 2016.
12. Tan JT, Coleman K, Norris S, Mapari J, Shastri S, Metz L. Health Technology Analysts Pty Ltd, Sydney, Australia, Johnson and Johnson Asia-Pacific. Surgical site infection in India: A systematic review of the incidence and economic burden (1995-2010). Available at www.aspjj.com/us/sites/www.aspjj.com.us/files/pdf/surgical-site-infection-in-india-pdf. Accessed on 8th June, 2016.
13. Efthimiou L, Skrepetis K. Prevention of Catheter-associated Urinary Tract Infections. Provisional chapter. Available at www.cdn.intechopen.com/pdfs-win/45151.pdf.
14. Catheter-associated Urinary Tract Infection (CAUTI). Factsheet. Wound and ostomy and continence Nurses society.
15. An epic guide 2008. Guide to elimination of Catheter-associated Urinary Tract Infections (CAUTIs). Available at www.apic.org/Resource/Elimination Guide Forum/c0790db8-2aca-4179-a7ae-676c27592de2/File/APIC-CAUTI-Guide.pdf.
16. Urinary Tract Infection [Catheter-associated Urinary Tract Infection (CAUTI) and Noncatheter-associated Urinary Tract Infection (UTI) and Other Urinary System Infection (USI)] Events. CDC. Device-associated-module. Available at www.cdc.gov/nhsn/pdfs/pscmanual/7psccauticurrent.pdf.
17. Wisplinghoff H, Bischoff T, Tallent SM, Seifert H, Wenzel RP, Edmond MB. Nosocomial Bloodstream Infections in US Hospitals: Analysis of 24,179 Cases from a Prospective Nationwide Surveillance Study. BSI in US hospitals. CID2004:39 (1August). Available at www.cid.oxfordjournals.org/content/39/3/309.fullpdf+html.
18. Marra AR, et al. Nosocomial bloodstream infections in Brazilian hospitals: Analysis of 2,563 cases from a Prospective Nationwide surveillance study. Journal of Clinical Microbiology; 2011.pp.1866-71.Available at www.jcm.asm.org/content/49/5/1866.full.
19. Johann RS. Epidemiology of early-onset bloodstream infection and implications for treatments. American Journal of Infection Control (AJIC). 2008;36(10):s171.e13-s171.e17. Available at www.ajicjournal.org/article/s0196-6553(08)00788-8/pdf.
20. Hospital-acquired Infection. From Wikipedia. Available at http//en.wikipedia.org/wiki/Hospital-acquired-Infection.
21. Guidelines for preventing healthcare-associated pneumonia, 2003. Recommendations of CDC and the healthcare infection control practices Advisory committee Taken from website:www.cdc.gov/hai/prevent/prevent-pubs.html. Accessed on 5/2/2014.
22. Tedja R. Hospital-acquired Healthcare-associated and Ventilator-associated Pneumonia. Cleveland Clinic. Center for continuing Education disease management. Available at www.clevelandclinicmeded.com/medicalpubs/disease-management/infectious-disease/healthcare-associated-pneumonia.
23. Patel Disha A, et al. Surveillance of Hospital-acquired Infection in Surgical wards in Tertiary Care Centre, Ahmedabad, Gujarat. National Journal of Community Medicine. 2011;12(3). Accessed from www.njcmindia.org/homedownload/157.
24. Oberoi L, et al. Changin Trends of Nosocomial Infections in Geriatric Patients in a Tertiary Care Hospital. JIMSA. 2012;25:4. Accessed from www.medind.nic.in/gov/t12/14/javt1214p233.pdf.
25. Saleem M, et al. Pattern of nosocomial infection among patients admitted in medical and surgical wards of a secondary care hospital in North India. An epidemiological evaluation. Indian Journal of Community Health. 2012;24:4. Accessed from www.lapsmupuk.org/journal/index.php/IJCH/article/view/363.

26. Malhotra S, Sharma S, Hans C. Prevalence of Hospital-acquired Infections in a tertiary care hospital in India. IJMMS. 2014;1(7):91-4. Accessed from www.internationalinventjournals.org/journals/.../malhotra%20et%20al.pdf.
27. Platt R, Goldmann DA, Hopkins CC. Epidemiology of nosocomial infection, Chapter 13. In: Gorbach SL, Bartlett JC, Blacklow NR (Eds). Infectious diseases, 2nd edition. WB Saunders Co; 1992.p.9.
28. CDC/NHSN Surveillance Definitions. Accessed from www.cdc.gov/nhsn/PDFS/psc manual/17 psc Nos .in/ Def_current pdf. On 22/9/2015.
29. Surveillance definitions for UTI recently modified in NHSN (as of Jan 2009)—NHSN Patient Safety Manual http://www.cdc.gov/nhsn/library.html.
30. Urinary Tract Infection [Catheter-associated Urinary Tract Infection (CAUTI) and Noncatheter-associated Urinary Tract Infection (UTI) and Other Urinary System Infection (USI)] Events www.cdc.gov/nhsn/PDFs/pscManual/7pscCAU accessed on 24/8/2015.

Chapter 2

Epidemiology of Nosocomial Infections

Chapter Outline

- Factors Affecting the Development of Hospital-acquired Infections
- Common Hospital-acquired Infections
- Microbiology of Hospital Infections
- Sources of Infection
- Modes of Transmission
- Etiological Agents
- Healthcare Workers and Transmission of Infection

FACTORS AFFECTING THE DEVELOPMENT OF HOSPITAL-ACQUIRED INFECTIONS

Whether nosocomial infection will develop or not will depend on various factors. These are:

Microbial Agent

Patient admitted to the hospital is exposed to a variety of microorganisms. But contact between the patient and the microorganism does not by itself necessarily lead to the development of clinical disease. There are other factors, which influence the nature and frequency of nosocomial infections. The likelihood of developing an infection will depend on the characteristic of the microorganism, especially its virulence, resistance to antimicrobial agents and inoculums of infective material.

Bacteria, viruses, fungi and parasites can all lead to nosocomial infections. Infection may be caused by a microorganism acquired from another person in the hospital (cross infection), or may be caused by patients' own endogenous flora (endogenous infection). Some organisms may be acquired from an inanimate object or substance recently contaminated from another human source (environmental infection).

In the past when basic hygiene practices and antibiotics were still not introduced into medical practice, most of the hospital infections were due to pathogens of external origin (food-borne and air-borne diseases, gas gangrene, tetanus, etc.), or were caused by organisms not present in the normal flora of the patients (e.g. diphtheria and tuberculosis). However, now the progress in antibiotic treatment of bacterial infections has considerably reduced mortality from infectious diseases. Most of the infections acquired in the hospital today are due to microorganisms common in the general population, in whom they cause milder disease than among hospital patients (e.g. *Staphylococcus aureus (S. aureus)*, *Coagulase-negative staphylococci*, *Enterococci*, *Enterobacteriaceae*).

Patient Susceptibility

Important factors as far as the patient is concerned, influencing the acquisition of infection are age, immune status, underlying disease and diagnostic and therapeutic procedure. At extremes of life, infancy and old age, there is a decreased resistance to infections. Patients with chronic diseases such as malignant tumors, leukemia, diabetes mellitus, chronic renal failure, acquired immunodeficiency syndrome, become susceptible to infections with opportunistic pathogens. These are organisms, which normally are innocuous, e.g. part of normal flora in the human, but may become pathogenic when the body's immunological defences are compromised. Immunosuppressive drugs or irradiation may also lower resistance to infection. Injuries to skin and mucus membrane may bypass natural defense mechanism and lead to an increased risk of infection. Malnutrition also increases the susceptibility of the patient to infection.

Environmental Factors

Healthcare settings are an environment where you have both infected persons and persons at increased risk of infection. Patients with infections or carriers of pathogenic microorganisms admitted to the hospital are the potential sources of infection for patients and staff. Patients who become infected in the hospital are a further source of infection. Crowded conditions in the hospital, frequent transfer of patients from one unit to another and concentration of patients who are highly susceptible to infection in one area (e.g. new born infants, burns patients, intensive care) all contribute to the development of nosocomial infections.

Microbial flora from the patients and carriers of pathogen may contaminate objects, devices and materials, which may subsequently come in contact with susceptible body sites of patients. In addition new infections associated with bacteria such as water-borne bacteria (atypical *Mycobacterium*) and/or viruses and parasites continue to be associated with hospital-acquired infections.

Bacterial Resistance

Most of the hospitalized patients receive antimicrobial drugs. This leads to selection of mutants and exchange of genetic resistance elements and thus antibiotics promote the emergence of multidrug-resistant strains of bacteria. Microorganisms in the normal human flora sensitive to the given drug are suppressed, whereas resistant strains persist and may become endemic in the hospital.

The widespread use of antimicrobials for therapy or prophylaxis is the major determinant of resistance. Antimicrobial agents are in some cases becoming less effective because of resistance. As an antimicrobial agent becomes widely used, bacteria resistant to this drug will develop eventually and may spread in the healthcare setting. Many strains of *Staphylococci*, *Pneumococci*, *Enterococci* and *Mycobacterium tuberculosis* are currently resistant to most or all antimicrobials to which they were sensitive at one time. So also, multidrug-resistant *Klebsiella* and *Pseudomonas aeruginosa* are prevalent in many hospitals, this problem is particularly critical in a developing country like ours where the more expensive second line antibiotics may not be available or affordable.

COMMON HOSPITAL-ACQUIRED INFECTIONS

The commonest type of nosocomial infection is urinary tract infection as mentioned earlier followed by surgical infections, lower respiratory tract infections, bacteremia and others.

Urinary Tract Infections

Occurrence

Urinary tract infection (UTI) is the most common nosocomial infections. They account for 39–40% of the total HAI infections.[1,2] Majority of these infections are asymptomatic and can be detected only by quantitative urine culture. About 80% of nosocomial UTIs are related to urethral catheterization, only 5–10% are related to genitourinary manipulation.[3]

Etiologic Agents

Principle etiologic agents are enteric gram-negative bacilli, most important being *E. coli.* More than 25% of the infections are due to *E. coli. Enterococci* and *Pseudomonas aeruginosa are* implicated in 10 to 20% of the infections.[2] *Staphylococcus aureus,* coagulase-negative staphylococci, *Enterobacter species, Klebsiella* species, *Serratia* are also known to cause infections. *Proteus and Pseudomonas* species are the organisms most commonly associated with biofilm growth on catheters.[4] Some of the infections are due to *Candida albicans.* MRSA is also responsible for some of the UTIs these days.[5]

Risk Factors

Majority of them (Nosocomial UTIs) result from:

- Instrumentation
  - Indwelling catheter drainage system
  - Cystoscopy
- Procedures
  - Nephrostomy
  - Creation of ileal bladder.

Most important risk factor—Duration of catheterization

Risk of infection increases by 1-5% for each day that the catheter remains in place.[6-8]

- Other risk factors:
  - Female sex
  - Impaired renal functions
  - Diabetes
  - Colonization of catheter drainage bag
  - Catheterization for purposes other than drainage, e.g. during surgery or measurement of urine output.

Systemic antibiotics appear to reduce the risk of infection for catheters that stay in place for very few days, but increase the risk if the catheter is in place for longer than 6 days.

Surgical Wound Infection

Occurrence

It varies depending on, who is carrying out the surveillance (See chapter on Surveillance). Among the infections detected during hospitalization, the overall risk is 1.2% for infections detected by combination of surveillance procedures used by the hospitals participating in the NNIS (national nosocomial infection survey), 4.1% for infections noted by especially trained reviewers, and 4.7% when prospective surveillance with telephone follow-up is added.[9] Some have quoted this to be up to 24%.[10]

Various studies from India from 2007 to 2013[11-14] have found the prevalence of SSi to vary between 7.44% and 39%. The most common isolates were *Escherichia coli* and *Staphylococcus aureus.* Significant determinants of SSI were found to be long stay in wards, diabetes, emergency surgery, pre-operative hospital stay and surgical wound class.

Etiologic Agents

Principal etiologic agent varies with the hospital's flora and the procedure, particularly with the anatomic site involved, but *Staphylococcus aureus* plays a major role in clean surgery. Other etiologic agent for wounds, skin sepsis is—*Escherichia coli (E. coli), Proteus* species, *Enterococcus,* anaerobes, *Staphylococcus epidermidis.* In burns—*S. aureus, Pseudomonas aeruginosa (P. aeruginosa), Acinetobacter and Streptococcus pyogenes (S. pyogenes) are commonly found.*

Risk Factors

There are four categories of procedures, based on a scoring system for risk of infection from wound contamination[15] (Also refer chapter on Surgical Site Infections).

- 2.9% risk of infection for clean procedures.
- 3.9% risk of infection for clean contaminated procedures.
- 8.5% risk of infection for procedures at contaminated site.
- 12.6% risk of infection for procedures that involve an infected site.

Pneumonia

Occurrence

Like surgical wound infections nosocomial pneumonia accounts for about 15–20% of HAIs.[16] Nosocomial pneumonia is reported in 0.6–11% of hospitalized patients.[17,18] The risk is high for patients in ICU; and among patients undergoing mechanical ventilation has been reported to be as high as 30%, so also it is high in patients who are unconscious or have chronic lung disease.[19]

Etiologic Agents

Gram-negative bacilli like *P. aeruginosa, Klebsiella* species, *Escherichia coli, Acinetobacter* species *and Haemophilus influenzae* and gram-positive cocci like *Staphylococcus aureus* (especially methicillin-resistant *S. aureus* (MRSA) and *Streptococcus pneumoniae* are the pathogens most frequently isolated from tracheal and bronchial secretions. Less common pathogens are *Serratia* species, *Legionella* species, influenza A virus, respratory syncitial virus (RSV), parainfluenza virus and adenovirus. Unusual causes of nosocomial pneumonia are *Enterobacter* species, *Stenotrophomonas maltophilia, Burkholderia cepacia,* oropharyngeal anaerobes (non-bacteroides fragilis). *Candida* species are an uncommon cause of hospital-acquired pneumonia, and cultures positive for these organisms more often reflect colonization). These organisms are commonly recovered from patients with ventilator-associated pneumonias. The recovery of a respiratory pathogen from respiratory secretions does not automatically establish it as a cause.[20] About 10% of patients with nosocomial pneumonia die as a result of infection despite treatment.[21]

Immunosuppressed patients are also at risk for a variety of special pathogens, including *Legionella* and fungi such as *Aspergillus.*

In case of HABP (Hospital-associated bacterial pneumonia) and VABP (Ventilator-associated bacterial pneumonia) organisms consistently present were *Staphylococcus aureus* (28%), *Pseudomonas aeruginosa* (21.8%), *Klebsiella* species (9.8%), *Escerichia coli* (6.9%), *Acinetobacter* species (6.8%) and *Enterobacter* species (6.3%) with lower prevalence rates of *Serratia* species, *Stenotrophomonas maltophilia* and community-acquired pathogens like *Pneumococci* and *Haemophilus influenzae.*[22]

Risk Factors

- Mechanical ventilation
- Aspiration
- Depressed level of consciousness
- Underlying chronic lung disease
- Thoracic or abdominal surgery
- Antimicrobial exposure
- Age greater than 70 years.

Bacteremia

Occurrence

This is the ultimate dreaded consequence of all serious hospital infections leading to septic shock. Bacteremia accounts for 5–7%

of nosocomial infections[23] and is secondary to respiratory, UTI and wound infections, but often because of intravascular catheter. More than half the patients with sepsis develop shock and mortality may raise up to 60-80%. Bacteremia is identified by a positive blood culture, however, it is important to differentiate between contaminants and true positive cultures.

Etiologic Agents

Most common etiologic agents are *Coagulase-negative—Staphylococci* and *S. aureus,* which are responsible for 40% of nosocomial infections. *E. coli, P. aeruginosa, Enterococci, Enterobacter, Klebsiella* and *Candida* each account for 5-8% of the reported incidence.[24] Other organisms reported recently are *Serratia marcescens, Proteus mirabilis, Propionibacterium acnes,*[25] *Acinetobacter baumannii* and *Klebsiella pneumoniae.*[26]

MICROBIOLOGY OF HOSPITAL INFECTIONS

Almost any pathogen can cause hospital infection, but those that survive in the hospital environment for long periods and develop resistance to antibiotics and disinfectants, are particularly important in this respect.

Initially *Streptococcus pyogenes* was the most important cause of hospital infection, but now it is hardly encountered, as it is highly susceptible to antibiotics.

In 1950s and 1960s *S. aureus* strains, resistant to multiple antibiotics and belonging to phage type 80/81 became important. *S. aureus* continues to be very common in hospital infection, but its original phage types have been replaced by others.

Recently, the enteric gram negative bacteria—*E. coli, Klebsiella, Enterobacter, Proteus* and *Serratia*—have become the most important group of hospital pathogens, particularly following dissemination of resistance factors amongst them, conferring multiple drug resistance.

During late 1970's multidrug resistant *Salmonella,* particularly *S. typhimurium* became a prominent hospital pathogen.

P. aeruginosa and other species of *Pseudomonas* have always been an important cause of hospital infection because of their intrinsic resistance to most antibiotics and ability to survive and even multiply at low temperatures and in disinfectant solutions. They also carry drug resistant plasmids.

Tetanus spores can survive in dust for a long time, and may sometimes contaminate cotton, suture material, plaster of Paris and other items used in hospitals. Hospital tetanus is usually a result of faulty sterilization techniques, or other lapses in sepsis.

Bacteria causing nosocomial infections can actually be divided into two groups:

1. *Commensal bacteria:* These are found as normal flora in the healthy human beings. They play an important role of preventing colonization of pathogenic microorganisms. Some of these commensals may cause infection if the natural host is compromised for example, cutaneous coagulase-negative staphylococci may cause intravascular infection and intestinal E. *coli* can cause UTI.
2. *Pathogenic bacteria:* These are more virulent and may cause sporadic or epidemic infections regardless of the host status for example anaerobic gram-positive rods like *Clostridium* can cause gas gangrene. Gram-positive bacteria like S. *aureus* (cutaneous bacteria that colonize the skin and nose of both hospital staff and patients) cause a wide variety of lung, bone, heart and blood stream infections and are frequently resistant to antibiotics. Beta hemolytic streptococci are also important.

Gram-negative bacteria (enterobacteriaceae) like *E. coli, Proteus, Klebsiella, Enterobacter, Serratia marcescens.* may colonize sites when the host defenses are compromised (catheter insertion, bladder catheter, cannula insertion) and cause serious infections (surgical site infections, lung infection, bacteremia, peritoneal infection). They may also be highly resistant.

Gram-negative organisms such as *Pseudomonas* species are often isolated from water and damp areas. They may colonize the digestive tract of hospitalized patients.

Some bacteria are a unique risk in hospitals, for example, *Legionella* species may cause pneumonia (sporadic or endemic) through inhalation of aerosols containing contaminated water (air conditioning, showers, therapeutic aerosols.)

Nowadays, the bacteria most commonly responsible for nosocomial infections are MRSA (Methicillin-resistant *S. aureus*), vancomycin-resistant enterococci and antibiotic resistant gram-negative bacilli.

HIV and hepatitis B and C viruses are important infections transmitted through blood and blood products. Screening of donors, and ensuring that the blood products are free of viable viruses has reduced this risk to a large extent. However, *HIV* escapes detection during window period. Screening for *HCV* antibody as practiced now is not satisfactory and done at few places.

Therefore, in view of the risk of transmission of known and unknown pathogens, it is safer to minimize blood transfusions and employ autologous transfusion, which will be safer. The use of shared syringes and needles, or syringes and needles not properly sterilized also carries the risk of transmission of these viruses. Possible routes of transmission of *hepatitis B, C viruses* and *HIV* are not only transfusions of blood, but also dialysis, injections, endoscopies, etc.

Viral diarrheas and chickenpox are often viral infections that spread in hospitals. *Cytomegalovirus, Herpes virus, Influenza virus, Enteroviruses, Arenovirus, Rotavirus and Ebola* may also cause hospital infections.

The range of hospital pathogens also include yeasts like *Candida albicans*, moulds like *Aspergillus and Mucor, Cryptococcus* and protozoa like *Giardia lamblia, Entamoeba histolytica, Pneumocystis carinii, Toxoplasma gondii, Sarcoptes scabiei* (scabies) is an ectoparasite, which can and has caused outbreaks in healthcare facilities.

SOURCES OF INFECTION (FIG. 2.1)

Endogenous

Many opportunistic infections are caused by the "patients own flora", which are not pathogenic under normal conditions, but only when there is an underlying disease, invasive diagnostic techniques, immunosuppressive therapy antibiotic therapy which may enable these organisms to reproduce, spread and implant itself at a site, where it produces an infection.

Exogenous

Hospital infections are mostly exogenous coming from the people around, environment, objects, etc.

Exogenous Sources

Contact with other patients and staff: People are by far the most important sources and reservoirs of infection including patients and hospital personnel suffering from infection or asymptomatic carriers.

Patients are often either colonized or infected with organisms that are disseminated by the hands of healthcare workers. In addition, the flora changes quickly during hospitalization to favor organisms less frequently found in the community, which tend to be more resistant to antibiotics and hence difficult to treat.

The extensive contact that patients have with healthcare workers and the high concentration of organisms that may be present in wound drainage, bladder catheter, drainage bags, and stool allows them to be efficient disseminators of this flora often to the hands of healthcare workers.

Example of organisms for which patients and healthcare workers may be reservoirs

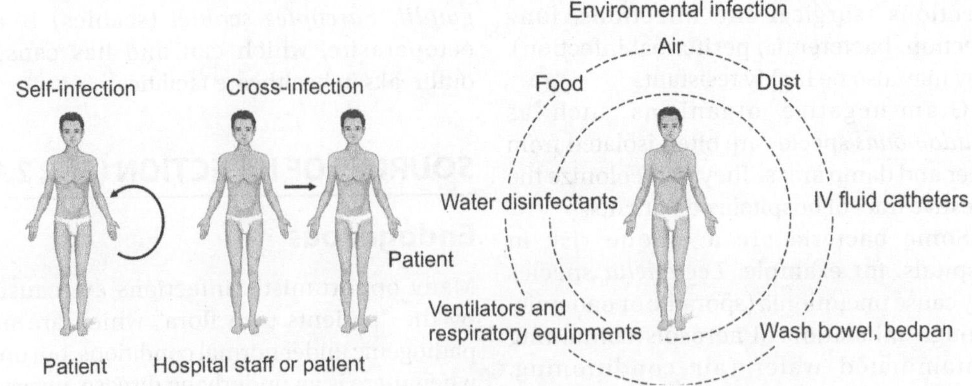

Fig. 2.1: Sources and methods of transmission of hospital-associated infection

include *S. aureus, Staphylococcus epidermidis (S. epidermidis)*, gram-negative bacilli, enterococci and large number of viruses, including hepatitis B virus, *Rotavirus* and *respiratory syncitial virus.*

Healthcare workers: Healthcare workers (HCW) often carry organisms that persist transiently on the skin, and less frequently colonization of the skin, gastrointestinal tract, respiratory tract and other mucous membranes also serve as reservoirs of infection.

Healthcare workers have been associated with nasal carriage of *S. aureus* and pharyngeal, rectal and vaginal carriage of group A streptococci. They may disseminate those infections by shedding colonized skin scales or generating aerosols. Certain conditions like symptomatic respiratory infections or skin rash appear to increase the likelihood of transmitting pathogens.

Inanimate objects: Inanimate objects are equipment, materials such as sanitary installation (bedpans, urinals) lights, table, blankets, and medical equipment like (endoscopes, catheters, needles, spatula and other instruments). Ventilating systems may be contaminated say by fungal spores, which may come from external sources. Recirculated air can be contaminated by organisms like *Aspergillus,* which colonize the insulation that lines ventilation ducts or air filters. *Legionella* can colonize central humidifiers from where they are disseminated through air.

Food and water contaminated by kitchen or other hospital staff or visitor may also be a source of infection. Coliforms are common in the moist environment such as fluids, in which they survive for long periods and sometime multiply in presence of minimum nutrients.

Water supplies especially hot water systems and environmental cooling systems can be colonized by *Legionella*. Ventilator reservoirs and room humidifiers can also become colonized especially by *Pseudomonas* species and other water loving species. Sink, drains and flower vases can become colonized with gram-negative bacilli, but the importance of these sites in propagating infections is often unclear.

Medical devices can be reservoirs of infecting pathogens; some of these may be contaminated during use and others during manufacture. There are a number of organisms, which can contaminate such devices, ranging from atypical mycobacterium colonizing prosthetic heart valves to the Jakob-Creutzfeldt agent contaminating implantable electrodes.

Hospital air: Because of increase in population especially in urban areas, there has been an overcrowding in hospitals, leading to an increase in bacterial count in the hospital air. Hospital air harbors gram-positive cocci derived from the body flora of hospital population and also other bacteria, which are more pathogenic and multidrug resistant.

Contaminated surfaces: Patient's secretions, excretions, blood and body fluids contaminate surfaces. Animals, and insects are also sources of hospital infection.

Contaminated solutions: Bacteria, which fix atmospheric nitrogen, may colonize dextrose solutions; lipids support the growth of many types of organisms, but have been especially associated with *Malassezia* and *S. epidermidis*. Even disinfectants can be colonized, for example, colonization of Benzalkonium chloride and iodophors by *Burkholderia cepacia* is well known.

MODES OF TRANSMISSION (FIG. 2.1)

There are four main routes of transmission of infections, the contact route, the aerial route, the oral route and the parenteral route.

Contact Route

Direct contact is probably the most important mode of spread of nosocomial infections.

Hands or Clothing

Hands and clothing of hospital personnel's' contain organisms received either from their own body or other patients. The hands of the staff are an important vehicle of transmission of hospital infection and hand washing by hospital persons, or use of gloves can make a significant contribution to control hospital-acquired infections.

Patients with comparable susceptibility to infection are housed in the same ward, e.g. urology, burns, nursery, where same staff looks after both infected and non-infected patients. Thus, there is adequate scope for transmission of microorganisms from one person to another by direct contact of hands and clothing of attendants. Important pathogens, which spread by hand contact, are *S. aureus, S. pyogenes, coliforms* (*E. coli*, and *Klebsiella* species) *Serratia* species and *Candida albicans*.

Inanimate Objects

Inanimate objects may serve as reservoirs of potentially pathogenic bacteria, which may spread without increasing its numbers, but when there is moisture, certain organisms (*P. aeruginosa*) multiply and so enhance the risk of infection.

Certain instruments (endoscopes, bronchoscopes, cystoscope) are difficult to disinfect because they do not withstand heating. Transmission of pathogenic organisms through these instruments may occur if not properly disinfected.

Oral Route and Feco-oral Route

Hospital food may contain gram-negative bacilli, which are most often antibiotic resistant (*P. aeruginosa, E. coli, Klebsiella* species and others). Although these bacteria may not cause gastroenteritis, they colonize the recipient's intestine and become established in the fecal flora of these patients.

Sometimes, contamination of the hands of healthcare workers can occur, who then carry the organisms to open wounds, urinary catheter systems, respiratory support equipment and to the mouth of the other patients.

Air-borne Route

From Patients and Hospital Personnel

Droplet nuclei, and droplets containing microorganisms that are a few micrometers in diameter coming from patients or the hospital personnel, are the most efficient disseminators of airborne infection.

Environmental Sources

i. *Dust:* Dust from bedding, floors, exudates dispersed from a wound during dressing and from the skin by natural shedding of skin scales. Commonly involved organisms are *Pseudomonas* species and *S. aureus*.

ii. *Aerosols:* Produced by nebulizers, humidifiers and air conditioning apparatus transmit certain pathogens (Coliforms, *Legionella*) to the respiratory tract if water in the instrument becomes contaminated.

Parenteral Route

With the introduction of screening tests, and use of disposable syringes and needles, transmission of infection by this route has become infrequent. However, certain infections are transmitted by blood transfusion or tissue donation, contaminated blood products like (Factor VIII), contaminated infusion fluids, and that resulting from sharp instruments.

Even though screening for *hepatitis B* and *HIV* infection, malaria and syphilis is carried out, rarely transmission of these infections can take place especially in rural areas where blood may not be screened before transfusion for these infections. So also some problems like non-A non-B hepatitis, other than *hepatitis C* remain. Transmission of HIV infection can also occur even after screening tests, if the donor is in the window period at that time. Blood transfusions can also transmit *Cytomegalovirus* infections which can be life- threatening for immunosuppressed patients, and also some bacterial infections.

Blood-borne transmission of infections to healthcare workers is also a problem at times.

Other Routes

Indwelling medical devices afford nosocomial pathogens direct access to normally sterile sites, particularly the lungs, urinary tract and blood stream. In addition surgical drains predispose to postoperative infection. In all of these cases organisms colonizing the skin or a mucosal surface are either dragged in when a device is inserted, migrate along the external surface of the device, or enter through an internal fluid lined channel.

ETIOLOGICAL AGENTS

Bacteria

S. aureus is the major cause of surgical wound and catheter entry site infections. The most common source of *S. aureus* infections is humans, although it can also be found in the environment. In most cases, human host carries the pathogen only transiently on hands, but contaminated hands are by far the main problem in transmission of *S. aureus* in hospital. Although persistent colonization of hospital staff occurs frequently (up to 50% in some studies), such colonization is rarely the source of nosocomial infection. When persons are colonized the major reservoir is anterior nares, it is also found on skin, especially of lower face and hands. The perineum and anus are occasionally colonized.

Therefore, evaluation of clusters of staphylococcal infections should focus attention first on identification of persons involved in care of infected patients and then reviewing their practice, rather than on search for a colonized individual or for an environmental source. Failure to use standard barrier precautions for care of wounds or to perform standard hand washing appear to cause the largest numbers of nosocomial staphylococcal infections. While organisms can be isolated from the environment or equipment, they are less likely to be the source, than is either another patient or an infected or colonized healthcare worker (HCW).

Coagulase-negative staphylococci, especially *S. epidermidis* are ubiquitous environmental and skin colonizing organisms. They rarely invade, except when they cause infections related to indwelling foreign bodies (from prosthesis to intravascular cannulas). Until recently, it has been difficult to distinguish different strains of *S. epidermidis,* so it was rarely possible to determine whether an infection arose from the hosts own flora or from cross infection. Application of newer technology such as plasmid fingerprinting, or endonuclease restriction enzyme mapping, indicates that cross infection plays an important role in introducing strains to patients.

Group A streptococcal infections are almost always the result of close contact with a colonized human. In community settings, the organism is transmitted principally by large respiratory droplets, and causes pharyngitis. In hospitals, the principal risk is wound infection, which follows transmission from pharyngeal and vaginal sites. The likelihood that a colonized healthcare worker is involved in transmission of nosocomial group A streptococcal infection is great enough, so much so that even a single case should prompt a search for additional cases and potential carriers.

There are two major groups of gram-negative bacillary infections. All of them propagate in moist environments. Enteric organisms such as *E. coli* are most likely to originate from a human source (urine or feces). Other non-enteric or water loving organisms, such as *Xanthomonas maltophila* and *Aeromonas hydrophila* can often be traced to a water source such as contaminated medical equipment.

The enteric gram-negative bacilli including organisms like *E. coli, Proteus and Klebsiella* are normal inhabitants of gastrointestinal tract, from where they colonize the perineum and introitus, thereby gaining access to the urinary tract. They are also among the early colonizers of the pharynx of hospitalized patients, and hence cause a large proportion of lower respiratory tract infections. This route is quite distinct from that taken by the non-enteric bacterial pneumonias.

Some strains of *Enterobacter* are able to live and grow in nitrogen poor fluids, for example, in 5% dextrose in water. Accordingly these organisms can play a disproportionate role in outbreaks of contaminated intravascular fluid systems. Conversely this provides a clue to the source of such infection when they cause bacteremia without an identifiable source.

Nonenteric gram-negative organisms such as *P. aeruginosa* and *Acinetobacter* may be found among normal flora, but less often and in smaller numbers than the enteric organisms.

Under appropriate selection pressure by antibiotics these minority organisms can proliferate, and become an endogenous source of infection. These organisms are also found in watery environments, ranging from sinks to irrigating solutions (Particularly if they are improperly stored).

Anaerobes are rarely documented as cause of nosocomial infections; although it is not clear whether this is a function of biology, or failure to culture. Outbreaks of infection with *Clostridium difficile*, have however been identified, and their ability to form hardy spores may make them more likely to persist in the environment. Presumably they can be transmitted either in the hands of HCWs or on fomites touched by patients.

Tuberculosis—transmitted by air-borne route, has its principal reservoir in infected patients. It is occasionally transmitted by HCW. On rare occasions endoscopes have been implicated in the transmission of tuberculosis.

Fungi

Aspergillus, a pathogen for immune-suppressed hosts is a nearly ubiquitous environmental agent. The principle issues in environmental control resolve around the need to prevent a large burden of organisms from accumulating and from being circulated in the hospital. This often requires attention to construction activities and ventilating equipment.

Candida albicans and other species have become important nosocomial pathogens. *Candida* commonly colonizes the GI tract and like *S. epidermidis* has been considered as an endogenous infection. Techniques that differentiate different strains indicate that cross infection is also an important problem.

Viruses

Patients and HCW are usually the source of nosocomial viral infections. Viral infections are commonly transferred between patients and employees, but are often unrecognized, partly because the lesser symptoms are not as well documented and also because viral cultures are obtained less frequently. Increased availability of viral cultures and other diagnostic tests should increase the recognition of these infections.

Respiratory viruses' especially *Respiratory syncitial virus* and *Rhinovirus* may be among the most common nosocomial infections. These appear to be transmitted by direct contact, although there is also evidence for respiratory spread of *Rhinovirus*. *Adenoviruses,* which are also transmitted by, direct contact or by transient colonization by fomites, can cause life-threatening infections among immunosuppressed patients. They also cause exposure epidemics of conjunctivitis among patients or HCW, who are exposed to contaminated equipment such as tonometers or the oculars of microscopes. In pediatrics some viral infections represent particular, problems. Transmission of RSV (*Respiratory syncitial virus*) from other infected children on the hands of HCW is a major mode of transmission. Contaminated fomites may also play a role. *RSV* infections can also be sustained by infected adult personnel who have symptoms of a common cold, who may be an important reservoir.

Common childhood respiratory diseases such as measles, rubella and chickenpox may provide truly airborne hazards to other susceptible patients and staff. Isolation is necessary for patients with these infections. Principally large droplets spread *Influenza virus,* a respiratory pathogen.

Enteric viruses such as *Rotaviruses* are another common cause of nosocomial infection. Hepatitis A and *Enteroviruses* have not been recognized to be major pathogens outside nurseries, probably because shedding of virus diminishes by the time symptoms prompt hospitalization.

HEALTHCARE WORKERS AND TRANSMISSION OF INFECTION

Healthcare workers are at risk both of acquiring infections from patients and transmitting their own illness to them. The epidemiology of infections in HCW is the same as for patients, although the emphasis and priorities differ. The same modes of spread operate; person-to-person contact may result in acquisition of nasal carriage with *S. aureus.* Most infections including respiratory infection, infectious diarrhea, and soft tissue infections such as boils, paronychia, and whitlows are not routinely identified, however, unless sought during a specific epidemiologic survey.

A few exposures are studied well enough to allow a specific estimate of risk, the tuberculosis conversion rate among general patient care employees in the US is about 1% per year, slightly higher than is expected in the population as a whole. Needle stick injuries involving transfer of blood from a hepatitis B antigen positive source result in a 23 to 37% seroconversion rate in susceptible persons.[27] Similar exposure to HIV infected blood carries a risk of about 0.3%.[28]

Some infections pose virtually no risk to employees. The risk of acquisition of *Cytomegalovirus* infection is not measurably greater for heavily exposed healthcare workers than for other personnel. Even pregnant employees can reasonably be expected to provide care for patients with mononucleosis or *Cytomegalovirus* infection, provided routine barrier precautions are used. *HIV* is transmitted infrequently when barrier techniques that are part of universal precautions are applied. These precautions should also reduce the risk of transmission of *hepatitis B,* although vaccination remains a principal prevention measure.

Some diseases in employees present sufficient risk to patients to require their exclusion from the workplace. Infections that require such attention include those that spread by respiratory droplets (e.g. pertusis or streptococcal infection of the throat), those spread by direct contact with lesions (adenoviral conjunctivitis, draining wounds) and those that spread by contact with diarrheal stools, and some diseases transmitted by an air-borne route (measles, rubella, chickenpox or tuberculosis). In epidemic situation, it may also be practical to identify influenza and to exclude infected personnel.

REFERENCES

1. Mims C, Palyfair J, Roitt I, Wakelin D, Williams R. Medical Microbiology, 2nd edn, Mosby International Ltd; 1999.p.482.
2. Gamor JS. CDC guidelines for prevention and control of nosocomial infections. Guidelines for prevention of surgical wound infections, 1985. Am J Infect Control. 1986;14:71-82.
3. Brusch JL, Bronze MS, et al. Catheter related urinary tract infection. Medscape (Drugs, Diseases and Procedures), Updated Jan 08 2013. Accessed from www.emedicine.medscape.com/article/2040035-overview.) on 18/8/2015.)
4. Brusch JL, Bronze MS, Cuervo Maldonado SI, Cortes Luna JA. Nosocomial Urinary Tract Infections. Accessed from www.cdn.intechopen.com/pdfs-wm/19326.pdf on 18/8/2015.
5. Platt R, Goldmann DA, Hopkins CC. Epidemiology of nosocomial infections. In: Gorbach SL, Bartlett JG, Blacklow NR (Eds). Infectious Diseases. WB Saunders Co; 1992.p.99.
6. Crook DWM, Bowler ICJ. Nosocomial infections. In: Weatherale DJ, Ledingham JGG, Warrel DA (Eds). Textbook of Medicine. Oxford University Press; 1996.pp.327-31.
7. Mukherjee S*, Nanivadekar AS. Nosocomial Infections—An Epidemiologic and Microbiologic Perspective—Guidelines for Antibiotic therapy. Net Address
8. Spelman DW. Hospital acquired infections. Med J Aust. 2002;176(6):286-91. Available at the Med J Aust 2002 ISSN: 0025-729x at www.mja.com.au. Accessed in Feb. 2004.
9. Nosocomial infection surveillance, 1984: MMWR CDC Surveill. 1986;35(ISS):17SS.
10. Haley RW, Culver DH, Margan WM, et al. identifying patients at high risk of surgical wound infection. A simple multivariate index of patient susceptibility and wound contamination. Am J Epidemiol. 1985;121:206.
11. Saxena A. Surgical site infection among postoperative patients of tertiary care centre in Central India—A prospective study. Asian Journal of Biomedical and Pharmaceutical Sciences. 2013;3:17. Accessed from www.jbiopharm.com/index.php/ajbps/article/view File/1871156
12. Apanga S, Adda J, Issahaku M, Amofa J, Mawufemor KRA, Bugr S. Postoperative Surgical Site Infection in a Surgical Ward of a Tertiary Care Hospital in Northern Ghana. Int J Res Health Sci [Internet]. 2014;2(1):207-12. Available from http://www.ijrhs.com/issues.php?val=Volume2&iss=Issue1
13. Patel S, Patel M, Patel S, Soni S, Kinariwala D, Vegad M. Surgical site infections: incidence and risk factors in a tertiary care hospital, western India (National Journal of Community Medicine Vol 3 Issue 2 April-June 2012). Accessed fromwww.njcm.org/home/download 238. On 13/8/2015.)
14. Kakati B, Kumar A, Gupta P, Sachan PK, Thakuria B. Surgical site abdominal wound infections: Experience at anorth Indian tertiary care hospital. JIACM. 2013;14(1):13-9. Accessed from www.medind.nic.in/jr/t13/i1/jact13I1p13pdf.)
15. Cruse PJE, Foord R. The epidemiology of wound infection. A 10-year prospective study of 62,939 wounds. Surg Clin North Am. 1980; 60:27.
16. Wilkin RT, Wenzel RP. Hospital acquired pneumonia. In: Remington JS, Swartz MN (Eds). Current Clinical Topics in Infectious Diseases. Cambridge, Massachusetts. Blackwell Science; 1996:pp.194-214.
17. Koran TC, White JW, Jarwis WR, et al. Nosocomial infection surveillance 1984. In Surveillance Summaries. 1985;35(ISS):17SS-29SS.
18. Leu HS, Kaiser DL, Mari M, et al. Hospital acquired pneumonia attributable mortality and morbidity. Am J Epidemiol. 1989;129:1258-67.
19. Maki DG. Nosocomial Bacteremia. An Epidemiologic Overview. Am J Med. 1981; 70:719.
20. Cunha BA, Brusch JL. Nosocomial and Healthcare-associated Pneumonia. Overview, Routes of Infection, Etiology and Pathophysiology (Medscape). Updated July 07 2015. Accessed from www.emedicine.medscape.com/article/234753-overview#a2. On 18/8/2015
21. Chandrasekar PH. Bacterial infections in hospitalized patients. Indian J Int Med. 1995; 5(Suppl 5): 3-11.

22. Jones RN. Microbial Etiologies of Hospital-Acquired Bacterial Pneumonia and Ventilator-Asoociated Pneumonia. CID (Clinical Infectious Diseases). 2010;51(S1):S81-S7. Accessed from www.cid.oxfordjournals.org/by me on August 11 2015.).
23. Ananthanarayan R, Jayaram Panikar CK. Hospital Infection; 5th edn, Orient Longman Ltd; 1999.p.584.
24. Grady CF, Lee VA. Hepatitis B immune globulin. Prevention of hepatitis from accidental exposures among medical personnel. New Eng J Med. 1975;293:106
25. Stephen Hugonnet, et al. Nosocomial bloodstream Infection and Clinical Sepsis. Emerging Infectious Diseases. Vol 10. No 1. Jan 2004. Accessed from www.nc.cdc.gov/eid/article/10/1/pdfs/03-407.pdf.on 18/8/2015.
26. Gahlot R, et al. Catheter-related bloodstrean infections. Int J Criti Illn Sci. 2014;4(2):162-7. Accessed from www. Ncbi.nim.nih.gov/pmc/articles/PMC 4093967/-
27. Updated US Public Health Service Guidelines for the management of occupational exposures to HBV, HCV and HIV and Recommendations for Post-exposure prophylaxis. Pg.3. from CDC MMWR Morbidity and Mortality Weekly Report June 29, 2001. Vol 50/No RR-11. US Dept of Health and Human Services CDC.Atlanta. From Net. www.cdc.gov/mmwr/preview/mmwrhtml/rr5011a1.htm-101k.
28. Updated US Public Health Service Guidelines for the management of occupational exposures to HBV, HCV and HIV and Recommendations for Post-exposure prophylaxis. Pg.7. from CDC MMWR Morbidity and Mortality Weekly Report June 29, 2001. Vol 50/No RR-11. US Dept of Health and Human Services CDC.Atlanta. From Net. www.cdc.gov/mmwr/preview/mmwrhtml/rr5011a1.htm-101k.

Chapter 3

Control of Hospital-acquired Infections

Chapter Outline

- Hospital-acquired Infection Control Committee
- Hospital-acquired Infection Control Team
- State Level Hospital-acquired Infection Control Board
- National Hospital-acquired Infection Control Central Board
- Role of Microbiology in Surveillance and Control
- Isolation Precaution Systems
- Limitations of Barrier Techniques
- Control of Epidemic Infections/Control of Outbreaks
- Investigations of Outbreaks
- Epidemiological Typing Techniques

INTRODUCTION

Controlling nosocomial infections is not easy. Any infection control officer would agree to this. It is easy to make policies, but difficult to implement them, therefore, persons working in this field should be watchful, non-interfering, ready to act, but patient. They must be bold enough to be critical, yet willing to accept criticism. They must be eager to teach, but willing to listen.

The prevention of HAI requires an organized management system. This can be achieved by creating a decision and policymaking body "the hospital-acquired infection control committee". This committee should be responsible for monitoring of HAI and implementation of control measures. A national network for hospital-acquired infections should be established to coordinate the infection control activities.

HOSPITAL-ACQUIRED INFECTION CONTROL COMMITTEE[1]

Every hospital must have a "hospital-acquired infection control committee" (HAICC). chaired by the medical superintendent of the hospital. Other members of the committee should be a microbiologist, one representative each from the clinical units, medical record officer; chief of nursing services and hospital-acquired infection control sister (HAICS).

A representative of supportive services (Central Sterile Supply Department—CSSD), dietetics department, laundry, operation theater (OT), house keeping, sanitation, etc. may be required to attend the meetings of HAICC, only when their agenda is being discussed. They may be grouped as invited members.

There must be a full time hospital-acquired infection control sister (HAICS). A microbiologist must be designated as "Infection control officer" who should be a member secretary of the committee.

The above committee must meet at least once every month to review the infection control activities. This should include reviewing the emergence of drug resistance, use of different antimicrobials, hospital environment, and sterilization and disinfection procedures. They must also review the incidence and type of infections and the antimicrobial sensitivity pattern of the prevalent pathogens.

There has been a tremendous increase in the use of presterilized disposable material. It is necessary to review how this disposable material is used and then discarded and disposed. It is also necessary to be aware of the misuse and reuse of these used and contaminated disposable material.

The concept of differentiating hospital waste from household waste does not exist in our country, it is necessary that this concept is developed, and hospital waste is taken care of properly. It has been noticed that blood and blood contaminated material like swabs; disposable needles, syringes, sponges, dressings, etc. are discarded and disposed off from the hospital with general waste. It is important that proper care is taken in their disposal to prevent blood-borne infections.

HOSPITAL-ACQUIRED INFECTION CONTROL TEAM[1]

The HAICC should have a small subordinate committee, which should be named "hospital-acquired infection control team (HAICT). This team should consist of three persons, the infection control officer (ICO), who is a microbiologist, infection control sister and a clinician.

The team should be responsible for surveillance activity. The members of the team should meet at least once a week. They should discuss the occurrence of different types of infections in the hospital, their etiological agents and antimicrobial sensitivity pattern. In case of outbreaks attempts must be made to find the source of infection and control this infection. They should also carry out periodical environmental survey for the carriage of pathogenic organisms by the health care workers. They should also draw guidelines aimed at reducing HAI in different areas like wards, OT's, injection rooms, blood collection centers, supportive services (e.g. kitchen and laundry), sterilization and disinfection procedures.

Special attention should also be paid by this team to disposal of hospital waste.

The findings and recommendations of the HAICT should be placed before HAICC for their approval. The medical superintendent who is the chairman of the HAICC should implement the recommendations accepted by HAICC. A policy for use of anti-microbial agents (antibiotics) should be formulated. This can be done only after keeping a close watch on the trends of antimicrobial resistance of hospital pathogens from time to time.

It is necessary to publish the analyzed data, so that necessary guidelines can be issued to different categories of staff. A continuous training program for all the categories should be held at the earliest for implementing the recommended procedures and practices according to the guidelines.

STATE LEVEL HOSPITAL-ACQUIRED INFECTION CONTROL BOARD[1]

A state level network of all the hospitals in a particular state should be formed. This "State level hospital infection control board" should be headed by the secretary of health services.

The director of health services or hospital should be the co-chairperson. All medical superintendents of the state hospitals should be members. A senior officer of the state health services should be designated as state coordinator of HAI control program, who should act as member secretary of the board.

NATIONAL HOSPITAL-ACQUIRED INFECTION CONTROL CENTRAL BOARD

A national level infection control program may also be developed. It should be through a similar committee at the national level. The "National hospital-acquired infection control board" should be chaired by the secretary health. The director general of health services should be co-chairperson. The other members of the board should be state coordinators of HAI control program or directors health services. A senior officer should be designated as national coordinator hospital-acquired infection control program at the national level, which should act as member secretary of the board.

A mechanism should be developed for the periodical assessment of the implementations of the recommendations of national HAICB and state HAICB. It may be feasible to implement a program by creating central and state coordinating institutions which should draw up national/state programs, and carry out research on various procedures for their cost-effectiveness and efficiency, draw up guidelines for all activities, publish the hospital manual, and regularly publish information and analytical data from various parts of the country which should emphasize the trends of infection and antimicrobial resistance.

Manpower development program must be developed and continuous in service training programs introduced for hospital-acquired infection control officers, hospital-acquired infection control nurses, microbiologists and all categories of hospital staff.

ROLE OF MICROBIOLOGY IN SURVEILLANCE AND CONTROL

Laboratory based surveillance is one of the important methods of surveillance to verify nosocomial infections. In the past, the problem was very few samples were cultured, however nowadays enough number of cultures are done. The real problem is that many of the organisms isolated from these cultures do not reflect infections, but only represent contaminants, saprophytes or normal components of microbial flora. However, a detailed review of this data by the epidemiologist will spot the emergence and spread of bacteria, that may later turn out to pose significant problems for the infection control team. Timely detection of bacteria that have acquired resistance to antibiotics that are generally used empirically at a given institution is particularly important, for example, it is easier to control a strain of amikacin resistant *Enterobacter* or of methicillin resistant *Staphylococcus aureus* if it has colonized only a few patients. Timely intervention by the HAICT will certainly prevent the spread of these organisms to other patients in the ward and perhaps to other areas of the hospital.

In India, surveillance for viral disease is still based mainly on clinical criteria, because few hospitals have clinical virology laboratories and therefore nosocomial viral infections are not documented. In advanced countries sensitive and rapid viral diagnostic tests have become commercially available for many of the viral agents that commonly cause nosocomial infections. The technologic revolution makes surveillance for nosocomial infections practically possible. Such viral surveillance is more essential for some areas of the hospital, such as infant wards, where respiratory syncitial virus (RSV) and rotavirus may account for the large majority of infections and considerable infection, related morbidity.

Nowadays, recently developed typing methods like plasmid typing, restriction nuclease analysis, DNA probe techniques, PCR may be required.

ISOLATION PRECAUTION SYSTEMS

Different types of isolation systems have been recommended:[2,3]

1. *CDC isolation systems:*
   a. Category-specific isolation system.
   b. Disease-specific isolation system.
2. *Body substance isolation system:* It was proposed by Harbor view medical center, Seattle and the university of California, San Diego.
3. *Universal precautions:* Now universal precautions have been made mandatory by OSHA (Occupational safety and health administration).

Traditional CDC Isolation Systems

Two isolation precautions systems have been defined and promoted by CDC.

a. Category-specific isolation system.
b. Disease-specific isolation system.

Category-specific Isolation System

In this system, diseases are grouped into six categories of isolation based on their usual modes of transmission. In each category, similar precautions are taken for all the diseases in that category. However, because many different diseases are grouped into six categories, unnecessary precautions will be applied to some diseases.

The six categories are:

1. Strict isolation.
2. Contact isolation.
3. Respiratory isolation.
4. Tuberculosis isolation.
5. Enteric precautions.
6. Drainage/secretion precautions.

No separate category for blood and body fluid precautions is required because of universal precautions.

1. Strict isolation: It is required for highly contagious or virulent infections. This includes infections, which spread by contact and air. This category is used for patients with pharyngeal diphtheria, Lassa fever, and other viral hemorrhagic fevers, pneumonic plague, varicella (chickenpox) and zoster that occurs in an immunocompromised host or is disseminated.

Precautions:

a. Private room—preferably with negative pressure ventilation. Doors should be closed.
b. Masks, gowns and gloves are indicated for all persons entering the room.
c. Hands must be washed after gloves are removed, and before taking care of another patient.
d. Articles contaminated with infectious material must be bagged, labeled and either discarded (that is incinerated or autoclaved) or decontaminated and reprocessed.

2. Contact isolation: This is for infections that can be spread only by close contact with patient. When feasible these patients should be put in a private room, or with other patients who have the same infection. This type of isolation is required for diseases like staphylococcal and streptococcal infections, patients colonized with *methicillin-resistant staphylococci* or multiply drug resistant gram-negative bacilli, children with acute respiratory infections like pharyngitis, pneumonias, newborn with gonococcal conjunctivitis, herpes simplex virus infections, patients with cutaneous diphtheria, infections like scabies, pediculosis, rubella, vaccinia.

Precautions:

a. Patient should be kept in a private room with anteroom and negative pressure.
b. Masks are suggested when personnel are likely to go within a few feet of a patient whose infection may be transmitted by droplet contact or direct contact.
c. Gown is worn if soiling of clothes is likely.

d. Gloves are worn when touching potentially infective material.
e. Hands must be washed after removing gloves and before taking care of another patient.
f. Articles contaminated with infective material are to be handled with care as described previously.

3. *Respiratory isolation:* It is preserved for patients with infections spread only by droplet contact, such as meningococcal infection, measles, *Haemophilus influenzae* epiglottitis, pneumonia, mumps and pertussis.

Precautions:

a. Private room is necessary with negative pressure ventilation.
b. Masks are indicated for close contact.
c. Gowns and gloves are not necessary.
d. Hands must be washed before taking care of the patient.
e. Articles contaminated with infective material are to be handled with care as described previously.

4. *Tuberculosis precautions:* This is a stricter form of respiratory isolation that recognizes the potential for spread of tuberculosis by air-borne droplet nuclei. With AIDS pandemic and re-emergence of tuberculosis often with multiply drug resistant tuberculosis, precautions have been updated.

Precautions:

a. Private room with anteroom and negative pressure ventilation. Doors of room should be kept closed.
b. Masks should be worn when entering the room. They should have a very good facial fit and filtration capability.
c. Gowns are worn if contamination of clothes is likely.
d. Gloves are not indicated.
e. Hands must be washed after touching the patient or contaminated articles and before taking care of another patient.
f. Contaminated or used articles should be thoroughly disinfected, cleaned and processed, or if disposable, safely discarded.

5. *Enteric isolation:* This is for infections that spread by direct or indirect contact with feces (feco-oral transmission. Infectious diarrhea due to *Entamoeba histolytica, Vibrio cholerae* and other *Vibrio* species, *Campylobacter, Cryptosporidium, Dientamoeba, Escherichia coli, Giardia, Salmonella, Shigella, Yersinia enterocolitica,* enteroviral infections (poliomyelitis, pleurodynia, viral meningitis), enterocolitis caused by *Staphylococcus aureus, Clostridium difficile,* hepatitis A.

Precautions:

a. Private room is necessary only for patients with incontinence or poor hygiene.
b. Gowns are indicated if soiling is likely.
c. Gloves are needed when touching feces or articles contaminated with feces.
d. Masks are not essential.
e. Hands must be washed after removing gloves and before taking care of another patient.
f. Articles contaminated with infective material are to be handled with care as described previously.

6. *Drainage secretion isolation system:* This is to prevent spread of infections that are spread by direct or indirect contact, with purulent infective material. Many minor draining infections fall into this category.

Precautions:

a. No private room is required.
b. Masks are not needed.
c. Gowns are required if soiling is likely.
d. Gloves used for contact with infective material.
e. Hands must be washed after removing gloves, before taking care of another patient.
f. Articles contaminated with infective material are to be handled with care.

Though this system is simple, infections with different modes of transmission are grouped together, sometimes with little logic, e.g. influenza and rubella are grouped together with staphylococcal wound infection in the contact isolation category.

Disease-specific Isolation System

This was introduced to provide a more logical approach to isolation based on epidemiology of individual pathogens. In the disease-specific isolation, each infectious disease is considered individually and only those precautions (private room, gloves, masks and gowns) are taken that will prevent transmission of a specific infectious agent, therefore this system would require a greater degree of clinical judgment than the category specific isolation system, and is difficult to apply to patients who do not yet have specific signs and symptoms that suggest a specific diagnosis.

The precautions manual published by CDC has been used in many hospitals as the starting point, but each hospital should develop its own precautions manual according to its requirement.

Body Substance Isolation

In 1987, an alternative system of isolation precautions were proposed by Harbor view medical center, Seattle and the university of California, San Diego.[4] It focuses on the isolation of all moist body substances (blood, feces, urine, sputum, saliva, wound drainage and other body fluids) from all patients. Additional precautions are taken for diseases that have airborne component of transmission. Body substance isolation includes the following precautions:

1. Gloves should be worn for anticipated contact with blood, secretions, mucous membranes, non-intact skin and moist body substances of all patients. Handwashing is not necessary when gloves are worn unless the hands become visibly soiled. Gloves should be changed before another patient is treated.
2. Gowns, plastic aprons, masks or goggles should be worn when secretions, blood or body fluids are likely to soil or splash on clothing, skin or face.
3. Soiled reusable items, linen, etc. should be stored in a leak proof container/bag. Double bagging is not necessary unless the outside of the bag is visibly soiled.
4. Needles (without recapping them) and sharp items should be placed in puncture resistant rigid containers.
5. Private rooms are indicated for patients with some diseases transmitted by the airborne route, e.g. pulmonary tuberculosis and other diseases listed in the "strict isolation category" of the CDC guidelines. Private rooms are also recommended for patients who soil articles in the environment with body substances.
6. HCW should be either immune or immunized against infectious microorganisms that are transmitted by airborne route. The diseases included are measles, mumps, rubella and varicella. They should also be immunized against tuberculosis, poliomyelitis, diphtheria and enteric fever. Nonimmune HCWs should not enter room of patients with these infections.

BSI has several advantages. It provides a barrier between the hands and nosocomial contaminants, so even if hand washing is neglected, there is a margin of safety. Compliance with gloving while personnel are in contact with patients should be much easier to monitor than handwashing. A single evidence in support of the BSI efficacy is provided by the study in an intensive (pediatric) care unit, in which procedures similar to BSI that is routine use of gloves and gowns for contact with patients significantly reduced nosocomial colonization and infection.[5]

On the other hand, implementation of BSI might also have a deleterious effect. Gloves may provide a false sense of security and result in even less handwashing. Care givers may even neglect changing gloves between patients and since some pathogens survive better on gloves than on skin [6] and since some bacteria may be difficult to remove from glove even if the care giver tries to wash the gloved hands, nosocomial transmission of organisms could be facilitated.[7]

Universal Precautions

Individual hospitals are free to select any of the general precaution systems described above. Universal precautions (UP) are now made mandatory by Occupational Safety and Health Administration (OSHA), largely to protect health care workers from blood-borne pathogens, especially the HIV and hepatitis B and C viruses. UP was originally designed to apply to CDC's previous blood and fluid precautions universally to all patients, but CDC recommendations[8] have broadened the scope of these guidelines to non-intact skin and mucosal surfaces and to many other body fluids such as pleural fluid, pericardial and cerebrospinal fluids and any other fluid that contains visible blood. Like BSI, UP relies on the use of barrier techniques. It is important to note that UP was implemented to protect personnel, not to prevent transmission of nosocomial pathogens from patient-to-patient. But if this is the message one gets, then HCWs may think of gloves only in terms of self-protection and may not worry about cross-infection and the importance of changing gloves between patient contacts. However, rigorous adherence to BSI might bring the focus back to patient while still protecting the personnel. Moreover, BSI would also protect workers concerned about microscopic amounts of blood in urine or feces or leukocytes present in draining wound, although there has been no evidence to date that such exposures are hazardous.

Whichever system of precautions or isolation is used, teaching and implementation are critical. It has been seen that open monitoring of compliance with surveillance procedures coupled with an intensive educational campaign will greatly increase the compliance rate.

LIMITATIONS OF BARRIER TECHNIQUES

Nosocomial infections caused by patient's own microbial flora (endogenous infection) are also important, but it must be emphasized that most of the times, these endogenous infections are not caused by the bacteria that these patients bring into the hospital, but rather by nosocomial strains that are acquired after admission and become a part of endogenous nosocomial flora. Pharyngeal colonization with gram-negative bacilli had been observed in 22% patients admitted to the intensive care unit just within 24 hours, so also skin may be colonized with gram-positive bacteria such as methicillin resistant *Staphylococcus aureus*.[9-11] Barrier precautions control the transmission of these pathogens and prevent subsequent colonization and infection of newly admitted patients. However, these barrier techniques have had very little impact on colonization and infection with some organisms such as *Pseudomonas*.[12] However, on detailed investigation, it was found that majority of the patients who were colonized with *Pseudomonas* actually brought these strains with them, although their bacteria may have become more resistant to antibiotics under the selection pressure of broad-spectrum therapy.[13,14] Similarly colonization and infection with *Enterobacter* in patients undergoing coronary artery surgery could be attributed to outgrowth of *Enterobacter* that had been present in small concentrations prior to surgery and emerged under selective pressure of cephalosporin prophylaxis.[15] Thus, intensive efforts to prevent cross-infection by using barrier techniques must be implemented, but never expected to eliminate all infections.

CONTROL OF EPIDEMIC INFECTIONS/CONTROL OF OUTBREAKS

Infections in the hospital can be prevented by implementation of appropriate policies, and control of sporadic and endemic nosocomial infections which should be included as part of day-to-day activity of the infection control program. So also control of antibiotic resistant bacteria and reinforcement of good techniques in the insertion and maintenance of urinary and intravenous catheters are important for controlling nosocomial infections.

There are many phases in control of outbreaks:

Phase 1: Confirm that an outbreak really exists, since false alarms are common.

Phase 2: Intensification of routine procedures. For this

a. Review current practices.
b. Check whether barrier techniques are used appropriately.
c. Correction of immediately apparent problems.

Phase 3: Case definition.

Every effort must be made to identify as many cases as possible as this facilitates both epidemiological investigation and outbreak control. Comprehensive case finding for many pathogens will require the detection of carriers as well as infected individuals. For this, the hospital microbiologist should be consulted for the most efficient screening techniques.

Knowledge regarding the spread of epidemic pathogen is necessary to narrow the focus of investigation and to come to a conclusion as early as possible, so that appropriate control measures can be taken immediately.

Although some outbreaks can be traced to a common source such as faulty air-handling system, an environmental reservoir, a carrier in the hospital staff, or a contaminated device or solution, most are attributable to a breakdown in the routine aseptic procedures and person-to-person spread. When person-to-person transmission is thought to be the principal source of the problem, appropriate precautions should be instituted and barrier techniques intensified.

The single most important intervention in such cases is cohorting all the patients who are either infected or colonized with the outbreak strain in one ward. Physical cohorting of the patients in the same location should be complemented by cohorting of caregivers if possible.

INVESTIGATIONS OF OUTBREAKS

Hospital-acquired Infections Outbreaks

These are defined as an increase in the number of hospital-acquired or healthcare facility-acquired cases of disease among patients or staff *over and above the expected number of cases**. (Two or three cases of a rare infection is considered as an outbreak.)

When an outbreak (epidemic) occurs, or when routine surveillance shows an increase in the incidence of infection, the infection control team, should initiate an investigation. There is no universally applicable routine for finding the cause of an outbreak, but in principle each investigation has an epidemiological element and a microbiological element.

Epidemiological Element

Definition of any Outbreak in Epidemiological Terms

This includes answering a number of questions like:

- How many people were affected?
- When were they admitted?
- When did they develop infection?
- Are they all in the same ward?
- Are they all treated by the same medical or surgical team?

Investigation of Outbreaks

- Identify the pathogen
- Identify the source
- Identify the mode of transmission
- To assess the relative risk associated with the factor under investigation and to formulate appropriate control strategies.

*The expected number of cases can be determined through ongoing disease surveillance. This involves systematic collection of numerator and denominator data using standardized case definitions and surveillance methods.[16]

Causative organism needs to be isolated in all patients involved in the outbreak.

It is the microbiology laboratory, which would attempt to isolate the causative organism and to show that all patients in the outbreak are infected with the same strain, i.e. strains that are indistinguishable (proved by typing methods).

The identity of the infecting organism provides clues to the possible source, e.g. an outbreak of wound infection with *S. aureus* is likely to be associated with contact spread from staff in the wards whereas an outbreak of *Salmonella* gastroenteritis is more likely to originate in the kitchen.

When the investigations are still going on, efforts must be made to contain the outbreak and prevent spread to other patients. Infected patients must be isolated and treated appropriately. Staff who are found to be infected or carriers must be suspended from duty until they have been treated. At the end of the investigation relevant procedures must be reviewed to try and prevent a similar outbreak occurring again.

Control measures of outbreak management

Types of transmission suspected	suggested action
Cross- transmission (transmission between individuals)	Patient isolation and barrier precautions determined by infectious agent(s)
Hand transmission	Improvements in hand washing; cohorting
Air-borne agent	Patient isolation with appropriate ventilation
Agent present in water, water-borne agent	Checking of water supply and all liquid containers Use of disposable devices
Food-borne agent	Elimination of the food at risk

EPIDEMIOLOGICAL TYPING TECHNIQUES

A number of typing methods are used to 'fingerprint' strains for epidemiological purposes.

In epidemiological studies of spread of infection and in the investigation of outbreaks both in the hospital and in the community, it is necessary to compare bacterial isolates to determine whether they belong to the same species, and if so whether they are distinct or of the same strain. In fact, it is not possible to say that two organisms are the same, only that they are indistinguishable. If the species is a regular member of the normal flora, or is found frequently in the environment, it is necessary to distinguish the outbreak strain from other strains of the same species not involved in the outbreak, but that may also be isolated during the course of the investigation.

A good typing technique must be:

- Discriminatory (i.e. able to show differences between strains of the same species)
- Reproducible (i.e. the same strains gives the same result when tested on different occasions and in different places)
- Have a high degree of typeability (i.e. capable of assigning a type to all strains)
- Ease of performance: To be widely useful, a typing method should be applicable to a broad range of microorganisms as well as inexpensive and technically easy
- Ease of interpretation: The typing tests must produce reproducible and unambiguous results that can be interpreted easily.

There are different typing methods:

Typing Methods[17]

It is sometimes important to analyze multiple isolates within a given species to determine whether they represent a single strain or multiple strains. If a species of bacteria is isolated and cultivated in the laboratory, it is known as a strain. A single isolate with distinctive characteristic(s) may also represent a strain.

Members of the same species that have small differences between them can be distinguished by additional methods. These species is then subdivided into subspecies, subgroups, biotypes, serotypes, variants, etc.

The process of differentiating strains based on their phenotypic and genotypic differences is known as 'typing'.

These typing methods are useful in hospital infection control, epidemiological studies, and understanding the pathogenesis of infection.

In hospital settings, they may be used to:
- Determine whether a set of isolates obtained from one patient represents a single infecting strain or multiple contaminants
- Determine whether a series of isolates obtained over time represents relapse of an infection due to single strain or separate episodes of disease due to different strains.

Types of typing methods:
1. Phenotypic techniques, those that detect characteristics expressed by the microorganism.
2. Genotypic techniques, those that involve direct DNA-based analysis of chromosomal or extrachromosomal genetic elements.[17]

Phenotypic Methods

Phenotypic properties are properties like shape, size, staining properties, biochemical properties, antigenic properties that can be measured without reference to the genome.

These phenotypic methods are limited by:
- Capacity of microorganisms to alter the expression of genes, which may occur spontaneously or in response to environmental stimuli. Cells, which are genetically indistinguishable, may have quite distinct phenotypes/phenotypic properties if growing under different conditions.
- Point mutations that may not bring considerable change in genotype can result in abnormal regulation or function responsible for a particular phenotype.
- Large fractions of strains are untypeable
  a. The ones which can be carried out in routine diagnostic laboratories like:
     1. Antibiotic susceptibility patterns
     2. Simple biotyping
  b. The ones which are specialized typing techniques are done in reference laboratories. These are:
     1. Serotyping
     2. Bacteriophage typing
     3. Bacteriocin typing
     4. Molecular typing techniques.

Antibiotic Susceptibility Patterns

This typing technique involves comparison of different isolates to a set of antibiotics. Isolates differing in their susceptibilities are considered as different strains. The identification of new or unusual pattern of antibiotic resistance among isolates cultured from multiple patients is often the first indication of an outbreak.[17]

These give a preliminary clue as to whether the two isolates are indistinguishable. However with this method, discrimination is poor, as many susceptibility patterns are common, and quite different strains may show the same pattern. Conversely, during an outbreak, strains may gain or lose plasmids carrying antibiotic resistance markers.

Advantages: Almost all strains are typeable. The technique has ease of performance and interpretation with fair amount of reproducibility.

Disadvantages: As a consequence of various genetic mechanisms, different strains may develop similar resistance pattern thus reducing the discriminating power. The susceptibility pattern of isolates taken over a period of time that represents the same strain may differ for one or more antibiotics due to acquisition of resistance.

Biotyping

This method involves the ability of the organism to grow on different substrates or produce different enzymes. Ideally the biochemical tests employed in a biotyping scheme should be different from those used to identify the organisms. Identification tests are done, because they 'lump' similar organisms together; biotyping tests are chosen because they split species into distinct strains. However, most of the diagnostic laboratories use profiles from multitest identification (often miniaturized) systems as biotypes.

Advantages: Most strains are typeable. The techniques are reproducible with relative ease of performance and interpretation.

Disadvantages: They have poor discriminatory power. Variation in gene expression is the most common reason for isolates that represent single strain to differ in one or more biochemical reactions. Point mutation too contributes to this problem.[17]

Serotyping

This technique distinguishes between strains by a difference in their antigenic structure, which is recognized by reaction with specific antigen, e.g. *Salmonella* is typed on basis of the 'O' somatic antigens and *H. flagellar* antigens. *S. pneumoniae, Neisseria meningitidis* and *Klebsiella aerogenes* can be typed on basis of their capsules (K) antigens and *S. pyogenes* on their M and T cell wall proteins. The established schemes use polyclonal antisera, but newer schemes based on monoclonal are being developed.

Serotyping requires the production and maintenance of appropriate banks of antisera, which is both time consuming and costly. It is therefore usually restricted to reference laboratories.

Advantages: Most strains are typeable. They have good reproducibility and ease of interpretation though some have ease of performance.

Disadvantages: Some methods of serotyping are technically demanding. There is dependency on good quality reagent from commercial sources. In-house preparation of reagents is a difficult process. Serotyping has poor discriminatory power due to large number of serotypes, cross reaction of antigens and untypeable nature of some strains.[17]

Bacteriophage Typing

Strains can be characterized by their pattern of resistance or susceptibility to a standard set of bacteriophages. This relies on the presence or absence of particular receptors on the bacterial surface that are used by the virus to bind to the bacterial wall. This method is used to type isolates of Staphylococcus aureus and Salmonella species. Such strains are referred as 'phage types'.[17]

In this method, the isolate to be typed is grown as a lawn culture on agar plates and exposed to standard series of phage suspensions. The method is important for typing *S. aureus, S. epidermidis* and *Salmonella typhi*, but has been applied to other organisms like *Pseudomonas aeruginosa.*

As with serotyping, phage typing requires the production, maintenance and testing of the standard phage suspensions and is usually carried out in reference laboratories rather than in hospital diagnostic laboratory.

Advantages: This technique has fair amount of reproducibility, discriminatory power and ease of interpretation.

Disadvantages: This technique requires maintenance of biologically active phages and hence is available only at reference centers. Even for the experienced worker, the technique is demanding. Many strains are non-typeable.[17]

Bacteriocin Typing

This method has been successfully used for *Pseudomonas aeruginosa* (pyocine typing) and *Shigella sonnei* (Colicine typing). In this method, the production of bacteriocins by the strain produces a pattern of inhibition of growth of a standard set of indicator strains, which can be used to assign the test strain to a type. Bacteriocins produced by a particular strain are usually only active against other strains of the same species. This method is potentially applied to any species that produces bacteriocins (and most do).

Advantages: This technique has fair amount of reproducibility, discriminatory power and ease of interpretation.

Disadvantages: This technique is available only at reference centers. Even for the experienced worker, the technique is demanding. Many strains are nontypeable.

Protein Typing[17]

Protein typing relies on major or minor differences in the range of proteins made by different strains. Variations in the types and structures of the proteins expressed by bacteria can be detected by several methods. The proteins, glycoproteins or polysaccharides are extracted from a culture of the strain, separated by sodium dodecyl sulfate-polyacrylamide gel electrophoresis and stained to compare with those of other strains. More-similar organisms display more-similar protein patterns.

In another method termed immunoblotting, the electrophoresed products are transferred to nitrocellulose membrane and then exposed to antisera raised against specific strain. The bound antibodies are then detected by enzyme-labeled anti-immunoglobulins.

These methods are currently employed for epidemiological studies of *Staphylococcus aureus* and *Clostridium difficile.*

Advantages: Almost all strains are typeable and techniques have good reproducibility and ease of interpretation.

Disadvantages: Since the patterns detected are very complex, comparisons among multiple strains are difficult and the interpretation becomes difficult. Methods employed are technically demanding and equipments are costly and hence are not available in all laboratories.

Multilocus Enzyme Electrophoresis (MLEE)[17]

Here, the isolates are analyzed for differences in the electrophoretic mobilities of a set of metablolic enzymes. Cell extracts containing soluble enzymes are electrophoresed in starch gels. Variations in the electrophoretic mobility of an enzyme, referred to as 'electromorph', typically reflect amino acid substitution that alter the charge of the protein.

Advantages: Almost all strains can be typed. The technique has excellent reproducibility and ease of interpretation.

Disadvantages: It is only moderately discriminatory for the epidemiological analysis of clinical isolates. It requires techniques and equipments that are not available in most laboratories.

Genotypic Methods[17]

These methods involve the study of the microbial DNA, the chromosome and plasmid, their composition, homology and presence or absence of specific genes. Originally performed only in research laboratories have now found their way into diagnostic laboratories. Due to their complexities and cost involved, they are however limited to few laboratories only.

Molecular Typing

This involves characterization of an organism's DNA—either chromosome or plasmid or total protein profile (i.e. all of the proteins in the cell encoded by the DNA). Plasmid profiles are only useful for species that carry variety of plasmids, and they suffer from the drawback that what is actually being characterized is the plasmid and not the organism containing it. Different gram-negative rods may acquire the same plasmids by conjugation between different species. However, this method has also been used to map the spread of antibiotic resistance plasmids among hospital pathogens.

Plasmid Analysis[17]

The number and sizes of plasmids carried by an isolate can be determined by preparing a plasmid extract and subjecting it to gel electrophoresis.

Advantages: Most strains are typeable and have good ease of interpretation.

Disadvantages: Reproducibility of this method suffers due to the existence of plasmid in different molecular forms such as supercoiled, nicked or linear, each of which migrate differently on electrophoresis. Since plasmids can be spontaneously lost or readily acquired, related strains can exhibit different plasmid profiles. Since certain genes are contained in transposons that can be readily acquired or deleted, the composition of plasmid DNA can change rapidly. Clinical isolates lacking plasmids are untypeable. Those strains with one or two plasmids provide poor discriminatory power.

Restriction Endonuclease Analysis (REA) of Chromosomal DNA[17]

A restriction endonuclease enzymatically cuts DNA at a specific nucleotide recognition sequence. The number and sizes of restriction fragments are influenced by the recognition sequence of enzyme and composition of DNA. Bacterial DNA is digested with endonucleases that have relatively frequent restriction sites, thereby generating hundreds of fragments ranging from ~0.5 to 50 kb in length. Such fragments can be separated by size using agarose gel electrophoresis. The pattern stained by ethidium bromide and examined under UV light. Different strains of the same species have different REA profiles because of variations in their DNA sequences.

Advantages: All the strains can by typed with good reproducibility.

Disadvantages: The complex profile consists of hundreds of bands that may be unresolved or overlapping thus making comparison difficult. The pattern may consist of bands generated from digestion of plasmids too. These reduce the ease of interpretation and discriminatory power.

PFGE of Chromosomal DNA[17]

This technique overcomes the limitations of REA. It is a variation of agarose gel electrophoresis in which the orientation of the electric field across the gel is changed periodically. This modification enables large fragments to be effectively separated by size.

Advantages: All the strains can by typed with good reproducibility. Restriction profiles are easily read and interpreted.

Disadvantages: The process takes 2–4 days and requires costly reagents and equipment besides being labor intensive.[17]

Southern Blot Analysis of RFLPs[17]

In contrast to REA of DNA, southern blot analyses detect only the particular restriction fragment. The DNA is digested by endonuclease, the fragments are separated by gel electrophoresis and the fragments transferred to nitrocellulose membranes. The fragments containing specific sequences are then detected by labeled DNA probes. Variations in the number and sizes of the fragments detected are referred to as restriction fragment length polymorphism (RFLP).

Ribotyping is the blotting of restriction enzyme digestion of 16s rRNA, 25s rRNA and one or more tRNAs. As the 16srRNA is so highly conserved, it is a very useful molecule for comparing relatedness of organisms over the course of evolution. Organisms are classified as separate species if their sequences show less than 98% homology and are classified as different genera if their sequences show less than 93% identity.

Advantages: All strains carrying loci homologous to probe are typeable. They are reproducible, have good ease of interpretation.

Disadvantages: The discriminatory power depends on the choice of probes. The process requires costly reagents and equipment besides being labor intensive.[17]

Nucleotide Sequence Analysis[17]

Genotype information at highest precision may be determined as DNA (or RNA) nucleotide-base sequences. RNA's are often sequenced either by converting the RNAs into DNA or by sequencing the DNA gene that gives rise to the RNA. By using Polymerase Chain Reaction (PCR) to amplify a known DNA segment and automated techniques to sequence the amplified product, it is possible to compare multiple isolates.

Advantages: This technique can apply on all strains; results are reproducible with ease in interpretation.

Disadvantages: The process requires costly reagents and equipment besides being labor intensive.[17]

REFERENCES

1. Shriniwas. Hospital acquired infections–Guidelines for control. Govt of India. Ministry of Health and Family Welfare. Nirman Bhavan, New Delhi. 1992.p.3.
2. Goldmann D, Platt R, Hopkins C. Control of hospital-acquired infections. In: Gorbach SL, Bartlett JG, Blacklow NR (Eds). Infectious Diseases. WB Saunders Co. 1992. pp.382-4.
3. *Agarwal DS. Guidelines for nosocomial infection—surveillence and control.
4. Lynch P, Jackson MM, Cummings MJ, Stamin WE. Rethinking the role of isolation precautions in the prevention of nosocomial infections. Ann Int Med. 1987;107:243.
5. Klein BS, Perloff WH, Maki DG. Reduction of nosocomial infection during paediatric intensive care by protective isolation. New Eng J Med. 1989;320:1714.
6. Hall CB, Douglas KG Jr, Geiman JM. Possible transmission by fomites of respiratory syncitial virus. J Infect Dis. 1980;141:98.
7. Doebbeling BN, Pfaller MA, Houstan AK, et al. Removal of nosocomial pathogens from the contaminated glove: Implications for glove reuse and handwashing. Ann Intern Med. 1988; 109:344.
8. Update: Universal precautions for prevention of transmission of Human immunodeficiency virus, Hepatitis virus and other blood borne pathogens in health care settings. MMWR. 1988; 24:377.
9. Johanson WG Jr, Pierce AK, Sanford JP, et al. Nosocomial respiratory infections with gram-negative bacilli. The significance of colonization of the respiratory tract. Ann Intern Med. 1972;77:701.
10. Selden R, Lee S, Wang WLL, et al. Nosocomial *Klebsiella* infections. Intestinal colonization as a reservoir. Am J Med. 1971;74:657.
11. Goldman DA, Leclair J, Macone A. Bacterial colonization of neonates admitted to an intensive care environment. J Pediatr. 1978; 93:288.
12. Weinstein RA, Kabins SA. Strategies for prevention and control of multiple drug resistant nosocomial infection. Am J Med. 1981;70:499.
13. Olson B, Weinstein RA, Nathen C, et al. Epidemiology of endemic *Pseudomonas aeruginosa*: Why infection control efforts failed? J Infect Dis. 1984;150:808.
14. Olson B, Weinstein RA, Nathen, et al. Occult amminoglycoside resistance in *Pseudomonas aeruginosa*: Epidemiology and implications for therapy and control. J Infect Dis. 1985;152:769.
15. Flynn DM, Weinstein RA, Nathan C, et al. Patient's endogenous flora as the source of nosocomial *Enterobacter* in cardiac surgery. J Infect Dis. 1987;156:363.
16. Healthcare-associated infections (HAI) outbreak investigation/notification protocol. West Virginia, Dept of Health. Human Resources Bureau for public Health. Accessed from www.dide.wv.gov. on 12/9/2015.
17. Shridhar Rao PN. Typing methods. Available at www.microrao.com/micronotes/typing.pdf. Accessed on 12/9/2015.

Chapter 4

Prevention of Hospital Infections

Chapter Outline

- Exclusion of Sources of Infection
- Breaking the Chain of Infection
- Enhancing the Host's Ability to Resist Infection by Boosting Immunity
- Appropriate use of Antibiotics
- Care of Invasive Devices
- Reducing the Risks of Postoperative Infections

There are three main strategies for preventing hospital infection. They are:

1. Excluding sources of infection from the hospital environment.
2. Interrupting the transmission of infection from source to the susceptible host.
3. Enhancing the host's ability to resist infection.

EXCLUSION OF SOURCES OF INFECTION[1]

Exclusion of inanimate sources of infection can be achieved but it can be difficult to avoid contamination by humans.

Exclusion of inanimate sources can be achieved in many ways, e.g. the provision of sterile instruments and dressings, sterile medicaments and intravenous fluids, use of blood and blood products screened for infectious agents, clean linen and uncontaminated food.

However, when human being is a source of infection, the task becomes more difficult. Hospitals must prevent patient contact with staff that are carriers of infection and relocate them to less hazardous positions. Staff must undergo health screening before employment and must have regular health check-ups. They should report any incidences of infection (e.g. infected cut, bout of diarrhea, etc.). Work restriction for personnel with selected infectious diseases is essential.

Infectious diseases where staffs contact with patient should be avoided:

- Diarrhea
- Hepatitis A
- Herpes simplex on hands (herpetic whitlow)
- *Streptococcus pyogenes* infections (e.g. sore throat, pyogenic infections)

- *Staphylococcus aureus* skin lesions
- Measles
- Mumps
- Whooping cough
- Rubella
- Varicella zoster infections
- Upper respiratory tract infections (high-risk patients).

However, healthy carriers, for example of virulent staphylococci are difficult to identify unless bacteriologic screening is undertaken which is not feasible on routine basis. In addition, hospital staff are sources of opportunistic organisms such as *Coagulase negative staphylococci* or enterobacteria, which are part of their normal flora and cannot be excluded.

BREAKING THE CHAIN OF INFECTION[1]

This is possible in two ways:

1. Breaking the structural chain: Hospital structure and equipment play a role in preventing air-borne spread of infection.
2. Breaking the human chain.

Breaking the Structural Chain

Ventilation Systems in Hospital Wards/ Operating Theaters/Rooms

Ventilation systems and airflow can play an important role in the dissemination of organisms by air-borne route.

Ventilation systems in operating theaters must be properly installed and maintained to prevent the entry of contaminated air and to minimize air currents carrying organisms from the staff in the operating room to the operation site. Ultraclean air is passed through high efficiency filters to remove bacteria and other particles and has been shown to contribute positively to a reduction in the number of postoperative wound infections developing after long orthopedic operations.

Wards comprising separate rooms have been shown to afford protection against airborne spread, and rooms with controlled ventilation are even better. However they neither prevent the carriage of organisms into the room on staff and their clothing, and some studies suggest that this is a more important route of transmission of infection than airborne spread. There is no doubt however that *Legionella* infection is acquired by airborne route and therefore air-conditioning systems should be so maintained so as to prevent multiplication of these organisms. Hospital-acquired *Aspergillus* infection has been attributed to dissemination of the spores in hospital air, especially when building work is going on in the locality.

Isolation of Patient

Isolating patients can also reduce airborne infections significantly. Patient isolation can be carried out in two ways:

a. Protective isolation: Protective isolation to protect a particularly susceptible patient from exposure to pathogens.
b. Source isolation: It protects the spread of pathogens from an infected patient to the others in the ward.

Isolation will also help to prevent the transmission of infection by other routes by limiting access to the patient and this will also help the staff in understanding the importance of contact in the spread of infection.

a. *Protective isolation:* Protective isolation can be provided in a single room in a ward. If possible appropriate positive pressure ventilation should be provided with airflow from the clean patient area out of the room. Staff entering the room or in contact with the patient should wear sterile gowns, gloves and masks to prevent organisms they are carrying or have picked up from other patients from coming in contact with the patient in protective isolation.
b. *Source isolation:* Ideally source isolation is arranged by accommodation in an

isolation unit in a separate building like tuberculosis sanatoria of the past. In general, source isolation is more often arranged in a separate ward or in a separate room of the main ward. To prevent air-borne transmission of organisms from patients' room to the ward, airflow should be from ward to isolation room.

In practice, it is difficult to maintain correct airflows without sophisticated designs, including double doors and air locks.

Breaking the Human Chain

Facilitation of Aseptic Behavior

A general state of cleanliness is essential in the hospital, so the staff should make a habit to practice good techniques. The design of the hospital facilities will affect the ease with which this can be done.

Bacteriologically effective hand washing is one of the most important ways of controlling hospital infection.

The hands of staff transfer the organisms to patients from septic lesions and healthy carrier sites of other patients. They can also transfer organisms from equipment contaminated by these sources and from carrier sites of the staff themselves.

Staff should therefore wash their hands:

- Before any procedure for which gloves or forceps are necessary
- After contact with an infected patient or one who is colonized with multiply resistant bacteria
- After touching infective material.

Soap and water are adequate in most circumstances, but when dealing with infected patients disinfectants are recommended. Drying hands after washing is important. A more prolonged and thorough scrub is required before commencing surgery.

It has been seen that there has been a disappointingly low compliance with the simple technique of hand washing. Therefore, training and regular reinforcement of appropriate behavior is essential.

ENHANCING THE HOST'S ABILITY TO RESIST INFECTION BY BOOSTING IMMUNITY[1]

Boosting immunity and reducing risk factors can enhance host resistance. Although attempts should be made to control and prevent hospital infection by removing sources of infection and preventing transmission from sources to susceptible hosts, these strategies may sometimes fail. So also they do not protect the host from endogenous infection. Therefore, a way could be adopted which would tilt the balance in favor of the host. This can be done by enhancing his/her ability to resist infection, both by boosting immunity and reducing personal risk factors. The following aspects should be considered:

- Boosting specific immunity by active or passive immunization
- The appropriate use of prophylactic antibiotics
- Care of invasive devices that breach the natural defenses, e. g. urinary catheter, intravenous lines.
- Attention to the risks predisposing to postoperative infection.

Boosting Immunity

Passive immunization provides short-term protection, but this is important especially in case of immunocompromised patients, because he/she may not be able to mount an antibody response. Passive immunization can also afford short-term protection in patients who are neutropenic as a result of cytotoxic therapy and whose white cell count should recover after successful treatment. With the advent of hepatitis B vaccine, it is recommended that all seronegative patients in dialysis units (and all staff) should be immunized.

Other immunizations for protection of hospital patients are summarized in Table 4.1.

Table 4.1: Immunizations for protection of hospital patients

	Active	Passive
1. Elderly (especially Those with multisystem disease)	Influenza vaccine	------
2. Prespleenectomy Prerenal or bone marrow transplant	Pneumococcal vaccine	-------
3. Hemodialysis patient	Pneumococcal vaccine Hepatitis B vaccine	---------
4. Infants born to HbsAg positive mothers	Hepatitis B vaccine	-------
5. Immunocompromised Exposed to varicella-zoster	Live attenuated VZ vaccine in trials	Zoster immune globulin within 3 days to prevent severe disease
6. Exposed to measles	-------------	Normal human immunoglobulin within 5 days

APPROPRIATE USE OF ANTIBIOTICS[1]

There are well-documented uses for prophylactic antibiotics, but antibiotics tend to be misused.

There are several well-documented uses for prophylactic antibiotics in dirty surgery and when the consequences of infection would be disastrous (e.g. in cardiac, neuro and transplant surgery). However, there is a tendency to misuse antibiotics.

- First by using them for too long, thereby increasing the selection pressure for the immergence of resistant organisms.
- By choosing inappropriate agents.

Treatment of patients and staff who are carriers of pathogens such as *S. aureus* or *S. pyogenes* has been used successfully to prevent endogenous infection, and to control outbreaks of infection with these organisms. Topical preparations of antibiotics such as bacitracin, neomycin and fucidin, have been used, but there is no doubt that the emergence of resistance is a problem. Pseudomonic acid (mupirocin), a fermentation product of *Pseudomonas fluorescens,* has been shown to be efficacious. It is unrelated to any other class of antibiotic, and is very effective against gram-positive cocci. In recent years, it has played an important role in eradicating carriage of MRSA but resistance is now beginning to emerge.

Gut contamination regimes and selective bowel decontamination to reduce the reservoir of potential pathogens in gut: Gut decontamination regimes to reduce the aerobic gram-negative flora of neutropenic patients have been practiced for sometime. More recently selective bowel decontamination (SBD) has been used especially in intensive care units (ICU). The aim to reduce the reservoir of potential pathogens in the gut by oral administration (or via a nasogastric tube) of a high concentration of mixture of antibiotics (Polymixin + Tobramycin+Amphotericin or a similar combination) to ICU patients throughout their stay in the unit. At present, there is still a controversy about the efficacy and safety of SBD.

CARE OF INVASIVE DEVICES[1]

Care of invasive devices is essential to reduce the risk of endogenous infection, e.g. from skin organisms, and of catheters from peri-urethral flora causing infection of bladder in catheterized patients.

Up to 35% of hospital-acquired bacteremias and majority candidemias are infusion related. They are derived mainly from vascular catheters. Most of the bacteremia associated with invasive devices are caused by patients' own skin flora, although this may be a more resistant flora acquired during patients' stay in the hospital, replacing his/her community acquired flora. *S. epidermidis* accounts for more than 50% of infections, but other aerobic bacteria including *S. aureus,* Enterococci, *Coryneforms, various* gram-negative rods and *Candida* are implicated. These infections are largely preventable if appropriate steps are taken.

REDUCING THE RISKS OF POSTOPERATIVE INFECTIONS[1]

Prevention of postoperative infection involves minimizing the risks. This can be done in the following ways:

- The preoperative length of stay in hospital should be kept at minimum.
- Intercurrent infections should be treated appropriately before surgery whenever possible.
- Operations should be kept to the minimum duration and associated with good operating techniques.
- Adequate debridement of dead and necrotic tissue is essential, together with adequate drainage, and maintenance or reestablishment of a good blood supply to provide the body's natural defenses with optimum working conditions.
- Prevention of pressure sores and stasis to minimize the risk of developing respiratory tract infection or UTI or good nursing techniques and active physiotherapy.

REFERENCE

1. Mims C, Playfair J, Roitt I, Wakelin D, Williams R. Medical Microbiology (2nd Edn). CV Mosby International Ltd; 1999.pp.485-90.

Chapter 5

Nosocomial Infection Surveillance

Chapter Outline

- Methods of Surveillance
- Statistical Analysis of the Data
- Health and Medical Surveillance
- Nosocomial Infection Rates

INTRODUCTION[1]

Surveillance (i.e. discovery and recording of infection) is defined as the continuous scrutiny of all aspects of occurrence and spread of a disease, which can be effectively controlled.

Surveillance of infection in hospital is essential for the following reasons:

- To detect changes in pattern of disease
- To recognize any unusual change in the level of incidence of disease
- To detect the existence of an outbreak, or an impending spread of an outbreak or to identify the appearance of a particularly dangerous organism
- To judge whether it is desirable to introduce special measures to control an existing outbreak, or an impending outbreak and to assess the efficacy of such measures
- To assess the efficacy of regular preventive measures used in the hospital
- To reduce the level of avoidable infection and to identify high-risk patients, so that selective measures can be introduced.

In short, without a surveillance system for nosocomial infections, control measures adopted by the hospital are unlikely to succeed.

Surveillance includes:

- Data collection
- Analysis of data
- Feedback of the results to medical and nursing staff and those involved in decision-making.

Surveillance and record keeping will therefore be useful to measure the effectiveness of an infection control program and to give an early indication of outbreaks.

However, calculating infection rates for the whole hospital should not be expected, as it is difficult, time consuming and not cost-effective. It will also not necessarily improve quality of control. Of course, it is true that a highly efficient surveillance and infection control system could reduce the infection by one third, and this has been proved by a study carried out in USA.[1]

Besides carrying out surveillance of infections in patients, surveillance of staff, the environment and equipment is also essential, but routine sampling of staff and environment is not generally recommended.

METHODS OF SURVEILLANCE

Collection of Data

a. Defining events to be surveyed or in other words having a clear idea of what is to be done.
   For example, finding the relation of pneumonia and endotracheal intubation in a particular patient, or labeling a UTI (Urinary tract infection to the indwelling catheter) and so on.
b. Collection of the data and analyzing the data, which is to be done by the ICN (Infection control nurse).
   Minimal data to be collected about infections is as follows:
   i. Essential data: patients name, age, sex, hospital registration number, ward number, date of admission, date of onset of infection, the site of infection, the organisms isolated and their antibiograms.
   ii. Additional information may be collected if it is essential for analysis, for example, primary diagnosis of the infected patient, severity of sepsis—mild, moderate or severe, names of attending physicians/surgeon and other staff, predisposing factors (e.g. surgery, antibiotic, steroid, immunosuppressive therapy, instrumentation like urinary catheterization, and use of respiratory therapy equipment or intravenous catheter). In case of surgery, the type of operation, classification of operation (clean, clean contaminated, contaminated), relation between onset of sepsis and number of days since operation, antimicrobials used to treat infection and mortality related to infection.

All this information is to be recorded on a card or form by ICN.

Methods of Surveillance of Infection in Patients

This can be done by daily visits to wards, microbiology laboratories rather than finding cases through completed infection report forms by physician or nurses.

Daily Scrutiny and Laboratory Reports and Correlation with Clinical Infection

Laboratory reports should enable the detection of those organisms, which are likely to spread and cause outbreaks and have to be routinely recorded, e.g.

i. *Streptococcus pyogenes, Salmonella* and *Shigella* species, enteropathogenic or toxigenic *E. coli, Mycobacterium tuberculosis, Pseudomonas aeruginosa, Neisseria meningitides, Legionella* species, rotavirus, RSV.
ii. Highly resistant strains of *Staphylococcus aureus* (resistant to methicillin, gentamicin, fusidic acid and mupirocin).
iii. Highly resistant strains of gram-negative bacilli (e.g. resistant to gentamicin, third generation cephalosporins, quinolones).
iv. Highly resistant *Enterococci* (e.g. resistant to vancomycin, β-lactamase-producing strains).
v. Strains showing unusual resistance (e.g. penicillin resistant *Streptococcus pneumoniae).*
vi. Blood culture isolates, CSF isolates.

Other infections to be routinely recorded are:

1. All infections from special baby care unit, intensive care unit, pediatric wards and high-risk areas.

2. Communicable diseases, e.g. food poisoning, diarrhea and vomiting, enteric fever, tuberculosis, childhood infectious diseases, diphtheria, legionellosis, meningitis).
3. Wound or other related infections (e.g. urinary tract infection).
4. The incidence of infection cannot be calculated from laboratory reports alone, as all infections may not be sampled bacteriologically, so also infectious agents may not be identified by a particular laboratory, and mere isolation of a pathogen does not mean infection, it needs clinical verification.

On Site Surveillance by ICN—Routine Visits to Wards

The infection control nurse should examine the records every morning and discuss the results with the infection control doctor. She must complete the necessary information on relevant infected patients by visiting the ward, and determine whether they are true clinical infections, and whether they are hospital acquired. Sometimes, it may happen that the ward staff do not send samples to the laboratory, in such cases, they should be encouraged to send samples from all patients with suspected infections. Special risk units (Intensive care units) should be visited regularly, even if none of the patients are known to be infected.

ICN should identify new infections, and follow the previously identified nosocomial infections. New patients may be identified by the ward staff themselves by review of temperature records or follow-up of suspicious laboratory reports.

Surveillance based on laboratory records and routine visits to wards detects 76% of infections as compared to continuous surveillance, but even then this method is time consuming and not cost effective. It is preferable to use selective method (e.g. by surveillance of certain wards only).

The surveyed wards can be rotated at regular intervals or monitored if there is a particular problem; but high-risk wards (e.g. ICU's, transplant units and special care baby units) should be routinely surveyed.

Inspection, documentation and sending samples from all visible infections must be done by ICN.

Post-discharge Follow-up

Since the average length of stay of patients in the hospital has been markedly reduced, some of the nosocomial infections may manifest only after discharge of the patient. This happens especially after surgery (surgical operations—surgical wound infection). It is thus essential to follow-up these patients for a month after operation say by calling them for a routine check up every week.

STATISTICAL ANALYSIS OF DATA[2]

Types of Rates

i. Incidence rates
ii. Prevalence rates

Incidence Rate

Calculating incidence:

Incidence rate is defined as the number of new cases occurring in a defined population during a specified period of time. It is given by the formula:

$$\frac{\text{Number of new cases of specific disease during a given time period}}{\text{Population at risk}} \times 1000$$

It will be seen from the above definition that incidence rate refers;

a. Only to new cases
b. During a given period (Usually one year)
c. In a specified population or population at risk unless other denominators are chosen.

Incidence measures the rate at which new cases are occurring in a population, it is not influenced by the duration of the disease. The use of incidence is generally restricted to acute conditions.

Use of incidence rate: Useful for taking action

- To control disease
- For research into etiology, pathogenesis. Distribution of disease
- Efficacy of therapeutic and preventive measures.

Prevalence Rate

Definition: The term "disease prevalence" refers specifically to all current cases (old and new) existing at a given point in time, or over a period of time in a given population.

Prevalence is of two types:

a. Point prevalence
b. Period prevalence

a. Point prevalence: Point prevalence of a disease is defined as the number of all current cases (old and new) of a disease at one point in time in relation to a defined population.

The point in point prevalence may for all practical purposes consist of a day, several days, or even a few weeks.

Point prevalence is given by the formula:

$$\frac{\text{No. of all current cases (old and new) of a specified disease existing at a given point in time}}{\text{Estimated population at the same point in time}} \times 100$$

When the term "prevalence rate" is used without any further qualification, it is taken to mean, "Point prevalence".

Point prevalence can be made specific for age, sex and other relevant factors or attributes.

b. Period prevalence: A less commonly used measure of prevalence is period prevalence. It measures the frequency all current cases (old and new) existing during a defined period of time (e.g. annual prevalence) expressed in relation to a defined population, it includes cases arising before, but extending into or through to the year as well as those cases arising during the year. Period prevalence is given by the formula.

$$\frac{\text{No. of all existing cases (old and new) of a specified disease existing at a given period of time interval}}{\text{Estimated mid-interval population at risk}} \times 100$$

The terms incidence and prevalence are illustrated in Figure 5.1.

Relation between prevalence and incidence: Prevalence depends on 2 factors (1) the incidence, (2) duration of illness. If we assume that the population is stable (1000) and incidence and duration are unchanging, the relationship between incidence and prevalence can be expressed as:

$$P = I \times D$$
$$= \text{(Incidence)} \times \text{(mean duration)}$$

Example (for a stable condition)
Incidence = 10 cases per 1000 population per year
Mean duration of disease = 5 years

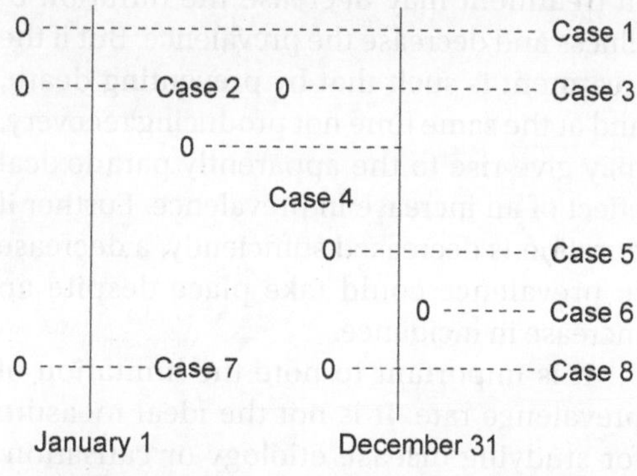

Fig. 5.1: Number of cases of disease beginning and developing and ending during a period of time.
Incidence would include cases—3,4,5,8
Point prevalence (Jan 1) cases—1,2,7
Point prevalence (Dec 31) cases—1,3,5,8
Period prevalence (Jan-Dec) cases—1,2,3,4,5,7 and 8

Prevalence = 10 × 5 = 50 per 1000 population conversely, it is possible to derive incidence and duration as follows:

Incidence = P/D

Duration = P/I

The above equation (P = I × D) shows that the longer the duration of the disease, the greater is the prevalence, e.g. tuberculosis has a high prevalence rate relative to incidence. This is because new cases of tuberculosis keep cropping up, throughout the year, while the old ones persist for months or years. On the other hand, if the disease is acute and of short duration either because of rapid recovery or death, the prevalence rate will be relatively low compared with the incidence rate. In some diseases (e.g. food poisoning), the disease is so short lived, that there are no old cases. Therefore, these have almost no prevalence. Therefore, decrease in prevalence may take place not only due to decrease in incidence, but also due to decrease in duration of illness due to rapid recovery or death.

When we see a change in prevalence from one time period to another, this can result from changes in incidence, changes in duration or both. For example, improvement in treatment may decrease the duration of illness and decrease the prevalence. But if the treatment is such that by preventing death, and at the same time not producing recovery, may give rise to the apparently paradoxical effect of an increase in prevalence. Further if duration is decreased sufficiently, a decrease in prevalence could take place despite an increase in incidence.

It is important to note the limitation of prevalence rate. It is not the ideal measure for studying disease etiology or causation. We have seen two factors that determine prevalence, namely incidence and duration. Incidence is related to the occurrence of disease and duration to the factors, which affect the course of disease. In other words, the element of durations reflects the prognostic factors, and incidence reflects the causal factors. Therefore, incidence rates should be optimally used in the formulation and testing of etiological hypothesis. When incidence rates are not available, prevalence rates (which are readily obtainable) may have to be used, but the contribution of duration element always has to be assessed.

Uses of prevalence

a. Helps to estimate the magnitude of health/disease in the community, and identify potential high-risk populations.
b. Prevalence rates are especially useful for administrative and planning purposes, e.g. hospital beds, man power needs, rehabilitation facility, etc.
c. Prevalence surveys are used to estimate antimicrobial usage pattern, to evaluate adherence to proper isolation practices, or to monitor the invasive procedure practices that carry high risk for infection.

Analysis of Data[3]

Comparing Patient Groups

Infection rates among different groups of patients are compared. Test of significance (e.g. Chi-square test, Fisher's exact test and Student's t-test) is applied to find out the difference if real. If the difference is real, further investigations are done to find the reason for difference and take necessary control measures.

Comparing Rates Over Time

The current infection rates can be compared with the past infection rates and the changes if any are examined. Further investigations then can be carried out if required.

Clusters

Screening for clustering can be done, e.g. patterns of antimicrobial sensitivity of particular pathogens in specific wards or service.

Appropriateness of Medical Care

If a hospitals' invasive device utilization in the ICU is higher than another hospital's ICU, a review of the appropriate use of device can be done. Similarly after comparing surgical wound infection rates of different hospitals, the risk factors can be further studied for appropriateness of medical/surgical care.

Interpretation

Analyzed data are interpreted to find if there is any change in the infection rate, e.g. no change or possible outbreak.

Reporting the Data

The data along with analysis and interpretation is supplied to administrator and concerned hospital staff. These reports are usually monthly. In case of outbreaks, these reports may be weekly or daily. The results may be in the form of tables or graphs. Graphic analysis has become easy now due to computer software. Infection control committee may decide to send this data to local health authorities or/and others.

Targeted Surveillance

The surveillance can be targeted towards specific infection problems in a hospital. This is especially useful in a large hospital with paucity of resources and infection control staff, e.g. it can be targeted for high-risk geographic areas, e.g. ICU, nursery or oncology unit. Another approach could be rotating surveillance. Surveillance is carried out in a specific area of the hospital for one month and another area is taken in the next month and so on. Thus, all areas of the hospital can be covered in a sequential manner in one year. The disadvantage is that the problems that arise in areas not under surveillance at a given time are missed.

A third alternative is to assign the level of surveillance efforts to various infection problems in the hospital on basis of priority levels. The priority may be determined according to incidence, duration of extra days stay in hospital or extra cost needed in caring for patients of each type of nosocomial infection (e.g. surgical wound infection, pneumonia, urinary tract infection, bacteremia). Accordingly the time and efforts can be alloted for surveillance of various types of infections. This approach utilizes resources for greatest possible nosocomial infection control program.

HEALTH AND MEDICAL SURVEILLANCE[3]

It is desirable to establish hospital staff health services which takes care of all aspects of health and illnesses in the hospital staff.

Pre-employment Medical Examination

All staff, i.e. medical, nursing, administrative, ancillary and supportive staff should undergo a medical checkup. It includes a history of past illnesses such as diarrheal diseases, sepsis, tonsillitis, chronic skin diseases, hepatitis, chickenpox and immunodeficient conditions. History should also determine the HCWs' immunization status. Physical examination, serology and routine laboratory tests are desirable. A base line serum sample (for future use) should be collected and stored. Special examination should include X-ray chest, cervical smear for women and ECG. Rubella antibody test should be done for all women of child-bearing age and if found negative immunization should be offered.

Continuing Surveillance

There is a need for continued surveillance of hospital staff:

- Special tests for staff particularly at risk, e.g. HbsAg detection for staff of renal dialysis unit. X-ray chest for staff of microbiology laboratory every year or two years.

- Examination of staff returning to work after absence due to illness particularly diarrhea, hepatitis, sepsis and to ensure that they are free from infection.
- Organizing clinical examination, laboratory tests and treatment for staff illnesses particularly, which are hospital acquired. In some cases, tests for carriers of pathogens amongst hospital staff has to be carried out and if found positive may have to be treated.
- Counseling, investigation and clinical examination of hospital staff exposed to needle stick injury or accidental injury due to sharps contaminated with blood or body fluids. Appropriate prophylaxis and treatment may have to be given for HBV, HIV exposure.
- Keeping accurate records of infections in the hospital staff.

Pregnancy

Pregnant HCWs should be made aware of the risk of themselves and their fetus of attending patients with viral infections. They should strictly observe all precautions and personal hygiene measure. They should not attend patients with cytomegalovirus, parvovirus, hepatitis, rubella (if HCW is rubella antibody negative) infections.

Vaccinations and Immunization

Appropriate immunization of HCWs not only protects them but also decreases the transmission of vaccine preventable infection to patients and avoids unnecessary work restrictions. An immunization program should be developed for hospital staff at initial employment, before posting to specific risk areas, booster doses at appropriate intervals, after accidental needle stick or 'sharps' injury and after attending to patients with particularly hazardous infectious agents, e.g. rabies.

Screening HCWs for susceptibility to infectious agents (HBV, rubella, measles) before vaccination may be cost-effective in certain situations. It is desirable to give vaccines for HBV (particularly those employed in renal dialysis unit, surgery or any invasive procedures), typhoid fever, BCG (Mantoux negative), rubella, cholera (in endemic regions), tetanus-diphtheria toxoid (if there is past history of full course of immunization, booster doses every 7–10 years), influenza (current strain), measles, mumps, poliomyelitis.

Work Restriction

Before a HCW is assigned duties his susceptibility status may be evaluated on the basis of past history of illnesses, immunization record and if need be by laboratory tests, e.g. HCW with past history of having suffered from chickenpox should care for chickenpox patients.

When HCW is suffering from certain diseases he/she should be excluded from direct contact with patients. These diseases are infectious conjunctivitis, diarrhea, Group A streptococcal infection, HAV infection, herpetic whitlow, measles, mumps, whooping cough, rubella, scabies skin lesions with *Staphylococcus aureus*, chickenpox, *Salmonella* carriers, eczema. It is advisable that if a HCW is suffering from HBV or HIV infection or carrier of HbsAg, he should not be involved in direct patient care.

Staff Health Service should also undertake the work of clearance for returns to work after recovery from an infectious condition.

Safety Training and Continuing Education

Training courses in biosafety measures should be organized by Infection Control Officer. This should include all categories of hospital staff. Therefore, they need different types of instructional courses. Training courses should be arranged at the time of employment and subsequently continuing education should be imparted.

1. HCWs should be told about the epidemiology, modes of transmission

and prevention of hospital-acquired infections. It should be stressed that HCWs can decrease the risk of acquiring or transmitting infection by rigorous adherence to infection control practices, e.g. careful hand washing, barrier precautions and universal precaution whenever exposure to blood and body fluids is likely to occur.

2. HCWs should be fully aware of hospital policies regarding measures to be taken after exposure or accidents. They should know how to deal with spillage of blood, body fluids and excretions from patients.
3. Adequate training should be given to staff about safe discard and handling of contaminated materials and instruments and disposal of infective hospital refuse.
4. Hospital administration must provide the appropriate equipments and materials for undertaking biosafety measures by HCWs.
5. A mechanism should be developed by infection control team to monitor the biosafety measures undertaken by HCWs. In case of lapses counseling, education, retraining and in certain instances disciplinary action may have to be taken. An all out effort should be made to motivate HCWs for strict observance of biosafety measures.

NOSOCOMIAL INFECTION RATES[4]

Rates—Numerators

- Number of infections
- Number of patients infected
- Note:
  - Infections caused by multiple organisms of similar origin at the same site = single infection
  - In a patient with a previously established nosocomial infection, a second nosocomial infection should be recorded in two situations
  - > the appearance of a clinical infection at a new and different site
  - > the appearance in culture of new and different organisms if deterioration of patient's condition.

Rates—Denominators

- Number of patients admitted (or discharged)
- Number of hospital days
- Number of device days.

Hospital Wide Rates

- Hospital wide nosocomial infection rate/100 admissions for a given period: month, quarter, year.

$$= \frac{\text{Number of nosocomial infections}}{\text{Number of patients admitted}} \times 100$$

In this rate, a patient with two infections is counted twice.

- Hospital wide patient infected rate/100 admissions for a given period: month, quarter, year.

$$= \frac{\text{No. of patients infected}}{\text{No. of patients admitted}} \times 100$$

In this rate, a patient with two infections is counted only once.

Ward-specific Rates

Ward	ICU

- Rate of infection/1000 HD

$$= \frac{\text{Number of infections}}{\text{Number of hospital days}} \times 1000$$

- Rate of patients infected/1000 HD

$$= \frac{\text{Number of patients infected}}{\text{Number of hospital days}} \times 1000$$

Procedure-specific Rates

- Surgical site infection rate:

$$= \frac{\text{Number of surgical site infections}}{\text{Number of patients operated upon}} \times 100$$

Device-specific Rates

How to Calculate a Device Associated Infection Rate

- Step 1: Decide on the time period for analysis.: month, quarter, six months, year.
- Step 2: Select patient population for analysis, e. g. type of ICU or a birth weight category.
- Step 3: Select infections to be used in numerator:
  - must be site-specific
  - must have occurred in selected patient population
  - date of onset must be during the selected time period.
- Step 4: Determine number of device days used as denominator.
  Device days = total number of days of exposure to device (central line, ventilator or urinary catheter) by all patients in selected population during selected time period.
- Step 5: Calculate device-associated infection rate (per 1000 device days) using the formula:

$$\text{Device-associated infection rate} = \frac{\text{Number of device-associated infections for specific site}}{\text{Number of device days}} \times 1000$$

Utilization Rate

- The device utilization rate (DUR) is the proportion of patient days for which a certain device is used
- DUR are specific to a certain device: catheter, IV line, ventilator
- DUR reflects the amount of devices used and is a reflection of the patient severity.

$$= \frac{\text{Number of device days}}{\text{Number of patient days}} \times 100$$

How to Calculate a Device Utilization Ratio

- Step 1: Decide on the time period for analysis: month, quarter, six months, year.
- Step 2: Select patient population for analysis, e.g. type of ICU or birth-weight category.
- Step 3: Determine the number of device days used as a numerator.
  Device days = total number of days of exposure to the device
  (central line, ventilator or urinary catheter) by all patients in the selected population during the selected time period.
- Note: Step 3 is the same as step 4 in the device day, but here it is used as a numerator.
- Step 4: Determine the number of patient-days which is used as denominator of DU ratio
- Patient-days = total number of days that patients are in ICU during the selected time period.
- Step 5: Calculate the DU ratio with the following formula:

$$\text{DU} = \frac{\text{Number of device days}}{\text{Number of patient days}}$$

- Example DU = 28/72 = 0.39 or 39% of patient-days were also central line days for the first week of the month.

REFERENCES

1. Surveillance, Records and Reports: In control of hospital infection. A Practical Handbook by Ayliffe GAJ, et al. 2002.pp.40-5.
2. Park K. Parks Textbook of Preventive and Social Medicine, 14th edn. Principles of epidemiology and epidemiologic methods; 1995.
3. Analysis in surveillance of nosocomial infections—Guidelines for Nosocomial infection—Surveillance and control by Agarwal DS, Microbiology Department, University of Medical Sciences, GTB Hospital, Delhi. WHO South East Asia Regional Office, New Delhi. Practical:
4. Nosocomial infection rates: Infectious Disease epidemiology section, Office of Public Health, Louisiana department of Health and Hospitals 800-256-2748. From www.oph,dhhluisiana. gov. accessed on 8th June 2015.

Chapter 6

Infection Control Responsibilities

Chapter Outline

- Role of Hospital Management
- Role of the Physician
- Role of Microbiologist
- Role of Pharmacist
- Role of Nursing Staff
- Role of Central Sterilization Services
- Role of Food Services
- Role of Laundry Services
- Role of Housekeeping Services
- Role of Maintenance
- Role of Infection Control Team

ROLE OF HOSPITAL MANAGEMENT[1]

They have to provide leadership by supporting the hospital infection program. They are responsible for:

- Establishing a multidisciplinary infection control committee.
- They have to identify and arrange for resources and apply the most appropriate methods to prevent infection.
- They must educate and train its staff regarding prevention of infection, disinfection and sterilization techniques.
- Delegate technical aspects of hospital hygiene to appropriate staff such as nursing, housekeeping, maintenance and clinical microbiology laboratory.
- Periodically review the status of nosocomial infections and effectiveness of the interventions to control them.
- Review, approve and implement policies approved by the infection control committee.
- Ensure that the infection control team has the authority to facilitate appropriate program function.
- Participate in outbreak investigation.

ROLE OF THE PHYSICIAN[1]

Role of the physician is very important. They are responsible for:

- Direct patient care using practices, which minimize infection.
- By following appropriate practice of hygiene (e.g. handwashing).
- Cooperating and serving with the HICC.
- Supporting the HI control team.

Specifically the physicians are responsible for:

- Protecting their own patients from other infected patients and from the hospital staff who may be infected.
- Obtaining appropriate microbiological specimens when an infection is present or suspected.
- Notifying cases of hospital acquired infection to the team, as well as the admission of infected patients.
- Complying with the recommendations of the antimicrobial use committee regarding use of antibiotics.
- Advising the patients, visitors and staff regarding techniques to prevent the transmission of infection.
- Institute appropriate treatment for any infections they themselves have, and taking steps to prevent such infections being transmitted to other individuals, especially patients.

ROLE OF MICROBIOLOGIST[1]

The microbiologist is responsible for the following:

- Handling patient and staff specimens, so as to come to an appropriate microbiological diagnosis.
- For developing guidelines for the appropriate collection, transport and handling of specimens.
- Ensuring that the laboratory practices meet appropriate standards.
- Ensuring safe laboratory practices to prevent infections in the staff.
- Performing antimicrobial susceptibility testing following internationally recognized methods and providing summary reports of prevalence of resistance.
- Monitoring sterilization, disinfection and the environment where necessary.
- Timely communication of the results to the infection control committee.
- Epidemiological typing of the hospital microorganisms where necessary.

ROLE OF HOSPITAL PHARMACIST[1]

- Obtaining, storing and distributing pharmaceutical preparations.
- Obtaining and storing vaccines or sera and making them available when necessary.
- Maintaining records of antibiotics distributed to the medical department.
- Providing the antimicrobial use committee and infection control committee with summary reports and trends of antimicrobial use.
- Having all the information regarding disinfectants, antiseptics, and other anti-infectious agents regarding:
  - Active properties in relation to concentration, temperature, length of action, antibiotic spectrum.
  - The toxic properties including sensitization or irritation of skin and mucosa.
  - Substances that are incompatible with antibiotics or reduce their potency.
  - Physical conditions which unfavourably affect potency during storage, temperature, light and humidity.
  - Harmful effect on materials.

The hospital pharmacist must also participate in the hospital sterilization and disinfection practices. He must;

- Develop guidelines for antiseptics, disinfectants and products used for washing and disinfecting hands.
- He must develop guidelines for reuse of equipment and patient materials.

- He must also participate in quality control of techniques used to sterilize equipment in the hospital including selection of hospital equipment (type of appliances) and monitoring.

ROLE OF NURSING STAFF[1]

Nursing staff is responsible for implementing patient care practices. Therefore, they should be familiar with practices to prevent the occurrence and spread of infections.

The senior nursing administration is responsible for:

- Participating in the Infection control committee.
- Promoting the development and improvement of nursing techniques. They should constantly review aseptic nursing policies with approval by the infection control committee.
- Developing training programs for members of the nursing staff.
- Supervising the implementation of techniques for prevention of infections in specialized areas such as the operation theater, ICU, maternity unit and newborns.
- Monitoring of nursing adherence to policies.

The nurse in charge of ward is responsible for:

- Maintaining the hygiene consistent with hospital policies and good nursing practices in the ward.
- Monitoring aseptic techniques, including handwashing, use of isolation.
- Promptly reporting an evidence of infection to the attending physician.
- Initiating patient isolation, and ordering culture specimens from any patient showing signs of a communicable disease, when the physician is not immediately available.
- Limiting the patient exposure to infections from visitors, hospital staff, other patients or equipment, used for diagnosis or treatment.
- Maintaining a safe and adequate supply of ward equipment, drugs and patient care supplies.

The nurse in charge of infection control is a member of the Infection control team and is responsible for:

- Identifying nosocomial infections.
- Investigation of the type of infection and infecting organism.
- Participating in training of personnel.
- Surveillance of hospital infections.
- Participating in investigation of outbreak.
- Development of infection control policy and review and approval of patient care policies relevant to infection control.
- Ensuring compliance to local and national regulations.
- Providing expert advice in matters relating to transmission of infections.

ROLE OF CENTRAL STERILIZATION SERVICES[1]

The central sterilization service serves all hospital areas including the operating theatres. An appropriately qualified individual must be responsible for management of the program. The day-to-day management can be delegated to a nurse or another individual with appropriate qualifications, experience and knowledge of medical devices.

The responsibilities of the CSS are to clean, decontaminate, test, prepare for use, sterilize and store aseptically all sterile hospital equipment. It works in collaboration with other hospital programs, to develop and monitor polices in cleaning and decontamination of:

- Reusable equipment.
- Contaminated equipment including:
  - Wrapping procedures according to type of sterilization.
  - Sterilization methods, according to the type of equipment.
  - Sterilization conditions (e.g. temperature, duration, pressure, humidity, etc).

The director of this service must:

- Oversee the use of different methods—physical, chemical and bacteriological to monitor the sterilization process.

- Ensure technical maintenance of the equipment according to national standards and manufacturers recommendations.
- Report any defect to administration, maintenance, infection control and other appropriate personnel.
- Maintain complete record of each autoclave run and ensure the long-term availability of records.
- Collect at regular intervals all outdated sterile units.
- Communicate if need be with the infection control committee, the nursing service, the operation theatre, the pharmacy, maintenance and other appropriate services.

ROLE OF FOOD SERVICES[1]

The director or incharge of kitchen (food service) must have knowledge of food supply, staff training, storage and preparation of foodstuffs use of equipment, etc. He is responsible for:

- Looking after the purchase of foodstuffs and the equipment used. He is also supposed to look after the cleaning procedures and maintain a high level of food safety.
- Ensure that all the equipment used and the working and storage areas are kept clean.
- Issuing written policies and instructions for handwashing, clothing responsibilities and daily disinfection duties.
- Ensuring that the methods used for storing, preparing and distributing food will avoid contamination by microorganisms.
- Using written instructions for the cleaning of dishes after use, including special instructions for infected or isolated patients where care has to be taken.
- Ensuring appropriate handling and disposal of waste.
- Establishing programs for training staff in food preparation, cleanliness and food safety.

ROLE OF THE LAUNDRY SERVICES[1]

The laundry is responsible for:

- Selection of the fabrics to be used in the hospital, developing polices for working clothes in each area, and maintaining appropriate supplies.
- Distribution of working clothes, and if necessary managing changing rooms.
- Developing polices for the collection and transport of dirty linen.
- Defining, where necessary, the method for disinfection of infected linen, either before it is taken to the laundry or in the laundry itself.
- Developing policies for the protection of clean linen from contamination during transport from the laundry to the area of use.
- Developing criteria for selection of site of laundry service:
  - Ensuring appropriate flow of linen, separation of clean and dirty areas.
  - Recommending washing conditions (e.g. temperature, duration).
  - Ensuring safety of laundry staff through prevention of exposure to sharps or laundry contaminated with potential pathogens.

ROLE OF HOUSEKEEPING SERVICE[1]

The housekeeping service is responsible for the regular and routine cleaning of all surfaces and maintaining a high level of hygiene in the facility. In collaboration with the infection control committee, it is responsible for:

- Classifying the different areas of the hospital according to the varying need for cleaning.
- Developing policies for appropriate cleaning techniques.
- Procedure, frequency, agents used, etc. for each type of rooms from highly contaminated to the most clean, and ensuring that these practices are followed.

- Developing policies for collection, transport and disposal of different types of waste (e.g. containers, frequency).
- Ensuring that liquid soap and paper towels, dispensers are replaced regularly, in places where these facilities are not available, supply of soap and hand dryer or at least clean towels are made available.
- Informing the maintenance service of any building problems requiring repair, cracks, defects in the sanitary or electrical equipment, etc.
- Caring for flowers and plants in public areas.
- Pest control (insects, rodents).
- Providing appropriate training for all new staff members and periodically for other employees and specific training when a new technique is introduced.
- Establishing methods for cleaning and disinfection of bedding (e.g. mattresses, pillows).
- Determining the frequency for the washing of curtains, screening curtains between beds, etc.
- Planning or renovations, new furnitures, including special patient beds to determine feasibility of cleaning.

There should be a continuing program for staff training. This program must stress personal hygiene, the importance of frequent and careful washing of hands, and cleaning methods (e.g. sequence of rooms, correct use of equipment, dilution of cleaning agents etc). Staff must also understand causes of contamination of premises, and how to limit this, including the method of action of disinfectants. The cleaning staff must also know to report to the staff health authorities, if they have a personal infection, especially infections of skin and gastrointestinal infections and respiratory infection.

ROLE OF MAINTENANCE[1]

Maintenance is responsible for:

- Collaborating with housekeeping, nursing staff or other appropriate groups in selecting equipment and ensuring early identification and prompt correction of any defect.
- Inspections and regular maintenance of plumbing, heating and refrigeration equipment, electrical fittings and air conditioning, records should be kept of this activity.
- Developing procedures for emergency repairs in essential departments.
- Ensuring environmental safety outside the hospital, e.g. waste disposal, water sources.

Additional special duties include:

- Participation in the choice of equipment if maintenance of the equipment requires technical assistance.
- Inspection, cleaning and regular replacement of the filters of all appliances for ventilation and humidifiers.
- Testing autoclaves (temperature, pressure, vacuum, recording mechanism) and regular maintenance (cleaning the inner chamber, emptying the tubes).
- Monitoring the recording thermometers of refrigerators in pharmacy stores, laboratories, blood blanks and kitchen.
- Regularly inspecting all surfaces—walls, floors, and ceilings, to ensure that they are kept smooth and washable.
- Repairing any opening or crack in partition walls or window frames.
- Maintaining hydrotherapy appliances.
- Notifying the infection control team/ committee if any interruption of service, such as plumbing or air-conditioning is anticipated.

ROLE OF INFECTION CONTROL TEAM (HOSPITAL HYGIENE SERVICE)[1]

The ICT is responsible for co-ordination of all infection control activities to ensure an effective infection control program. The team is responsible for:

- Organizing an epidemiological surveillance program for nosocomial infections.

- Participating with pharmacy in developing a program for supervising the use of anti-infective drugs.
- Ensuring that patient care activities are appropriate to the level of patient risk.
- Checking the efficacy of the methods of disinfection and sterilization and the efficacy of systems developed to improve hospital cleanliness.
- Participating in development and provision of teaching programs for the medical, nursing and allied health personnel, as well as all other categories of staff.
- Providing expert advice, analysis and leadership in outbreak investigation and control.
- Participating in the development and operation of regional and national infection control initiatives.
- This team may also provide assistance for smaller institutions and undertake research in hospital hygiene and infection control at the local, national or international level.

REFERENCE

1. Ducel G, Fabry J, Nicolle L. Prevention of Hospital-acquired Infections, 2nd edn, WHO; 2002.pp.10-4.

Chapter 7

Sterilization

Chapter Outline

- Steam Sterilization
- Low-temperature Sterilization Technologies
- Other Sterilization Methods
- Sterilizing Practices
- Recommendations for Disinfection and Sterilization in Healthcare Facilities
- Performance Indicators

INTRODUCTION[1]

Sterilization is required for all materials coming in contact with tissues underneath the skin and mucosa of the body, e.g. needles, sharps, instruments, gauze pieces and dressing. Some of these materials are single use items (guaze pieces, dressings, catheters, etc.) to be sterilized before use and then disposed off, while reusable items are required to be sterilized before every use. Heat treatment is a simple and foolproof method of sterilization if properly carried out and appropriately monitored.

Most medical and surgical devices used in healthcare facilities are made of materials that are heat stable and therefore undergo heat sterilization (primarily steam sterilization). However, since 1950, there has been an increase in medical devices and instruments made of materials (e.g. plastics) that require low temperature sterilization. Ethylene oxide gas has been used since the 1950s for heat- and moisture-sensitive medical devices. Within the past 15 years, a number of new, low temperature sterilization systems (e.g. hydrogen peroxide gas plasma, peracetic acid immersion, ozone) have been developed and are being used to sterilize medical devices. This chapter reviews sterilization technologies used in healthcare and makes recommendations for their optimum performance in the processing of medical devices.

Medical devices that have contact with sterile body tissues or fluids are considered critical items. These items should be sterile when used because any microbial contamination could result in disease transmission. Such items include surgical instruments, biopsy forceps, and implanted medical devices. If these items are heat resistant, the recommended sterilization process is steam sterilization, because it has the largest margin of safety due to its reliability, consistency, and lethality. However, reprocessing heat- and moisture-sensitive items requires use of a low temperature sterilization technology (e.g. ethylene oxide, hydrogen peroxide gas plasma, peracetic acid). A summary of the advantages and disadvantages for commonly used sterilization technologies is presented in Table 7.1.

Table 7.1: Summary of advantages and disadvantages of commonly used sterilization

Sterilization method	Advantages	Disadvantages
Steam	• Nontoxic to patient, staff, environment • Cycle easy to control and monitor. Rapidly microbicidal • Least affected by organic/inorganic soils among sterilization processes listed • Rapid cycle time • Penetrates medical packing, device lumens	• Deleterious for heat-sensitive instruments • Microsurgical instruments damaged by repeated exposure • May leave instruments wet, causing them to rust • Potential for burns
Hydrogen peroxide gas plasma	• Safe for the environment • Leaves no toxic residuals • Cycle time is 28–75 minutes (varies with model type) and no aeration necessary • Used for heat- and moisture-sensitive items since process temperature <50°C • Simple to operate, install, and monitor • Compatible with most medical devices • Only requires electrical outlet	• Cellulose (paper), linens and liquids cannot be processed • Sterilization chamber size from 1.8–9.4 ft^3 total volume (varies with model type) • Some endoscopes or medical devices with long or narrow lumens cannot be processed • Requires synthetic packaging (polypropylene wraps, polyolefin pouches) and special container tray • Hydrogen peroxide may be toxic at levels greater than 1 ppm TWA
100% ethylene oxide (ETO)	• Penetrates packaging materials, device lumens • Single-dose cartridge and negative-pressure chamber minimizes the potential for gas leak and ETO exposure • Simple to operate and monitor • Compatible with most medical materials	• Requires aeration time to remove ETO residue • Sterilization chamber size from 4.0–7.9 ft^3 total volume (varies with model type) • ETO is toxic, a carcinogen, and flammable • ETO emission regulated by states but catalytic cell removes 99.9% of ETO and converts it to CO_2 and H_2O • ETO cartridges should be stored in flammable liquid storage cabinet • Lengthy cycle/aeration time
ETO mixtures 8.6% ETO/91.4% HCFC 10% ETO/90% HCFC 8.5% ETO/91.5% CO_2	• Penetrates medical packaging and many plastics • Compatible with most medical materials • Cycle easy to control and monitor	• CFC (inert gas that eliminates explosion hazard) banned in 1995 • Potential hazards to staff and patients • Lengthy cycle/aeration time • ETO is toxic, a carcinogen, and flammable
Peracetic acid	• Rapid cycle time (30–45 minutes) • Low temperature (50–55°C liquid immersion sterilization • Environmental friendly by products • Sterilant flows through endoscope which facilitates salt, protein and microbe removal	• Point-of-use system, no sterile storage • Biological indicator may not be suitable for routine monitoring • Used for immersible instruments only • Some material incompatibility (e.g. aluminum anodized coating becomes dull) • One scope or a small number of instruments processed in a cycle • Potential for serious eye and skin damage (concentrated solution) with contact

Source: Rutala.[30]
Abbreviations: CFC, chlorofluorocarbon; HCFC, hydrochlorofluorocarbon

STEAM STERILIZATION[1]

Of all the methods available for sterilization, moist heat in the form of saturated steam under pressure is the most widely used and the most dependable. Steam sterilization is nontoxic, inexpensive, rapidly microbicidal, sporicidal, and rapidly heats and penetrates fabrics. Like all sterilization processes, steam sterilization has some deleterious effects on some materials, including corrosion and combustion of lubricants associated with dental handpieces; reduction in ability to transmit light associated with laryngoscopes; and increased hardening time (5-6 fold) with plaster-cast.

The basic principle of steam sterilization, as accomplished in an autoclave, is to expose each item to direct steam contact at the required temperature and pressure for the specified time. Thus, there are four parameters of steam sterilization: steam, pressure, temperature, and time. Pressure serves as a means to obtain the high temperatures necessary to quickly kill microorganisms. Specific temperatures must be obtained to ensure the microbicidal activity. The two common steam-sterilizing temperatures are 121°C (250°F) and 132°C (270°F). These temperatures (and other high temperatures) must be maintained for a minimal time to kill microorganisms. Recognized minimum exposure periods for sterilization of wrapped healthcare supplies are 30 minutes at 121°C (250°F) in a gravity displacement sterilizer or 4 minutes at 132°C (270°C) in a prevacuum sterilizer (Table 7.2). At constant temperatures, sterilization times vary depending on the type of item (e.g. metal versus rubber, plastic, items with lumens), whether the item is wrapped or unwrapped, and the sterilizer type.

Gravity Displacement Autoclave[1]

The two basic types of steam sterilizers (autoclaves) are the gravity displacement autoclave and the high-speed prevacuum sterilizer. In the former, steam is admitted at the top or the sides of the sterilizing chamber and, because the steam is lighter than air, forces air out from the bottom of the chamber through the drain vent. The gravity displacement autoclaves are primarily used to process laboratory media, water, pharmaceutical products, regulated medical waste, and nonporous articles whose surfaces have direct steam contact. For gravity displacement sterilizers the penetration time into porous items is prolonged because of incomplete air elimination. This point is illustrated with the decontamination of 10 lbs of microbiological waste, which requires at least 45 minutes at 121°C because the entrapped air remaining in a load of waste greatly retards steam permeation and heating efficiency.

High-speed Prevacuum Sterilizer[1]

The high-speed prevacuum sterilizers are similar to the gravity displacement sterilizers

Table 7.2: Minimum cycle times for steam sterilization cycles

Type of sterilizer	Item	Exposure time at 250°F (121°C)	Exposure time at 270°F (132°C)	Drying time
Gravity displacement	Wrapped instruments	30 minutes	15 minutes	15–30 minutes
	Textile packs	30 minutes	25 minutes	15 minutes
	Wrapped utensils	30 minutes	15 minutes	15–30 minutes
Dynamic-air-removal (e.g. prevacuum)	Wrapped instruments		4 minutes	20–30 minutes
	Textile packs		4 minutes	5–20 minutes
	Wrapped utensils		4 minutes	20 minutes

Source: Association for the Advancement of Medical Instrumentation.[31,32]

except they are fitted with a vacuum pump (or ejector) to ensure air removal from the sterilizing chamber and load before the steam is admitted. The advantage of using a vacuum pump is that there is nearly instantaneous steam penetration even into porous loads.

The Bowie-Dick test is used to detect air leaks and inadequate air removal and consists of folded 100% cotton surgical towels that are clean and preconditioned. A commercially available Bowie-Dick type test sheet should be placed in the center of the pack. The test pack should be placed horizontally in the front, bottom section of the sterilizer rack, near the door and over the drain, in an otherwise empty chamber and run at 134°C for 3.5 minutes. The test is used each day the vacuum type steam sterilizer is used, before the first processed load. Air that is not removed from the chamber will interfere with steam contact. Smaller disposable test packs (or process challenge devices) have been devised to replace the stack of folded surgical towels for testing the efficacy of the vacuum system in a prevacuum sterilizer. These devices are 'designed to simulate product to be sterilized and to constitute a defined challenge to the sterilization process'. They should be representative of the load and simulate the greatest challenge to the load. Sterilizer vacuum performance is acceptable if the sheet inside the test pack shows a uniform color change. Entrapped air will cause a spot to appear on the test sheet, due to the inability of the steam to reach the chemical indicator. If the sterilizer fails the Bowie-Dick test, do not use the sterilizer until it is inspected by the sterilizer maintenance personnel and passes the Bowie-Dick test.

Steam Flush-Pressure Pulsing Process[1]

Another design in steam sterilization is a steam flush-pressure pulsing process, which removes air rapidly by repeatedly alternating a steam flush and a pressure pulse above atmospheric pressure. Air is rapidly removed from the load as with the prevacuum sterilizer, but air leaks do not affect this process because the steam in the sterilizing chamber is always above atmospheric pressure. Typical sterilization temperatures and times are 132°C to 135°C with 3 to 4 minutes exposure time for porous loads and instruments.

Like other sterilization systems the steam cycle is monitored by mechanical, chemical, and biological monitors. Steam sterilizers usually are monitored using a printout (or graphically) by measuring temperature, the time at the temperature, and pressure. Typically, chemical indicators are affixed to the outside and incorporated into the pack to monitor the temperature or time and temperature. The effectiveness of steam sterilization is monitored with a biological indicator containing spores of *Geobacillus stearothermophilus* (formerly *Bacillus stearothermophilus*). Positive spore test results are a relatively rare event[2] and can be attributed to operator error, inadequate steam delivery, or equipment malfunction.

Portable (Table-top) Steam Sterilizers[1]

Portable (table-top) steam sterilizers are used in outpatient, dental, and rural clinics. These sterilizers are designed for small instruments, such as hypodermic syringes and needles and dental instruments. The ability of the sterilizer to reach physical parameters necessary to achieve sterilization should be monitored by mechanical, chemical, and biological indicators.

Mode of Action

Moist heat destroys microorganisms by the irreversible coagulation and denaturation of enzymes and structural proteins. In support of this fact, it has been found that the presence of moisture significantly affects the coagulation temperature of proteins and the temperature at which microorganisms are destroyed.

Uses

Steam sterilization should be used whenever possible on all critical and semicritical items that are heat and moisture resistant (e.g. steam sterilizable respiratory therapy and anesthesia equipment), even when not essential to prevent pathogen transmission. Steam sterilizers also are used in healthcare facilities to decontaminate microbiological waste and sharps containers, but additional exposure time is required in the gravity displacement sterilizer for these items.

Flash Sterilization[1]

'Flash' steam sterilization was originally defined by Underwood and Perkins as sterilization of an unwrapped object at 132°C for 3 minutes at 27–28 lbs. of pressure in a gravity displacement sterilizer.[3] Currently, the time required for flash sterilization depends on the type of sterilizer and the type of item (i.e. porous vs non-porous items)(Table 7.3). Although the wrapped method of sterilization is preferred for the reasons listed below, correctly performed flash sterilization is an effective process for the sterilization of critical medical devices. Flash sterilization is a modification of conventional steam sterilization (either gravity, prevacuum, or steam-flush pressure-pulse) in which the flashed item is placed in an open tray or is placed in a specially designed, covered, rigid container to allow for rapid penetration of steam. Historically, it is not recommended as a routine sterilization method because of the lack of timely biological indicators to monitor performance, absence of protective packaging following sterilization, possibility for contamination of processed items during transportation to the operating rooms, and the sterilization cycle parameters (i.e. time, temperature, pressure) are minimal. To address some of these concerns, many healthcare facilities have done the following: placed equipment for flash sterilization in close proximity to operating rooms to facilitate aseptic delivery to the point of use (usually the sterile field in an ongoing surgical procedure); extended the exposure time to ensure lethality comparable to sterilized wrapped items (e.g., 4 minutes at 132°C); used biological indicators that provide results in 1 hour for flash-sterilized items; and used protective packaging that permits steam penetration. Further, some rigid, reusable sterilization container systems have been designed and validated by the container manufacturer for use with flash cycles. When sterile items are open to air, they will eventually become contaminated. Thus, the longer a sterile item is exposed to air, the greater the number of micro-organisms that will settle on it. Sterilization cycle parameters for flash sterilization are shown in (Table 7.3).

Table 7.3: Examples of flash steam sterilization parameters

Type of sterilizer	Load configuration	*Temperature*	*Time*
Gravity displacement	Nonporous items only (i.e. routine metal instruments, no lumens)	132°C (270°F)	3 minutes
	Nonporous and porous items (e.g. rubber or plastic items, items with lumens) sterilized together	132°C (270°F)	10 minutes
Prevacuum	Nonporous items only (i.e. routine metal instruments, no lumens)	132°C (270°F)	3 minutes
	Nonporous and porous items (e.g. rubber or plastic items, items with lumens) sterilized together	132°C (270°F)	4 minutes
Steam-flush pressure-pulse	Nonporous or mixed nonporous/porous items	132° (270°F) Manufacturers' instruction	4 minutes

Source: Association for the Advancement of Medical instrumentations.[33,34]

Use of Flash Sterilization

Flash sterilization is considered acceptable for processing cleaned patient-care items that cannot be packaged, sterilized, and stored before use. It also is used when there is insufficient time to sterilize an item by the preferred package method. Flash sterilization should not be used for reasons of convenience, as an alternative to purchasing additional instrument sets, or to save time. Because of the potential for serious infections, flash sterilization is not recommended for implantable devices (i.e. devices placed into a surgically or naturally formed cavity of the human body); however, flash sterilization may be unavoidable for some devices (e.g. orthopedic screw, plates). If flash sterilization of an implantable device is unavoidable, record-keeping (i.e. load identification, patient's name/hospital identifier, and biological indicator result) is essential for epidemiological tracking (e.g. of surgical site infection, tracing results of biological indicators to patients who received the item to document sterility), and for an assessment of the reliability of the sterilization process (e.g. evaluation of biological monitoring records and sterilization maintenance records noting preventive maintenance and repairs with dates).

LOW-TEMPERATURE STERILIZATION TECHNOLOGIES[1]

Ethylene Oxide

Ethylene oxide (EtO) has been widely used as a low-temperature sterilant since the 1950s. It has been the most commonly used process for sterilizing, temperature- and moisture-sensitive medical devices and supplies in healthcare institutions. Two types of EtO sterilizers are available, mixed gas and 100% EtO. Until 1995, ethylene oxide sterilizers combined EtO with a chlorofluorocarbon (CFC) stabilizing agent, most commonly in a ratio of 12% EtO mixed with 88% CFC (referred to as 12/88 EtO).

For several reasons, healthcare personnel have been exploring the use of new low-temperature sterilization technologies as CFCs were phased out in December 1995 Act because of scientific evidence linking them to destruction of the earth's ozone layer and because of concerns that EtO exposure represents an occupational hazard.

Alternative technologies to EtO with chlorofluorocarbon that are currently available and cleared by the FDA for medical equipment include 100% EtO or EtO with a different stabilizing gas, such as carbon dioxide or hydrochlorofluorocarbons (HCFC); immersion in peracetic acid; hydrogen peroxide gas plasma; and ozone. Technologies under development for use in healthcare facilities, include vaporized hydrogen peroxide, vapor phase peracetic acid, gaseous chlorine dioxide, ionizing radiation, or pulsed light.

While it is apparent that all technologies will have limitations (Table 7.4) understanding the limitations imposed by restrictive device designs (e.g. long, narrow lumens) is critical for proper application of new sterilization technology. For example, the development of increasingly small and complex endoscopes presents a difficult challenge for current sterilization processes. This occurs because microorganisms must be in direct contact with the sterilant for inactivation to occur. Factors shown to affect the efficacy of sterilization are shown in (Table 7.5).

Ethylene Oxide 'Gas' Sterilization

EtO is a colorless gas that is flammable and explosive. The four essential parameters (operational ranges) are: gas concentration (450–1200 mg/L); temperature (37–63°C); relative humidity (40–80%) (water molecules carry EtO to reactive sites); and exposure time (1–6 hours). These influence the effectiveness of EtO sterilization. Within certain limitations, an increase in gas concentration and temperature may shorten the time necessary for achieving sterilization.

Table 7.4: Characteristics of an ideal low-temperature sterilization process

High efficacy: The agent should be virucidal, bactericidal, tuberculocidal, fungicidal and sporicidal
Rapid activity: Ability to quickly achieve sterilization
Strong penetrability: Ability to penetrate common medical-device packaging materials and penetrate into the interior of device lumens
Material compatibility: Produces only negligible changes in the appearance or the function of processed items and packaging materials even after repeated cycling
Nontoxic: Presents no toxic health risk to the operator or the patient and poses no hazard to the environment
Organic material resistance: Withstands reasonable organic material challenge without loss of efficacy
Adaptability: Suitable for large or small (point of use) installations
Monitoring capability: Monitored easily and accurately with physical, chemical, and biological process monitors
Cost effectiveness: Reasonable cost for installation and for routine operation

Source: Modified from Schneider.[35]

Table 7.5: Factors affecting the efficacy of sterilization

Factors	Effect
Cleaning 1	Failure to adequately clean instrument results in higher bioburden, protein load, and salt concentration. These will decrease sterilization efficacy
Bioburden1	The natural bioburden of used surgical devices is 10^0 to 10^3 organisms (primarily vegetative bacteria), which is substantially below the 10^5-10^6 spores used with biological indicators
Pathogen type	Spore-forming organisms are most resistant to sterilization and are the test organisms required for FDA clearance. However, the contaminating microflora on used surgical instruments consists mainly of vegetative bacteria
Protein1	Residual protein decreases efficacy of sterilization. However, cleaning appears to rapidly remove protein load
Salt1	Residual salt decreases efficacy of sterilization more than does protein load. However, cleaning appears to rapidly remove salt load
Biofilm accumulation 1	Biofilm accumulation reduces efficacy of sterilization by impairing exposure of the sterilant to the microbial cell
Lumen length	Increasing lumen length impairs sterilant penetration. May require forced flow through lumen to achieve sterilization
Lumen diameter	Decreasing lumen diameter impairs sterilant penetration. May require forced flow through lumen to achieve sterilization
Restricted flow	Sterilant must come into contact with microorganisms. Device designs that prevent or inhibit this contact (e.g. sharp bends, blind lumens) will decrease sterilization efficacy
Device design and construction	Materials used in construction may affect compatibility with different sterilization processes and affect sterilization efficacy. Design issues (e.g. screws, hinges) will also affect sterilization efficacy

Source: Alfa and Rutala[36,37]

[1]Factor only relevant for reused surgical/medical devices

The main disadvantages associated with EtO are the lengthy cycle time, the cost, and its potential hazards to patients and staff; the main advantage is that it can sterilize heat- or moisture-sensitive medical equipment without deleterious effects on the material used in the medical devices. Acute exposure to EtO may result in irritation (e.g. to skin, eyes, gastrointestinal or respiratory tracts) and central nervous system depression. Chronic inhalation has been linked to the formation of cataracts, cognitive impairment, neurologic dysfunction, and disabling polyneuropathies. Occupational exposure in healthcare facilities has been linked to hematologic changes and an increased risk of spontaneous abortions and various cancers. EtO should be considered a known human carcinogen.

The basic EtO sterilization cycle consists of five stages (i.e. preconditioning and humidification, gas introduction, exposure, evacuation, and air washes) and takes approximately 2 1/2 hours excluding aeration time. Mechanical aeration for 8 to 12 hours at 50 to 60°C allows desorption of the toxic EtO residual contained in exposed absorbent materials. Most modern EtO sterilizers combine sterilization and aeration in the same chamber as a continuous process. These EtO models minimize potential EtO exposure during door opening and load transfer to the aerator. Ambient room aeration also will achieve desorption of the toxic EtO but requires 7 days at 20°C.

The use of EtO evolved when few alternatives existed for sterilizing heat- and moisture-sensitive medical devices; however, favorable properties account for its continued widespread use. Two EtO gas mixtures are available to replace EtO-chlorofluorocarbon (CFC) mixtures for large capacity, tank-supplied sterilizers. The EtO carbon dioxide (CO_2) mixture consists of 8.5% EtO and 91.5% CO_2. This mixture is less expensive than EtO-hydrochlorofluorocarbons (HCFC), but a disadvantage is the need for pressure vessels rated for steam sterilization, because higher pressures (28-psi gauge) are required. The other mixture, which is a drop-in CFC replacement, is EtO mixed with HCFC. HCFCs are approximately 50-fold less damaging to the earth's ozone layer than are CFCs. The EPA will begin regulation of HCFC in the year 2015 and will terminate production in the year 2030. Two companies provide EtO-HCFC mixtures as drop-in replacement for CFC-12; one mixture consists of 8.6% EtO and 91.4% HCFC, and the other mixture is composed of 10% EtO and 90% HCFC.[4] An alternative to the pressurized mixed gas EtO systems is 100% EtO. The 100% EtO sterilizers using unit-dose cartridges eliminate the need for external tanks.

EtO is absorbed by many materials. For this reason, following sterilization the item must undergo aeration to remove residual EtO. Guidelines have been promulgated regarding allowable EtO limits for devices that depend on how the device is used, how often, and how long in order to pose a minimal risk to patients in normal product use. EtO toxicity has been established in a variety of animals. Exposure to EtO can cause eye pain, sore throat, difficulty in breathing and blurred vision. Exposure can also cause dizziness, nausea, headache, convulsions, blisters, vomiting and coughing. In a variety of in vitro and animal studies, EtO has been demonstrated to be carcinogenic. EtO has been linked to spontaneous abortion, genetic damage, nerve damage, peripheral paralysis, muscle weakness, and impaired thinking and memory. Occupational exposure in healthcare facilities has been linked to an increased risk of spontaneous abortions and various cancers. Injuries (e.g. tissue burns) to patients have been associated with EtO residues in implants used in surgical procedures. Residual EtO in capillary flow dialysis membranes has been shown to be neurotoxic in vitro.

Mode of action: The microbicidal activity of EtO is considered to be the result of alkylation of protein, DNA, and RNA. Alkylation, or the replacement of a hydrogen atom with an alkyl group, within cells prevents normal cellular metabolism and replication.

Microbicidal activity: EtO inactivates all microorganisms although bacterial spores (especially *B. atrophaeus*) are more resistant than other microorganisms. For this reason *B. atrophaeus* is the recommended biological indicator.

Like all sterilization processes, the effectiveness of EtO sterilization can be altered by lumen length, lumen diameter, inorganic salts, and organic materials. For example, although EtO is not used commonly for reprocessing endoscopes, several studies have shown failure of EtO in inactivating contaminating spores in endoscope channels or lumen test units and residual EtO levels averaging 66.2 ppm even after the standard degassing time. Failure of EtO also has been observed when dental handpieces were contaminated with *Streptococcus mutans* and exposed to EtO.[5] It is recommended that dental handpieces be steam sterilized.

Uses: EtO is used in healthcare facilities to sterilize critical items (and sometimes semicritical items) that are moisture or heat sensitive and cannot be sterilized by steam sterilization.

Hydrogen Peroxide Gas Plasma[1]

Gas plasmas have been referred to as the fourth state of matter (i.e. liquids, solids, gases, and gas plasmas). Gas plasmas are generated in an enclosed chamber under deep vacuum using radiofrequency or microwave energy to excite the gas molecules and produce charged particles, many of which are in the form of free radicals. A free radical is an atom with an unpaired electron and is a highly reactive species. The proposed mechanism of action of this device is the production of free radicals within a plasma field that are capable of interacting with essential cell components (e.g. enzymes, nucleic acids) and thereby disrupt the metabolism of microorganisms. The type of seed gas used and the depth of the vacuum are two important variables that can determine the effectiveness of this process.

In the late 1980s the first hydrogen peroxide gas plasma system for sterilization of medical and surgical devices was field-tested. According to the manufacturer, the sterilization chamber is evacuated and hydrogen peroxide solution is injected from a cassette and is vaporized in the sterilization chamber to a concentration of 6 mg/L. The hydrogen peroxide vapor diffuses through the chamber (50 minutes), exposes all surfaces of the load to the sterilant, and initiates the inactivation of microorganisms. An electrical field created by a radiofrequency is applied to the chamber to create a gas plasma. Microbicidal free radicals (e.g. hydroxyl and hydroperoxyl) are generated in the plasma. The excess gas is removed and in the final stage (i.e. vent) of the process the sterilization chamber is returned to atmospheric pressure by introduction of high-efficiency filtered air. The by-products of the cycle (e.g. water vapor, oxygen) are nontoxic and eliminate the need for aeration. Thus, the sterilized materials can be handled safely, either for immediate use or storage. The process operates in the range of 37–44°C and has a cycle time of 75 minutes. If any moisture is present on the objects the vacuum will not be achieved and the cycle aborts.

A newer version of the unit improves sterilizer efficacy by using two cycles with a hydrogen peroxide diffusion stage and a plasma stage per sterilization cycle. This revision, which is achieved by a software modification, reduces total processing time from 73 to 52 minutes. The manufacturer believes that the enhanced activity obtained with this system is due in part to the pressure changes that occur during the injection and diffusion phases of the process and to the fact that the process consists of two equal and consecutive half cycles, each with a separate injection of hydrogen peroxide. The biological indicator used with this system is *Bacillus atrophaeus* spores. The newest version of the unit, which employs a new vaporization system that removes most of the water from the hydrogen peroxide, has a cycle time from 28–38 minutes.

Penetration of hydrogen peroxide vapor into long or narrow lumens has been addressed outside the United States by the use of a diffusion enhancer. This is a small, breakable glass ampoule of concentrated hydrogen peroxide (50%) with an elastic connector that is inserted into the device lumen and crushed immediately before sterilization.

The diffusion enhancer has been shown to sterilize bronchoscopes contaminated with *Mycobacteria tuberculosis*.

Mechanism of action: This process inactivates microorganisms primarily by the combined use of hydrogen peroxide gas and the generation of free radicals (hydroxyl and hydroproxyl free radicals) during the plasma phase of the cycle.

Range of activity: This process has the ability to inactivate a broad range of microorganisms, including resistant bacterial spores. Like all sterilization processes, the effectiveness can be altered by lumen length, lumen diameter, inorganic salts, and organic materials.

Uses: Materials and devices that cannot tolerate high temperatures and humidity, such as some plastics, electrical devices, and corrosion-susceptible metal alloys, can be sterilized by hydrogen peroxide gas plasma. This method has been compatible with most (>95%) medical devices and materials tested.

Peracetic Acid Sterilization

Peracetic acid is a highly biocidal oxidizer that maintains its efficacy in the presence of organic soil. Peracetic acid removes surface contaminants (primarily protein) on endoscopic tubing. An automated machine using peracetic acid to sterilize medical, surgical, and dental instruments chemically (e.g. endoscopes, arthroscopes) was introduced in 1988. The sterilant, 35% peracetic acid, and an anticorrosive agent are supplied in a single-dose container. The container is punctured at the time of use, immediately prior to closing the lid and initiating the cycle. The concentrated peracetic acid is diluted to 0.2% with filtered water (0.2 μm) at a temperature of approximately 50°C. The diluted peracetic acid is circulated within the chamber of the machine and pumped through the channels of the endoscope for 12 minutes, decontaminating exterior surfaces, lumens, and accessories. Interchangeable trays are available to permit the processing of up to three rigid endoscopes or one flexible endoscope. Connectors are available for most types of flexible endoscopes for the irrigation of all channels by directed flow. Rigid endoscopes are placed within a lidded container, and the sterilant fills the lumens either by immersion in the circulating sterilant or by use of channel connectors to direct flow into the lumen(s) (see below for the importance of channel connectors). The peracetic acid is discarded via the sewer and the instrument rinsed four times with filtered water. Concern has been raised that filtered water may be inadequate to maintain sterility. Clean filtered air is passed through the chamber of the machine and endoscope channels to remove excess water. As with any sterilization process, the system can only sterilize surfaces that can be contacted by the sterilant. For example, bronchoscopy-related infections occurred when bronchoscopes were processed using the wrong connector. Investigation of these incidents revealed that bronchoscopes were inadequately reprocessed when inappropriate channel connectors were used and when there were inconsistencies between the reprocessing instructions provided by the manufacturer of the bronchoscope and the manufacturer of the automatic endoscope reprocessor. The importance of channel connectors to achieve sterilization was also shown for rigid lumen devices.

The manufacturers suggest the use of biological monitors (*G. stearothermophilus* spore strips) both at the time of installation and routinely to ensure effectiveness of the process. The manufacturer's clip must be used to hold the strip in the designated spot in the machine as a broader clamp will not allow the sterilant to reach the spores trapped under it. The use of biological monitors designed to monitor either steam sterilization or EtO for a liquid chemical sterilizer has been questioned for several reasons including spore wash-off from the filter paper strips which may cause less valid monitoring. The processor is equipped with a conductivity probe that will automatically abort the cycle if the buffer system is not detected in a fresh container of the peracetic acid solution. A chemical monitoring strip that detects that the active ingredient is >1500 ppm is available for routine use as an additional process control.

Mechanism of action: Only limited information is available regarding the mechanism of action of peracetic acid, but it is thought to function as other oxidizing agents, i.e. it denatures proteins, disrupts cell wall permeability, and oxidizes sulfhydryl and sulfur bonds in proteins, enzymes, and other metabolites.

Range of activity: Peracetic acid will inactivate gram-positive and gram-negative bacteria, fungi, and yeasts and viruses.

Uses: This automated machine is used to chemically sterilize medical (e.g. gastrointestinal endoscopes) and surgical (e.g. flexible endoscopes) instruments. Lumened endoscopes must be connected to an appropriate channel connector to ensure that the sterilant has direct contact with the contaminated lumen.

OTHER STERILIZATION METHODS[1]

Ionizing Radiation

Sterilization by ionizing radiation, primarily by cobalt 60 gamma rays or electron accelerators, is a low-temperature sterilization method that has been used for a number of medical products (e.g. tissue for transplantation, pharmaceuticals, medical devices). Because of high sterilization costs, this method is an unfavorable alternative to EtO and plasma sterilization in healthcare facilities but is suitable for large-scale sterilization.

Dry-Heat Sterilizers

This method should be used only for materials that might be damaged by moist heat or that are impenetrable to moist heat (e.g. powders, petroleum products, sharp instruments). The advantages for dry heat include the following: it is nontoxic and does not harm the environment; a dry heat cabinet is easy to install and has relatively low operating costs; it penetrates materials; and it is noncorrosive for metal and sharp instruments. The disadvantages for dry heat are the slow rate of heat penetration and microbial killing makes this a time-consuming method. In addition, the high temperatures are not suitable for most materials.

The most common time-temperature relationships for sterilization with hot air sterilizers are 170°C (340°F) for 60 minutes, 160°C (320°F) for 120 minutes, and 150°C (300°F) for 150 minutes. *B. atrophaeus* spores should be used to monitor the sterilization process for dry heat because they are more resistant to dry heat than are *G. stearothermophilus* spores. The primary lethal process is considered to be oxidation of cell constituents.

There are two types of dry-heat sterilizers: the static-air type and the forced-air type. The static-air type is referred to as the oven-type sterilizer as heating coils in the bottom of the unit cause the hot air to rise inside the chamber via gravity convection. This type of dry-heat sterilizer is much slower in heating, requires longer time to reach sterilizing temperature, and is less uniform in temperature control throughout the chamber than is the forced-air type. The forced-air or mechanical convection sterilizer is equipped with a motor-driven blower that circulates heated air throughout the chamber at a high velocity, permitting a more rapid transfer of energy from the air to the instruments.

Liquid Chemicals

Several liquid chemical sterilants are used for sterilization of medical devices. The indicated contact times range from 3 to 12 hours.

One of the differences between thermal and liquid chemical processes for sterilization of devices is the accessibility of microorganisms to the sterilant. Heat can penetrate barriers, such as biofilm, tissue, and blood, to attain organism kill, whereas liquids cannot adequately penetrate these barriers. In addition, the viscosity of some liquid chemical sterilants impedes their access to organisms in the narrow lumens and mated surfaces of devices. Another limitation to sterilization of devices with liquid chemical germicides is the post-processing environment of the device. Devices cannot be wrapped or adequately contained during processing in a liquid chemical sterilant to maintain sterility following processing and during storage. Furthermore, devices may require rinsing following exposure to the liquid chemical sterilant with water that typically is not sterile. Therefore, due to the inherent limitations of using liquid chemical sterilants, their use should be restricted to reprocessing critical devices that are heat-sensitive and incompatible with other sterilization methods.

Performic Acid

Performic acid is a fast-acting sporicide that was incorporated into an automated endoscope reprocessing system.[6]

Filtration

Although filtration is not a lethality-based process, this technology is used to remove bacteria from thermolabile pharmaceutical fluids that cannot be purified by any other means. In order to remove bacteria, the membrane pore size (e.g. 0.22 μm) must be smaller than the bacteria and uniform throughout. Some investigators have appropriately questioned whether the removal of microorganisms by filtration really is a sterilization method because of slight bacterial passage through filters, viral passage through filters, and transference of the sterile filtrate into the final container under aseptic conditions entail a risk of contamination.

Microwave

Microwaves are used in medicine for disinfection of soft contact lenses, dental instruments, dentures, milk, and urinary catheters for intermittent self-catheterization. However, microwaves must only be used with products that are compatible (e.g. do not melt). Microwaves are radiofrequency waves, which are usually used at a frequency of 2450 MHz. The microwaves produce friction of water molecules in an alternating electrical field. The intermolecular friction derived from the vibrations generates heat and some authors believe that the effect of microwaves depends on the heat produced while others postulate a nonthermal lethal effect. The initial reports showed microwaves to be an effective microbicide. The microwaves produced by a 'home-type' microwave oven (2.45 GHz) completely inactivate bacterial cultures, mycobacteria, viruses, and *G. stearothermophilus* spores within 60 seconds to 5 minutes depending on the challenge organism. Another study confirmed these results but also found that higher power microwaves in the presence of water may be needed for sterilization complete destruction of *Mycobacterium bovis* was obtained with 4 minutes of microwave exposure (600W, 2450 MHz).[7] The effectiveness of microwave ovens for different sterilization and disinfection purposes should be tested and demonstrated as test conditions affect the results (e.g. presence of water, microwave power). Sterilization of metal instruments can be accomplished but requires certain precautions. Of concern is that home-type microwave ovens may not have even distribution of microwave energy over the entire dry device (there may be hot and cold spots on solid medical devices); hence there may be areas that are not sterilized or disinfected. The use of microwave ovens to disinfect intermittent-use catheters also has been suggested.

Glass Bead 'Sterilizer'

Glass bead 'sterilization' uses small glass beads (1.2–1.5 mm diameter) and high temperature (217°C–232°C) for brief exposure times (e.g.

45 seconds) to inactivate microorganisms. These devices have been used for several years in the dental profession.

Vaporized Hydrogen Peroxide (VHP)

Hydrogen peroxide solutions have been used as chemical sterilants for many years. However, the VHP was not developed for the sterilization of medical equipment until the mid-1980s. One method for delivering VHP to the reaction site uses a deep vacuum to pull liquid hydrogen peroxide (30–35% concentration) from a disposable cartridge through a heated vaporizer and then, following vaporization, into the sterilization chamber. A second approach to VHP delivery is the flow-through approach in which the VHP is carried into the sterilization chamber by a carrier gas such as air using either a slight negative pressure (vacuum) or slight positive pressure. Applications of this technology include vacuum systems for industrial sterilization of medical devices and atmospheric systems for decontaminating for large and small areas. VHP offers several appealing features that include rapid cycle time (e.g. 30–45 minutes); low temperature; environmentally safe by-products [H_2O, oxygen (O_2)]; good material compatibility; and ease of operation, installation and monitoring. VHP has limitations including that cellulose cannot be processed; nylon becomes brittle; and VHP penetration capabilities are less than those of EtO.

Ozone

Ozone has been used for years as a drinking water disinfectant. Ozone is produced when O_2 is energized and split into two monatomic (O_1) molecules. The monatomic oxygen molecules then collide with O_2 molecules to form ozone, which is O_3. Thus, ozone consists of O_2 with a loosely bonded third oxygen atom that is readily available to attach to, and oxidize, other molecules. This additional oxygen atom makes ozone a powerful oxidant that destroys microorganisms but is highly unstable (i.e. half-life of 22 minutes at room temperature).

The ozone process is compatible with a wide range of commonly used materials including stainless steel, titanium, anodized aluminum, ceramic, glass, silica, PVC, teflon, silicone, polypropylene, polyethylene and acrylic. In addition, rigid lumen devices of the following diameter and length can be processed: internal diameter (ID): >2 mm, length ≤25 cm; ID >3 mm, length ≤47 cm; and ID >4 mm, length ≤60 cm.

The process is safe for use by the operator because there is no handling of the sterilant, no toxic emissions, no residue to aerate, and low operating temperature means there is no danger of an accidental burn. The cycle is monitored using a self-contained biological indicator and a chemical indicator.

A gaseous ozone generator was investigated for decontamination of rooms used to house patients colonized with MRSA. The results demonstrated that the device tested would be inadequate for the decontamination of a hospital room.

Formaldehyde Steam

Low temperature steam with formaldehyde is used as a low temperature sterilization method in many countries. The process involves the use of formalin, which is vaporized into a formaldehyde gas that is admitted into the sterilization chamber. A formaldehyde concentration of 8–16 mg/L is generated at an operating temperature of 70–75°C. The sterilization cycle consists of a series of stages that include an initial vacuum to remove air from the chamber and load, followed by steam admission to the chamber with the vacuum pump running to purge the chamber of air and to heat the load, followed by a series of pulses of formaldehyde gas, followed by steam. Formaldehyde is removed from the sterilizer and load by repeated alternate evacuations and flushing with steam and air.

This system has some advantages, e.g. the cycle time for formaldehyde gas is faster than that for EtO and the cost per cycle is relatively low. However, EtO is more penetrating and operates at lower temperatures than do steam/formaldehyde sterilizers. Low-temperature steam formaldehyde sterilization has been found effective against vegetative bacteria, mycobacteria, *B. atrophaeus* and *G. stearothermophilus* spores and *Candida albicans*.

Formaldehyde vapor cabinets also may be used in healthcare facilities to sterilize heat-sensitive medical equipment. Commonly, there is no circulation of formaldehyde and no temperature and humidity controls. The release of gas from paraformaldehyde tablets (placed on the lower tray) is slow and produces a low partial pressure of gas. The microbicidal quality of this procedure is unknown.

Reliable sterilization using formaldehyde is achieved when performed with a high concentration of gas, at a temperature between 60° and 80°C and with a relative humidity of 75–100%.

Studies indicate that formaldehyde is a mutagen and a potential human carcinogen. The permissible exposure limit for formaldehyde in work areas is 0.75 ppm measured as a 8-hour TWA (Time weighed average). The OSHA standard includes a 2 ppm STEL (i.e. maximum exposure allowed during a 15 minute period). As with the EtO standard, the formaldehyde standard requires that the employer conduct initial monitoring to identify employees who are exposed to formaldehyde at or above the action level or STEL. If this exposure level is maintained, employers may discontinue exposure monitoring until there is a change that could affect exposure levels or an employee reports formaldehyde-related signs and symptoms.

Gaseous Chlorine Dioxide

A gaseous chlorine dioxide system for sterilization of healthcare products was developed in the late 1980s. Chlorine dioxide is not mutagenic or carcinogenic in humans. As the chlorine dioxide concentration increases, the time required to achieve sterilization becomes progressively shorter. For example, only 30 minutes were required at 40 mg/L to sterilize the 10^6 *B. atrophaeus* spores at 30° to 32°C.

Vaporized Peracetic Acid

The sporicidal activity of peracetic acid vapor at 20, 40, 60, and 80% relative humidity and 25°C was determined on *Bacillus atrophaeus* spores on paper and glass surfaces. Appreciable activity occurred within 10 minutes of exposure to 1 mg of peracetic acid per liter at 40% or higher relative humidity.

Infrared Radiation

An infrared radiation prototype sterilizer was investigated and found to destroy *B. atrophaeus* spores. Some of the possible advantages of infrared technology include short cycle time, low energy consumption, no cycle residuals, and no toxicologic or environmental effects. This may provide an alternative technology for sterilization of selected heat-resistant items.

STERILIZING PRACTICES

Overview

The delivery of sterile products for use in patient care depends not only on the effectiveness of the sterilization process but also on the unit design, decontamination, disassembling and packaging of the device, loading the sterilizer, monitoring, sterilant quality and quantity, and the appropriateness of the cycle for the load contents, and other aspects of device reprocessing. Healthcare personnel should perform most cleaning, disinfecting, and sterilizing of patient-care supplies in a central processing department in order to more easily control quality. The aim of central processing is the orderly processing of medical and surgical instruments to protect patients from infections while minimizing risks to staff and preserving the value of the items being reprocessed. Healthcare facilities should promote the same level of efficiency and safety in the preparation of supplies in other areas (e.g. operating room, respiratory therapy) as is practiced in central processing.

Ensuring consistency of sterilization practices requires a comprehensive program that ensures operator competence and proper methods of cleaning and wrapping instruments, loading the sterilizer, operating the sterilizer, and monitoring of the entire process. Furthermore, care must be consistent from an infection prevention standpoint in all patient-care settings, such as hospital and outpatient facilities.

Sterilization Cycle Verification

A sterilization process should be verified before it is put into use in healthcare settings. All steam, EtO, and other low-temperature sterilizers are tested with biological and chemical indicators upon installation, when the sterilizer is relocated, redesigned, after major repair and after a sterilization failure has occurred to ensure they are functioning prior to placing them into routine use. Three consecutive empty steam cycles are run with a biological and chemical indicator in an appropriate test package or tray. Each type of steam cycle used for sterilization (e.g. vacuum-assisted, gravity) is tested separately. In a prevacuum steam sterilizer three consecutive empty cycles are also run with a Bowie-Dick test. The sterilizer is not put back into use until all biological indicators are negative and chemical indicators show a correct end-point response. Biological and chemical indicator testing is also done for ongoing quality assurance testing of representative samples of actual products being sterilized and product testing when major changes are made in packaging, wraps, or load configuration. Biological and chemical indicators are placed in products, which are processed in a full load. When three consecutive cycles show negative biological indicators and chemical indicators with a correct end point response, you can put the change made into routine use. Items processed during the three evaluation cycles should be quarantined until the test results are negative.

Physical Facilities

The central processing area(s) ideally should be divided into at least three areas: decontamination, packaging, and sterilization and storage. Physical barriers should separate the decontamination area from the other sections to contain contamination on used items. In the decontamination area reusable contaminated supplies (and possibly disposable items that are reused) are received, sorted, and decontaminated. The recommended airflow pattern should contain contaminates within the decontamination area and minimize the flow of contaminates to the clean areas. The American Institute of Architects[8] recommends negative pressure and no fewer than six air exchanges per hour in the decontamination area and 10 air changes per hour with positive pressure in the sterilizer equipment room. The packaging area is for inspecting, assembling, and packaging clean, but not sterile, material. The sterile storage area should be a limited access area with a controlled temperature (may be as high as 75°F) and relative humidity (30–60% in all works areas except sterile storage, where the relative humidity should not exceed 70%). The floors and walls should be constructed of materials capable of withstanding chemical agents used for cleaning or disinfecting. Ceilings and wall surfaces should be constructed of non-shedding materials.

Cleaning

As repeatedly mentioned, items must be cleaned using water with detergents or enzymatic cleaners before processing.

Cleaning reduces the bioburden and removes foreign material (i.e. organic residue and inorganic salts) that interferes with the sterilization process by acting as a barrier to the sterilization agent. Surgical instruments are generally presoaked or prerinsed to prevent drying of blood and tissue. Precleaning in patient-care areas may be needed on items that are heavily soiled with feces, sputum, blood, or other material. Items sent to central processing without removing gross soil may be difficult to clean because of dried secretions and excretions. Cleaning and decontamination should be done as soon as possible after items have been used.

Several types of mechanical cleaning machines (e.g. utensil washer-sanitizer, ultrasonic cleaner, washer-sterilizer, dishwasher, washer-disinfector) may facilitate cleaning and decontamination of most items. This equipment often is automated and may increase productivity, improve cleaning effectiveness, and decrease worker exposure to blood and body fluids. Delicate and intricate objects and heat- or moisture-sensitive articles may require careful cleaning by hand. All used items sent to the central processing area should be considered contaminated (unless decontaminated in the area of origin), handled with gloves (forceps or tongs are sometimes needed to avoid exposure to sharps), and decontaminated by one of the aforementioned methods to render them safer to handle. Items composed of more than one removable part should be disassembled. Care should be taken to ensure that all parts are kept together, so that reassembly can be accomplished efficiently.

Investigators have described the degree of cleanliness by visual and microscopic examination. One study found 91% of the instruments to be clean visually but, when examined microscopically, 84% of the instruments had residual debris. Sites that contained residual debris included junctions between insulating sheaths and activating mechanisms of laparoscopic instruments and articulations and grooves of forceps. More research is needed to understand the clinical significance of these findings and how to ensure proper cleaning.

Personnel working in the decontamination area should wear household-cleaning-type rubber or plastic gloves when handling or cleaning contaminated instruments and devices. Face masks, eye protection such as goggles or full-length faceshields, and appropriate gowns should be worn when exposure to blood and contaminated fluids may occur (e.g. when manually cleaning contaminated devices). Contaminated instruments are a source of microorganisms that could inoculate personnel through nonintact skin on the hands or through contact with the mucous membranes of eyes, nose, or mouth. Reusable sharps that have been in contact with blood present a special hazard. Employees must not reach with their gloved hands into trays or containers that hold these sharps to retrieve them. Rather, employees should use engineering controls (e.g. forceps) to retrieve these devices.

Packaging

Once items are cleaned, dried, and inspected, those requiring sterilization must be wrapped or placed in rigid containers and should be arranged in instrument trays/baskets according to the guidelines.These guidelines state that hinged instruments should be opened; items with removable parts should be disassembled unless the device manufacturer provide specific instructions to the contrary; complex instruments should be prepared and sterilized according to device manufacturer's instructions; devices with concave surfaces should be positioned to facilitate drainage of water; heavy items should be positioned not to damage delicate items; and the weight of the instrument set should be based on the design and density of the instruments and the distribution of metal mass. While there is no longer a specified sterilization weight limit for surgical sets, heavy metal mass is a cause of wet packs (i.e. moisture inside the case and tray after completion of the sterilization cycle). Other parameters that may influence drying are the density of the wraps and the design of the set.

There are several choices in methods to maintain sterility of surgical instruments, including rigid containers, peel-open pouches (e.g. self-sealed or heat-sealed plastic and paper pouches), roll stock or reels (i.e. paper-plastic combinations of tubing designed to allow the user to cut and seal the ends to form a pouch) and sterilization wraps (woven and nonwoven). Healthcare facilities may use all of these packaging options. The packaging material must allow penetration of the sterilant, provide protection against contact contamination during handling, provide an effective barrier to microbial penetration, and maintain the sterility of the processed item after sterilization. An ideal sterilization wrap would successfully address barrier effectiveness, penetrability (i.e. allows sterilant to penetrate), aeration (e.g. allows EtO to dissipate), ease of use, drapeability, flexibility, puncture resistance, tear strength, toxicity, odor, waste disposal, linting, cost, and transparency. Unacceptable packaging for use with EtO [e.g. foil, polyvinylchloride, and polyvinylidene chlorine (kitchen-type transparent wrap)] or hydrogen peroxide gas plasma (e.g. linens and paper) should not be used to wrap medical items.

In central processing, double wrapping can be done sequentially or nonsequentially (i.e. simultaneous wrapping). Wrapping should be done in such a manner to avoid tenting and gapping. The sequential wrap uses two sheets of the standard sterilization wrap, one wrapped after the other. This procedure creates a package within a package. The nonsequential process uses two sheets wrapped at the same time so that the wrapping needs to be performed only once. This latter method provides multiple layers of protection of surgical instruments from contamination and saves time since wrapping is done only once. Multiple layers are still common practice due to the rigors of handling within the facility even though the barrier efficacy of a single sheet of wrap has improved over the years. Written and illustrated procedures for preparation of items to be packaged should be readily available and used by personnel when packaging procedures are performed.

Loading

All items to be sterilized should be arranged so all surfaces will be directly exposed to the sterilizing agent. Thus, loading procedures must allow for free circulation of steam (or another sterilant) around each item. Historically, it was recommended that muslin fabric packs should not exceed the maximal dimensions, weight, and density of 12 inches wide × 12 inches high × 20 inches long, 12 lbs, and 7.2 lbs per cubic foot, respectively. Due to the variety of textiles and metal/plastic containers on the market, the textile and metal/plastic container manufacturer and the sterilizer manufacturers should be consulted for instructions on pack preparation and density parameters.[9]

There are several important basic principles for loading a sterilizer: allow for proper sterilant circulation; perforated trays should be placed so the tray is parallel to the shelf; nonperforated containers should be placed on their edge (e.g. basins); small items should be loosely placed in wire baskets; and peel packs should be placed on edge in perforated or mesh bottom racks or baskets.[10]

Storage

Studies in the early 1970s suggested that wrapped surgical trays remained sterile for varying periods depending on the type of material used to wrap the trays. Safe storage times for sterile packs vary with the porosity of the wrapper and storage conditions (e.g. open versus closed cabinets). Heat-sealed, plastic peel-down pouches and wrapped packs sealed in 3-mil (3/1000 inch) polyethylene overwrap have been reported to be sterile for as long as 9 months after sterilization. The

3-mil polyethylene is applied after sterilization to extend the shelf life for infrequently used items. Supplies wrapped in double-thickness muslin comprising four layers, or equivalent, remain sterile for at least 30 days. Any item that has been sterilized should not be used after the expiration date has been exceeded or if the sterilized package is wet, torn, or punctured.

Although some hospitals continue to date every sterilized product and use the time-related shelf-life practice, many hospitals have switched to an event-related shelf-life practice. This latter practice recognizes that the product should remain sterile until some event causes the item to become contaminated (e.g. tear in packaging, packaging becomes wet, seal is broken). Event-related factors that contribute to the contamination of a product include bioburden (i.e. the amount of contamination in the environment), air movement, traffic, location, humidity, insects, vermin, flooding, storage area space, open/closed shelving, temperature, and the properties of the wrap material. There are data that support the event-related shelf-life practice.[11-13] One study examined the effect of time on the sterile integrity of paper envelopes, peel pouches, and nylon sleeves. The most important finding was the absence of a trend toward an increased rate of contamination over time for any pack when placed in covered storage.[12] Another evaluated the effectiveness of event-related outdating by microbiologically testing sterilized items. During the 2-year study period, all of the items tested were sterile.[13] Thus, contamination of a sterile item is event-related and the probability of contamination increases with increased handling.[14]

Following the sterilization process, medical and surgical devices must be handled using aseptic technique in order to prevent contamination. Sterile supplies should be stored far enough from the floor (8 to 10 inches), the ceiling [5 inches unless near a sprinkler head (18 inches from sprinkler head)], and the outside walls (2 inches) to allow for adequate air circulation, ease of cleaning, and compliance with local fire codes (e.g. supplies must be at least 18 inches from sprinkler heads). Medical and surgical supplies should not be stored under sinks or in other locations where they can become wet. Sterile items that become wet are considered contaminated because moisture brings with it microorganisms from the air and surfaces. Closed or covered cabinets are ideal but open shelving may be used for storage. Any package that has fallen or been dropped on the floor must be inspected for damage to the packaging and contents (if the items are breakable). If the package is heat-sealed in impervious plastic and the seal is still intact, the package should be considered not contaminated. If undamaged, items packaged in plastic need not be reprocessed.

Monitoring

The sterilization procedure should be monitored routinely by using a combination of mechanical, chemical, and biological indicators to evaluate the sterilizing conditions and indirectly the microbiologic status of the processed items. The mechanical monitors for steam sterilization include the daily assessment of cycle time and temperature by examining the temperature record chart (or computer printout) and an assessment of pressure via the pressure gauge. The mechanical monitors for EtO include time, temperature, and pressure recorders that provide data via computer printouts, gauges, and/or displays. Generally, two essential elements for EtO sterilization (i.e. the gas concentration and humidity) cannot be monitored in healthcare EtO sterilizers.

Chemical indicators are convenient, inexpensive, and indicate that the item has been exposed to the sterilization process. In one study, chemical indicators were more likely than biological indicators to inaccurately indicate sterilization at marginal sterilization times (e.g. 2 minutes).[15] Chemical indicators should be used in conjunction with biological indicators, but based on current studies should not replace them because they indicate sterilization at marginal sterilization time and because only a biological indicator consisting of resistant spores can measure the microbial killing power of the sterilization process. Chemical indicators are affixed on the outside of each pack to show that the package has been processed through a sterilization cycle, but these indicators do not prove sterilization has been achieved. Preferably, a chemical indicator also should be placed on the inside of each pack to verify sterilant penetration. Chemical indicators usually are either heat- or chemical-sensitive inks that change color when one or more sterilization parameters (e.g. steam-time, temperature, and/or saturated steam; EtO-time, temperature, relative humidity and/or EtO concentration) are present. Chemical indicators have been grouped into five classes based on their ability to monitor one or multiple sterilization parameters. If the internal and/or external indicator suggests inadequate processing, the item should not be used. An air-removal test (Bowie-Dick Test) must be performed daily in an empty dynamic-air-removal sterilizer (e.g. prevacuum steam sterilizer) to ensure air removal.

Biological indicators are recognized by most authorities as being closest to the ideal monitors of the sterilization process because they measure the sterilization process directly by using the most resistant microorganisms (i.e. *Bacillus* spores), and not by merely testing the physical and chemical conditions necessary for sterilization. Since the *Bacillus* spores used in biological indicators are more resistant and present in greater numbers than are the common microbial contaminants found on patient-care equipment, the demonstration that the biological indicator has been inactivated strongly implies that other potential pathogens in the load have been killed.

An ideal biological monitor of the sterilization process should be easy to use, be inexpensive, not be subject to exogenous contamination, provide positive results as soon as possible after the cycle so that corrective action may be accomplished, and provide positive results only when the sterilization parameters (e.g. steam-time, temperature, and/or saturated steam; EtO-time, temperature, relative humidity and/or EtO concentration) are inadequate to kill microbial contaminates.

Biological indicators are the only process indicators that directly monitor the lethality of a given sterilization process. Spores used to monitor a sterilization process have demonstrated resistance to the sterilizing agent and are more resistant than the bioburden found on medical devices. *B. atrophaeus* spores (10^6) are used to monitor EtO and dry heat, and *G. stearothermophilus* spores (10^5) are used to monitor steam sterilization, hydrogen peroxide gas plasma, and liquid peracetic acid sterilizers. *G. stearothermophilus* is incubated at 55–60°C, and *B. atrophaeus* is incubated at 35–37°C. Steam and low temperature sterilizers (e.g. hydrogen peroxide gas plasma, peracetic acid) should be monitored at least weekly with the appropriate commercial preparation of spores. If a sterilizer is used frequently (e.g. several loads per day), daily use of biological indicators allows earlier discovery of equipment malfunctions or procedural errors and thus minimizes the extent of patient surveillance and product recall needed in the event of a positive biological indicator. Each load should be monitored if it contains implantable objects. If feasible, implantable items should not be used until the results of spore tests are known to be negative.

Originally, spore-strip biological indicators required up to 7 days of incubation to detect viable spores from marginal cycles (i.e. when few spores remained viable). The next generation of biological indicator was self-contained in plastic vials containing a spore-coated paper strip and a growth media in a crushable glass ampoule. This indicator had a maximum incubation of 48 hours but significant failures could be detected in ≤24 hours. A rapid-readout biological indicator that detects the presence of enzymes of *G. stearothermophilus* by reading a fluorescent product produced by the enzymatic breakdown of a nonfluorescent substrate has been marketed for the more than 10 years. Studies demonstrate that the sensitivity of rapid-readout tests for steam sterilization (1 hour for 132°C gravity sterilizers, 3 hours for 121°C gravity and 132°C vacuum sterilizers) parallels that of the conventional sterilization-specific biological indicators and the fluorescent rapid readout results reliably predict 24- and 48-hour and 7-day growth. The rapid-readout biological indicator is a dual indicator system as it also detects acid metabolites produced during growth of the *G. stearothermophilus* spores. This system is different from the indicator system consisting of an enzyme system of bacterial origin without spores.

A new rapid-readout EtO biological indicator has been designed for rapid and reliable monitoring of EtO sterilization processes. The rapid-readout EtO biological indicator detects the presence of *B. atrophaeus* by detecting a fluorescent signal indicating the activity of an enzyme present within the *B. atrophaeus* organism, beta-glucosidase. The fluorescence indicates the presence of an active spore-associated enzyme and a sterilization process failure. This indicator also detects acid metabolites produced during growth of the *B. atrophaeus* spore. As per manufacturer's data, the enzyme always was detected whenever viable spores were present. This was expected because the enzyme is relatively EtO resistant and is inactivated at a slightly longer exposure time than the spore. The rapid-readout EtO biological indicator can be used to monitor 100% EtO, and EtO-HCFC mixture sterilization cycles. It has not been tested in EtO-CO_2 mixture sterilization cycles.

The standard biological indicator used for monitoring full-cycle steam sterilizers does not provide reliable monitoring for flash sterilizers. Biological indicators specifically designed for monitoring flash sterilization are now available, and studies comparing them have been published.

Since sterilization failure can occur (about 1% for steam),[16] a procedure to follow in the event of positive spore tests with steam sterilization has been provided by CDC and the Association of periOperative Registered Nurses (AORN). The 1981 CDC recommendation is that 'objects, other than implantable objects, do not need to be recalled because of a single positive spore test unless the steam sterilizer or the sterilization procedure is defective.' The rationale for this recommendation is that single positive spore tests in sterilizers occur sporadically. They may occur for reasons such as slight variation in the resistance of the spores,[17] improper use of the sterilizer, and laboratory contamination during culture (uncommon with self-contained spore tests). If the mechanical (e.g. time, temperature, pressure in the steam sterilizer) and chemical (internal and/or external) indicators suggest that the sterilizer was functioning properly, a single positive spore test probably does not indicate sterilizer malfunction but the spore test should be repeated immediately. If the spore tests remain positive, use of the sterilizer should be discontinued until it is serviced. Similarly, AORN states that a single positive spore test does not necessarily indicate a sterilizer failure. If the test is positive, the sterilizer should immediately be rechallenged for proper use and function. Items, other than implantable ones, do not necessarily need to be recalled unless a sterilizer malfunction is found. If a sterilizer malfunction is discovered, the items must be considered nonsterile, and the items from the suspect load(s) should be recalled, insofar as possible, and reprocessed. A suggested protocol for management of positive biological indicators is shown in (Table 7.6). A more conservative approach also has been recommended in which any positive spore test is assumed to represent sterilizer malfunction and requires that all materials processed in that sterilizer, dating from the sterilization cycle having the last negative

Table 7.6: Suggested protocol for management of positive biological indicator in a steam sterilizer[38]

1. Take the sterilizer out of service. Notify area supervisor and infection control department
2. Objects, other than implantable objects, do not need to be recalled because of a single positive spore test unless the sterilizer or the sterilization procedure is defective. As soon as possible, repeat biological indicator test in three consecutive sterilizer cycles. If additional spore tests remain positive, the items should be considered nonsterile, and supplies processed since the last acceptable (negative) biological indicator should be recalled. The items from the suspect load(s) should be recalled and reprocessed
3. Check to ensure the sterilizer was used correctly (e.g. verify correct time and temperature setting). If not, repeat using appropriate settings and recall and reprocess all inadequately processed items
4. Check with hospital maintenance for irregularities (e.g. electrical) or changes in the hospital steam supply (i.e., from standard ≥97% steam, <3% moisture). Any abnormalities should be reported to the person who performs sterilizer maintenance (e.g. medical engineering, sterilizer manufacturer)
5. Check to ensure the correct biological indicator was used and appropriately interpreted. If not, repeat using appropriate settings If steps 1 through 5 resolve the problem
6. If all three repeat biological indicators from three consecutive sterilizer cycles (step 2 above) are negative, put the sterilizer back in service If one or both biological indicators are positive, do one or more of the following until problem is resolved
7. A. Request an inspection of the equipment by sterilizer maintenance personnel B. Have hospital maintenance inspect the steam supply lines C. Discuss the abnormalities with the sterilizer manufacturer D. Repeat the biological indicator using a different manufacturer's indicator If step 7 does not resolve the problem Close sterilizer down until the manufacturer can assure that it is operating properly. Retest at that time with biological indicators in three consecutive sterilizer cycles

Source: Modified from Bryce.[38]

biologic indicator to the next cycle showing satisfactory biologic indicator challenge results, must be considered nonsterile and retrieved, if possible, and reprocessed. This more conservative approach should be used for sterilization methods other than steam (e.g. EtO, hydrogen peroxide gas plasma). However, no action is necessary if there is strong evidence for the biological indicator being defective or the growth medium contained a *Bacillus* contaminant.

If patient-care items were used before retrieval, the infection control professional should assess the risk of infection in collaboration with central processing, surgical services, and risk management staff. The factors that should be considered include the chemical indicator result (e.g. nonreactive chemical indicator may indicate temperature not achieved); the results of other biological indicators that followed the positive biological indicator (e.g. positive on Tuesday, negative on Wednesday); the parameters of the sterilizer associated with the positive biological indicator (e.g. reduced time at correct temperature); the time-temperature chart (or printout); and the microbial load associated with decontaminated surgical instruments (e.g. 85% of decontaminated surgical instruments have less than 100 CFU). The margin of safety in steam sterilization is sufficiently large that there is minimal infection risk associated with items in a load that show spore growth, especially if the item was properly cleaned and the temperature was achieved (e.g. as shown by acceptable chemical indicator or temperature chart). There are no published studies that document disease transmission via a nonretrieved surgical instrument following a sterilization cycle with a positive biological indicator.

False-positive biological indicators may occur from improper testing or faulty indicators. The latter may occur from improper storage, processing, product contamination, material failure, or variation in resistance of spores. Gram stain and subculture of a positive biological indicator may determine if a contaminant has created a false-positive result. However, in one incident, the broth used as growth medium contained a contaminant, *B. coagulans,* which resulted in broth turbidity at 55°C. Testing of paired biological indicators from different manufacturers can assist in assessing a product defect. False-positive biological indicators due to extrinsic contamination when using self-contained biological indicators should be uncommon. A biological indicator should not be considered a false-positive indicator until a thorough analysis of the entire sterilization process shows this to be likely.

The size and composition of the biological indicator test pack should be standardized to create a significant challenge to air removal and sterilant penetration and to obtain interpretable results. There is a standard 16-towel pack recommended by AAMI (Association for the Advancement of Medical Instrumentation) for steam sterilization.[18-20] consisting of 16 clean, preconditioned, reusable absorbent surgical towels each of which is approximately 16 inches by 26 inches. Each towel is folded lengthwise into thirds and then folded widthwise in the middle. One or more biological indicators are placed between the eight and ninth towels in the approximate geometric center of the pack. When the towels are folded and placed one on top of another, to form a stack (approximately 6 inch height) it should weigh approximately 3 pounds and should have a density of approximately 11.3 pounds per cubic foot. This test pack has not gained universal use as a standard pack that simulates the actual in-use conditions of steam sterilizers. Commercially available disposable test packs that have been shown to be equivalent to the AAMI 16 towel test pack also may be used. The test pack should be placed flat in an otherwise fully loaded sterilizer chamber, in the area least favorable to sterilization (i.e. the area representing the greatest challenge to the biological indicator). This area is normally in the front, bottom section of the sterilizer, near the drain. A control biological indicator from the lot used for testing should be left unexposed to the sterilant, and then incubated to verify the presterilization viability of the test spores and proper incubation. The most conservative approach would be to use a control for each run; however, less frequent use may be adequate (e.g. weekly). There also is a routine test pack for EtO where a biological indicator is placed in a plastic syringe with plunger, then placed in the folds of a clean surgical towel, and wrapped. Alternatively, commercially available disposal test packs that have been shown to be equivalent to the AAMI test pack may be used. The test pack is placed in the center of the sterilizer load. Sterilization records (mechanical, chemical, and biological) should be retained for a time period in compliance with standards (e.g. Joint Commission for the Accreditation of Healthcare Facilities requests 3 years) and state and federal regulations.

Periodic infection control rounds to areas using sterilizers to standardize the sterilizer's use may identify correctable variances in operator competence; documentation of sterilization records, including chemical and biological indicator test results; sterilizer maintenance and wrapping; and load numbering of packs. These rounds also may identify improvement activities to ensure that operators are adhering to established standards.

RECOMMENDATIONS FOR DISINFECTION AND STERILIZATION IN HEALTHCARE FACILITIES[1]

Rationale

The ultimate goal of the Recommendations for Disinfection and Sterilization in Health-Care Facilities, 2008, is to reduce rates of health-care associated infections through appropriate use of both disinfection and sterilization. Each recommendation is categorized according to scientific evidence, theoretical rationale, applicability, and federal regulations. The CDC system for categorizing recommendations is defined in the following (Rankings) section.

Rankings

Category IA: Strongly recommended for implementation and strongly supported by well-designed experimental, clinical, or epidemiologic studies.

Category IB: Strongly recommended for implementation and supported by some experimental, clinical, or epidemiologic studies, and by a strong theoretical rationale.

Category IC: Required by state or federal regulations. Because of state differences, readers should not assume that the absence of an *IC* recommendation implies the absence of state regulations.

Category II: Suggested for implementation and supported by suggestive clinical or epidemiologic studies or by a theoretical rationale.

No recommendation: Unresolved issue. These include practices for which insufficient evidence or no consensus exists regarding efficacy.

Recommendations

Occupational

a. Inform each worker of the possible health effects of his or her exposure to infectious agents [e.g. hepatitis B virus (HBV), hepatitis C virus, human immunodeficiency virus (HIV)], and/or chemicals (e.g. EtO, formaldehyde). The information should be consistent with Occupational Safety and Health Administration (OSHA) requirements and identify the areas and tasks in which potential exists for exposure (*Category II, IC*).
b. Educate healthcare workers in the selection and proper use of personal protective equipment (PPE) (*Category II, IC*).
c. Ensure that workers wear appropriate PPE to preclude exposure to infectious agents or chemicals through the respiratory system, skin, or mucous membranes of the eyes, nose, or mouth. PPE can include gloves, gowns, masks, and eye protection. The exact type of PPE depends on the infectious or chemical agent and the anticipated duration of exposure. The employer is responsible for making such equipment and training available (*Category II, IC*).
d. Establish a program for monitoring occupational exposure to regulated chemicals (e.g. formaldehyde, EtO) that adheres to state and federal regulations (*Category II, IC*).
e. Exclude healthcare workers with weeping dermatitis of hands from direct contact with patient-care equipment (*Category IB*).

Cleaning of Patient-care Devices

a. In hospitals, perform most cleaning, disinfection, and sterilization of patient-care devices in a central processing department in order to more easily control quality (*Category II*).
b. Meticulously clean patient-care items with water and detergent, or with water and enzymatic cleaners before high-level disinfection or sterilization procedures (*Category IB*).
   - Remove visible organic residue (e.g. residue of blood and tissue) and inorganic salts with cleaning. Use cleaning agents that are capable of removing visible organic and inorganic residues (*Category IB*).
   - Clean medical devices as soon as practical after use (e.g. at the point of use) because soiled materials become dried onto the instruments. Dried or baked materials on the instrument make the removal process more difficult and the disinfection or sterilization process less effective or ineffective (*Category IB*).

c. Perform either manual cleaning (i.e. using friction) or mechanical cleaning (e.g. with ultrasonic cleaners, washer-disinfector, washer-sterilizers) (*Category IB*).
d. If using an automatic washer/disinfector, ensure that the unit is used in accordance with the manufacturer's recommendations (*Category IB*).
e. Ensure that the detergents or enzymatic cleaners selected are compatible with the metals and other materials used in medical instruments. Ensure that the rinse step is adequate for removing cleaning residues to levels that will not interfere with subsequent disinfection/sterilization processes (*Category II*).
f. Inspect equipment surfaces for breaks in integrity that would impair either cleaning or disinfection/sterilization. Discard or repair equipment that no longer functions as intended or cannot be properly cleaned, and disinfected or sterilized (*Category II*).

Indications for Sterilization, High-level Disinfection, and Low-level Disinfection

a. Before use on each patient, sterilize critical medical and surgical devices and instruments that enter normally sterile tissue or the vascular system or through which a sterile body fluid flows (e.g. blood). See recommendation 7 g for exceptions (*Category IA*).
b. Provide, at a minimum, high-level disinfection for semicritical patient-care equipment (e.g. gastrointestinal endoscopes, endotracheal tubes, anesthesia breathing circuits, and respiratory therapy equipment) that touches either mucous membranes or nonintact skin (*Category IA*).
c. Perform low-level disinfection for noncritical patient-care surfaces (e.g. bedrails, over-the-bed table) and equipment (e.g. blood pressure cuff) that touch intact skin (recommendation 5 g) (*Category II*).

Selection and Use of Low-level Disinfectants for Noncritical Patient-care Devices

a. Process noncritical patient-care devices using a disinfectant and the concentration of germicide listed in Table 7.7.
b. Disinfect noncritical medical devices (e.g. blood pressure cuff) with an EPA (Environmental Protection Act)-registered hospital disinfectant using the label's safety precautions and use directions. Most EPA-registered hospital disinfectants have a label contact time of 10 minutes. However, multiple scientific studies have demonstrated the efficacy of hospital disinfectants against pathogens with a contact time of at least 1 minute. By law, all applicable label instructions on EPA-registered products must be followed (*Category IB*).
c. Ensure that, at a minimum, noncritical patient-care devices are disinfected when visibly soiled and on a regular basis (such as after use on each patient or once daily or once weekly) (*Category II*).
d. If dedicated, disposable devices are not available, disinfect noncritical patient-care equipment after using it on a patient who is on contact precautions before using this equipment on another patient (*Category IB*).

Cleaning and Disinfecting Environmental Surfaces in Healthcare Facilities

a. Clean housekeeping surfaces (e.g. floors, tabletops) on a regular basis, when spills

Table 7.7: Dilutions of household bleach and chlorine ppm

Bleach solution	Dilution	Chlorine (ppm)
5.25–6.15%	None	52,500–61,500
	1:10	5,250–6,150
	1:100	525–615
	1:1000	53–62

occur, and when these surfaces are visibly soiled (*Category II*).

b. Disinfect (or clean) environmental surfaces on a regular basis (e.g. daily, three times per week) and when surfaces are visibly soiled (*Category II*).

c. Follow manufacturers' instructions for proper use of disinfecting (or detergent) products—such as recommended use-dilution, material compatibility, storage, shelf-life, and safe use and disposal (*Category II*).

d. Clean walls, blinds, and window curtains in patient-care areas when these surfaces are visibly contaminated or soiled (*Category II*).

e. Prepare disinfecting (or detergent) solutions as needed and replace these with fresh solution frequently (e.g. replace floor mopping solution every three patient rooms, change no less often than at 60-minute intervals), according to the facility's policy (*Category IB*).

f. Decontaminate mop heads and cleaning cloths regularly to prevent contamination (e.g. launder and dry at least daily) (*Category II*).

g. Use a one-step process and an EPA-registered hospital disinfectant designed for housekeeping purposes in patient care areas where (1) uncertainty exists about the nature of the soil on the surfaces (e.g. blood or body fluid contamination versus routine dust or dirt); or (2) uncertainty exists about the presence of multidrug resistant organisms on such surfaces. See 5n for recommendations requiring cleaning and disinfecting blood-contaminated surfaces (*Category II*).

h. Detergent and water are adequate for cleaning surfaces in nonpatient-care areas (e.g. administrative offices) (*Category II*)

i. Do not use high-level disinfectants/liquid chemical sterilants for disinfection of non-critical surfaces (*Category IB*).

j. Wet-dust horizontal surfaces regularly (e.g. daily, three times per week) using clean cloths moistened with an EPA-registered hospital disinfectant (or detergent). Prepare the disinfectant (or detergent) as recommended by the manufacturer (*Category II*).

k. Disinfect noncritical surfaces with an EPA-registered hospital disinfectant according to the label's safety precautions and use directions. Most EPA-registered hospital disinfectants have a label contact time of 10 minutes. However, many scientific studies have demonstrated the efficacy of hospital disinfectants against pathogens with a contact time of at least 1 minute (*Category II, IC*).

l. Do not use disinfectants to clean infant bassinets and incubators while these items are occupied. If disinfectants (e.g. phenolics) are used for the terminal cleaning of infant bassinets and incubators, thoroughly rinse the surfaces of these items with water and dry them before these items are reused (*Category IB*).

m. Promptly clean and decontaminate spills of blood and other potentially infectious materials (*Category IB, IC*).

n. For site decontamination of spills of blood or other potentially infectious materials (OPIM), implement the following procedures. Use protective gloves and other PPE (e.g. when sharps are involved use forceps to pick up sharps, and discard these items in a puncture-resistant container) appropriate for this task. Disinfect areas contaminated with blood spills using an tuberculocidal agent, a germicide (i.e. with specific label claims for HIV or HBV) or freshly diluted hypochlorite solution (*Category II, IC*). If sodium hypochlorite solutions are selected use a 1:100 dilution (e.g. 1:100 dilution of a 5.25–6.15% sodium hypochlorite provides 525–615 ppm available chlorine) to decontaminate nonporous surfaces after a small spill (e.g. <10 mL) of either blood or OPIM. If a spill involves large amounts (e.g. >10 mL) of blood or OPIM, or involves a culture spill in the laboratory, use a 1:10 dilution for the first application of hypochlorite solution before cleaning in order to reduce the risk of infection during the cleaning process in the event of a sharp injury. Follow this decontamination process with a terminal disinfection, using a 1:100 dilution of sodium hypochlorite (*Category IB, IC*).

o. If the spill contains large amounts of blood or body fluids, clean the visible matter with disposable absorbent material, and discard the contaminated materials in appropriate, labeled container (*Category II, IC*).
p. Use protective gloves and other PPE appropriate for this task (*Category II, IC*).
q. In units with high rates of endemic *Clostridium difficile* infection or in an outbreak setting, use dilute solutions of 5.25%–6.15% sodium hypochlorite (e.g. 1:10 dilution of household bleach) for routine environmental disinfection.
r. If chlorine solution is not prepared fresh daily, it can be stored at room temperature for up to 30 days in a capped, opaque plastic bottle with a 50% reduction in chlorine concentration after 30 days of storage [e.g. 1000 ppm chlorine (approximately a 1:50 dilution) at day 0 decreases to 500 ppm chlorine by day 30] (*Category IB*).

Disinfectant Fogging

a. Do not perform disinfectant fogging for routine purposes in patient-care areas (*Category II*).

High-level Disinfection of Endoscopes

a. To detect damaged endoscopes, test each flexible endoscope for leaks as part of each reprocessing cycle. Remove from clinical use any instrument that fails the leak test, and repair this instrument (*Category II*).
b. Immediately after use, meticulously clean the endoscope with an enzymatic cleaner that is compatible with the endoscope. Cleaning is necessary before both automated and manual disinfection (*Category IA*).
c. Disconnect and disassemble endoscopic components (e.g. suction valves) as completely as possible and completely immerse all components in the enzymatic cleaner. Steam sterilize these components if they are heat stable (*Category IB*).
d. Flush and brush all accessible channels to remove all organic (e.g. blood, tissue) and other residue. Clean the external surfaces and accessories of the devices by using a soft cloth or sponge or brushes. Continue brushing until no debris appears on the brush (*Category IA*).
e. Use cleaning brushes appropriate for the size of the endoscope channel or port (e.g. bristles should contact surfaces). Cleaning items (e.g. brushes, cloth) should be disposable or, if they are not disposable, they should be thoroughly cleaned and either high-level disinfected or sterilized after each use (*Category II*).
f. Discard enzymatic cleaners (or detergents) after each use because they are not microbicidal and, therefore, will not retard microbial growth (*Category IB*).
g. Process endoscopes (e.g. arthroscopes, cystoscope, laparoscopes) that pass through normally sterile tissues using a sterilization procedure before each use; if this is not feasible, provide at least high-level disinfection. High-level disinfection of arthroscopes, laparoscopes, and cytoscopes should be followed by a sterile water rinse (*Category IB*).
h. Phase out endoscopes that are critical items (e.g. arthroscopes, laparoscopes) but cannot be steam sterilized. Replace these endoscopes with steam sterilizable instruments when feasible (*Category II*).
i. Mechanically clean reusable accessories inserted into endoscopes (e.g. biopsy forceps or other cutting instruments) that break the mucosal barrier (e.g. ultrasonically clean biopsy forceps) and then sterilize these items between each patient (*Category IA*).

j. Use ultrasonic cleaning of reusable endoscopic accessories to remove soil and organic material from hard-to-clean areas (*Category II*).
k. Process endoscopes and accessories that contact mucous membranes as semicritical items, and use at least high-level disinfection after use on each patient (*Category IA*).
l. Use an FDA-cleared sterilant or high-level disinfectant for sterilization or high-level disinfection (Table 7.7) (*Category IA*).
m. After cleaning, use formulations containing glutaraldehyde, glutaraldehyde with phenol/phenate, ortho-phthalaldehyde, hydrogen peroxide, and both hydrogen peroxide and peracetic acid to achieve high-level disinfection followed by rinsing and drying (*Category IB*).
n. Extend exposure times beyond the minimum effective time for disinfecting semicritical patient-care equipment cautiously and conservatively because extended exposure to a high-level disinfectant is more likely to damage delicate and intricate instruments such as flexible endoscopes (*Category IB*).
o. Federal regulations are to follow the FDA-cleared label claim for high-level disinfectants. The FDA-cleared labels for high-level disinfection with >2% glutaradehyde at 25°C range from 20–90 minutes, depending upon the product based on three-tier testing which includes AOAC sporicidal tests, simulated use testing with mycobacterial and in use testing (*Category IC*).
p. Several scientific studies and professional organizations support the efficacy of >2% glutaraldehyde for 20 minutes at 20°C; that efficacy assumes adequate cleaning prior to disinfection, whereas the FDA-cleared label claim incorporates an added margin of safety to accommodate possible lapses in cleaning practices.
q. When using FDA-cleared high-level disinfectants, use manufacturers' recommended exposure conditions. Certain products may require a shorter exposure time (e.g. 0.55% ortho-phthalaldehyde for 12 minutes at 20°C, 7.35% hydrogen peroxide plus 0.23% peracetic acid for 15 minutes at 20°C) than glutaraldehyde at room temperature because of their rapid inactivation of mycobacteria or reduced exposure time because of increased mycobactericidal activity at elevated temperature (e.g. 2.5% glutaraldehyde at 5 minutes at 35°C) (*Category IB*).
r. Select a disinfectant or chemical sterilant that is compatible with the device that is being reprocessed. Avoid using reprocessing chemicals on an endoscope if the endoscope manufacturer warns against using these chemicals because of functional damage (with or without cosmetic damage) (*Category IB*).
s. Completely immerse the endoscope in the high-level disinfectant, and ensure all channels are perfused. As soon as is feasible, phase out nonimmersible endoscopes (*Category IB*).
t. After high-level disinfection, rinse endoscopes and flush channels with sterile water, filtered water, or tapwater to prevent adverse effects on patients associated with disinfectant retained in the endoscope (e.g. disinfectant induced colitis). Follow this water rinse with a rinse with 70–90% ethyl or isopropyl alcohol (*Category IB*).
u. After flushing all channels with alcohol, purge the channels using forced air to reduce the likelihood of contamination of the endoscope by waterborne pathogens and to facilitate drying (*Category IB*).
v. Hang endoscopes in a vertical position to facilitate drying (*Category II*).
w. Store endoscopes in a manner that will protect them from damage or contamination (*Category II*).
x. Sterilize or high-level disinfect both the water bottle used to provide intraprocedural flush solution and its connecting tube at least once daily. After sterilizing or high-level disinfecting

the water bottle, fill it with sterile water (*Category IB*).

y. Maintain a log for each procedure and record the following: patient's name and medical record number (if available), procedure, date, endoscopist, system used to reprocess the endoscope (if more than one system could be used in the reprocessing area), and serial number or other identifier of the endoscope used (*Category II*).

z. Design facilities where endoscopes are used and disinfected to provide a safe environment for healthcare workers and patients. Use air-exchange equipment (e.g. the ventilation system, out-exhaust ducts) to minimize exposure of all persons to potentially toxic vapors (e.g. glutaraldehyde vapor). Do not exceed the allowable limits of the vapor concentration of the chemical sterilant or high-level disinfectant (e.g. OSHA) (*Category IB, IC*).

aa. Routinely test the liquid sterilant/high-level disinfectant to ensure minimal effective concentration of the active ingredient. Check the solution each day of use (or more frequently) using the appropriate chemical indicator (e.g. glutaraldehyde chemical indicator to test minimal effective concentration of glutaraldehyde) and document the results of this testing. Discard the solution if the chemical indicator shows the concentration is less than the minimum effective concentration. Do not use the liquid sterilant/high-level disinfectant beyond the reuse-life recommended by the manufacturer (e.g. 14 days for *ortho*-phthalaldehyde) (*Category IA*).

bb. Provide personnel assigned to reprocess endoscopes with device-specific reprocessing instructions to ensure proper cleaning and high-level disinfection or sterilization. Require competency testing on a regular basis (e.g. beginning of employment, annually) of all personnel who reprocess endoscopes (*Category IA*).

cc. Educate all personnel who use chemicals about the possible biologic, chemical, and environmental hazards of performing procedures that require disinfectants (*Category IB, IC*).

dd. Make PPE (e.g. gloves, gowns, eyewear, face mask or shields, respiratory protection devices) available and use these items appropriately to protect workers from exposure to both chemicals and micro-organisms (e.g. HBV) (*Category IB, IC*).

ee. If using an automated endoscope reprocessor (AER), place the endoscope in the reprocessor and attach all channel connectors according to the AER manufacturer's instructions to ensure exposure of all internal surfaces to the high-level disinfectant/chemical sterilant (*Category IB*).

ff. If using an AER, ensure the endoscope can be effectively reprocessed in the AER. Also, ensure any required manual cleaning/disinfecting steps are performed (e.g. elevator wire channel of duodenoscopes might not be effectively disinfected by most AERs) (*Category IB*).

gg. Review the FDA advisories and the scientific literature for reports of deficiencies that can lead to infection because design flaws and improper operation and practices have compromised the effectiveness of AERs (*Category II*).

hh. Develop protocols to ensure that users can readily identify an endoscope that has been properly processed and is ready for patient use (*Category II*).

ii. Do not use the carrying case designed to transport clean and reprocessed endoscopes outside of the healthcare environment to store an endoscope or to transport the instrument within the healthcare environment (*Category II*).

jj. No recommendation is made about routinely performing microbiologic testing of either endoscopes or rinse water for quality assurance purposes (*Unresolved Issue*).

kk. If environmental microbiologic testing is conducted, use standard microbiologic techniques (*Category II*).

ll. If a cluster of endoscopy-related infections occurs, investigate potential routes of transmission (e.g. person-to-person, common source) and reservoirs (*Category IA*).

mm. Report outbreaks of endoscope-related infections to persons responsible for institutional infection control and risk management (*Category IB, II*).

nn. No recommendation is made regarding the reprocessing of an endoscope again immediately before use if that endoscope has been processed after use according to the recommendations in this guideline (*Unresolved Issue*).

oo. Compare the reprocessing instructions provided by both the endoscope's and the AER's manufacturer's instructions and resolve any conflicting recommendations (*Category IB*).

Management of Equipment and Surfaces in Dentistry

a. Dental instruments that penetrate soft tissue or bone (e.g. extraction forceps, scalpel blades, bone chisels, periodontal scalers, and surgical burs) are classified as critical and should be sterilized after each use or discarded. In addition, after each use, sterilize dental instruments that are not intended to penetrate oral soft tissue or bone (e.g. amalgam condensers, air-water syringes) but that might contact oral tissues and are heat-tolerant, although classified as semicritical. Clean and, at a minimum, high-level disinfect heat-sensitive semicritical items (*Category IA*).

b. Noncritical clinical contact surfaces, such as uncovered operatory surfaces (e.g. countertops, switches, light handles), should be barrier-protected or disinfected between patients with an intermediate-disinfectant (i.e. EPA-registered hospital disinfectant with a tuberculocidal claim) or low-level disinfectant (i.e. EPA-registered hospital disinfectant with HIV and HBV claim) (*Category IB*).

c. Barrier protective coverings can be used for noncritical clinical contact surfaces that are touched frequently with gloved hands during the delivery of patient care, that are likely to become contaminated with blood or body substances, or that are difficult to clean. Change these coverings when they are visibly soiled, when they become damaged, and on a routine basis (e.g. between patients). Disinfect protected surfaces at the end of the day or if visibly soiled (*Category II*).

Processing Patient-care Equipment Contaminated with Blood-borne Pathogens (HBV, Hepatitis C Virus, HIV), Antibiotic-resistant Bacteria (e.g. Vancomycin-resistant Enterococci, Methicillin-resistant *Staphylococcus aureus*, Multidrug-resistant Tuberculosis), or Emerging Pathogens (e.g. *Cryptosporidium, Helicobacter pylori, Escherichia coli O157:H7, Clostridium difficile, Mycobacterium tuberculosis*, Severe Acute Respiratory Syndrome Coronavirus), or Bioterrorist Agents

a. Use standard sterilization and disinfection procedures for patient-care equipment (as recommended in this guideline), because these procedures are adequate to sterilize or disinfect instruments or devices contaminated with blood or other body fluids from persons infected with bloodborne pathogens or emerging pathogens, with the exception of prions. No changes in these procedures for cleaning, disinfecting, or sterilizing are necessary for removing bloodborne and emerging pathogens other than prions (*Category IA*).

Disinfection Strategies for Other Semicritical Devices

a. Even if probe covers have been used, clean and high-level disinfect other semicritical devices such as rectal probes, vaginal probes, and cryosurgical probes with a product that is not toxic to staff, patients, probes, and retrieved germ cells (if applicable). Use a high-level disinfectant at the FDA-cleared exposure time (See Recommendations 7o and 11e for exceptions) (*Category IB*).

b. When probe covers are available, use a probe cover or condom to reduce the level of microbial contamination (*Category II*). Do not use a lower category of disinfection or cease to follow the appropriate disinfectant recommendations when using probe covers because these sheaths and condoms can fail (*Category IB*).

c. After high-level disinfection, rinse all items. Use sterile water, filtered water or tapwater followed by an alcohol rinse for semicritical equipment that will have contact with mucous membranes of the upper respiratory tract (e.g. nose, pharynx, esophagus) (*Category II*).

d. There is no recommendation to use sterile or filtered water rather than tapwater for rinsing semicritical equipment that contact the mucous membranes of the rectum (e.g. rectal probes, anoscope) or vagina (e.g. vaginal probes) (*Unresolved Issue*).

e. Wipe clean tonometer tips and then disinfect them by immersing for 5–10 minutes in either 5,000 ppm chlorine or 70% ethyl alcohol. None of these listed disinfectant products are FDA-cleared high-level disinfectants (*Category II*).

Disinfection by Healthcare Personnel in Ambulatory Care and Home Care

a. Follow the same classification scheme described above (i.e. that critical devices require sterilization, semicritical devices require high-level disinfection, and noncritical equipment requires low-level disinfection) in the ambulatory-care (outpatient medical/surgical facilities) setting because risk for infection in this setting is similar to that in the hospital setting (*Category IB*).

b. When performing care in the home, clean and disinfect reusable objects that touch mucous membranes (e.g. tracheostomy tubes) by immersing these objects in a 1:50 dilution of 5.25%–6.15% sodium hypochlorite (household bleach) (3 minutes), 70% isopropyl alcohol (5 minutes), or 3% hydrogen peroxide (30 minutes) because the home environment is, in most instances, safer than either hospital or ambulatory care settings because person-to-person transmission is less likely (*Category II*).

c. Clean noncritical items that would not be shared between patients (e.g. crutches, blood pressure cuffs) in the home setting with a detergent or commercial household disinfectant (*Category II*).

Microbial Contamination of Disinfectants

a. Institute the following control measures to reduce the occurrence of contaminated disinfectants: (1) prepare the disinfectant correctly to achieve the manufacturer's recommended use-dilution; and (2) prevent common sources of extrinsic contamination of germicides (e.g. container contamination or surface contamination of the healthcare environment where the germicide are prepared and/or used) (*Category IB*).

Flash Sterilization

a. Do not flash sterilize implanted surgical devices unless doing so is unavoidable (*Category IB*).

b. Do not use flash sterilization for convenience, as an alternative to purchasing additional instrument sets, or to save time (*Category II*).

c. When using flash sterilization, make sure the following parameters are met: (1) clean the item before placing it in the sterilizing container (that are FDA cleared for use with flash sterilization) or tray; (2) prevent exogenous contamination of the item during transport from the sterilizer to the patient; and (3) monitor sterilizer function with mechanical, chemical, and biologic monitors (*Category IB*).

d. Do not use packaging materials and containers in flash sterilization cycles unless the sterilizer and the packaging material/container are designed for this use (*Category IB*).

e. When necessary, use flash sterilization for patient-care items that will be used immediately (e.g. to reprocess an inadvertently dropped instrument) (*Category IB*).

f. When necessary, use flash sterilization for processing patient-care items that cannot be packaged, sterilized, and stored before use (*Category IB*).

Methods of Sterilization

a. Steam is the preferred method for sterilizing critical medical and surgical instruments that are not damaged by heat, steam, pressure, or moisture (*Category IA*).

b. Cool, steam- or heat-sterilized items before they are handled or used in the operative setting (*Category IB*).

c. Follow the sterilization times, temperatures, and other operating parameters (e.g. gas concentration, humidity) recommended by the manufacturers of the instruments, the sterilizer, and the container or wrap used, and that are consistent with guidelines published by government agencies and professional organizations (*Category IB*).

d. Use low-temperature sterilization technologies (e.g. EtO, hydrogen peroxide gas plasma) for reprocessing critical patient-care equipment that is heat or moisture sensitive (*Category IA*).

e. Completely aerate surgical and medical items that have been sterilized in the EtO sterilizer (e.g. polyvinylchloride tubing requires 12 hours at 50°C, 8 hours at 60°C) before using these items in patient care (*Category IB*).

f. Sterilization using the peracetic acid immersion system can be used to sterilize heat-sensitive immersible medical and surgical items (*Category IB*).

g. Critical items that have been sterilized by the peracetic acid immersion process must be used immediately (i.e. items are not completely protected from contamination, making long-term storage unacceptable) (*Category II*).

h. Dry-heat sterilization (e.g., 340°F for 60 minutes) can be used to sterilize items (e.g. powders, oils) that can sustain high temperatures (*Category IB*).

i. Comply with the sterilizer manufacturer's instructions regarding the sterilizer cycle parameters (e.g. time, temperature, concentration) (*Category IB*).

j. Because narrow-lumen devices provide a challenge to all low-temperature sterilization technologies and direct contact is necessary for the sterilant to be effective, ensure that the sterilant has direct contact with contaminated surfaces (e.g. scopes processed in peracetic acid must be connected to channel irrigators) (*Category IB*).

Packaging

a. Ensure that packaging materials are compatible with the sterilization process (*Category IB*).

b. Ensure that packaging is sufficiently strong to resist punctures and tears to provide a barrier to microorganisms and moisture (*Category IB*).

Monitoring of Sterilizers

a. Use mechanical, chemical, and biologic monitors to ensure the effectiveness of the sterilization process (*Category IB*).
b. Monitor each load with mechanical (e.g. time, temperature, pressure) and chemical (internal and external) indicators. If the internal chemical indicator is visible, an external indicator is not needed (*Category II*).
c. Do not use processed items if the mechanical (e.g. time, temperature, pressure) or chemical (internal and/or external) indicators suggest inadequate processing (*Category IB*).
d. Use biologic indicators to monitor the effectiveness of sterilizers at least weekly with an FDA-cleared commercial preparation of spores (e.g. *Geobacillus stearothermophilus* for steam) intended specifically for the type and cycle parameters of the sterilizer (*Category IB*).
e. After a single positive biologic indicator used with a method other than steam sterilization, treat as nonsterile all items that have been processed in that sterilizer, dating from the sterilization cycle having the last negative biologic indicator to the next cycle showing satisfactory biologic indicator results. These nonsterile items should be retrieved if possible and reprocessed (*Category II*).
f. After a positive biologic indicator with steam sterilization, objects other than implantable objects do not need to be recalled because of a single positive spore test unless the sterilizer or the sterilization procedure is defective as determined by maintenance personnel or inappropriate cycle settings. If additional spore tests remain positive, consider the items nonsterile and recall and reprocess the items from the implicated load(s) (*Category II*).
g. Use biologic indicators for every load containing implantable items and quarantine items, whenever possible, until the biologic indicator is negative (*Category IB*).

Load Configuration

a. Place items correctly and loosely into the basket, shelf, or cart of the sterilizer so as not to impede the penetration of the sterilant (*Category IB*).

Storage of Sterile Items

a. Ensure the sterile storage area is a well-ventilated area that provides protection against dust, moisture, insects, and temperature and humidity extremes (*Category II*).
b. Store sterile items so the packaging is not compromised (e.g. punctured, bent) (*Category II*).
c. Label sterilized items with a load number that indicates the sterilizer used, the cycle or load number, the date of sterilization, and, if applicable, the expiration date (*Category IB*).
d. The shelf life of a packaged sterile item depends on the quality of the wrapper, the storage conditions, the conditions during transport, the amount of handling, and other events (moisture) that compromise the integrity of the package. If event-related storage of sterile items is used, then packaged sterile items can be used indefinitely unless the packaging is compromised (see f and g below) (*Category IB*).
e. Evaluate packages before use for loss of integrity (e.g. torn, wet, punctured). The pack can be used unless the integrity of the packaging is compromised (*Category II*).
f. If the integrity of the packaging is compromised (e.g. torn, wet, or punctured), repack and reprocess the pack before use (*Category II*).
g. If time-related storage of sterile items is used, label the pack at the time of sterilization with an expiration date.

Once this date expires, reprocess the pack (*Category II*).

Quality Control

a. Provide comprehensive and intensive training for all staff assigned to reprocess semicritical and critical medical/surgical instruments to ensure they understand the importance of reprocessing these instruments. To achieve and maintain competency, train each member of the staff that reprocesses semicritical and/or critical instruments as follows: (1) provide hands-on training according to the institutional policy for reprocessing critical and semicritical devices; (2) supervise all work until competency is documented for each reprocessing task; (3) conduct competency testing at beginning of employment and regularly thereafter (e.g. annually); and (4) review the written reprocessing instructions regularly to ensure they comply with the scientific literature and the manufacturers' instructions (*Category IB*).
b. Compare the reprocessing instructions (e.g. for the appropriate use of endoscope connectors, the capping/noncapping of specific lumens) provided by the instrument manufacturer and the sterilizer manufacturer and resolve any conflicting recommendations by communicating with both manufacturers (*Category IB*).
c. Conduct infection control rounds periodically (e.g. annually) in high-risk reprocessing areas (e.g. the gastroenterology clinic, central processing); ensure reprocessing instructions are current and accurate and are correctly implemented. Document all deviations from policy. All stakeholders should identify what corrective actions will be implemented (*Category IB*).
d. Include the following in a quality control program for sterilized items: a sterilizer maintenance contract with records of service; a system of process monitoring; air-removal testing for prevacuum steam sterilizers; visual inspection of packaging materials; and traceability of load contents (*Category II*).
e. For each sterilization cycle, record the type of sterilizer and cycle used; the load identification number; the load contents; the exposure parameters (e.g. time and temperature); the operator's name or initials; and the results of mechanical, chemical, and biological monitoring (*Category II*).
f. Retain sterilization records (mechanical, chemical, and biological) for a time period that complies with standards (e.g. 3 years), statutes of limitations, and state and federal regulations (*Category II, IC*).
g. Prepare and package items to be sterilized so that sterility can be achieved and maintained to the point of use. Consult the Association for the Advancement of Medical Instrumentation or the manufacturers of surgical instruments, sterilizers, and container systems for guidelines for the density of wrapped packages (*Category II*).
h. Periodically review policies and procedures for sterilization (*Category II*).
i. Perform preventive maintenance on sterilizers by qualified personnel who are guided by the manufacturer's instruction (*Category II*).

Reuse of Single-use Medical Devices

a. Adhere to the FDA enforcement document for single-use devices reprocessed by hospitals. FDA considers the hospital that reprocesses a single-use device as the manufacturer of the device and regulates the hospital using the same standards by which it regulates the original equipment manufacturer (*Category II, IC*).

PERFORMANCE INDICATORS

1. Monitor adherence to high-level disinfection and/or sterilization guidelines for endoscopes on a regular basis. This monitoring should include ensuring the proper training of persons performing reprocessing and their adherence to all endoscope reprocessing steps, as demonstrated by competency testing at commencement of employment and annually.
2. Develop a mechanism for the occupational health service to report all adverse health events potentially resulting from exposure to disinfectants and sterilants; review such exposures; and implement engineering, work practice, and PPE to prevent future exposures.
3. Monitor possible sterilization failures that resulted in instrument recall. Assess whether additional training of personnel or equipment maintenance is required.

GLOSSARY

Action level: Concentration of a regulated substance (e.g. ethylene oxide, formaldehyde) within the employee breathing zone, above which OSHA requirements apply.

Activation of a sterilant: Process of mixing the contents of a chemical sterilant that come in two containers. (small vial with the activator solution; container of the chemical) Keeping the two chemicals separate until use extends the shelf life of the chemicals.

Aeration: Method by which ethylene oxide (EtO) is removed from EtO-sterilized items by warm air circulation in an enclosed cabinet specifically designed for this purpose.

Biologic indicator: Device for monitoring the sterilization process. The device consists of a standardized, viable population of microorganisms (usually bacterial spores) known to be resistant to the sterilization process being monitored. Biologic indicators are intended to demonstrate whether conditions were adequate to achieve sterilization. A negative biologic indicator does not prove that all items in the load are sterile or that they were all exposed to adequate sterilization conditions.

Bleach: Household bleach (5.25% or 6.00%–6.15% sodium hypochlorite depending on manufacturer) usually diluted in water at 1:10 or 1:100. Approximate dilutions are 1.5 cups of bleach in a gallon of water for a 1:10 dilution (~6,000 ppm) and 0.25 cup of bleach in a gallon of water for a 1:100 dilution (~600 ppm) (see Table 7.7).

Bowie-Dick test: Diagnostic test of a sterilizer's ability to remove air from the chamber of a prevacuum steam sterilizer. The air-removal or Bowie-Dick test is not a test for sterilization.

Ceiling limit: Concentration of an airborne chemical contaminant that should not be exceeded during any part of the workday. If instantaneous monitoring is not feasible, the ceiling must be assessed as a 15-minute time-weighted average exposure.

Central processing or central service department: The department within a health-care facility that processes, issues, and controls professional supplies and equipment, both sterile and nonsterile, for some or all patient-care areas of the facility.

Challenge test pack: Pack used in installation, qualification, and ongoing quality assurance testing of health-care facility sterilizers.

Chemical indicator: Device for monitoring a sterilization process. The device is designed to respond with a characteristic chemical or physical change to one or more of the physical conditions within the sterilizing chamber. Chemical indicators are intended to detect potential sterilization failures that could result from incorrect packaging, incorrect loading of the sterilizer, or malfunctions of the sterilizer. The "pass" response of a chemical indicator does not prove the item accompanied by the indicator is necessarily sterile. The Association for the Advancement of Medical Instrumentation has defined five classes of chemical indicators: *Class 1* (process indicator); *Class 2* (Bowie-Dick test indicator); *Class 3* (single-parameter indicator); *Class 4* (multi-parameter indicator); and *Class 5* (integrating indicator).

Contact time: The time a disinfectant is in direct contact with the surface or item to be disinfected. For surface disinfection, this period is framed by the application to the surface until complete drying has occurred.

Control, positive: Biologic indicator, from the same lot as a test biologic indicator, that is left unexposed to the sterilization cycle and then incubated to verify the viability of the test biologic indicator.

D value: Time or radiation dose required to inactivate 90% of a population of the test microorganism under stated exposure conditions.

EPA Registration Number or EPA Registration No.: A hyphenated, two- or three-part number assigned by EPA to identify each germicidal product registered within the United States. The first number is the company identification number, the second is the specific product number, and the third (when present) is the company identification number for a supplemental registrant.

Exposure time: Period in a sterilization process during which items are exposed to the sterilant at the specified sterilization parameters. For example, in a steam sterilization process, exposure time is the period during which items are exposed to saturated steam at the specified temperature.

Flash sterilization: Process designed for the steam sterilization of unwrapped patient-care items for immediate use (or placed in a specially designed, covered, rigid container to allow for rapid penetration of steam.

General disinfectant: EPA-registered disinfectant labeled for use against both gram-negative and gram-positive bacteria. Efficacy is demonstrated against both *Salmonella choleraesuis* and *Staphylococcus aureus*. Also called broad-spectrum disinfectant.

Huck towel: All-cotton surgical towel with a honey-comb weave; both warp and fill yarns are tightly twisted. Huck towels can be used to prepare biologic indicator challenge test packs.

Implantable device: According to FDA, 'device that is placed into a surgically or naturally formed cavity of the human body if it is intended to remain there for a period of 30 days or more'.

Minimum effective concentration (MEC): The minimum concentration of a liquid chemical germicide needed to achieve the claimed microbicidal activity as determined by dose-response testing. Sometimes used interchangeably with minimum recommended concentration.

Muslin: Loosely woven (by convention, 140 threads per square inch), 100% cotton cloth. Formerly used as a wrap for sterile packs or a surgical drape. Fabric wraps used currently consist of a cotton-polyester blend.

One-step disinfection process: Simultaneous cleaning and disinfection of a noncritical surface or item.

Pasteurization: Process developed by Louis Pasteur of heating milk, wine, or other liquids to 65–77°C (or the equivalent) for approximately 30 minutes to kill or markedly reduce the number of pathogenic and spoilage organisms other than bacterial spores.

Parametric release: Declaration that a product is sterile on the basis of physical and/or chemical process data rather than on sample testing or biologic indicator results.

Permissible exposure limit (PEL): Time-weighted average maximum concentration of an air contaminant to which a worker can be exposed, according to OSHA standards. Usually calculated over 8 hours, with exposure considered over a 40-hour work week.

Prions: These are transmissible pathogenic agents that cause a variety of neurodegenerative diseases of humans and animals, including sheep and goats, bovine spongiform encephalopathy in cattle, and Creutzfeldt-Jakob disease in humans. They are unlike any other infectious pathogens because they are composed of an abnormal conformational isoform of a normal cellular protein, the prion protein (PrP). Prions are extremely resistant to inactivation by sterilization processes and disinfecting agents.

Process challenge device (PCD): These are items designed to simulate product to be sterilized and to constitute a defined challenge to the sterilization process and used to assess the effective performance of the process. A PCD is a challenge test pack or test tray that contains a biologic indicator, a Class 5 integrating indicator, or an enzyme-only indicator.

QUAT: This is an abbreviation for quaternary ammonium compound, a surface-active, water-soluble disinfecting substance that has four carbon atoms linked to a nitrogen atom through covalent bonds.

Recommended exposure limit (REL): It is the occupational exposure limit recommended by NIOSH (National Institute for Occupational Safety and Health) as being protective of worker health and safety over a working lifetime. Frequently expressed as a 40-hour time-weighted-average exposure for up to 10 hours per day during a 40-work week.

Reprocess: This is a method to ensure proper disinfection or sterilization; can include: cleaning, inspection, wrapping, sterilizing, and storing.

Sanitizer: This is an agent that reduces the number of bacterial contaminants to safe levels as judged by public health requirements. Commonly used with substances applied to inanimate objects. According to the protocol for the official sanitizer test, a sanitizer is a chemical that kills 99.999% of the specific test bacteria in 30 seconds under the conditions of the test.

Shelf life: This is the length of time an undiluted or use dilution of a product can remain active and effective. Also refers to the length of time a sterilized product (e.g. sterile instrument set) is expected to remain sterile.

Spaulding classification: This is the strategy for reprocessing contaminated medical devices. The system classifies a medical device as critical, semicritical, or noncritical on the basis of risk to patient safety from contamination on a device. The system also established three levels of germicidal activity (sterilization, high-level disinfection, and low-level disinfection) for strategies with the three classes of medical devices (critical, semicritical, and noncritical).

Spore strip: This is a paper strip impregnated with a known population of spores that meets the definition of biological indicators.

Steam sterilization, dynamic air removal type: These are one of two types of sterilization cycles in which air is removed from the chamber and the load by a series of pressure and vacuum excursions (prevacuum cycle) or by a series of steam flushes and pressure pulses above atmospheric pressure (steam-flush-pressure-pulse cycle).

Sterile or sterility: It is the state of being free from all living microorganisms. In practice, usually described as a probability function, e.g. as the probability of a microorganism surviving sterilization being one in one million.

Sterility assurance level (SAL): It is the probability of a viable microorganism being present on a product unit after sterilization. Usually expressed as 10^{-6}; a SAL of 10^{-6} means $\leq 1/1$ million chance that a single viable microorganism is present on a sterilized item. A SAL of 10^{-6} generally is accepted as appropriate for items intended to contact compromised tissue (i.e. tissue that has lost the integrity of the natural body barriers). The sterilizer manufacturer is responsible for ensuring the sterilizer can achieve the desired SAL. The user is responsible for monitoring the performance of the sterilizer to ensure it is operating in conformance to the manufacturer's recommendations.

Sterilizer, gravity-displacement type: This is a type of steam sterilizer in which incoming steam displaces residual air through a port or drain in or near the bottom (usually) of the sterilizer chamber. Typical operating temperatures are 121–123°C (250–254°F) and 132–135°C (270–275°F).

Sterilizer, prevacuum type: This is a type of steam sterilizer that depends on one or more pressure and vacuum excursions at the beginning of the cycle to remove air. This method of operation results in shorter cycle times for wrapped items because of the rapid removal of air from the chamber and the load by the vacuum system and because of the usually higher operating temperature [132–135°C (270–275°F); 141–144°C (285–291°F)]. This type of sterilizer generally provides for shorter exposure time and accelerated drying of fabric loads by pulling a further vacuum at the end of the sterilizing cycle.

Sterilizer, steam-flush pressure-pulse type: This is a type of sterilizer in which a repeated sequence consisting of a steam flush and a pressure pulse removes air from the sterilizing chamber and processed materials using steam at above atmospheric pressure (no vacuum is required). Like a prevacuum sterilizer, a steam-flush pressure-pulse sterilizer rapidly removes air from the sterilizing chamber and wrapped items; however, the system is not susceptible to air leaks because air is removed with the sterilizing chamber pressure at above atmospheric pressure. Typical operating temperatures are 121–123°C (250–254°F), 132–135°C (270–275°F), and 141–144°C (285–291°F).

Surfactant: Agent that reduces the surface tension of water or the tension at the interface between water and another liquid; a wetting agent found in many sterilants and disinfectants.

Tabletop steam sterilizer: A compact gravity-displacement steam sterilizer that has a chamber volume of not more than 2 cubic feet and that generates its own steam when distilled or deionized water is added.

Time-weighted average (TWA): An average of all the concentrations of a chemical to which a worker has been exposed during a specific sampling time, reported as an average over the sampling time. For example, the permissible exposure limit for ethylene oxide is 1 ppm as an 8-hour TWA. Exposures above the ppm limit are permitted if they are compensated for by equal or longer exposures below the limit during the 8-hour workday as long as they do not exceed the ceiling limit; short-term exposure limit; or, in the case of ethylene oxide, excursion limit of 5 ppm averaged over a 15-minute sampling period.

Tuberculocide: An EPA-classified hospital disinfectant that also kills *Mycobacterium tuberculosis* (tubercle bacilli).

Use-life: The length of time a diluted product can remain active and effective. The stability of the chemical and the storage conditions (e.g. temperature and presence of air, light, organic matter, or metals) determine the use-life of antimicrobial products.

Table 7.8: Decreasing order of resistance of microorganisms to disinfection and sterilization and the level of disinfection or sterilization.

Resistant	Level
Prions (Creutzfeldt-Jakob Disease)	Prion reprocessing
Bacterial spores (*Bacillus atrophaeus*)	Sterilization
Coccidia (*Cryptosporidium*)	
Mycobacteria (*M. tuberculosis, M. terrae*)	High
Nonlipid or small viruses (polio, coxsackie)	Intermediate
Fungi (*Aspergillus, Candida*)	
Vegetative bacteria (*S. aureus, P. aeruginosa*)	Low
Lipid or medium-sized viruses (HIV, herpes, hepatitis B)	
Susceptible	

Source: Russell and Favero[39,40]

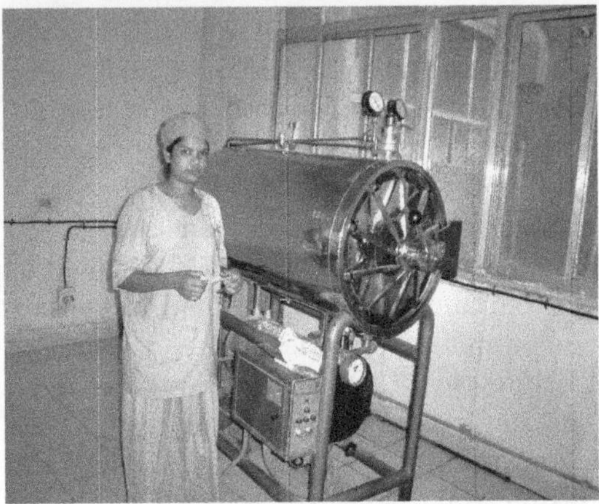

Fig. 7.1: Autoclave machine

Source: Association for the Advancement of Medical Instrumentation;[21-25] Association of perioperating Registered Nurses (AORN),[26] American Hospital Association,[27] and Block.[28,29]

REFERENCES

1. Rutala WA, Weber DJ. The Healthcare Infection Control Practices Advisory Committee (HICPAC). CDC Guideline for Disinfection and Sterilization in Healthcare facilities, 2008. accessed www. 11th Nov 2014.
2. Gurevich I, Jacobsen E, Cunha BA. Pseudoautoclave failure caused by differences in spore test steam sensitivities. Am J Infect Control. 1996;24:402-4.
3. Rutala WA. Disinfection and flash sterilization in the operating room. J Ophthal Nurs Technol. 1991;10:106-15.
4. Anonymous. Ethylene oxide sterilization: How hospitals can adapt to the changes. Health Devices. 1994;23:485-92.
5. Parker HH, Johnson RB. Effectiveness of ethylene oxide for sterilization of dental handpieces. J Dent. 1995;23:113-5.
6. Rutala WA, Weber DJ. New disinfection and sterilization methods. Emerg Inf Dis. 2001;7:348-53.
7. Rosaspina S, Salvatorelli G, Anzanel D. The bactericidal effect of microwaves on Mycobacterium bovis dried on scalpel blades. J Hosp Infect. 1994;26:45-50.
8. American Institute of Architects. Guidelines for design and construction of hospital and health care facilities. Washington, DC: The American Institute of Architects Press; 2001.
9. Association for the Advancement of Medical Instrumentation. Comprehensive guide to steam sterilization and sterility assurance in health care facilities, ANSI/AAMI ST79; 2006.
10. Ninemeier JD. Central service technical manual. Chicago: International Association of Healthcare Central Service Materiel Management; 1998.
11. Klapes NA, Greene VW, Langholz AC. Microbial contamination associated with routine aseptic practice. J Hosp Infect. 1987;10:299-304.
12. Butt WE, Bradley DV Jr, Mayhew RB, Schwartz RS. Evaluation of the shelf life of sterile instrument packs. Oral Surg Med Pathol. 1991;72:650- 4.
13. Webster J, Lloyd W, Ho P, Burridge C, George N. Rethinking sterilization practices: Evidence for event-related outdating. Infect Control Hosp Epidemiol. 2003;24:622-4.
14. Widmer AF, Houston A, Bollinger E, Wenzel RP. A new standard for sterility testing for autoclaved surgical trays. J Hosp Infect. 1992;21:253-60.
15. Rutala WA, Gergen MF, Weber DJ. Evaluation of a rapid readout biological indicator for flash sterilization with three biological indicators and three chemical indicators. Infect Control Hosp Epidemiol. 1993;14:390-4.
16. Kleinegger CL, Yeager DL, Huling JK, Drake DR. The effects of contamination on biological monitoring. Infect Control Hosp Epidemiol. 2001;22:391-2.
17. Centers for Disease Control. False-positive results of spore tests in ethylene oxide sterilizers-Wisconsin. MMWR. 1981;30:238-40.
18. Association for the Advancement of Medical Instrumentation. Steam sterilization and sterility assurance in health care facilities. ANSI/AAMI ST46.Arlington, VA, 2002:ANSI/AAMI ST46;2002.
19. Association for the Advancement of Medical Instrumentation. Comprehensive guide to steam sterilization and sterility assurance in health care facilities, ANSI/AAMI ST79;2006.
20. Association for the Advancement of Medical Instrumentation. Good hospital practice: steam sterilization and sterility assurance. Arlington, VA: AAMI;1988.
21. Association for the Advancement of Medical Instrumentation. Good hospital practice: Steam sterilization and sterility assurance. AAMI. Arlington, VA;1993.
22. Association for the Advancement of Medical Instrumentation. Flash sterilization: Steam sterilization of patient care items for immediate use. AAMI. Arlington, VA;1996.
23. Association for the Advancement of Medical Instrumentation. Steam sterilization and sterility assurance in health care facilities. ANSI/AAMI ST46. Arlington, VA, 2002:ANSI/AAMI ST46;2002.
24. Association for the Advancement of Medical Instrumentation. Ethylene oxide sterilization in health care facilities: Safety and effectiveness. AAMI. Arlington, VA;1999.
25. Association for the Advancement of Medical Instrumentation. Comprehensive guide to steam sterilization and sterility assurance in health care facilities, ANSI/AAMI ST79; 2006.
26. Association of Operating Room Nurses. Recommended practices for sterilization in perioperative practice settings. 2000 Standards,

Recommended Practices, and Guidelines. Denver, CO: AORN; 2000:347-58.

27. Cokendolpher JC, Haukos JF. The Practical Application of Disinfection and Sterilization in Health Care Facilities. Chicago: American Hospital Association; 1996.
28. Block SS. Disinfection, sterilization, and preservation. Philadelphia: Lippincott Williams and Wilkins; 2001.
29. Block SS. Definition of terms. In: Block SS (Ed). Disinfection, sterilization, and preservation. Philadelphia: Lippincott Williams and Wilkins, 2001.pp.19-28.
30. Rutala WA, Weber DJ. Clinical effectiveness of low-temperature sterilization technologies. Infect. Control Hosp. Epidemiol 1998;19:798-804.
31. Association for the Advancement of Medical Instrumentation. Steam sterilization and sterility assurance in health care facilities. ANSI/AAMI ST46.Arlington, VA, 2002:ANSI/AAMI ST46;2002.
32. Association for the Advancement of Medical Instrumentation. Comprehensive guide to steam sterilization and sterility assurance in health care facilities, ANSI/AAMI ST79;2006.
33. Association for the Advancement of Medical Instrumentation. Flash sterilization: Steam sterilization of patient care items for immediate use. AAMI. Arlington, VA; 1996.
34. Association for the Advancement of Medical Instrumentation. Comprehensive guide to steam sterilization and sterility assurance in health care facilities, ANSI/AAMI ST79; 2006.
35. Schneider PM. Low-temperature sterilization alternatives in the 1990s. Tappi J. 1994;77:115-9.
36. Alfa MJ. Flexible endoscope reprocessing. Infect. Control Steril Technol. 1997;3:26-36.
37. Rutala WA, Weber DJ. Clinical effectiveness of low-temperature sterilization technologies. Infect. Control Hosp Epidemiol. 1998;19:798-804.
38. Bryce EA, Roberts FJ, Clements B, MacLean S. When the biological indicator is positive: investigating autoclave failures. Infect Control Hosp Epidemiol. 1997;18:654-6.
39. Favero MS, Bond WW. Chemical disinfection of medical and surgical materials. In: Block SS (Ed). Disinfection, sterilization, and preservation. Philadelphia: Lippincott Williams & Wilkins; 2001.pp.881-917.
40. Russell AD. Bacterial resistance to disinfectants: present knowledge and future problems. J Hosp Infect. 1998;43:S57-68.

Chapter 8

Disinfection

Chapter Outline

- Definitions
- A Rational Approach to Disinfection and Sterilization
- Selection and Use of Disinfectants
- Changes Since 1981
- Problems with Disinfection and Sterilization of Healthcare Equipment
- Endoscopes
- Tonometers, Diaphragm Fitting Rings and Cryosurgical Instruments
- Dental Instruments
- Disinfection of Devices Contaminated with HBV, HIV or *M. tuberculosis*
- Disinfection in Hemodialysis Unit
- Inactivation of *Clostridium difficile*
- OSHA Blood-borne Pathogen Standard
- Emerging Pathogens
- Inactivation of Bioterrorist Agents
- Inactivation of Creutzfeldt-Jakob Disease Agent
- Toxicologic and Environmental Concerns
- Disinfection in Ambulatory Care, and Home Care
- Susceptibility of Antibiotic Resistant Bacteria to Disinfectants
- Surface Disinfection: Is Surface Disinfection Necessary?
- Contact Times for Surface Disinfectants
- Air Disinfection
- Microbial Contamination of Disinfectants
- Factors Affecting the Efficacy of Disinfection and Sterilization
- Cleaning
- Disinfection
- Type of Chemical Disinfectants
- Formulation of a Disinfectant Policy
- Testing of Disinfectants

INTRODUCTION

Everyone is aware of the fact that sterilization and disinfection of items used for patient care is necessary to prevent transmission of infection in the hospitals. It is also a known fact that infections have occurred following improper processing of patient care items. Hospital policies must identify whether disinfection or sterilization is indicated on the basis of each item intended for use since it is unnecessary to sterilize all patient care items. The Association for Professionals in Infection Control and Epidemiology (APIC) have prepared guidelines for the selection and use of disinfectants, which are discussed in the following part of this chapter.

Initially it is important to define certain terms, which are being used frequently, appropriate definitions have been given by APIC.[1]

DEFINITIONS

Sterilization

Sterilization is the complete elimination or destruction of all forms of microbial life (i.e. including spores). It is accomplished in the hospital by either physical or chemical processes. Steam under pressure, dry heat, and low temperature sterilization processes [ethylene oxide (EtO) gas, plasma sterilization] and liquid chemicals are the principal sterilizing agents used. The term sterilization is intended to convey an absolute meaning, not a relative one.

Disinfection

Disinfection is a process, which eliminates many or all-pathogenic microorganisms with the exception of bacterial spores, from inanimate objects. This can be achieved by the use of liquid chemicals or wet pasteurization. The efficacy of disinfection is affected by a number of factors, each of which may nullify or limit the efficacy of the process. Some of the factors which affect disinfection efficacy are the previous cleaning of the object, the organic load on the object, the type and level of microbial contamination, the concentration of and the exposure time to the germicide, the physical configuration of the object (crevices, hinges, lumens) presence of biofilms, and the temperature and pH of the disinfection process, and in some cases, relative humidity of the sterilization process (e.g., ethylene oxide).

Unlike sterilization, disinfection is not sporicidal. A few disinfectants will kill spores with prolonged exposure times (3–12 hours); these are called chemical sterilants. At similar concentrations but with shorter exposure periods (e.g. 20 minutes for 2% glutaraldehyde), these same disinfectants will kill all microorganisms except large numbers of bacterial spores; they are called high-level disinfectants. Low-level disinfectants can kill most vegetative bacteria, some fungi, and some viruses in a practical period of time ($\leq$10 minutes). Intermediate-level disinfectants might be cidal for mycobacteria, vegetative bacteria, most viruses, and most fungi but do not necessarily kill bacterial spores. Germicides differ markedly, primarily in their antimicrobial spectrum and rapidity of action.[2]

The levels of disinfection are defined as sterilization, high-level disinfection, intermediate-level disinfection and low- level disinfection.

High-level Disinfection

It can be expected to destroy all micro-organisms, with the exception of high numbers of bacterial spores.

Intermediate-level Disinfection

Inactivates *Mycobacterium tuberculosis*, vegetative bacteria, most viruses, most fungi, but it does not necessarily kill bacterial spores.

Low-level Disinfection

It can kill most bacteria, some viruses, some fungi, but it cannot be relied on to kill resistant microorganisms such as tubercle bacilli or bacterial spores.

- **Cleaning**: It is the removal of all foreign material (e.g. soil, oraganic material, lubricants) from objects. It is normally accomplished with water, mechanical action, and detergents or enzymatic products. Failure to remove foreign material from an object before a disinfection or sterilization process is likely to render the process ineffective. Meticulous physical cleaning must precede disinfection and sterilization procedures. Thorough cleaning is essential before high-level disinfection and sterilization because inorganic and organic materials that remain on the surfaces of instruments interfere with the effectiveness of these processes.[2]
- **Decontamination**: Removes pathogenic microorganisms from objects so they are safe to handle, use or discard.
- **Germicide:** It is an agent that destroys microorganisms particularly pathogenic organisms ('germs'). Other agents designated with the suffix-cide (e.g. virucide, fungicide, bactericide, sporicide, tuberculocide) destroy the microorganisms identified by the prefix for, e.g. bactericide is an agent that kills bacteria.
- **Chemical sterilants**: Chemicals used for the purpose of destroying all forms of microbial life, including fungal and bacterial spores are called chemical sterilants. These same chemical sterilants may be part of high-level disinfection process when used for shorter periods.
- **Antiseptics**: Chemicals that kill microorganisms on living skin or mucous membranes.
- **Bactericidal:** Chemical agents capable of killing bacteria. Similarly agents that are virucidal, fungicidal or sporicidal are agents capable of killing these organisms.
- **Bacteriostatic:** Chemical agents that inhibit the growth of bacteria but do not necessarily kill them.

A RATIONAL APPROACH TO DISINFECTION AND STERILIZATION

More than 30 years ago, Earle H Spaulding devised a rational approach to disinfection and sterilization of patient-care items and equipment. This classification scheme is so clear and logical that it has been retained, refined, and successfully used by infection control professionals and others when planning methods for disinfection or sterilization. Spaulding believed the nature of disinfection could be understood readily if instruments and items for patient care were categorized as critical, semicritical, and noncritical according to the degree of risk for infection involved in use of the items.

Classification of Patient Care Instruments and Items

Instruments and items for patient care are divided into three categories on the basis of degree of risk of infection involved in the use of items. The three categories of items are critical, semi-critical and non-critical.

Critical Items

Critical items are objects that enter sterile tissue or the vascular system. These items present a high-risk of infection if the item is contaminated with any microorganism, including bacterial spores. Critical items must be sterile. This category includes surgical instruments, cardiac and urinary catheters, implants and needles, and ultrasound probes used in sterile body cavities. Items in this category should be purchased as sterile or be sterilized by steam under pressure if possible. If heat labile, the object may be treated with EtO or other low temperature sterilization processes or by chemical sterilants. These chemical sterilants include ≥2.4% glutaraldehyde-based formulations, 0.95% glutaraldehyde with 1.64% phenol/phenate,

7.5% stabilized hydrogen peroxide, 7.35% hydrogen peroxide with 0.23% peracetic acid, 0.2% peracetic acid, and 0.08% peracetic acid with 1.0% hydrogen peroxide. Chemical sterilants can be relied on to produce sterility only if adequate cleaning precedes treatment and if proper guidelines with regard to organic load, contact time and temperature and PH are met.

Semicritical Items

Semicritical items are those objects that come in contact with mucous membranes or skin that is not intact. These items must be free from all microorganisms with the exception of high numbers of bacterial spores. Intact mucous membranes are generally resistant to infection by common bacterial spores but are susceptible to other organisms such as bacteria, tubercle bacilli and viruses.

Respiratory therapy and anaesthesia equipment, endoscopes, laryngoscope blades, esophageal manometry probes, cystoscopes, anorectal manometry catheters, and cervical diaphragm fitting rings are included in this category. Semicritical items generally require high-level disinfection with wet pasteurization or chemical disinfectant Glutaraldehyde, hydrogen peroxide, ortho-phthalaldehyde, peracetic acid with hydrogen peroxide are dependable high-level disinfectants. When a disinfectant is selected for use with certain patient-care items, the chemical compatibility after extended use with the items to be disinfected also must be considered.

High-level disinfection traditionally is defined as complete elimination of all microorganisms in or on an instrument, except for small numbers of bacterial spores. The FDA definition of high-level disinfection is a sterilant used for a shorter contact time to achieve a 6-log10 kill of an appropriate *Mycobacterium* species. Cleaning followed by high-level disinfection should eliminate enough pathogens to prevent transmission of infection.[2]

Laparoscopes and arthroscopes entering sterile tissue ideally should be sterilized between patients. However, this equipment sometimes undergoes only high-level disinfection between patients.[2] As with flexible endoscopes, these devices can be difficult to clean and high-level disinfect or sterilize because of intricate device design (e.g. long narrow lumens, hinges). Meticulous cleaning must precede any high-level disinfection or sterilization process. Although sterilization is preferred, no reports have been published of outbreaks resulting from high-level disinfection of these scopes when they are properly cleaned and high-level disinfected. Newer models of these instruments can withstand steam sterilization. These items should be preferably sterilized rather than high-level disinfected.

Rinsing endoscopes and flushing channels with sterile water, filtered water, or tap water will prevent adverse effects associated with disinfectant retained in the endoscope (e.g. disinfectant-induced colitis). Items can be rinsed and flushed using sterile water after high-level disinfection to prevent contamination with organisms in tap water, such as nontuberculous mycobacteria, *Legionella*, or gram-negative bacilli such as *Pseudomonas*. Alternatively, tapwater or filtered water (0.2 μ filter) rinse should be followed by an alcohol rinse and forced air drying. Forced-air drying markedly reduces bacterial contamination of stored endoscopes, most likely by removing the wet environment favorable for bacterial growth. After rinsing, items should be dried and stored (e.g. packaged) in a manner that protects them from recontamination.

Some items that may come in contact with nonintact skin for a brief period of time (i.e. hydrotherapy tanks, bed side rails) are usually considered noncritical surfaces and are disinfected with intermediate-level disinfectants (i.e. phenolic, iodophor, alcohol, chlorine). Since hydrotherapy tanks have been associated with spread of infection, some facilities have chosen to disinfect them with recommended levels of chlorine.

In the past, high-level disinfection was recommended for mouthpieces and spirometry tubing (e.g. glutaraldehyde) but cleaning the interior surfaces of the spirometers was considered unnecessary. This was based on a study that showed that mouthpieces and spirometry tubing become contaminated with microorganisms but there was no bacterial contamination of the surfaces inside the spirometers. Filters have been used to prevent contamination of this equipment distal to the filter; such filters and the proximal mouthpiece are changed between patients.

Noncritical Items

Noncritical items are items, which come in contact with intact skin but not with mucous membrane. Intact skin acts as an effective barrier to most microorganisms, and sterility is not critical. Noncritical items are divided into noncritical patient care items and noncritical environmental surfaces Noncritical patient-care items are bedpans, blood pressure cuffs, crutches and computer. Noncritcal environmental surfaces include bed rails, some food utensils, bedside tables, patient furniture and floors. Most noncritical reusable items may be disinfected where they are used and do not need to be transported to central processing area. There is very little risk of transmitting infectious agents to patients by means of noncritical items, however these items could contribute to secondary transmission by contaminating hands of health care workers or by contact with medical equipment that subsequently comes in contact with patients. Mops and reusable cloths are regularly used to clean environmental surfaces but if they are not cleaned and disinfected adequately and if the disinfectant-water mixture is not changed regularly (e.g. after every three to four rooms, at no longer than 60 minute intervals), the mopping procedure can spread heavy microbial contamination throughout the health care facility. Instead frequent laundering has found to provide acceptable decontamination of heavily contaminated mops, but chemical decontamination with a phenolic was less effective. Hence laundering of mops is therefore recommended. Single use disposable towels impregnated with a disinfectant also can be used for low-level disinfection when spot cleaning of non-critical surfaces is needed disinfectants used are sodium hypochlorite, ethyl or isopropyl alcohol, phenolic agent, iodophore and quaternary ammonium compounds.

SELECTION AND USE OF DISINFECTANTS

Selection Criteria

Usually disinfectants are 'cidal' in that they kill the susceptible potential pathogenic agents. The selection of a disinfectant should be based on the function the disinfectant is expected to perform. Ideally, a disinfectant should be broad spectrum (eliminates bacteria, viruses, protozoa, fungi and spores), nonirritating, nontoxic, noncorrosive and inexpensive. Selection decisions should include effectiveness against the potential pathogenic agent, safety to people, impact on equipment, the environment, and expense.

Disinfectant effectiveness depends on many factors. These include:

- Type of contaminating microorganism. Each disinfectant has unique antimicrobial attributes.
- Degree of contamination. This determines the quality of disinfectant required and time of exposure.
- Amount of proteinaceous material present. High protein based materials absorb and neutralize some chemical disinfectants.
- Presence of organic matter and other compounds such as soaps may neutralize some disinfectants.
- Chemical nature of disinfectant. It is important to understand the mode of action in order to select the appropriate disinfectant.
- Concentration and quantity of disinfectant. It is important to choose the proper concentration and quantity of

disinfectant that is best suited to each situation.

- Contact time and temperature. Sufficient time and appropriate temperature must be allowed for action of the disinfectant and may depend on the degree of contamination and organic matter load.
- Residual activity and effects on fabric and metal should be considered for specific situations.
- Application temperature, pH and interactions with other compounds must be considered.
- Toxicity to the environment and relative safety to people that may be exposed.
- Cost.

CHANGES SINCE 1981

CDC has made certain changes in the choice of disinfectants.

1. Formaldehyde-alcohol has been deleted as a chemical sterilant and high-level disinfectant, because with the exception of dialysis equipment, it no longer has a role in disinfection strategies. It is corrosive, irritating, toxic and not commonly used.
2. Second, several new chemical sterilants have been added, including hydrogen peroxide, peracetic acid and peracetic acid and hydrogen peroxide in combination.
3. The chemical sterilant chlorine di-oxide is no longer used, as it is not commercially available, since it caused leaks in dialyzer membranes.
4. 3% phenolics and ioidophores have been deleted as high level disinfectants because they have not been proved to be effective against bacterial endospores, *M. tuberculosis* and some fungi.
5. Isopropyl and ethyl alcohols have also been excluded as high level disinfectants because of their inability to inactivate bacterial spores and because of the inability of isopropyl alcohol to inactivate hydrophilic viruses (i.e. poliovirus, coxsackievirus).
6. A 1:16 dilution of 2% glutaraldehyde—7.05% phenol—1.2% sodium phenate (which contains 0.13% glutaraldehyde, 0.44% phenol and 0.075% sodium phenate when diluted) has been deleted as high-level disinfectant because of numerous scientific publications that demonstrate a lack of bactericidal activity in the presence of organic matter, a lack of fungicidal, tuberculocidal and sporicidal activity and reduced virucidal activity.
7. The exposure time required to achieve high-level disinfection has been changed from 10–30 minutes to 12 minutes.[2] A glutaraldehyde and an ortho-phthalaldehyde have an FDA-cleared label claim of 5 minutes when used at 35°C and 25°C, respectively, in an automated endoscope reprocessor with FDA-cleared capability to maintain the solution at the appropriate temperature.[2]

PROBLEMS WITH DISINFECTION AND STERILIZATION OF HEALTHCARE EQUIPMENT

It is not as simple as it sounds to make the right choice of disinfectant even after considering the categories of risk to patients. A number of problems may not be considered while making the choice of disinfectant, e.g. processing complicated medical equipment, which is often heat labile or problems of inactivating certain types of infectious agents [prions such as Creutzfeldt-Jakob disease (CJD) agent]. Thus, in some situations, choosing a method of disinfection remains difficult, even after consideration of the categories of risk to patients. This is especially true for a few medical devices (e.g. arthroscopes and laparoscopes) in the critical category because of controversy about whether they should be sterilized or high-level disinfected. Heat-stable scopes (e.g. many rigid scopes) should be steam sterilized. Some of these items cannot be steam sterilized because they are heat-sensitive; additionally, sterilization using ethylene oxide (EtO) can be too time-consuming for routine use between patients (new technologies, such as hydrogen peroxide gas plasma and peracetic acid reprocessor, provide faster cycle times). However, evidence that sterilization of these items improves patient care by reducing the infection risk is lacking. Many newer models of these instruments can withstand steam sterilization, which for critical items is the preferred method.

Ideally biopsy forceps or other cutting instruments that break the mucosal barrier and laparoscopes, arthroscopes, and other scopes that enter normally sterile tissue should be subjected to a sterilization process before each use. This is also true for flexible endoscopes, which may be heat labile. They are included in the semi critical category and are processed by high-level disinfection, but when this is used in the gastrointestinal tract for a patient with bleeding esophageal varices or used with a sterile biopsy forceps then high-level disinfection which is used for this category should ensure that the desired level of infection is achieved and all microorganisms with the exception of a high number of bacterial spores have been removed from the endoscope, so that it should not pose an infection risk. Infection with spore-forming bacteria has not been reported from appropriately high-level disinfected endoscopes.

Therefore, the controversy regarding whether we should sterilize or high-level disinfect these patient care items still remains.

ENDOSCOPES

Physicians use endoscopes to diagnose and treat numerous medical disorders. Even though endoscopes represent a valuable diagnostic and therapeutic tool in modern medicine and the incidence of infection associated with their use reportedly is very low (about 1 in 1.8 million procedures), more healthcare-associated outbreaks have been linked to contaminated endoscopes than to any other medical device. To prevent the spread of health-care-associated infections, all heat-sensitive endoscopes (e.g., gastrointestinal endoscopes, bronchoscopes, nasopharygoscopes) must be properly cleaned and, at a minimum, subjected to high-level disinfection after each use. High-level disinfection can be expected to destroy all microorganisms, although when high numbers of bacterial spores are present, a few spores might survive.

Because of the types of body cavities they enter, flexible endoscopes acquire high levels of microbial contamination (bioburden) during each use. Cleaning reduces the level of microbial contamination by 4–6 log. Using human immunodeficiency virus (HIV)—contaminated endoscopes, several investigators have shown that cleaning completely eliminates the microbial contamination on the scopes. Similarly, other investigators found that EtO sterilization or soaking in 2% glutaraldehyde for 20 minutes was effective only when the device first was properly cleaned.[2]

FDA maintains a list of cleared liquid chemical sterilants and high-level disinfectants that can be used to reprocess heat-sensitive medical devices, such as flexible endoscopes (http://www.fda.gov/cdrh/ode/germlab.html). At this time, the FDA-cleared and marketed formulations include: ≥2.4% glutaraldehyde, 0.55% ortho-phthalaldehyde (OPA), 0.95% glutaraldehyde with 1.64% phenol/phenate, 7.35% hydrogen peroxide with 0.23% peracetic acid, 1.0% hydrogen peroxide with 0.08% peracetic acid, and 7.5% hydrogen peroxide. These products have excellent antimicrobial activity; however, some oxidizing chemicals (e.g. 7.5% hydrogen peroxide) reportedly have caused cosmetic and functional damage to endoscopes. Users should check with device manufacturers for information about germicide compatibility with their device. Professionals should review the scientific literature for newly available data regarding human safety or materials compatibility.

EtO sterilization of flexible endoscopes is infrequent because it requires a lengthy processing and aeration time (e.g., 12 hours) and is a potential hazard to staff and patients. The two products most commonly used for reprocessing endoscopes in the United States are glutaraldehyde and an automated, liquid chemical sterilization process that uses peracetic acid. The American Society for Gastrointestinal Endoscopy (ASGE) recommends glutaraldehyde solutions that do not contain surfactants because the soapy residues of surfactants are difficult to remove during rinsing. Ortho-phthalaldehyde has begun to replace glutaraldehyde in many health-care facilities because it has several potential advantages over glutaraldehyde: is not known to irritate the eyes and nasal passages, does not require activation or exposure monitoring, and has a 12-minute high-level disinfection claim in the United States.

High-level disinfection is used for endoscopes. This can be done by immersion in 2% glutaraldehyde for $\geq$ 20 minutes at 20°C which is adequate between patient procedures. Flexible endoscopes are difficult to disinfect and easy to damage because of their intricate design and delicate materials. Meticulous cleaning must precede any sterilization or high-level disinfection of these instruments. Failure to perform good cleaning can result in sterilization or disinfection failure and outbreaks of infection can occur.

Nosocomial infections have been reported due to gastrointestinal endoscopy and bronchoscopy. The clinical spectrum ranged from asymptomatic colonization to death. *Salmonella* species and *Pseudomonas aeruginosa* were identified as causative agents in infections transmitted by gastrointestinal endoscopy, whereas *M. tuberculosis,* atypical *mycobacteria* and *P. aeruginosa* were the most common infection transmitted by bronchoscopy. Major reasons for transmission were inadequate cleaning, improper selection of disinfecting agent and failure to follow recommended cleaning and disinfection procedures.

Automated endoscope reprocessors (AER) offer several advantages. As the reprocessing steps are standardized and automated, the likelihood that an essential reprocessing step will be skipped is reduced, so also the personnel exposure to high-level disinfectants or chemical sterilants is reduced. Failure of AERs has been linked to outbreaks of infections or colonization. Outbreaks involving removable endoscope parts, such as suction valves and endoscopic accessories designed to be inserted through flexible endoscopes such as biopsy forceps emphasize the importance of cleaning to remove all foreign matter before high-level disinfection or sterilization. Some types of valves are now available as single-use, disposable products (e.g. bronchoscope valves) or steam sterilizable products (e.g. gastrointestinal endoscope valves).

AERs need further development and redesign, as do endoscopes, so that they do not represent a potential source of infectious agents. Endoscopes employing disposable components (e.g. protective barrier devices or sheaths) might provide an alternative to conventional liquid chemical high-level disinfection/sterilization. Another new technology is a swallowable camera-in-a-capsule that travels through the digestive tract and transmits color pictures of the small intestine to a receiver worn outside the body. This capsule currently does not replace colonoscopies.

Published recommendations for cleaning and disinfecting endoscopic equipment should be strictly followed. Unfortunately, audits have shown that personnel do not consistently adhere to guidelines on reprocessing and outbreaks of infection continue to occur.

Therefore certain recommendations have been made for cleaning and disinfection of endoscopic equipment. They are as follows:

1. Clean: Mechanically clean internal and external surfaces, including brushing internal channels and flushing each internal channel with water and a detergent or enzymatic cleaners (leak

testing is recommended for endoscopes before immersion).

2. Disinfect: Immerse endoscope in high-level disinfectant (or chemical sterilant) and perfuse (eliminates air pockets and ensures contact of the germicide with the internal channels) disinfectant into all accessible channels, such as the suction/biopsy channel and air/water channel and expose for a time recommended for specific products.
3. Rinse: Rinse the endoscope and all channels with sterile water, filtered water (commonly used with AERs) or tap water (i.e. high-quality potable water).
4. Dry: Rinse the insertion tube and inner channels with alcohol, and dry with forced air after disinfection and before storage.

Store

The endoscope should be stored in a way that prevents recontamination and promotes drying.

Although the debate regarding high level disinfection versus sterilization of laparoscopes and arthroscopes still remains unsettled, until reports of well designed randomized clinical trials are available, the CDC and APIC guidelines should be considered as appropriate, i.e. laparoscopes, arthroscopes and other scopes that enter normally sterile tissue should be subjected to a sterilization procedure before each use; if this is not feasible, they should receive at least high level disinfections.

TONOMETERS, DIAPHRAGM FITTING RINGS AND CRYOSURGICAL INSTRUMENTS

As per CDC recommendations to prevent transmission of viruses (e.g. herpes simplex, adenovirus 8 and HIV) by tonometer tips, the instrument should be wiped clean and disinfected for 5–10 minutes with 3% hydrogen peroxide, 500-ppm chlorine, 70% ethyl alcohol or 70% isopropyl alcohol. However recent data suggests that 3% hydrogen peroxide and 70% isopropyl alcohol are not effective against adenovirus capable of causing epidemic keratoconjunctivitis and similar viruses and should not be used for disinfecting applanation tonometers. Structural damage to Schiotz tonometers has been observed with a 1:10 sodium hypochlorite (5,000 ppm chlorine)and 3% hydrogen peroxide. Preliminary studies suggest that wiping the tonometer tip with an alcohol wipe and then allowing the alcohol to evaporate might be effective in eliminating HSV, HIV and adenovirus, but still further studies are needed before this decontamination procedure can be recommended. Since this decontamination procedure is short and simple, swabbing the tonometer tip with alcohol is often practiced, but there have been two reports of this decontamination procedure being associated with epidemic keratoconjunctivitis by adenovirus.

Diaphragm fitting rings should be washed with soap and water and followed by immersion in 70% alcohol for 15 minutes. This method is adequate to inactivate HIV 1, HBV and HSV but does not ensure the inactivation of all other relevant viruses.

Vaginal probes used in sonographic scanning should be high level disinfected after each use however as an alternative a condom can be used to cover the vaginal probe during the procedure but a new condom should be used with each new patient. Although most manufacturers recommend use of 2% glutaraldehyde for high level disinfection of contaminated transvaginal transducers, this agent has been questioned as it might shorten the life of the transducer and might have toxic effects on the gametes and embryos. High level disinfection with hydrogen peroxide that is not toxic to staff, patients, probes and retrieved cells should be used till alternative procedures become available. Other probes such as rectal, cryosurgical and transesophageal probes or devices should be high-level disinfected between patients.

DENTAL INSTRUMENTS

The dental instruments that normally penetrate soft tissue or bone (e.g. forceps, scalpels, bone chisels, scalers and surgical burs) are classified as critical and must be sterilized or discarded after each use. Instruments that do not penetrate oral soft tissues or bone (e.g. amalgam, condensers, air/water syringes) but may come in contact with oral tissues are classified as semi-critical and should also be sterilized after each use. Chemical disinfection is not recommended for critical or semi critical dental instruments that can be heat sterilized. Heat stable dental instruments and materials can be sterilized by autoclave, chemical (formaldehyde) vapor and dry heat (e.g. 320°F for 2 hours). If a semicritical item is heat sensitive, it should at a minimum be processed with high-level disinfection. ETO may not be an effective means of sterilization because it may be difficult to ensure that the internal portions of the hand pieces are adequately cleaned and dried beforehand.

The CDC has divided noncritical surfaces in dental offices into clinical contact and housekeeping. Clinical contact surfaces are surfaces that might be touched frequently with gloved hands during patient care or that might become contaminated with blood or other potentially infectious material and subsequently contact instruments, hands, gloves or devices (e.g. light handles, switches, dental X-ray equipment, chair-side computers). Barrier protective coverings (e.g. clear plastic wraps) can be used for these surfaces, particularly those that are difficult to clean (e.g. light handles ,chair switches). The coverings should be changed when visibly soiled or damaged and routinely (e.g. between patients). Protected surfaces should be disinfected at the end of each day or if contamination is evident, if not barrier protected, these surfaces should be disinfected between patients with an intermediate level disinfectant.

Most housekeeping surfaces need to be cleaned only with a detergent and water or a hospital disinfectant, depending on the nature of the surface and the type and degree of contamination. When housekeeping surfaces are visibly contaminated by blood or body substances, however, prompt removal and surface disinfection is a sound infection control practice.

DISINFECTION OF DEVICES CONTAMINATED WITH HBV, HIV, OR *M. TUBERCULOSIS*

Semi-critical devices may be contaminated by blood from patients infected with HIV or HBV or by respiratory secretions from a patient with pulmonary tuberculosis; it was a problem whether these contaminated devices should be sterilized or high-level disinfection done. CDC recommends that high-level disinfection is appropriate because experiments have demonstrated the effectiveness of high-level disinfectants to inactivate these and other pathogens Therefore, endoscopes and other semi critical devices should be managed in the same way regardless of whether the patient is infected with *M. tuberculosis*, HIV or HBV.

DISINFECTION IN HEMODIALYSIS UNIT

Hemodialysis systems include hemodailysis machines, water supply, water treatment systems and distribution systems. During hemodialysis patients have acquired blood borne viruses and pathogenic bacteria. Cleaning and disinfection are important components of infection control in hemodailysis center. EPA and FDA regulate disinfectants used to reprocess hemodialyzers, hemodialysis machines and water treatment systems.

Noncritical surfaces (dialysis bed or chair, counter tops, external surfaces of dialysis machines and equipment (scissors, hemostats, clamps, blood pressure cuffs, stethoscopes) should be disinfected with an disinfectant unless the item is visibly contaminated with blood; in that case a tuberculocidal agent (or a disinfectant with specific label claims for HBV and HIV) or a 1:100 dilution of hypochlorite solution (500–600 ppm of free chlorine) should be used. Hemodialyzers are disinfected with per acetic acid, formaldehyde, glutaraldehyde, heat pasteurization with citric acid and chlorine containing compounds. Hemodialysis systems are usually disinfected by chlorine based disinfectants (e.g. sodium hypochlorite), acqueous formaldehyde, heat pasteurization, ozone or peracetic acid. All products must be used according to the manufacturer's recommendations. Some dialysis systems use hot-water disinfection to control microbial contamination.

INACTIVATION OF *CLOSTRIDIUM DIFFICILE*

Dilute solutions of hypochlorite for routine environmental disinfection of rooms of patients with *C. difficile* associated diarrhea or colitis have been recommended, however, this seems unnecessary since patients without symptoms constitute an important reservoir within the hospital and that person to person transmission is the principal means of transmission between patients. Therefore handwashing, barrier precautions and meticulous environmental cleaning may be equally effective in preventing the spread of *C. difficile*. Contaminated endoscopes such as colon scopes and thermometers can serve as vehicles of transmission. But data demonstrates that 2% glutaraldehyde and peracetic acid reliably kills *C. difficile* spores with short exposure times of 5 to 20 minutes. Ortho-pthaladehyde and ≥0.2% peracetic (Rutala)acid also can inactivate $\geq 10^4$ *C. difficile* spores in 10–12 minutes at 20°C.

OSHA BLOOD-BORNE PATHOGEN STANDARD

In December 1991, OSHA declared a standard entitled 'Occupational Exposure to Blood borne Pathogens' to eliminate or minimize occupational exposure to bloodborne pathogens. One component of this requirement is that all equipment and environmental and working surfaces be cleaned and decontaminated with an appropriate disinfectant after contact with blood or other potentially infectious material. OSHA has suggested the use of a tuberculocidal agent also effective against HIV and HBV. Studies demonstrate that for large blood spills a 1:10 final dilution of hypochlorite solution should be used to inactivate bloodborne viruses to minimize risk of infection to HCWs from percutaneous injury during cleanup.

EMERGING PATHOGENS [*CRYPTOSPORIDIUM, HELICOBACTER PYLORI, ESCHERICHIA COLI* O157:H7, ROTAVIRUS, HUMAN PAPILLOMAVIRUS, NOROVIRUS, SEVERE ACUTE RESPIRATORY SYNDROME (SARS), CORONAVIRUS]

All the above pathogens including HIV, HCV, multidrug-resistant *M. tuberculosis* and non-tuberculous mycobacteria (e.g. *M. chelonae*) are of a growing concern. However with a few exceptions mentioned later all these pathogens are susceptible to currently available chemical disinfectants and sterilants.

Most disinfectants like ethyl alcohol, glutaraldehyde, 5.25 % hypochlorite, peracetic acid, ortho-pthalaldehyde, phenol, povidone-iodine and QACs do not completely inactivate *Cryptosporidium*. The only chemicals and sterilants which can inactivate these are 6% and 7.5% hydrogen peroxide. Sterilization methods like steam and ETO and hydrogen peroxide gas plasma can fully inactivate *C. parvum*. Although most disinfectants are ineffective against *C. parvum*, current cleaning and disinfection practices appear satisfactory to prevent health-care associated transmission, e.g. endoscopes are unlikely to be an important vehicle for transmiting *C. parvum*, beca use the results of bacterial studies indicate mechanical cleaning will remove approximillately 10^4 organisms and drying results in a rapid loss of *C. parvum* viability.

Cleaning with soap and water, immersion in 70% ethanol for 3 minutes, instillation of 70% ethanol, instillation of 30 mL of 83% methanol are all ineffective for removing *H. pylori* from endoscopes. Cleaning followed by use of 2% glutaraldehyde (or automated peracetic acid) has been demonstrated by culture to be effective in eliminating *H. pylori*.

Outbreak of health care-associated rotavirus-gastroenteritis in paediatric unit has been reported. The transmission is from person to person through the hands of health care workers. Prolonged survival of rotavirus on environmental surfaces and hands has been demonstrated. Rotavirus suspended in feces can survive longer. Vectors have included hands,fomites,air,water and food. Products with demonstrated efficacy were 95% ethanol, 70% isopropanol, some phenolics, 2% glutaraldehyde, 0.35% peracetic acid and some quarternary ammonium compounds.

Much data does not exist on inactivation of HPV by alcohol or other disinfectants because in vitro replication of the virus has not been achieved. Similarly little is known about inactivation of noroviruses (members of the family Calciviridae and important cause of gastroenteritis in humans), because they cannot be grown in tissue culture. Improper disinfection of environmental surfaces contaminated with faeces or vomitus is believed to play a role in the spread of noroviruses.

Disinfectants effective against corona-viruses (SARS virus) were found to be sodium hypochlorite, 70% ethyl alcohol and Povidone iodine (1% iodine). Because SARS virus is stable in faeces and urine at room temperature for at least 1–2 days, surfaces might be a possible source of contamination and lead to infection with SARS coronavirus and should be disinfected. Until more precise information is available, environments in which SARS patients are housed should be considered heavily contaminated and the rooms and equipment should be thoroughly disinfected daily and after the patient is discharged. A 1:100 dilution of household bleach and water should be used for surface disinfection and disinfection on non-critical patient care equipment. High level disinfection and sterilization of semi-critical and crirical medical devices respectively ,does not need to be altered for patients with known or suspected SARS.

Free living ameba can be pathogenic and can harbor agents of pneumonia such as *Legionella pneumophila*. Limited studies have shown that 2% glutaraldehyde and peracetic acid do not completely inactivate *Acanthamoeba polyphaga* in a 20 minute exposure time for high-level disinfection. If ameba are found to contaminate instruments and fascilitate infection, longer immersion times or other disinfectants may need to be considered.

INACTIVATION OF BIOTERRORIST AGENTS

There are presently concerns of biological terrorism. These agents include *B. anthrax* causing anthrax), *Yersinia pestis* (plague), variola major (small pox), *Clostridium botulinum* toxin (botulism), *Francisella tularensis* (tularemia), filoviruses (Ebola hemorrhagic fever, marburg hemorrhagic fever) and arenaviruses (Lassa fever), junin (Argentine hemorrhagic fever) and related viruses.

Susceptibiltiy of these agents to germicides in vitro is similar to that of other related pathogens. Many of these agents are stable enough in the environment that contaminated environmental surfaces or fomites could lead to transmission of agents such as *B. anthracis*,

F. tularensis, variola major, *C. botulinum* toxin and *C. burnetti*. Data suggest that current disinfection and sterilization practices are appropriate for managing patient care equipment and environmental surfaces when potentially contaminated patients are evaluated and/or admitted in a healthcare facility after exposure to a bioterrorist agent.

In instances where healthcare facility is the site of bioterrorist attack, environmental decontamination might require special procedures (e.g. chlorine dioxide gas for *B. anthracis* spores). The only theoretical concern is the possibility that a bioterrorist agent could be engineered to be less susceptible to disinfection and sterilization processes.

INACTIVATION OF CREUTZFELDT-JAKOB DISEASE AGENT

This is the only infective agent, which needs a unique decontamination. CJD is a degenerative neurologic disorder with an incidence rate of one new case in 1 million people per year. Infectivity is dependent on the tissue, with the brain, spinal cord and eye suspected to have highest infectivity. It has been transmitted iatrogenically by means of implanted brain electrodes that were disinfected with ethanol and formaldehyde after use on a patient known to have CJD.Iatrogenic transmission has also been observed in recipients of contaminated human growth hormone, gonadotropin, corneal, pericardial and dura mater grafts. This is because of the highly resistant population of prions, which resist normal inactivation methods. Steam sterilization for at least 30 minutes at a temperature of 132°C (121°C is ineffective) in a gravity displacement sterilizer has been recommended as the preferred method for the treatment of contaminated material. When a prevaccum sterilizer is used, 18 minutes at 134° to 138°C has been found to be effective. Immersion in 1N sodium hydroxide (which is caustic for 1 hour at room temperature) followed by steam sterilization at 121°C for 30 minutes is an alternative procedure for critical and semi-critical items. Because noncritical patient care items or surfaces (e.g. autopsy tables, floors) have not been involved in disease transmission, these surfaces may be disinfected with either bleach (undiluted or upto 1:10 dilution) or 1 N sodium hydroxide at room temperature for 15 minutes or less. A formalin-formic acid procedure is required for inactivating virus activity in tissue samples from patients with CJD.

TOXICOLOGIC AND ENVIRONMENTAL CONCERNS

Germicides can be associated with health hazards varying from mucous membrane irritation to death, later involving accidental ingestion by mentally disturbed patients.

Some water and sewer jurisdictions have excluded the disposal of certain chemical germicides (e.g. glutaraldehyde, formaldehyde, phenol) by means of sewer system. These rules are intended to minimize environmental harm.

If hospitals exceed the maximum allowable concentration for a given chemical (e.g. ≥5 mg/L) they have three options. First they can use alternative products. For example they can change from glutaraldehyde to another disinfectant for high-level disinfection or from phenolics to quaternary ammonium compounds for low-level disinfection. Second the hospitals can collect the disinfectant and dispose it off as a hazardous chemical. Third they can use a commercially available small-scale treatment system that may neutralize glutaraldehyde with glycine.

Disinfection by heat rather than chemicals should be used for instruments and ventilation therapy equipment.

The disadvantages of chemical disinfection include toxic side effects for the patient caused by chemical residues, on the instrument or object; occupational exposure to toxic chemicals and the danger of recontamination by rinsing the instrument with microbially contaminated tap water.

DISINFECTION IN AMBULATORY CARE AND HOME CARE

Since increasing number of patients are now being cared for in ambulatory care and home settings, and many of these might have communicable disease or immunocompromising condition or invasive devices, therefore adequate disinfection in these settings is necessary to provide a safe patient environment. Because the ambulatory -care settings (i.e. outpatient facility) provides the same risk for infection as the hospital the Spaulding scheme of classification described in this guideline should be followed.

The home environment should be much safer than hospitals or ambulatory care. Epidemics should not be a problem, and cross-infection should be rare. The healthcare provider is responsible for providing the responsible family member information about infection-control procedures to follow in the home, including hand hygiene, proper cleaning and disinfection of equipment, and safe storage of cleaned and disinfected devices. Among the products recommended for home disinfection of reusable objects are bleach, alcohol, and hydrogen peroxide. APIC recommends that reusable objects (e.g. tracheostomy tubes) that touch mucous membranes be disinfected by immersion in 70% isopropyl alcohol for 5 minutes or in 3% hydrogen peroxide for 30 minutes. Additionally, a 1:50 dilution of 5.25–6.15% sodium hypochlorite (household bleach) for 5 minutes should be effective. Noncritical items (e.g. blood pressure cuffs, crutches) can be cleaned with a detergent. Blood spills should be handled according to OSHA regulations as previously described (see section on OSHA Blood-borne Pathogen Standard). In general, sterilization of critical items is not practical in homes but theoretically could be accomplished by chemical sterilants or boiling. Single-use disposable items can be used or reusable items sterilized in a hospital.

SUSCEPTIBILITY OF ANTIBIOTIC RESISTANT BACTERIA TO DISINFECTANTS

As with antibiotics, reduced susceptibility (or acquired 'resistance') of bacteria to disinfectants can arise by either chromosomal gene mutation or acquisition of genetic material in the form of plasmids or transposons. When changes occur in bacterial susceptibility that renders an antibiotic ineffective against an infection previously treatable by that antibiotic, the bacteria are referred to as 'resistant.' In contrast, reduced susceptibility to disinfectants does not correlate with failure of the disinfectant because concentrations used in disinfection still greatly exceed the cidal level. Thus, the word 'resistance' when applied to these changes is incorrect, and the preferred term is 'reduced susceptibility' or 'increased tolerance.' No data are available that show that antibiotic-resistant bacteria are less sensitive to the liquid chemical germicides than antibiotic-sensitive bacteria at currently used germicide contact conditions and concentrations.

There is a growing concern of antibiotic resistance amongst bacteria. Of special concern is the increased incidence of infections caused by methicillin-resistant *S. aureus*, vancomycin-resistant *Enterococcus* and multiple drug resistant *M. tuberculosis* and gram-negative bacilli.

Chromosal-mediated antibiotic resistance may confer resistance to broad classes of antibiotics [e.g. methicillin-resistant *S. aureus* (MRSA) exhibits resistance to all penicillins and cephalosporins]. Plasmid mediated resistance may also include multiple drugs. For these reasons, it is also possible that antibiotic-resistant bacteria may also exhibit cross-resistance to antiseptics and disinfectants.

There is ample evidence in literature of plasmid-mediated resistance to antiseptics and disinfectants.

However, these observations have no clinical relevance because even for the more reistant strains the concentrations of disinfectants used in practice are much higher than the observed minimum inhibitory concentrations (MIC's). For example, phenolics are used as surface disinfectants at concentrations of approxiamately 400 ppm and quaternary ammonium compounds at concentrations of approximately 500 ppm. Resistant bacterial strains described in literature have exhibited MIC's less than 15 ppm (micrograms/mL) for phenolics and quarternary ammonium compounds.

In fact Rutala et al.[3] found antibiotic resistant hospital strains of common nosocomial pathogens (e.g. *P. aeruginosa, Klebsiella pneumoniae, E. coli, S. aureus, S. epidermidis, and Enterocococcus)* to be equally susceptible to disinfectants as antibiotic sensitive strains by use of use-dilution. Other investigators have also been unable to demonstrate a relationship between antibiotic resistance and germicide resistance when the disinfectants are used at the manufacturer's use-dilution. Thus It is observed that vancomycin-resistant enterococci (VRE) MRSA and MDR-TB are as sensitive to commonly used disinfectants as drug-sensitive strains at use concentrations.

For these reasons CDC does not recommend any special strategies or germicides with higher potencies for cleaning noncritical surfaces in rooms of patients who are infected with multi-antibiotic resistant organisms such as vancomycin- resistant enterococci. Any registered germicidal detergent is appropriate for the purpose. Lastly, does the use of antiseptics or disinfectants facilitate the development of disinfectant-tolerant organisms? Evidence and reviews indicate enhanced tolerance to disinfectants can be developed in response to disinfectant exposure. However, the level of tolerance is not important in clinical terms because it is low and unlikely to compromise the effectiveness of disinfectants of which much higher concentrations are used.

The issue of whether low-level tolerance to germicides selects for antibiotic-resistant strains is unsettled but might depend on the mechanism by which tolerance is attained. For example, changes in the permeability barrier or efflux mechanisms might affect susceptibility to both antibiotics and germicides, but specific changes to a target site might not. Some researchers have suggested that use of disinfectants or antiseptics (e.g. triclosan) could facilitate development of antibiotic-resistant microorganisms. There is no evidence that using antiseptics or disinfectants selects for antibiotic-resistant organisms in nature or that such mutants survive in nature.[4] In addition, the action of antibiotics and the action of disinfectants differ fundamentally. Antibiotics are selectively toxic and generally have a single target site in bacteria, thereby inhibiting a specific biosynthetic process. Germicides generally are considered nonspecific antimicrobials because of a multiplicity of toxic-effect mechanisms or target sites and are broader spectrum in the types of microorganisms against which they are effective.

The rotational use of disinfectants in some environments (e.g. pharmacy production units) has been recommended and practiced in an attempt to prevent development of resistant microbes. There have been only rare case reports that appropriately used disinfectants have resulted in a clinical problem arising from the selection or development of nonsusceptible microorganisms.

SURFACE DISINFECTION: IS SURFACE DISINFECTION NECESSARY?

The effective use of disinfectants is part of a multibarrier strategy to prevent healthcare-associated infections. Surfaces are considered noncritical items because they contact intact skin. Use of noncritical items or contact with noncritical surfaces carries little risk of causing an infection in patients or staff. Thus, the routine use of germicidal chemicals to disinfect hospital floors and other noncritical items is controversial.[5,6] A 1991 study expanded the Spaulding scheme by dividing the noncritical environmental surfaces into housekeeping surfaces and medical equipment surfaces.[7] The classes of disinfectants used on housekeeping and medical equipment surfaces can be similar. However, the frequency of decontaminating can vary (see recommendations). Medical equipment surfaces (e.g. blood pressure cuffs, stethoscopes, hemodialysis machines, and X-ray machines) can become contaminated with infectious agents and contribute to the spread of healthcare-associated infections. For this reason, noncritical medical equipment surfaces should be disinfected with an low- or intermediate-level disinfectant.

Environmental surfaces (e.g. bedside table) also could potentially contribute to cross-transmission by contamination of healthcare personnel from hand contact with contaminated surfaces, medical equipment, or patients.

Of the seven reasons to use a disinfectant on noncritical surfaces, five are particularly noteworthy and support the use of a germicidal detergent.

1. Hospital floors become contaminated with microorganisms from settling airborne bacteria: by contact with shoes, wheels, and other objects; and occasionally by spills. The removal of microbes is a component in controlling health-care-associated infections. In an investigation of the cleaning of hospital floors, the use of soap and water (80% reduction) was less effective in reducing the numbers of bacteria than was a phenolic disinfectant (94–99.9% reduction).[8] However, a few hours after floor disinfection, the bacterial count was nearly back to the pretreatment level.
2. Detergents become contaminated and result in seeding the patient's environment with bacteria. Investigators have shown that mop water becomes increasingly dirty during cleaning and becomes contaminated if soap and water is used rather than a disinfectant. For example, in one study, bacterial contamination in soap and water without a disinfectant increased from 10 CFU/mL to 34,000 CFU/mL after cleaning a ward, whereas contamination in a disinfectant solution did not change (20 CFU/mL).[9] Contamination of surfaces close to the patient that are frequently touched by the patient or staff (e.g. bed rails) could result in patient exposures.
3. The CDC isolation guideline recommends that noncritical equipment contaminated with blood, body fluids, secretions, or excretions be cleaned and disinfected after use. The same guideline recommends that, in addition to cleaning, disinfection of the bedside equipment and environmental surfaces (e.g. bedrails, bedside tables, carts, commodes, door-knobs, and faucet handles) is indicated for certain pathogens, e.g. enterococci, which can survive in the inanimate environment for prolonged periods.[10]
4. OSHA requires that surfaces contaminated with blood and other potentially infectious materials (e.g. amniotic, pleural fluid) be disinfected.
5. Using a single product throughout the facility can simplify both training and appropriate practice.

Reasons also exist for using a detergent alone on floors because noncritical surfaces contribute minimally to endemic healthcare-associated infections,[11] and no differences have been found in healthcare-associated infections rates when floors are cleaned with detergent rather than disinfectant. Because housekeeping surfaces are associated with the lowest risk for disease transmission, some researchers have suggested that either detergents or a disinfectant/detergent could be used. Regardless of whether a detergent or disinfectant is used on surfaces in a health-care facility, surfaces should be cleaned routinely and when dirty or soiled to provide an aesthetically pleasing environment and to prevent potentially contaminated objects from serving as a source for health-care-associated infections.[12]

Several investigators have recognized heavy microbial contamination of wet mops and cleaning cloths and the potential for spread of such contamination. They have shown that wiping hard surfaces with contaminated cloths can contaminate hands, equipment, and other surfaces. If reusable cleaning cloths or mops are used, they should be decontaminated regularly to prevent surface contamination during cleaning with subsequent transfer of organisms from these surfaces to patients or equipment by the hands of healthcare workers. Some hospitals have begun using a new mopping technique involving microfiber materials to clean floors. Microfibers are densely constructed, polyester and polyamide (nylon) fibers, that are approximately 1/16 the thickness of a human hair. The positively charged microfibers attract dust (which has a negative charge) and are more absorbent than a conventional, cotton-loop mop. Microfiber materials also can be wet with disinfectants, such as quaternary ammonium compounds. In one study, the microfiber system tested demonstrated superior microbial removal compared with conventional string mops when used with a detergent cleaner (94% vs 68%). The use of a disinfectant did not improve the microbial elimination demonstrated by the microfiber system (95% vs 94%). However, use of disinfectant significantly improved microbial removal when a conventional string mop was used (95% vs 68%)(WA Rutala, unpublished data, August 2006). The microfiber system also prevents the possibility of transferring microbes from room to room because a new microfiber pad is used in each room (Table 8.1).

CONTACT TIMES FOR SURFACE DISINFECTANTS

An important issue concerning use of disinfectants for noncritical surfaces in health-care settings is that the contact time specified on the label of the product is often too long to be practically followed. The labels of most products for use against HBV, HIV, or *M. tuberculosis* specify a contact time of 10 minutes. Such a long contact time is not

Table 8.1: Epidemiologic evidence associated with the use of surface disinfectants or detergents on noncritical environmental surfaces[54]

Justification for use of disinfectants for noncritical environmental surfaces
• Surfaces may contribute to transmission of epidemiologically important microbes (e.g. vancomycin-resistant enterococci, methicillin-resistant *S. aureus*, viruses)
• Disinfectants are needed for surfaces contaminated by blood and other potentially infective material
• Disinfectants are more effective than detergents in reducing microbial load on floors
• Detergents become contaminated and result in seeding the patient's environment with bacteria
• Disinfection of noncritical equipment and surfaces is recommended for patients on isolation precautions by the centers for disease control and prevention
• Advantage of using a single product for decontamination of noncritical surfaces, both floors and equipment
• Some newer disinfectants have persistent antimicrobial activity
Justification for using a detergent on noncritical environmental surfaces
• Noncritical surfaces contribute minimally to endemic healthcare-associated infections
• No difference in healthcare-associated infection rates when floors are cleaned with detergent versus disinfectant
• No environmental impact issues with disposal
• No occupational health exposure issues
• Lower costs
• Use of antiseptics/disinfectants selects for antibiotic-resistant bacteria (?)
• More aesthetically pleasing floor

Source: Rutala[54]

practical for disinfection of environmental surfaces in a health-care setting because most health-care facilities apply a disinfectant and allow it to dry (~1 minute). Multiple scientific papers have demonstrated significant microbial reduction with contact times of 30 to 60 seconds.[13-16]

Ideally, product users should consider and use products that have the shortened contact time.

AIR DISINFECTION

Disinfectant spray-fog techniques for antimicrobial control in hospital rooms has been used. This technique of spraying of disinfectants is an unsatisfactory method of decontaminating air and surfaces and is not recommended for general infection control in routine patient-care areas.[10]

MICROBIAL CONTAMINATION OF DISINFECTANTS

Contaminated disinfectants and antiseptics have been occasional vehicles of health-care infections and pseudoepidemics for more than 50 years. High-level disinfectants/ liquid chemical sterilants have not been associated with outbreaks due to intrinsic or extrinsic contamination. Members of the genus *Pseudomonas* (e.g. *P. aeruginosa*) are the most frequent isolates from contaminated disinfectants—recovered from 80% of contaminated products. Their ability to remain viable or grow in use-dilutions of disinfectants is unparalleled. This survival advantage for *Pseudomonas* results presumably from their nutritional versatility, their unique outer membrane that constitutes an effective barrier to the passage of germicides, and/or efflux systems.[17]

In most of the reports that describe illness associated with contaminated disinfectants, the product was used to disinfect patient-care equipment, such as cystoscopes, cardiac catheters, and thermometers. Germicides used as disinfectants that were reported to have been contaminated include chlorhexidine, quaternary ammonium compounds and phenolics.

The following control measures should be instituted to reduce the frequency of bacterial growth in disinfectants and the threat of serious healthcare-associated infections from the use of such contaminated products. First, some disinfectants should not be diluted; those that are diluted must be prepared correctly to achieve the manufacturers' recommended use-dilution. Second, infection-control professionals must learn from the literature what inappropriate activities result in extrinsic contamination (i.e. at the point of use) of germicides and train users to prevent recurrence. Common sources of extrinsic contamination of germicides in the reviewed literature are the water to make working dilutions, contaminated containers, and general contamination of the hospital areas where the germicides are prepared and/ or used. Third, stock solutions of germicides must be stored as indicated on the product label.

FACTORS AFFECTING THE EFFICACY OF DISINFECTION AND STERILIZATION

The activity of germicides against microorganisms depends on a number of factors, some of which are intrinsic qualities of the organism, others of which are the chemical and external physical environment. Awareness of these factors should lead to better use of disinfection and sterilization processes and will be briefly reviewed.

Number and Location of Microorganisms

All other conditions remaining constant, the larger the number of microbes, the more time a germicide needs to destroy all of them. This reinforces the need for scrupulous cleaning of medical instruments before disinfection and sterilization. Reducing the number of microorganisms that must be inactivated through meticulous cleaning, increases the margin of safety when the germicide is used according to the labeling and shortens the exposure time required to kill the entire microbial load.

The location of microorganisms also must be considered when factors affecting the efficacy of germicides are assessed. Medical instruments with multiple pieces must be disassembled and equipment such as endoscopes that have crevices, joints, and channels are more difficult to disinfect than are flat-surface equipment because penetration of the disinfectant of all parts of the equipment is more difficult. Only surfaces that directly contact the germicide will be disinfected, so there must be no air pockets and the equipment must be completely immersed for the entire exposure period.

Innate Resistance of Microorganisms

Microorganisms vary greatly in their resistance to chemical germicides and sterilization processes (Fig. 8.1).[18] Intrinsic resistance mechanisms in microorganisms to disinfectants vary. For example, spores are resistant to disinfectants because the spore coat and cortex act as a barrier, mycobacteria have a waxy cell wall that prevents disinfectant entry, and gram-negative bacteria possess an outer membrane that acts as a barrier to the uptake of disinfectants. The most resistant microbial subpopulation controls the sterilization or disinfection time. That is, to destroy the most resistant types of microorganisms (i.e. bacterial spores), the user needs to employ exposure times and a concentration of germicide needed to achieve complete destruction. Except for prions, bacterial spores possess the highest innate resistance to chemical germicides, followed by coccidia (e.g. *Cryptosporidium*), mycobacteria (e.g. *M. tuberculosis*), nonlipid or small viruses (e.g. poliovirus, and coxsackievirus), fungi (e.g. *Aspergillus,* and *Candida*), vegetative bacteria (e.g. *Staphylococcus,* and *Pseudomonas*) and lipid or medium-size viruses (e.g. herpes, and HIV). The germicidal resistance exhibited by the gram-positive and gram-negative bacteria is similar with some exceptions (e.g. *P. aeruginosa* which shows greater resistance to some disinfectants).

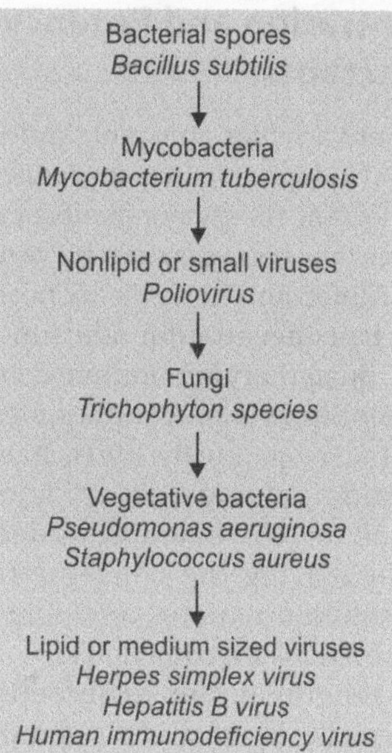

Fig. 8.1: Showing descending order of resistance to germicidal chemicals (This is considered a rough guide to general susceptibility of microorganisms to disinfectants)

Rickettsiae, Chlamydiae, and mycoplasma cannot be placed in this scale of relative resistance because information about the efficacy of germicides against these agents is limited. Because these microorganisms contain lipid and are similar in structure and composition to other bacteria, they can be predicted to be inactivated by the same germicides that destroy lipid viruses and vegetative bacteria. A known exception to this supposition is *Coxiella burnetti,* which has demonstrated resistance to disinfectants.[19]

Concentration and Potency of Disinfectants

With other variables constant, and with one exception (iodophors), the more concentrated the disinfectant, the greater its efficacy and the shorter the time necessary to achieve microbial kill. All disinfectants however are not similarly affected by concentration adjustments. For example, quaternary ammonium compounds and phenol have a concentration exponent of 1 and 6, respectively; thus, halving the concentration of a quaternary ammonium compound requires doubling its disinfecting time, but halving the concentration of a phenol solution requires a 64-fold (i.e. 26) increase in its disinfecting time.

The length of the disinfection time depends on the potency of the germicide.

Physical and Chemical Factors

Several physical and chemical factors also influence disinfectant procedures: temperature, pH, relative humidity, and water hardness.

For example, the activity of most disinfectants increases as the temperature increases, but some exceptions exist. Furthermore, too great an increase in temperature causes the disinfectant to degrade and weakens its germicidal activity and thus might produce a potential health hazard.

An increase in pH improves the antimicrobial activity of some disinfectants (e.g. glutaraldehyde, quaternary ammonium compounds) but decreases the antimicrobial activity of others (e.g. phenols, hypochlorites, and iodine). The pH influences the antimicrobial activity by altering the disinfectant molecule or the cell surface.

Relative humidity is the single most important factor influencing the activity of gaseous disinfectants/sterilants, such as EtO, chlorine dioxide, and formaldehyde.

Water hardness (i.e. high concentration of divalent cations) reduces the rate of kill of certain disinfectants because divalent cations (e.g. magnesium, calcium) in the hard water interact with the disinfectant to form insoluble precipitates.

Organic and Inorganic Matter

Organic matter in the form of serum, blood, pus, or fecal or lubricant material can interfere with the antimicrobial activity of disinfectants in at least two ways. Most commonly, interference occurs by a chemical reaction between the germicide and the organic matter resulting in a complex that is less germicidal or non-germicidal, leaving less of the active germicide available for attacking microorganisms. Chlorine and iodine disinfectants, in particular, are prone to such interaction. Alternatively, organic material can protect microorganisms from attack by acting as a physical barrier.

Protection by inorganic contaminants of microorganisms to all sterilization processes results from occlusion in salt crystals. This further emphasizes the importance of meticulous cleaning of medical devices before any sterilization or disinfection procedure because both organic and inorganic soils are easily removed by washing.

Duration of Exposure

Items must be exposed to the germicide for the appropriate minimum contact time. Multiple investigators have demonstrated the effectiveness of low-level disinfectants against vegetative bacteria (e.g. *Listeria, E. coli, Salmonella*, VRE, MRSA), yeasts (e.g. *Candida*), mycobacteria (e.g. *M. tuberculosis*), and viruses (e.g. poliovirus) at exposure times of 30–60 seconds.[20,21]

All lumens and channels of endoscopic instruments must contact the disinfectant. Air pockets interfere with the disinfection process, and items that float on the disinfectant will not be disinfected. The disinfectant must be introduced reliably into the internal channels of the device. Certain contact times have proved reliable but, in general, longer contact times are more effective than shorter contact times.

Biofilms

Microorganisms may be protected from disinfectants by production of thick masses of cells and extracellular materials, or biofilms. Biofilms are microbial communities that are tightly attached to surfaces and cannot be easily removed. Once these masses form, microbes within them can be resistant to disinfectants by multiple mechanisms, including physical characteristics of older biofilms, genotypic variation of the bacteria, microbial production of neutralizing enzymes, and physiologic gradients within the biofilm (e.g. pH). Bacteria within biofilms are up to 1,000 times more resistant to antimicrobials than are the same bacteria in suspension.[22] Although new decontamination methods are being investigated for removing biofilms, chlorine and monochloramines can effectively inactivate biofilm bacteria.[23,24] Investigators have hypothesized that the glycocalyx-like cellular masses on the interior walls of polyvinyl chloride pipe would protect embedded organisms from some disinfectants and be a reservoir for continuous contamination. Biofilms have been found in whirlpools,[25] dental unit waterlines,[26] and numerous medical devices (e.g. contact lenses, pacemakers, hemodialysis systems, urinary catheters, central venous catheters, endoscopes.[22,24,27,28] Their presence can have serious implications for immunocompromised patients and patients who have indwelling medical devices. Some enzymes[22,29,30] and detergents[22] can degrade biofilms or reduce numbers of viable bacteria within a biofilm.

CLEANING

Cleaning is the removal of foreign material (e.g. soil, and organic material) from objects and is normally accomplished using water with detergents or enzymatic products. Thorough cleaning is required before high-level disinfection and sterilization because inorganic and organic materials that remain on the surfaces of instruments interfere with the effectiveness of these processes. Also, if soiled materials dry or bake onto the instruments, the removal process becomes more difficult and the disinfection or sterilization process less effective or ineffective. Surgical instruments should be presoaked or rinsed to prevent drying of blood and to soften or remove blood from the instruments.

Cleaning is done manually in use areas without mechanical units (e.g. ultrasonic cleaners or washer-disinfectors) or for fragile or difficult-to-clean instruments. With manual cleaning, the two essential components are friction and fluidics. Friction (e.g. rubbing/scrubbing the soiled area with a brush) is an old and dependable method. Fluidics (i.e. fluids under pressure) is used to remove soil and debris from internal channels after brushing and when the design does not allow passage of a brush through a channel. When a washer-disinfector is used, care should be taken in loading instruments: hinged instruments should be opened fully to allow adequate contact with the detergent solution; stacking of instruments in washers should be avoided; and instruments should be disassembled as much as possible.

The most common types of mechanical or automatic cleaners are ultrasonic cleaners, washer-decontaminators, washer-disinfectors, and washer-sterilizers. Ultrasonic cleaning removes soil by cavitation and implosion in which waves of acoustic energy are propagated in aqueous solutions to disrupt the bonds that hold particulate matter to surfaces. Bacterial contamination can be present in used ultrasonic cleaning solutions (and other used detergent solutions). Even though ultrasound alone does not significantly inactivate bacteria, sonication can act synergistically to increase the cidal efficacy of a disinfectant. Users of ultrasonic cleaners should be aware that the cleaning fluid could result in endotoxin contamination of surgical instruments, which could cause severe inflammatory reactions. Washer-sterilizers are modified steam sterilizers that clean by filling the chamber with water and detergent through which steam passes to provide agitation. Instruments are subsequently rinsed and subjected to a short steam-sterilization cycle. Another washer-sterilizer employs rotating spray arms for a wash cycle followed by a steam sterilization cycle at 285°F. Washer-decontaminators/disinfectors act like a dishwasher that uses a combination of water circulation and detergents to remove soil. These units sometimes have a cycle that subjects the instruments to a heat process (e.g. 93°C for 10 minutes). Washer-disinfectors are generally computer-controlled units for cleaning, disinfecting, and drying solid and hollow surgical and medical equipment. Studies have shown that manual and mechanical cleaning of endoscopes achieves approximately a 4-log 10 reduction of contaminating organisms. Thus, cleaning alone effectively reduces the number of microorganisms on contaminated equipment. When manual methods were compared with automated methods for cleaning reusable accessory devices used for minimally invasive surgical procedures, the automated method was more efficient for cleaning biopsy forceps and ported and nonported laparoscopic devices.

For instrument cleaning, a neutral or near-neutral pH detergent solution commonly is used because such solutions generally provide the best material compatibility profile and good soil removal.

Enzymes, usually proteases, sometimes are added to neutral pH solutions to assist in removing organic material. Enzymes in these formulations attack proteins that make up a large portion of common soil (e.g. blood, pus). Cleaning solutions also can contain lipases (enzymes active on fats) and amylases (enzymes active on starches). Enzymatic cleaners are not disinfectants, and proteinaceous enzymes can be inactivated by germicides. As with all chemicals, enzymes must be rinsed from the equipment or adverse reactions (e.g. fever, residual amounts of high-level disinfectants, proteinaceous residue) could result. Enzyme solutions should be used in accordance with manufacturer's instructions, which include proper dilution of the enzymatic detergent and contact with equipment for the amount of time specified on the label. Detergent enzymes can result in asthma or other allergic effects in users.

Neutral pH detergent solutions that contain enzymes are compatible with metals and other materials used in medical instruments and are the best choice for cleaning delicate medical instruments, especially flexible endoscopes. Alkaline-based cleaning agents are used for processing medical devices because they efficiently dissolve protein and fat residues however, they can be corrosive.

Although the effectiveness of high-level disinfection and sterilization mandates effective cleaning, no 'real-time' tests exist that can be employed in a clinical setting to verify cleaning. All instruments should be individually inspected and be visibly clean.

DISINFECTION

Many disinfectants are used alone or in combinations (e.g. hydrogen peroxide and peracetic acid) in the health-care setting. These include alcohols, chlorine and chlorine compounds, formaldehyde, glutaraldehyde, ortho-phthalaldehyde, hydrogen peroxide, iodophors, peracetic acid, phenolics, and quaternary ammonium compounds.

In most instances, a given product is designed for a specific purpose and is to be used in a certain manner. Therefore, users should read labels carefully to ensure the correct product is selected for the intended use and applied efficiently.

Disinfectants are not interchangeable, and incorrect concentrations and inappropriate disinfectants can result in excessive costs. Because occupational diseases among cleaning personnel have been associated with use of several disinfectants (e.g. formaldehyde, glutaraldehyde, and chlorine), precautions (e.g. gloves and proper ventilation) should be used to minimize exposure. Asthma and reactive airway disease can occur in sensitized persons exposed to any airborne chemical, including germicides. The preferred method of control is elimination of the chemical (through engineering controls or substitution) or relocation of the worker.

TYPES OF CHEMICAL DISINFECTANTS

Most of the hospitals have their own policy for the use of disinfectants, but it is still possible to find that inappropriate disinfectants are used at inadequate or inappropriate concentrations. There is a tendency to use expensive and ineffective disinfectant, when cheaper or more effective agents are available, or when a disinfectant is not required at all. A disinfectant policy will certainly increase the cost effectiveness of disinfectants in hospital.

The following overview of the performance characteristics of each provides users with sufficient information to select an appropriate disinfectant for any item and use it in the most efficient way.

Following disinfectants are commonly used in hospitals.

i. Alcohols
ii. Chlorine and chlorine compounds
iii. Aldehydes
  a. Formaldehyde
  b. Para formaldehyde
  c. Glutaraldehyde
iv. Oxidizing agents
  a. Hydrogen peroxide
  b. Plasma sterilization
v. Iodine and Iodophors
vi. Peracetic acid
vii. Phenolics
viii. Quaternary ammonium compounds

Alcohols

Examples are the two water-soluble chemical compounds, ethyl alcohol (ethanol), isopropyl alcohol (isopropanol). These are bactericidal rather than bacteriostatic against vegetative forms of bacteria; they also are tuberculocidal, fungicidal, and virucidal but do not destroy bacterial spores. Their cidal activity drops sharply when diluted below 50% concentration and the optimum bactericidal concentration is 60 to 90%, hence usually used in a concentration of 70%. They are rapidly acting disinfectants and are mainly used as skin antiseptics.

Advantages: Their advantage is that they evaporate rapidly leaving the treated surfaces dry.

Disadvantages:

1. They have a poor penetrative power, and their activity is lower in presence of proteins.
2. Alcohols are flammable and hence must be stored in a cool well-ventilated area.
3. They also evaporate rapidly making extended exposure time difficult to achieve unless the items are immersed.
4. They damage the shellac mountings of lensed instruments.
5. Tend to swell and harden rubber and certain plastic tubing after prolonged and repeated use, bleach rubber and plastic tiles.
6. Damage tonometer tips (by deterioration of the glue) after the equivalent of 1 working year of routine use.
7. Tonometer biprisms soaked in alcohol for 4 days developed rough front surfaces that potentially could cause corneal damage; this appeared to be caused by weakening of the cementing substances used to fabricate the biprisms.
8. Corneal opacification has been reported when tonometer tips were swabbed with alcohol immediately before measurement of intraocular pressure.

Mechanism of action and range of activity: They act by denaturating bacterial proteins. They are active against vegetative forms of bacteria, fungi, viruses, mycobacterium, but not against bacterial spores. Ethanol and isopropanol are more effective than absolute alcohol. Isopropanol is preferred to ethanol because it is a better solvent, more bactericidal and less volatile.

Uses:

1. To disinfect oral or rectal thermometer, scissors , stethoscopes, hospital pagers.
2. Rapid disinfection of smooth clean surfaces (e.g. trolley tops; thermometer probes and electrical/ electronic equipment) that cannot be safely immersed in an aqueous disinfectant.
3. Commonly used for skin disinfection (e.g. without additives for treating skin prior to injection). With addition of 1% glycerol or other suitable emollients, 60–70% alcohol rubbed on hand until skin is dry, is an effective agent for the rapid disinfection of physically clean hands, especially if hand washing facilities are unsuitable or not readily available. The addition of non-volatile antiseptics (e.g. chlorhexidine, povidone-iodine, triclosan) may provide residual antiseptic action on skin.
4. It is occasionally used to disinfect external surfaces of equipment (e.g. stethoscopes, ventilators, manual ventilation bags, cardiopulmonary resuscitation manikins, ultrasounds and medication preparation areas.
5. Methyl alcohol is effective against fungal spores and is used for treating cabinets and incubators affected by them. The inside of the chambers are wiped with liberal amounts of methanol. A pad moistened with methanol and a dish of water (to ensure humidity) is kept inside and the incubator is left at working temperature for several hours. However it must be remembered that methyl alcohol vapor is toxic and inflammable.

Alcohols are not recommended for sterilizing medical and surgical materials, because of their lack of action on spore and inability to penetrate protein rich material. Fatal postoperative wound infections with *Clostridium* have occurred when alcohols were used to sterilize surgical instruments contaminated with bacterial spores.

Ethyl alcohol and isopropyl alcohol therefore are not high-level disinfectants because of their inability to inactivate bacterial spores and because of isopropyl alcohol's inability to kill hydrophilic viruses (e.g. echovirus, Coxsackie's viruses).

Chlorine and Chlorine Compounds

Hypochlorites are the most widely used of the chlorine disinfectants. They are available in two forms (1) liquid, e.g. sodium hypochlorite and (2) solid-calcium hypochlorite, sodium dichloroisocyanurate. The most prevalent chlorine products are aqueous solutions of 5.25%–6.15% sodium hypochlorite, usually called household bleach.

Alternative compounds that release chlorine and are used in the health-care setting include demand-release chlorine dioxide, sodium dichloroisocyanurate, and chloramine-T.

The advantage of these compounds over the hypochlorites is that they retain chlorine longer and therefore exerts a more prolonged bactericidal effect. Sodium dichloroisocyanurate tablets are also stable, and the microbicidal activity of solutions prepared from these tablets may be greater than that of sodium hypochlorite solutions containing the same total available chlorine.

Another product chlorine dioxide was also available, but this product has been voluntarily removed from the market because its use was found to cause dialyzer membrane leaks, which allowed bacteria to migrate from the dialysis fluid side of the dialyzer to the blood side in cellulose-based membranes.

For surface disinfection in laboratory and healthcare settings,the CDC recommends the use of household bleach diluted to approximately 5,000 parts per million (ppm)

Table 8.2: Dilutions of household bleach and chlorine ppm: Preparation of various chlorine concentrations[50]

	Desired chlorine concentration			
	5,000 ppm	1,000 ppm	500 ppm	100 ppm
Dilution of bleach (5.25% NaOCL) prepared fresh for use within 24 hours	1:10* (0.5%)	1:50 (0.1%)	1:100 (0.05%)	1:500 (0.01%)
Dilution of bleach (5.25% NaOCL) prepared fresh and used for 1–30 days	1:5**	1:25	1:50	1:250

*To achieve a 1:10 dilution adds one part of bleach to nine parts of water.
** To achieve 1:5 dilution add one part of bleach to four parts of water.

available chlorine. Stock household bleach is 5.25% sodium hypochlorite equal to approximately 50,000 ppm available chlorine, therefore, it must be diluted to 10% with water (or expressed as a ratio, 9 parts water to 1 part bleach) to arrive at the recommended 5,000 ppm strength (Table 8.2).

Start with	Sodium hypochlorite	Available chlorine
Regular household bleach	5.25% NaChl	50,000 ppm AvChl
Dilute 1 part bleach to 9 parts water	0.525% NaChl	5,000 ppm AvChl

Therefore, if you use 5.25% household bleach:

- 1:10 dilution = 0.5% = 5,000 ppm
- 1:50 dilution = 0.1% = 1,000 ppm
- 1:100 dilution = 0.05% = 500 ppm
- 1:200 dilution = 0.025% = 200 ppm
- 1:500 dilution = 0.01% = 100 ppm

Low concentrations of free chlorine have biocidal effects on mycoplasma (25 ppm) and vegetative bacteria (<1 ppm) within seconds in presence of organic matter. A concentration of 100 ppm will kill 99.9% of bacillus subtlis spores within 5 minutes, and will destroy fungal agents in less than 1 hour. Higher concentrations (1000 ppm) of chlorine are required to kill *M. tuberculosis*.

Advantages:

1. They are cheap and fast acting.
2. They have a broad spectrum of antimicrobial activity. They are effective against bacteria, viruses, fungi, and bacterial spores. They are particularly recommended for use where special hazards of viral infection exist (e.g. Hepatitis B virus or HIV virus).
3. Do not leave toxic residues, are unaffected by water hardness, remove dried or fixed organisms and biofilms from surfaces, and have a low incidence of serious toxicity.

Disadvantages:

1. They are unstable, readily inactivated by organic matter (e.g. pus, dirt, blood, etc).
2. They are corrosive to metals in high concentrations (>500 ppm), and may damage material like plastics, rubber, some metals and fabrics.
3. Discolor or 'bleach' fabrics.
4. Release toxic chlorine gas when mixed with ammonia or acid (e.g. household cleaning agents), and relative stability.
5. Sodium hypochlorite at the concentration used in household bleach (5.25–6.15%) can produce ocular irritation or oropharyngeal, esophageal, and gastric burns.
6. They are not compatible with some detergents and so should not be mixed with them, and should not also be mixed with acids including acidic body fluids, such as urine, as the free chlorine produced may be harmful particularly in a confined place.
7. Solutions must be stabilized by alkali or sodium chloride.
8. When hypochlorite comes in contact with formaldehyde, carcinogen bis-chloromethyl ether is formed and the

animal carcinogen trihalomethane is produced when hot water is hyperchlorinated.

Superoxidized Water

The microbicidal activity of a new disinfectant, 'superoxidized water,' has been examined. The concept of electrolyzing saline to create a disinfectant or antiseptics is appealing because the basic materials of saline and electricity are inexpensive and the end product (i.e. water) does not damage the environment. The main products of this water are hypochlorous acid (e.g. at a concentration of about 144 mg/L) and chlorine. As with any germicide, the antimicrobial activity of superoxidized water is strongly affected by the concentration of the active ingredient (available free chlorine). Although superoxidized water is intended to be generated fresh at the point of use, when tested under clean conditions the disinfectant was effective within 5 minutes when 48 hours old. Unfortunately, the equipment required to produce the product can be expensive because parameters such as pH, current, and redox potential must be closely monitored. The solution is nontoxic to biologic tissues.

Mechanism of action: Disinfection of all chlorine compounds is due to release of free chlorine. When hypochlorites are added to water, the chlorine reacts with water to form hypochlorous acid, which is a strong oxidizing agent and effective disinfectant.

The microbicidal activity of chlorine is largely attributable to undissociated hypochlorous acid (HOCL). The dissociation of hypochlorous acid to the less microbicidal form (hypochlorite ion, OCL) is dependent on pH. As the pH increases, more hypochlorite ion is formed, and microbicidal activity decreases.

The exact mechanism by which free chlorine destroys microorganisms has not been elucidated. Inactivation by chlorine can result from a number of factors: oxidation of sulfhydryl enzymes and amino acids; ring chlorination of amino acids; loss of intracellular contents; decreased uptake of nutrients; inhibition of protein synthesis; decreased oxygen uptake; oxidation of respiratory components; decreased adenosine triphosphate production; breaks in DNA; and depressed DNA synthesis. The actual microbicidal mechanism of chlorine might involve a combination of these factors or the effect of chlorine on critical sites.

Uses: Because household bleach contains 5.25%–6.15% sodium hypochlorite, or 52,500–61,500 ppm available chlorine, a 1:1,000 dilution provides about 53–62 ppm available chlorine, and a 1:10 dilution of household bleach provides about 5,250–6,150 ppm., and 1:100 dilution provides 525–615 ppm.

Note:

1. Used in disinfection of swimming pools, water supplies, feeding bottles, food and dairy industries.
2. Inorganic chlorine solution is used for disinfecting tonometer heads and for spot disinfection of countertops and floors.
3. A 1:10 (5,000 ppm) or 1:100 (500 ppm) dilution of 5.25–6.15% sodium hypochlorite (household bleach) can be used for decontamination of blood spills. For small spills of blood (i.e. drops of blood) on noncritical surfaces, the area can be disinfected with a 1:100 dilution of 5.25–6.15% sodium hypochlorite or an tuberculocidal disinfectant. Because hypochlorites and other germicides are substantially inactivated in the presence of blood, large spills of blood require that the surface be cleaned before an tuberculocidal disinfectant or a 1:10 (final concentration) solution of household bleach is applied. CDC recommends a contact time of 20 minutes for decontamination of spills,[30a] while some others say a minimum contact time of 10 minutes is essential.[30b]
4. At least 500 ppm of available chlorine for 10 minutes is recommended for decontamination of cardiopulmonary resuscitation training manikins.
5. Other uses in healthcare include its use as an irrigating agent in endodontic

treatment, dental appliances and as a disinfectant for laundry.

6. Used in hydrotherapy tanks, chloramine T and hypochlorites have been used to disinfect hydrotherapy equipment.
7. Used for regulated medical waste before disposal.
8. Used in the water distribution system in hemodialysis centers and hemodialysis machines.

Hypochlorite solutions in tap water at pH 8.0 or greater are stable for a period of 1 month when stored at room temperature (23°C). In closed opaque plastic containers. During one month at room temperature, the free available chlorine levels of solutions in opened and closed polyethylene containers are reduced maximally to 40% to 50% of the original concentration. Therefore if one wishes to have a solution containing 500 ppm of available chlorine at day 30, a solution initially containing 1000 ppm should be prepared. If stored in a brown bottle, there is no decomposition of the sodium hypochlorite solution (see Table 8.2).

Various chlorine releasing compounds have been used in different concentrations in clean contaminated and grossly contaminated conditions (Table 8.3).

Aldehydes

Formaldehyde

Is used as a disinfectant and a sterilant in both its liquid form and its gaseous state.

Liquid form: Formaldehyde is sold and used principally as a water-based solution called formalin which is 35% formaldehyde by weight. The aqueous solution is a bactericide, tuberculocide, fungicide, virucide, and sporicide.

OSHA has indicated that formaldehyde should be handled in the work place as a potential carcinogen, and an employee exposure standard should be set for formaldehyde that limits an 8-hour time-weighted average exposure to a concentration of 0.75 ppm. The standard includes a second permissible exposure limit in the form of a short-term exposure limit (STEL) of 2 ppm that is the maximum exposure allowed during a 15-minute period. Ingestion of formaldehyde can be fatal, and long-term exposure to low levels in the air or on the skin can cause asthma-like respiratory problems and skin irritation, such as dermatitis and itching. For this reason employee should have limited direct contact with formaldehyde. These considerations limit the role of formaldehyde in sterilization and disinfection processes.

Mechanism of action: Formaldehyde inactivates microorganisms by alkylating the amino and sulfhydryl groups of proteins and the ring nitrogen atoms of purine bases.

Advantages and disadvantages: Although formaldehyde-alcohol is a chemical sterilant and formaldehyde is a high-level disinfectant, uses of formaldhyde in hospital are limited by its irritating fumes and the pungent odor

Table 8.3: Concentrations/dilutions of chlorine releasing compounds to be used in clean contaminated and grossly contaminated conditions[51,52]

Sl. No.	Disinfectant	Clean contaminated	Grossly contaminated
1.	Sodium hypochlorite	0.1% (1000 ppm) 1 g/L	1% (10,000 ppm) 10 g/L
2.	Liquid bleach (usually 5% available chlorine)	20 mL/L (1000 ppm)	200 mL/L. (5000 ppm)
3.	Calcium hypochlorite (usually 70% available chlorine)	1.4 g/L	14 g/L
4.	NaDCC (usually 60% available chlorine-monostable, available as 1.5 g tablet)	1.7 g/L	17 g/L
5.	Chloramine (slow chlorine release-more stable than 1 and 2–25% available chlorine)	2.0 g/L	20 g/L

that is apparent at very low levels (<1 ppm). When it is used direct employee exposure is generally limited, but significant exposures have been documented for employees of renal transplant units and students in gross anatomy laboratory.

Uses:

1. For preparing viral vaccines (e.g. poliovirus, influenza).
2. Preservation of anatomical specimens.
3. As an embalming agent.
4. 10% formalin containing half percent sodium tetraborate is used to sterilize clean metal instruments.
5. Disinfection of hemodialyzers that are reused on the same patient: for this if formaldehyde is used at room temperature, then CDC recommends a concentration of 4% with a minimum exposure time of 24 hours.
6. Aqueous formaldehyde solutions (1% to 2%) have been used to disinfect the internal fluid pathways of dialysis machines.

To prevent health hazard to patients undergoing dialysis, the dialysis equipment must be thoroughly rinsed and tested for residual formaldehyde before use.

Other disinfectants that are available for dialysis systems are chlorine-based disinfectants, glutaraldehyde-based disinfectants, per acetic acid with hydrogen peroxide. Some dialysis systems use hot water for control of microbial contamination.

Formaldehyde gas: Formaldehyde gas is used for sterilizing instruments, heat sensitive catheters, or other articles likely to be damaged by heat such as clothing, woolen blankets, mattresses, respiratory and other heat-sensitive instruments, furniture and books. It is also used for fumigation of operation theatres, wards, sick rooms, and laboratories.

The gas is irritant and toxic when inhaled. Surfaces, which have been disinfected, give an irritant vapour for some time after disinfection. This can be nullified by exposure to ammonia vapor after disinfection has been completed. But in view of the health hazards due to formalin as stated earlier, one should not go for use of formaldehyde if other better alternatives are available.

Paraformaldehyde

This is a solid polymer of formaldehyde, which may be vaporized by heat for the gaseous decontamination of laminar flow biologic safety cabinets when maintenance work or filter changes require access to the sealed portion of the cabinet.

Glutaraldehyde

Is a saturated dialdehyde. It has gained acceptance as a high-level disinfectant and sterilant. Aqueous solutions are acidic and generally in this state are not sporicidal. Only when the solution is 'activated', (made alkaline) by alkalizing agents to a Ph of 7.5 to 8.0 does the solution become sporicidal. Once activated these solutions have a shelf life of minimally 14 days because of the polymerization of the glutaraldehyde molecules at alkaline pH levels. This polymerization blocks the active sites (aldehyde groups) of the glutaraldehyde molecules that are responsible for its biocidal activity.

Novel glutaraldehyde formulations (e.g. glutaraldehyde-phenate, potentiated acid glutaraldehyde, stabilized alkaline glutaraldehyde) have been produced that have overcome the problem of rapid loss of stability (e.g. use life 28 to 30 days) while generally maintaining excellent microbicidal activity. It should be remembered however that antimicrobial activity is dependent not only on age but also on use conditions such as dilution and organic stress.

Advantage:

1. Excellent microbicidal properties.
2. Activity in presence of organic matter (20% bovine serum).
3. Non-corrosive action on endoscopic equipment, thermometers and rubber or plastic equipment.
4. Non-coagulation of proteinaceous material.

Mechanism of action: The microbicidal activity is a consequence of its alkylation of sulfhydryl, hydroxyl, carboxyl, and amino groups of microorganisms, which alters RNA, DNA and protein synthesis.

Range of action: The in vitro inactivation of microorganisms by glutaraldehydes has been extensively investigated and reviewed.[31,32] Several investigators have shown that 2% aqueous solution of glutaraldehyde, buffered to a PH of 7.5 to 8.5 with sodium bicarbonate, were effective in killing vegetative bacteria in less than 2 minutes; *M.tuberculosis*, fungi and viruses in less then 10 minutes; and spores of *Bacillus* and *Clostridium* species in 3 hours,[33-35] spores of *Clostridium difficile* are more rapidly killed (e.g 20 minutes) by 2% glutaraldehyde. Concern has been raised about the mycobactericidal power of glutaraldehyde. On the basis of several studies, it has been decided that 20 minutes at room temperature with 2% glutaraldehyde is the minimum exposure time to reliably kill organisms such as *M. tuberculosis* that are resistant to disinfectants. A time of 60 mins should be used to kill oocysts of *Cryptosporidium.*

Uses: Glutaraldehyde is mainly used as a high-level disinfectant.

1. It is used as a high-level disinfectant for medical equipment such as endoscopes, respiratory therapy equipment, dialyzers, transducers, anesthesia equipment, spirometry tubing and hemodialysis proportioning and dialysate delivery systems, and reuse of laparoscopic disposable plastic trocars.
2. It is non-corrosive to metals and does not damage lensed instruments, rubber or plastics.

It should not be used for noncritical surfaces; it is too toxic and expensive for this application.

Dilution of glutaraldehyde commonly occurs during use, the concentration may fall to less than 1% by four days; therefore a check should be kept on the dilution of glutaraldehyde when in use. Test strips are available for determining whether an effective concentration of active ingredients (e.g. glutaraldehyde) is present despite repeated use and dilution. The glutaraldehyde test kits have been preliminarily evaluated for efficacy and range. And most test strips are constructed to indicate a concentration above 1.5%. The frequency of testing should be based on how frequently the solutions are used (e.g. if used daily test daily; used weekly, test before use; used 30 times per day, test each 10th use), but the strips should not be used to extend the use life beyond the expiration date). Data suggest the chemicals in the test strip deteriorate with time and a manufacturer's expiration date should be placed on the bottles. The bottle of test strips should be dated when opened and used for the period of time indicated on the bottle (e.g. 120 days). The results of test strip monitoring should be documented. The concentration should be considered unacceptable or unsafe when the test indicates a dilution below the product's minimum effective concentration (MEC) (generally to ≤1.0%–1.5% glutaraldehyde) by the indicator not changing color. The solution should be considered unsafe when a dilution of 1% glutaraldehyde or lower is measured.

It has been reported that proctitis can be caused by glutaraldehyde exposure from residual endoscopes solution contaminating the air-water channel and is preventable by thorough endoscope rinsing. Similarly keratopathy was reported to be caused by ophthalmic instruments that were inadequately rinsed after soaking in 2% glutaraldehyde.

Healthcare workers can become exposed to elevated levels of glutaraldehyde vapor when equipment is processed in poorly ventilated rooms, when spills occur or when there are open immersion baths. Acute or chronic exposure can result in skin irritation or dermatitis, mucous membrane irritation (eye, nose, mouth), or pulmonary symptoms. Epistaxis, allergic contact dermatitis, asthma, and rhinitis also have been reported in health-care workers exposed to glutaraldehyde.

Glutaraldehyde exposure should be monitored to ensure a safe work. In these situations the glutaraldehyde level in the air could reach its ceiling limit of 0.05 ppm. Engineering and work control practice that may be used to combat these problems include the following; improved ventilation (7 to 15 air exchanges per hour); use of ducted exhaust hoods or ductless fume hoods with absorbents for glutaraldehyde vapor, tight fitting lids on immersion bath; and personal protective equipment [e.g. gloves (nitrite rubber, butyl rubber, polyethylene), goggles] to minimize skin or mucous membrane contact. Some workers have been fitted with a half face respirator with organic vapor 'filters' or offered a type 'C' supplied air respirator with a full face piece operated in a positive pressure mode. In general, engineering controls are preferred over work-practice and administrative controls because they do not require active participation by the healthcare worker. If glutaraldehyde disposal through the sanitary sewer system is restricted, sodium bisulfate can be used to neutralize the glutaraldehyde and make it safe for disposal.

Ortho-phthalaldehyde

Ortho-phthalaldehyde (OPA) is a high-level disinfectant that received FDA clearance in October 1999. It contains 0.55% 1,2 benzenedicarboxaldehyde (OPA). OPA solution is a clear, pale-blue liquid with a pH of 7.5.

Mode of action: Preliminary studies on the mode of action of OPA suggest that both OPA and glutaraldehyde interact with amino acids, proteins, and microorganisms. However, OPA is a less potent cross-linking agent. This is compensated for by the lipophilic aromatic nature of OPA that is likely to assist its uptake through the outer layers of mycobacteria and gram-negative bacteria. OPA appears to kill spores by blocking the spore germination process.

Studies have demonstrated excellent microbicidal activity in vitro. For example, OPA has superior mycobactericidal activity (5-log10 reduction in 5 minutes) to glutaraldehyde. OPA showed good activity against the mycobacteria tested, including the glutaraldehyde-resistant strains.

Uses: OPA has several potential advantages over glutaraldehyde.

1. It has excellent stability over a wide pH range (pH 3–9).
2. It is not a known irritant to the eyes and nasal passages, does not require exposure monitoring, has a barely perceptible odor, and requires no activation.
3. OPA, like glutaraldehyde, has excellent material compatibility.

Disadvantages:

1. A potential disadvantage of OPA is that it stains proteins gray (including unprotected skin) and thus must be handled with caution. However, skin staining would indicate improper handling that requires additional training and/or personal protective equipment (e.g. gloves, eye and mouth protection, and fluid-resistant gowns).
2. OPA residues remaining on inadequately water-rinsed transesophageal echocardiogram probes can stain the patient's mouth. Meticulous cleaning, using the correct OPA exposure time (e.g., 12 minutes) and copious rinsing of the probe with water should eliminate this problem. The results of one study provided a basis for a recommendation that rinsing of instruments disinfected with OPA will require at least 250 mL of water per channel to reduce the chemical residue to a level that will not compromise patient or staff safety (<1 ppm).[36] Personal protective equipment should be worn when contaminated instruments, equipment, and chemicals are handled. In addition, equipment must be thoroughly rinsed to prevent discoloration of a patient's skin or mucous membrane.

Oxidizing Agents

Hydrogen Peroxide

The literature contains several accounts of the properties, germicidal effectiveness, and potential uses for stabilized hydrogen peroxide in the healthcare setting. Published reports have ascribed good bactericidal, virucidal, tuberculocidal, and sporicidal and fungicidal properties.

Mechanism of action: Hydrogen peroxide works by the production of destructive hydroxyl free radicals. These can attack membrane lipids, DNA and other essential cell components. Catalase, produced by aerobic organisms and facultative anaerobes that possess cytochrome systems, can protect cells from metabolically produced hydrogen peroxide by degrading hydrogen peroxide to water and oxygen. This defense is overwhelmed by the concentrations used for disinfection.

Microbicidal activity: Hydrogen peroxide is active against a wide range of micro-organisms, including bacteria, yeasts, fungi, viruses, and spores A 7% stabilized hydrogen peroxide proved to be sporicidal (6 hours of exposure), mycobactericidal (20 minutes), fungicidal (5 minutes) at full strength, virucidal (5 minutes) and bactericidal (3 minutes) at a 1:16 dilution. Synergistic sporicidal effects were observed when spores were exposed to a combination of hydrogen peroxide (5.9–23.6%) and peracetic acid.[37] Concentrations of hydrogen peroxide from 6% to 25% show promise as chemical sterilants. The product marketed as a sterilant is a premixed, ready-to-use chemical that contains 7.5% hydrogen peroxide and 0.85% phosphoric acid (to maintain a low pH).[38]

A new, rapid-acting 13.4% hydrogen peroxide formulation has demonstrated sporicidal, mycobactericidal, fungicidal, and virucidal efficacy.

Under normal conditions, hydrogen peroxide is extremely stable when properly stored (e.g. in dark containers). The decomposition or loss of potency in small containers is less than 2% per year at ambient temperatures.

Uses: Commercially available 3% hydrogen peroxide is a stable and effective disinfectant when used on inanimate surfaces.

i. It has been used in concentrations ranging from 3% to 6 % for the disinfection of soft contact lenses (3% for 2–3 hours), tonometer biprisms and ventilators not protected by filters. Corneal damage from a hydrogen peroxide-disinfected tonometer tip that was not properly rinsed has been reported.
ii. It has also been added to urinary drainage bag, although this reduced the microbial contamination of the bag, it did not reduce the incidence of catheter-associated bacteriuria.

Concentrations of hydrogen peroxide from 6% to 25% have promise as chemical sterilants.

A chemical irritation resembling pseudomembranous colitis caused by either 3% hydrogen peroxide or a 2% glutaraldehyde has been reported.[39] As with other chemical sterilants, dilution of the hydrogen peroxide must be monitored by regularly testing the minimum effective concentration (i.e. 7.5–6.0%).

Frequent use has been associated with corrosion of certain metals. They are less corrosive than hypochlorites and may have a role in the disinfection of laboratory equipment and environmental surfaces where the infection risk is low.

Plasma Sterilization

Plasma is any gas that consists of electrons, ions or neutral particles; several devices are required for the formation of low temperature plasma, which include a closed chamber, a deep vaccum and a chemical processor from which to derive the plasma. In addition to above a source of electromagnetic energy (such as radiofrequency energy) is required which creates an electromagnetic field.

The electromagnetic field interacts with the chemical disinfectant (H_2O_2 or a mixture of H_2O_2 + per acetic acid) that induces the plasma. The resulting UV radiation cause rapid destruction of vegetative organisms including spores.

Two commercial plasma sterilizers Sterrad 100S and Plazlyte Sterilizer are now in use in United States. Sterilization of surgical instruments containing longer and narrower lumens, such as those used in urologic, laproscopic and arthroscopic procedures including single stainless steel lumens ($\geq$3 mm and <400 mm in length) are done.

Iodine and Iodophors

Iodine

Iodine solutions or tinctures have been used by health professionals primarily as antiseptics on skin or tissue. Iodophors, on the other hand, have been used both as antiseptics and disinfectants.

Iodophor

An iodophor is a combination of iodine and a solubilizing agent or carrier; the resulting complex provides a sustained-release reservoir of iodine and releases small amounts of free iodine in aqueous solution. The best-known and most widely used iodophor is povidone-iodine, a compound of polyvinylpyrrolidone with iodine. This product and other iodophors retain the germicidal efficacy of iodine but unlike iodine generally are nonstaining and relatively free of toxicity and irritancy.

'Free' iodine (I_2) contributes to the bactericidal activity of iodophors and dilutions of iodophors demonstrate more rapid bactericidal action than does a full-strength povidone-iodine solution. The reason for the observation that dilution increases bactericidal activity is unclear, but dilution of povidone-iodine might weaken the iodine linkage to the carrier polymer with an accompanying increase of free iodine in solution. Therefore, iodophors must be diluted according to the manufacturers' directions to achieve antimicrobial activity.

Iodine is used as an aqueous or alcoholic solution. It is mainly used for disinfection of skin. It is active against tubercle bacilli and a number of viruses. It has moderate action against spores. Like chlorine-releasing compounds organic matter also inactivates it.

Usually a 1% solution of iodine in 70% alcohol is used, which is an effective preoperative skin antiseptic. Skin reactions may occur in some individuals, and for this reason 0.5% alcoholic chlorhexidine or alcoholic iodophor solution is preferred.

Mechanism of action: Iodine is able to penetrate the cell walls of microorganisms quickly. It is believed that iodine's lethal effects result from a disruption of protein and nucleic acid structure and synthesis.

Range of activity: Iodophors are bactericidal, virucidal, and mycobactericidal but may require prolonged contact time to kill certain fungi and bacterial spores.

Uses:

1. Iodophors are used mainly for hand disinfection for example [povidone-iodine (PVP-I), betadine], detergent preparations or surgical scrubs. These contain 7% PVP-I (equivalent to 0.7% available iodine) and are effective for this purpose. Alcoholic preparations containing 10% PVP-I (1% available iodine) are suitable for preoperative preparation of the skin at the operation site. Iodine is the only antiseptic which has been shown to be having a useful sporicidal action on the skin. When applied as an iodophor, it can be left on the skin long enough to remove a large proportion of *Clostridium perfringens* spores when these are present, but property is of uncertain value.
2. Besides their use as antiseptics iodophors have been used for the disinfection of blood culture bottles and medical equipment such as hydrotherapy tanks, thermometers and endoscopes. Antiseptic iodophors are not suitable for use as

hard surface disinfectants because of concentration differences.

Iodophors formulated as antiseptics contain less free iodine than do those formulated as disinfectants. Iodine or iodine-based antiseptics should not be used on silicone catheters because they can adversely affect the silicone tubing.

Peracetic Acid

Peracetic acid or peroxyacetic acid, in low concentrations (0.001–0.2%) is rapidly effective against all microorganisms including bacterial spores. It is rapidly bactericidal, virucidal and mycobactericidal (within 5 minutes) and sporicidal (within 10 minutes).

Advantage: A special advantage is that its decomposition products (i.e. acetic acid, water, oxygen, hydrogen peroxide) are not harmful and do not leave any residues. It remains effective in the presence of organic matter and it is sporicidal even at low temperatures.

Disadvantage: It can corrode copper, bronze, brass, plain steel and galvanized iron, but additives and pH modifications can reduce these effects. Peracetic acid is considered unstable, particularly when diluted. For example, a 1% solution looses half its strength through hydrolysis in 6 days, whereas 40% peracetic acid looses 1 to 2% of the activity per month.

Mechanism of action: It is believed to function in the same manner as other oxidizing agents. It denaturates proteins, disrupts the cell wall permeability and oxidizes sulfhydryl and sulfur bonds in proteins, enzymes and other metabolites.

Uses: An automated machine using peracetic acid to chemically sterilize medical (e.g., endoscopes, arthroscopes), surgical, and dental instruments is used.[40-42] The sterilant, 35% peracetic acid, is diluted to 0.2% with filtered water at 50°C.

Peracetic Acid and Hydrogen Peroxide

A chemical sterilant is available that contains 0.23% peracetic acid plus 7.35% hydrogen peroxide.

Range of activity: The bactericidal properties of peracetic acid and hydrogen peroxide have been demonstrated.[43] This combination of peracetic acid and hydrogen peroxide inactivates all microorganisms except bacterial spores within 20 minutes.

The combination of peracetic acid and hydrogen peroxide has been used for disinfecting hemodialyzers.

Phenolics

Phenol has occupied a prominent place in the field of hospital disinfection since its initial use as a germicide by Lister in his pioneering work on antiseptic surgery. In the past 30 years, however, work has concentrated on the numerous phenol derivatives or phenolics and their antimicrobial properties. Phenol derivatives originate when a functional group (e.g. alkyl, phenyl, benzyl, halogen) replaces one of the hydrogen atoms on the aromatic ring. Two phenol derivatives commonly found as constituents of hospital disinfectants are ortho-phenylphenol and ortho-benzyl-para-chlorophenol. The antimicrobial properties of these compounds and many other phenol derivatives are much improved over those of the parent chemical. Phenolics are absorbed by porous materials, and the residual disinfectant can irritate tissue. In 1970, depigmentation of the skin was reported to be caused by phenolic germicidal detergents containing para-tertiary butylphenol and para-tertiary amylphenol.

Phenol derivatives are called phenolics. Phenol (carbolic acid) is the most commonly used phenol. Others are Lysol, Cresol, Stericol, Hycolin, and Clearsol.

Mechanism of action: At higher concentrations phenol acts as a gross protoplasmic poison.

It penetrates and disrupts the cell wall and precipitates the cell proteins. Lower concentrations of phenol and higher molecular weight phenol derivatives cause bacterial death by the inactivation of essential enzyme systems and leakage of essential metabolites from the cell wall.

Range of action: Commercial phenolic detergents are not sporicidal, but are tuberculocidal, fungicidal, virucidal and bactericidal at their recommended use dilutions.

Advantages: They are stable and not inactivated in the presence of organic matter.

Disadnantages: They are too corrosive for some instruments and they are too toxic to be applied to the skin.

Use: They are used as general-purpose disinfectants in hospitals, as organic matter does not easily inactivate them. They are usually used in two concentrations.

1. 1% concentration-at, which it is bactericidal.
2. 0.5% it is used for preservation of sera and vaccines.
   i. Many phenolic germicides are used as disinfectants on environmental surfaces (e.g. bedside tables, bedrails, and laboratory surfaces) and noncritical medical devices. Phenolics are not FDA-cleared as high-level disinfectants for use with semicritical items but could be used to preclean or decontaminate critical and semicritical devices before terminal sterilization or high level disinfection.
   ii. Use of phenolics in nurseries has been associated with hyperbilirubinemia in infants. If phenolics are used to clean nursery floors, they must be diluted according to the recommendations on the product label. Based on these observations, phenolics should not be used to clean infant bassinets and incubators during stay of an infant. If phenolics are used to terminally clean the infant bassinets and incubators, the surfaces should be rinsed thoroughly with water and dried before they are reused. However since use of phenolics in infant nurseries has been associated with hyperbilirubinemia even when used at manufacturer's recommended use dilution, its use in infant nurseries remains questionable.

Phenol Derivatives

a. ***Chlorophenols and chloroxyenols***: For example, dettol (chloroxylenol)
   1. These are less toxic and non-irritant.
   2. Organic matter however readily inactivates them.
   3. Higher concentrations are required (2.5–5%).
   4. These are mainly active against gram-positive bacteria, but less active against gram-negative bacteria.
   5. Most of them are not active against mycobacteria, spores, but may have a good fungicidal property.
   6. Various combinations of these are used in control of pyogenic cocci in surgical and neonatal units in hospitals.
b. ***Cresols:*** (methylphenols) It is used as solutions of cresols in soap (lysol). It is cheaper but toxic to skin or tissues and mainly used for preliminary steriliztion of infected glassware in laboratory, disinfection of excreta, cleaning floors of wards and operation rooms in hospitals.
c. ***Chlorhexidine:*** (hibitane) this is a useful skin antiseptic highly effective against vegetative gram-positive organisms, but less active against gram-negative bacilli. It has a good fungicidal activity, but shows little or no activity against tubercle bacilli, enveloped viruses and bacterial spores.

It is relatively nontoxic, but inactivated by soaps. Its use in hospitals should be restricted to procedures involving contact with skin or mucus membranes. It is too expensive for environmental use.

Use: Detergent solutions containing 4% chlorhexidine gluconate are available. These have been found to be highly effective for the disinfection of surgeon's hands prior to operating, and they have a good persistent effect due to residuals left on the skin after rinsing and drying.

Savlon is a combination of chlorhexidine and cetrimide, the hospital concentration contains 1.5% cetrimide and 1.5% chlorhexidine. It is usually used at a concentration of 1%. At this concentration the antimicrobicidal activity of chlorhexidine is poor, but cetremide is a good cleansing agent and enhances the activity of chlorhexidine.

Savlon is used in burns, wounds, as bladder irrigant, for surgical instruments and preoperative disinfection for skin.

Hexachlorophene (Halogenated Bisphenol)

Range of action: This compound is highly active against gram-positive organisms, but less effective against gram-negative ones.

It is relatively insoluble in water and alcohol, but can be incorporated in soaps or detergent solutions without loss of activity, or can be used in powder form.

Advantage: It has a good residual effect on the skin.

Disadvantage: These solutions are prone to contamination with gram-negative bacteria, unless a preservative is added in the formulation. Potentially neurotoxic levels may occur in blood if emulsions or other preparations of hexachlorophene are repeatedly and extensively applied to the body surface of babies. Therefore this product although very effective, is now infrequently used in hospitals and can only be obtained for use on medical advice.

Use:

1. It may be used for hand washing of staff during staphylococcal outbreak.
2. It may be used for surgical hand disinfection.
3. Hexachlorophene dusting powder can be used for umbilical stump of neonates, as this does not attain toxic levels. It is very effective in the control of staphylococcal infection and may have a role in hospital practice.
4. It may also be applied to the groin and buttock regions of MRSA carriers.

Triclosan

Triclosan containing products have properties similar to those of hexachlorophene, but they show no toxicity to neonates. They are widely used as alternatives to hexachlorophene in hand rubs, soaps and bath concentrates. In use concentrations are in the range of 0.3% to 2%.

Triclosan containing products are often used for the treatment of MRSA carriers, as they are better tolerated than some other antiseptic containing detergents.

Quaternary Ammonium Compounds

These have enjoyed the wide use as disinfectants and until recently as antiseptics. The first compound to be commercially available was benzalkonium chloride. It was acclaimed for its good microbicidal activity and detergent action. Common environmental factors such as hard water, soap, anionic residues and proteinaceous soils were subsequently found to reduce the effectiveness of benzalkonium chloride. CDC later recommended the elimination of such solutions from being used as antiseptics on the skin and in tissues, because of several outbreaks of infections associated with in use contamination. So also few reports of nosocomial infections were associated with contaminated quaternary ammonium compounds used to disinfect patient care supplies or equipment such as cystoscopes or cardiac catheters.

The QACs' are good cleansing agents, but materials such as cotton and guaze pads make them less microbicidal because these materials may absorb the active ingredients. As with several other disinfectants (e.g. phenolics, iodophors) gram-negative bacteria can survive or grow in them.

Some of the chemical names of quaternary ammonium compounds used in healthcare are alkyl dimethyl benzyl ammonium chloride, alkyl didecyl dimethyl ammonium chloride, and dialkyl dimethyl ammonium chloride. The newer quaternary ammonium compounds (i.e. fourth generation), referred to as twin-chain or dialkyl quaternaries (e.g. didecyl dimethyl ammonium bromide and dioctyl dimethyl ammonium bromide), purportedly remain active in hard water and are tolerant of anionic residues.

A few case reports have documented occupational asthma as a result of exposure to benzalkonium chloride.

Mechanism of action: The bactericidal action of QACs has been attributed to inactivation of energy producing enzymes, denaturation of essential cell proteins, and disruption of cell membrane.

Range of action: QACs are fungicidal, bactericidal, and virucidal against lipophilic viruses (enveloped viruses); they are not sporicidal and generally are not tuberculocidal or virucidal against hydrophilic (non-enveloped viruses) viruses. The poor mycobactericidal activities of quaternary ammonium compounds have been demonstrated.

Products available: The common compounds are cetyltrimethylammonium bromide (cetavlon or cetrimide), benzalkonium chloride (Saniquad).

Uses: QACs are bacteriostatic rather than bactericidal at higher dilutions. Their use in hospitals is limited because of their narrrow spectrum of activity, but they may be used for cleaning wounds. They are also used in ordinary environmental sanitation of noncritical surfaces such as floors, furniture and walls.

Disadvantage: QACs can also be contaminated with gram-negative bacilli. Incorporating a chelating agent enhances the activity of QACs against gram-negative bacilli. More recently QACs have been introduced which show reasonable activity against *Pseudomonas aeruginosa* although their activity against virus's and mycobacteria has yet to be established.

Table 8.4 shows the various concentrations of phenol and QACs that can be used for disinfection of clean contaminated and grossly contaminated conditions.

Table 8.4: Concentrations of different disinfectants to be used in clean contaminated and grossly contaminated conditions[51]

Sl. No.	Disinfectant	Clean contaminated	Grossly contaminated
Phenols			
1.	Phenol (carbolic acid)	5%	10%
2.	Cresol	2.5%	5%
3.	Lysol (saponified cresol)	2.5%	2.5%
4.	Choroxylenol (4.8 % v/v marketed as dettol)	4%	10%
Diguanides			
1.	Chlorhexidine (1.5 % v/v hibitane)	5%	5–10%
2.	Savlon (chlorhexidine 1.5% and cetrimide 1.5%) now used as 1% solution	1%	1%
Quaternary ammonium compounds			
1.	Cetrimide (cetavlon)		
2.	Benzalkonium chloride	2%	2%
Aqueous solution of 4% chlorhexidine gluconate with detergent can be used			
Alcoholic solution of chorhexidine gluconate, i.e. 0.5% chlorhexidine in isopropanol or 60% ethanol or 70% ethanol with emollient can be used			

Miscellaneous Inactivating Agents

Other Germicides

Several compounds have antimicrobial activity but for various reasons have not been incorporated as health-care disinfectants. These include mercurials, sodium hydroxide, β-propiolactone, chlorhexidine gluconate, cetrimide-chlorhexidine, glycols (triethylene and propylene), and the Tego disinfectants.

A peroxygen-containing formulation had marked bactericidal action when used as a 1% weight/volume solution and virucidal activity at 3%, but did not have mycobactericidal activity at concentrations of 2.3% and 4% and exposure times ranging from 30 to 120 minutes. It also required 20 hours to kill *B. atrophaeus* spores. A powder-based peroxygen compound for disinfecting contaminated spill was strongly and rapidly bactericidal.

In preliminary studies, nanoemulsions (composed of detergents and lipids in water) showed activity against vegetative bacteria, enveloped viruses and *Candida*. This product represents a potential agent for use as a topical biocidal agent.

New disinfectants that require further evaluation include glucoprotamin,[44] tertiary amines and a light-activated antimicrobial coating. Several other disinfection technologies might have potential.

Metals as Microbicides

The anti-infective activity of some heavy metals has been known since long. Heavy metals such as silver have been used for prophylaxis of conjunctivitis of the newborn, topical therapy for burn wounds, and bonding to indwelling catheters, and the use of heavy metals as antiseptics or disinfectants is again being explored. Metals such as silver, iron, and copper could be used for environmental control, disinfection of water, or reusable medical devices or incorporated into medical devices (e.g. intravascular catheters). Preliminary data suggest metals are effective against a wide variety of microorganisms.

Clinical uses of other heavy metals include copper-8-quinolinolate as a fungicide against *Aspergillus*, copper-silver ionization for *Legionella* disinfection, organic mercurials as an antiseptic (e.g. mercurochrome) and preservative/disinfectant [e.g. thiomerosal (currently being removed from vaccines)] in pharmaceuticals and cosmetics.

Ultraviolet Radiation

The wavelength of ultraviolet radiation (UV) radiation ranges from 328 nm to 210 nm (3280 A to 2100 A). Its maximum bactericidal effect occurs at 240–280 nm. Mercury vapor lamps emit more than 90% of their radiation at 253.7 nm, which is near the maximum microbicidal activity. Inactivation of micro-organisms results from destruction of nucleic acid through induction of thymine dimers. UV radiation has been employed in the disinfection of drinking water, air, titanium implants, and contact lenses. Bacteria and viruses are more easily killed by UV light than are bacterial spores. UV radiation has several potential applications, but unfortunately its germicidal effectiveness and use is influenced by organic matter; wavelength; type of suspension; temperature; type of microorganism; and UV intensity, which is affected by distance and dirty tubes. The application of UV radiation in the healthcare environment (i.e. operating rooms, isolation rooms, and biologic safety cabinets) is limited to destruction of airborne organisms or inactivation of microorganisms on surfaces.

Pasteurization

Pasteurization is not a sterilization process; its purpose is to destroy all pathogenic microorganisms. However, pasteurization does not destroy bacterial spores. The time-temperature relation for hot-water pasteurization is generally 70°C (158°F) for 30 minutes. The water temperature and time should be monitored as part of a quality-assurance program. Pasteurization of respiratory therapy and anesthesia equipment is a recognized alternative to chemical disinfection.

Flushing- and Washer-Disinfectors

Flushing- and washer-disinfectors are automated and closed equipment that clean and disinfect objects from bedpans and washbowls to surgical instruments and anesthesia tubes. Items such as bedpans and urinals can be cleaned and disinfected in flushing-disinfectors. They have a short cycle of a few minutes. They clean by flushing with warm water, possibly with a detergent, and then disinfect by flushing the items with hot water or with steam. Because this machine empties, cleans, and disinfects, manual cleaning is eliminated, fewer disposable items are needed, and fewer chemical germicides are used.

Surgical instruments and anesthesia equipment are more difficult to clean. They are run in washer-disinfectors on a longer cycle of approximately 20–30 minutes with a detergent. These machines also disinfect by hot water at approximately 90°C.

Ethylene Oxide

Reprocessing of heat-labile medical equipment is a major problem in hospitals. Ethylene oxide (ETO) has been the sterilant of choice for sterilizing heat-labile medical equipment.

Until recently EtO sterilizers combined EtO with a chlorofluorocarbon (CFC) stabilizing agent most commonly in the ratio of 12% EtO mixed with 88% CFC (Referred to as 12/88 EtO). Now alternative technologies to EtO with CFC include the following; 100% EtO, EtO with a different stabilizing gas such as carbon dioxide or hydrochlorofluorocarbon; vaporized hydrogen peroxide; gas plasmas; ozone and chlorine dioxide.

Advantage: EtO is extremely penetrative non-corrosive and an effective sterilizing agent.

Disadvantage: It is toxic, irritant, mutagenic and a suspected carcinogen. It is explosive when mixed with air at concentrations higher than 3%. It is also odorless and leaks may therefore go unnoticed.

Use:

1. Despite these disadvantages EtO is widely used for sterilizing heat-sensitive items, e.g. plastic and rubber items, blankets, pharmaceutical products (crude drugs and powders), fabrics, glass, metal and paper, surfaces, some food stuffs and tobacco.
2. It is specially used for sterilizing heart lung machines, respirators, sutures, dental equipment, books, etc. It is unsuitable for fumigation of rooms because of its explosive property.

Use of EtO for sterilization: EtO is usually used at 55°C to 60°C at about 33% humidity. EtO is explosive except when mixed with another gas, e.g. carbon dioxide or nitrogen in the ratio 1:10. These arrangements require expensive equipment and are not easily possible. This is rather difficult and requires monitoring (spore test-*Bacillus subtilis* strain globigii, variety niger).

During a typical cycle air is removed from the load, by creating a vacuum and the chamber and its contents are heated to the desired temperature (37°C or 55°C). As air removal reduces the humidity, which is an essential prerequisite for sterilization, sub atmospheric steam is introduced to rehumidify the load. Gas is then introduced from a cylinder, or single-use canister and the temperature and pressure are maintained for the sterilization period. Finally gas is removed and the chamber and its contents are flushed with filtered air. The holding time is dependent on the temperature and, pressure, humidity and gas concentration. The design of the sterilizers is therefore related to these parameters and the requirements of the user. (i.e. temperature/pressure tolerance of the items processed, size of load, time available for processing, etc.)

Types of sterilizers:

1. Subatmospheric type: It is the most commonly used EtO sterilizers in the hospital in UK. They utilize pure EtO, but the risk is minimal as the entire cycle is below atmospheric pressure. These sterilizers are much smaller than high-pressure models, but they may be used to sterilize items, which are sensitive to high pressures (e.g. flexible fibre optic endocscopes.).
2. High-pressure type: Commonly used in industrial process. By adopting a high pressure (5.5 bar), it is possible to maintain lethal concentration of the used mixtures of EtO and inert substances (e.g. carbon dioxide). This reduces the risk of flammability or explosion, but the high pressure increases the risk of leaks.

Effectiveness of EtO as a sterilizing agent may be influenced by other factors (e.g. the presence of salt crystals and packaging). All items must therefore be scrupulously clean. For packaging, paper, polypropylene or polythene bags are suitable, but nylon must not be used. Packages should be heat sealed or sealed with tape. Indicator tape on packaging should be used to indicate the items, which have been processed. The sterilizing process must be controlled by spore tests or supplemented by indicator tests.

EtO and its residues are toxic and irritant and therefore the materials exposed to it must be thoroughly aerated before use. Aeration time is dependent on the absorbency of the items processed, the temperature, and the air-exchange rates in the storage facility. Those with high capacity sterilizers should use a separate aeration room with exhaust ventilation and open shelving to allow good air circulation. Very absorbent items or those required soon after sterilization may be aerated in a heated exhaust-ventilated cabinet. Aeration at 55°C greatly enhances the elution of EtO, and consequently much shorter aeration periods may be used. Where practicable, aeration is carried out in the chamber itself in order to protect staff from exposure, during removal of the load. For aeration outside the chamber, a temperature of 55°C for 24 hours, or 3 to 7 days at room temperature, is normally considered to be adequate.

As much concern is expressed about the toxicity of EtO, the health and safety executive[45] has adopted a control limit of exposure of individuals at work to 1 ppm EtO over an 8 hour time-weighted averaged period. Exposure can be minimized by installing the sterilizer in a separate exhaust-ventilated suite of rooms, by carrying out aeration in the chamber, and by installing an exhaust hood above the sterilizer door. It is recommended that access to the sterilizer, plant room and aeration facility be restricted to trained personnel who are fully conversant with the hazards associated with the process and emergency procedures. Notices on emergency procedures should be clearly displayed in the work area.

Irradiated articles should not be subsequently treated with EtO unless they are known to be safe after such treatment.

Table 8.5 shows the properties of an ideal disinfectant and Table 8.6 shows the comparison of the characterstics of selected chemicals used as high level disinfectants or chemical sterilants. Table 8.7 shows the summary of advantages and disadvantages of chemical agents used as chemical sterilants or as high level disinfectants.

Table 8.5: Properties of an ideal disinfectant[53]

Broad spectrum: should have a wide antimicrobial spectrum
Fast acting: should produce a rapid kill
Not affected by environmental factors: should be active in the presence of organic matter (e.g. blood, sputum, feces) and compatible with soaps, detergents, and other chemicals encountered in use
Nontoxic: should not be harmful to the user or patient

Contd...

Contd...

Surface compatibility: should not corrode instruments and metallic surfaces and should not cause the deterioration of cloth, rubber, plastics, and other materials
Residual effect on treated surfaces: should leave an antimicrobial film on the treated surface
Easy to use with clear label directions
Odorless: should have a pleasant odor or no odor to facilitate its routine use
Economical: should not be prohibitively high in cost
Solubility: should be soluble in water
Stability: should be stable in concentrate and use-dilution
Cleaner: should have good cleaning properties
Environmentally friendly: should not damage the environment on disposal

Source: Modified from Molinari[53]

Table 8.6: Comparison of the characteristics of selected chemicals used as high-level disinfectants or chemical sterilants[55]

	HP (7.5%)	PA (0.2%)	Glut (>2.0%)	OPA (0.55%)	HP/PA (7.35%/0.23%)
HLD Claim	30 m @ 20°C	NA	20-90 m @ 20°-25°C	12 m @ 20°C, 5 m @ 25°C in AER	15m @ 20°C
Sterilization Claim	6 h @ 20°C	12m @ 50-56°C	10 h @ 20 to 25°C	None	3 h @ 20°C
Activation	No	No	Yes (alkaline glut)	No	No
Reuse Life[1]	21d	Single use	14-30 d	14d	14d
Shelf Life Stability[2]	2 y	6 mo	2 y	2 y	2 y
Disposal Restrictions	None	None	Local[3]	Local[3]	None
Materials Compatibility	Good	Good	Excellent	Excellent	No data
Monitor MEC[4]	Yes (6%)	No	Yes (1.5% or higher)	Yes (0.3% OPA)	No
Safety	Serious eye damage (safety glasses)	Serious eye and skin damage (conc soln)[5]	Respiratory	Eye irritant, stains skin	Eye damage
Processing	Manual or automated	Automated	Manual or automated	Manual or automated	Manual
Organic material resistance	Yes	Yes	Yes	Yes	Yes
OSHA exposure limit	1 ppm TWA	None	None[6]	None	HP-1 ppm TWA
Cost profile (per cycle)[7]	+ (manual), ++ (automated)	+++++ (automated)	+ (manual), ++ (automated)	++ (manual)	++ (manual)

Source: Modified form Rutala[55]

Abbreviations: HLD, high-level disinfectant; HP, hydrogen peroxide; PA, peracetic acid; glut, glutaraldehyde; PA/HP, peracetic acid and hydrogen peroxide; OPA, ortho-phthalaldehyde (FDA cleared as a high-level disinfectant, included for comparison to other chemical agents used for high-level disinfection); m, minutes; h, hours; NA, not applicable; TWA, time-weighted average for a conventional 8-hour workday.

[1]number of days a product can be reused as determined by re-use protocol

[2]time a product can remain in storage (unused)

[3]no US EPA regulations but some states and local authorities have additional restrictions

[4]MEC, minimum effective concentration is the lowest concentration of active ingredients at which the product is still effective

[5]Conc soln, concentrated solution

[6]The ceiling limit recommended by the American Conference of Governmental Industrial Hygienists is 0.05 ppm.

[7]Per cycle cost profile considers cost of the processing solution (suggested list price to healthcare facilities in August 2001) and assumes maximum use life (e.g., 21 days for hydrogen peroxide, 14 days for glutaraldehyde), 5 reprocessing cycles per day, 1-gallon basin for manual processing, and 4-gallon tank for automated processing. + = least expensive; +++++ = most expensive

Table 8.7: Summary of advantages and disadvantages of chemical agents used as chemical sterilants[1] or as high-level disinfectants[55]

Sterilization method	Advantages	Disadvantages
Peracetic Acid/ Hydrogen Peroxide	No activation required odor or irritation not significant	Materials compatibility concerns (lead, brass, copper, zinc) both cosmetic and functional Limited clinical experience Potential for eye and skin damage
Glutaraldehyde	Numerous use studies published Relatively inexpensive Excellent materials compatibility	Respiratory irritation from glutaraldehyde vapor Pungent and irritating odor Relatively slow mycobactericidal activity Coagulates blood and fixes tissue to surfaces Allergic contact dermatitis Glutaraldehyde vapor monitoring recommended
Hydrogen Peroxide	No activation required May enhance removal of organic matter and organisms No disposal issues No odor or irritation issues Does not coagulate blood or fix tissues to surfaces Inactivates *Cryptosporidium* Use studies published	Material compatibility concerns (brass, zinc, copper, and nickel/silver plating) both cosmetic and functional Serious eye damage with contact
Ortho-phthalaldehyde	Fast acting high-level disinfectant No activation required Odor not significant Excellent materials compatibility claimed Does not coagulate blood or fix tissues to surfaces claimed	Stains skin, mucous membranes, clothing, and environmental surfaces Repeated exposure may result in hypersensitivity in some patients with bladder cancer More expensive than glutaraldehyde Eye irritation with contact Slow sporicidal activity
Peracetic Acid	Rapid sterilization cycle time (30–45 minutes) Low temperature (50–55°C) liquid immersion sterilization Environmental friendly by-products (acetic acid, O_2, H_2O) Fully automated Single-use system eliminates need for concentration testing Standardized cycle May enhance removal of organic material and endotoxin No adverse health effects to operators under normal operating conditions Compatible with many materials and instruments Does not coagulate blood or fix tissues to surfaces Sterilant flows through scope facilitating salt, protein, and microbe removal Rapidly sporicidal Provides procedure standardization (constant dilution, perfusion of channel, temperatures, exposure)	Potential material incompatibility (e.g. aluminum anodized coating becomes dull) Used for immersible instruments only Biological indicator may not be suitable for routine monitoring One scope or a small number of instruments can be processed in a cycle More expensive (endoscope repairs, operating costs, purchase costs) than high-level disinfection Serious eye and skin damage (concentrated solution) with contact Point-of-use system, no sterile storage

Source: Modified from Rutala[52–55]

[1]All products effective in presence of organic soil, relatively easy to use, and have a broad spectrum of antimicrobial activity (bacteria, fungi, viruses, bacterial spores, and mycobacteria). The above characteristics are documented in the literature; contact the manufacturer of the instrument and sterilant for additional information. All products listed above are FDA-cleared as chemical sterilants except OPA, which is an FDA-cleared high-level disinfectant.

FORMULATION OF A DISINFECTANT POLICY

Disinfectant policy should be formulated by the " Hospital Infection Control Committee", who would then decide on the types of disinfectants to be used in their hospital. This requires consultation between the microbiologist, infection control doctor, infection control nurse, pharmacist, supplies officer and representative of the medical, nursing and domestic staff. The hospital pharmacist, who can check whether they are in agreement with the hospital policy, should approve all requests for disinfectants. The selection of a disinfectant depends on many factors like:

a. Intended use of the disinfectant whether for medical equipment, environment, skin and mucous membranes
b. Range of activity
c. Speed of action
d. Inactivation by organic material
e. Compatibility with items processed and processing equipment
f. Safety to user
g. Stability
h. Cost.

Principles

1. Make a list of all the purposes for which disinfectants are used. Select the disinfectants, which you require for your hospital, and then place orders, making sure that the list is complete.
2. While making the list of disinfectants to be ordered, select the smallest practicable number of disinfectants, i.e. one routine disinfectant for each field of use (e.g. the environment, skin and equipment) plus an alternative disinfectant if patients or staff are sensitive to routine disinfectants, and for use when routine disinfectant is unavailable or inappropriate for a particular purpose, or for instruments which may be damaged by the disinfectant.
3. Do not use chemical disinfectants (a) when heat can reasonably be used as alternative, (b) when sterilization is required, (c) when thorough cleaning alone is adequate, (d) or if single-use equipment can be used economically.

After selection of the appropriate disinfectant, distribute the disinfectants, with the necessary supply equipment and personal protective equipment for measuring and preparing the disinfectants at the site of use. Adequate instructions are to be given regarding:

a. The correct disinfectant and concentration to be used for each task.
b. The shelf life of the disinfectant at the concentration supplied, the type of container to be used, and the frequency with which the solution should be changed.
c. Substances or materials, which will react with or neutralize the disinfectant.
d. An assessment of toxicity or risks to employees using the disinfectant, with the measures required for protection of employees. Personnel should also be informed about the personal safety measures, whether rubber gloves should be worn, how the product can be safely opened and prepared, how the disinfectant should be disposed off and what should be done if the product comes into contact with the skin or the eyes.

The policy must be monitored to ensure that it is effective and continues to be so. Occasional in-use tests and chemical estimations of concentrations may be required.

Recommended Disinfectants and Use of Dilutions

For most environmental requirements in the hospital, chlorine-releasing agent and a phenolic disinfectant should be sufficient.

Hypochlorites and chlorine-releasing agents may be incorporated in a powder for cleaning baths, toilets, and wash-basins. Solutions (1,000 ppm of av Cl_2) may be used for disinfecting clean surfaces, and when necessary for food preparation area. Chlorine-releasing agents should be used if disinfection of virus-contaminated material is required. However routine or too frequent use can cause extensive corrosion and damage to equipment and some surfaces, in which case other less corrosive antiviral agent is required. Higher concentrations of chlorine (10,000 ppm) are recommended in the presence of organic material, e.g. blood or body fluid spillages.

A clear phenolic disinfectant (phenol, lysol, cresol, stericol, hycolin, clearsol) is often chosen as one of the disinfectants for routine use as 1% concentration. This concentration is used for light contamination. It provides a reasonable margin of safety and should be used unless otherwise indicated. The strong concentrations (i.e. twofold) should be used for heavily contaminated areas or if contamination with *Mycobacterium tuberculosis* is likely. Disinfection by heat or use of single-use items is particularly important for dealing with contamination by *Mycobacterium tuberculosis*. Phenolics are usually not suitable for use against viruses, and the increasing anxiety about HIV is responsible for a reduction in their routine use.

Narrow spectrum or expensive disinfectants are mainly used for clinical purposes and are not recommended for general environmental use, but may sometimes be required for special equipment. After thorough cleaning with detergent and water items may be immersed in alcohol or cleaned and disinfected using a disposable alcohol-impregnated wipe. This is preferable to the use of glutaraldehyde. NaDCC compound tends to be less corrosive than hypochlorites.

Instruments: It is always good to purchase heat tolerant instruments. However for heat-labile instruments, glutaraldehyde may be used. Other alternatives are peracetic acid.

Skin: Antiseptics containing chlorhexidine, povidone-iodine and triclosan are used for disinfection of skin, i.e. hands and the operation site. Alcohol is also widely used, especially when hand-washing facilities are either unavailable or unsuitable. However in most instances soap and water are sufficient.

Dilution and Distribution of Disinfectants

The disinfectants used must be prepared properly with the correct dilution because too low a concentration and ineffective cleaning (of the instrument/equipment before treating with disinfectant) are the commonest cause of failure of a disinfectant to kill organisms, and survival of contaminants in the disinfectants is unlikely, if it is used at the recommended in-use dilution.

For this there are two alternatives (1) the pharmacist should supply the departments with containers of disinfectants already prepared at the correct use-dilution, or (2) the departments should prepare their own solutions from the undiluted disinfectant. For this the staff must be trained to prepare the in-use dilution, and explain them the drawback of not using the correct concentration.

Containers must be thoroughly washed and properly disinfected by heat before refilling. If heating is not possible, thorough drying after washing should be adequate, as this will kill most bacteria that are likely to be present. Corks must not be used. Containers should have plastic closures, which can be easily cleaned. The strong disinfectant solutions require careful handling in order to avoid damage to the skin of the operator. Gloves and plastic apron should be worn and eye protection is necessary if splashing is likely.

TESTING OF DISINFECTANTS

There are different tests, which can be used for testing of disinfectants. They can be placed in three categories:

1. Those for the routine quality control of production batches of a standard formulation and for the control of purchasing (e.g. the Rideal-Walker and the Chick-Martin and other phenol coefficient tests.)[46]

2. Use dilution tests, which suggests a practical use dilution for a disinfectant under defined conditions (Capacity tests e.g. Kelsey and Sykes test 1969).[47]
3. In-use tests to evaluate the efficiency of disinfectant under practical (field) conditions and uses (Kelsey and Maurer, 1966; Betty Croshaw, 1981).[48,49]

Phenol Coefficient Tests

Also called as manufacturers tests as they do them for assessing the efficacy of the disinfectants produced. In this test similar quantities of organisms are added to increasing dilutions of phenol, and of the disinfectant to be tested. In UK the organisms used are *S. typhi* and in USA the organisms used are *S. typhi, S. aureus*, and *P. aeruginosa*. For testing two methods are used, i.e. Rideal-Walker and Chick-Martin. In the later but not the former, a source of organic matter (e.g. 2% killed yeast suspension, or 20% inactivated horse serum or 3% dried human faeces) is used to simulate natural conditions. The dilution of the disinfectant under question, which kills the organisms in a given time, is divided by the dilution of phenol, which kills the organisms at the same time. This gives the phenol coefficient. A phenol coefficient of 1.0 means that the disinfectant in question has the same effectiveness as, and a coefficient of <1.0 means it is less effective than phenol, and a coefficient of >1.0 means, it is more effective than phenol.

Capacity Tests (Kelsey and Sykes Test)

Capacity tests are designed to simulate the natural conditions under which the disinfectants are used in the hospitals. In this test instead of addition of a large inoculum of the test organism, additions are made in increments with or without organic matter. This gives a measure of the capacity of the disinfectant to cope with successive bacterial invasions. Test organisms (*S. aureus, E. coli, P. aeruginosa and Proteus vulgaris*) in both clean (test bacteria in broth) and dirty (bacteria in 20% inactivated horse serum or 2% yeast suspension) conditions are added to the disinfectant in 3 successive lots at 0, 10 and 20 minutes. Each addition remains in contact with the disinfectant for 8 minutes, and therefore samples are transferred at 8, 18 and 28 minutes respectively to a recovery medium. The disinfectant is judged on its overall performance that is its ability to kill bacteria as judged by recovery on subculture and not by comparison with phenol.

In-use Test[48,49]

The in-use tests are performed to check the end results of disinfection. Samples are taken from the disinfectant dilutions in use in the hospital for any purpose such as thermometer, cheatle forceps, laboratory discard jar, mop fluid etc. The object is to determine whether the fluids contain living bacteria and in what numbers.

Procedure

Step 1: Transfer 1 mL of the disinfectant fluid into a tube containing 9 mL of the diluent. Diluents used for different groups of disinfectants are: 'In-use' test diluents.

Diluent	Disinfectant group
1. Nutrient broth Alcohols	Aldehydes Hypochlorites Phenolics
2. Nutrient broth + Tween 80, 3% w/v	Hypochlorites + detergent Iodophors Phenolic + detergent QACs Diguanides

Step 2: The 1.0 mL sample is added to 9.0 mL of diluent in a sterile universal container. The diluent should be selected according to the group to which the disinfectant belongs.

Step 3: Place 0.02 mL (20 microlit) of the diluted disinfectant solution on 10 different areas on the surface of well-dried nutrient agar plates in duplicate.

Step 4: Incubate one plate at 37°C for 3 days and the other at room temperature for 7 days.

Results

Read the test as showing failure of disinfection if there is growth in more than five drops on either plate.

REFERENCES

1. Guidelines for selection and use of disinfectants: APIC Guidelines for Infection Control Practice. Am J Infection Control. 1990; 18:99-113.
2. Rutala WA, Weber DJ. Healthcare Infection Control Practices Advisory Committee (HICPAC). CDC Guideline for Disinfection and Sterilization in Healthcare Facilities; 2008.
3. Rautala WA, Stiegel MM, Sarubbi FA, Weber DJ. Ineffectiveness of disinfectants against hospital strains of bacteria. Infect Control Hosp Epidemiol (in press). Quoted by Ref. 1.
4. Russell AD, Maillard JY. Reaction and response-relationship between antibiotic resistance and resistance to antiseptics and disinfectants. Am J Infect Control. 2000;28:204-6.
5. Ruden H, Daschner F. Should we routinely disinfect floors? J Hosp Infect. 2002;51:309.
6. Cozad A, Jones RD. Disinfection and the prevention of infectious disease. Am J Infect Control. 2003;31:243-54.
7. Favero MS, Bond WW. Chemical disinfection of medical and surgical materials. In: Block SS (Ed). Disinfection, sterilization, and preservation. Philadelphia: Lea and Febiger; 1991.pp.617-41.
8. Ayliffe GAJ, Collins DM, Lowbury EJL. Cleaning and disinfection of hospital floors. Brit Med J. 1966;2:442-5.
9. Ayliffe GA, Collins BJ, Lowbury EJ, Babb JR, Lilly HA. Ward floors and other surfaces as reservoirs of hospital infection. J Hyg (Lond). 1967;65:515-36.
10. Garner JS. Guideline for isolation precautions in hospitals. The Hospital Infection Control Practices Advisory Committee. Infect Control Hosp Epidemiol. 1996;17:53-80.
11. Maki DG, Alvarado CJ, Hassemer CA, Zilz MA. Relation of the inanimate hospital environment to endemic nosocomial infection. N Engl J Med. 1982;307:1562-6.
12. Griffith CJ, Cooper RA, Gilmore J, Davies C, Lewis M. An evaluation of hospital cleaning regimes and standards. J Hosp Infect. 2000;45:19-28.
13. Sattar SA, Lloyd-Evans N, Springthorpe VS, Nair RC. Institutional outbreaks of rotavirus diarrhoea: potential role of fomites and environmental surfaces as vehicles for virus transmission. J Hyg (Lond). 1986;96:277-89.
14. Best M, Kennedy ME, Coates F. Efficacy of a variety of disinfectants against Listeria spp. Appl Environ Microbiol. 1990;56:377-80.
15. Mbithi JN, Springthorpe VS, Sattar SA. Chemical disinfection of hepatitis A virus on environmental surfaces. Appl Environ Microbiol. 1990;56:3601-4.
16. Rice EW, Clark RM, Johnson CH. Chlorine inactivation of *Escherichia coli* O157:H7. Emerg Infect Dis. 1999;5:461-3.
17. Chuanchuen R, Karkhoff-Schweizer RR, Schweizer HP. High-level triclosan resistance in *Pseudomonas aeruginosa* is solely a result of efflux. Am J Infect Control. 2003;31:124-7.
18. Newman KA, Tenney JH, Oken HA, Moody MR, Wharton R, Schimpff SC. Persistent isolation of an unusual Pseudomonas species from a phenolic disinfectant system. Infect Control. 1984;5(5):219-22.
19. Russell AD. Bacterial resistance to disinfectants: Present knowledge and future problems. J Hosp Infect. 1998;43:S57-S68.
20. Scott GH, Williams JC. Susceptibility of *Coxiella burnetii* to chemical disinfectants. Ann NY Acad Sci. 1990;590:291-6.
21. Sattar SA, Lloyd-Evans N, Springthorpe VS, Nair RC. Institutional outbreaks of rotavirus diarrhoea: potential role of fomites and environmental surfaces as vehicles for virus transmission. J Hyg (Lond). 1986;96:277-89.
22. Vickery K, Pajkos A, Cossart Y. Removal of biofilm from endoscopes: Evaluation of detergent efficiency. Am J Infect Control. 2004;32:170-6.
23. LeChevallier MW, Cawthon CD, Lee RG. Inactivation of biofilm bacteria. Appl Environ Microbiol. 1988;54:2492-9.
24. Marion-Ferey K, Pasmore M, Stoodley P, Wilson S, Husson GP, Costerton JW.

Biofilm removal from silicone tubing: an assessment of the efficacy of dialysis machine decontamination procedures using an in vitro model. J Hosp Infect. 2003;53:64-71.
25. Price D, Ahearn DG. Incidence and persistence of *Pseudomonas aeruginosa* in whirlpools. J Clin Microbiol. 1988;26:1650-4.
26. Anonymous. Dental Unit Waterlines: Approaching the Year 2000. ADA Council on Scientific Affairs. JADA. 1999;130:1653-64.
27. Donlan RM, Costerton JW. Biofilms: Survival mechanisms of clinically relevant mirocorganisms. Clin Microbiol Rev. 2002;15:167-93.
28. Donlan RM. Biofilms: a source of infection? In: Rutala WA (Ed). Disinfection, sterilization and antisepsis: Principles and practices in healthcare facilities. Washington, DC: Association for Professional in Infection Control and Epidemiology; 2001.pp.219-26.
29. Loukili NH, Zink E, Grandadam S, Bientz M, Meunier O. Effectiveness of detergent-disinfecting agents on *Escherichia coli* 54127 biofilm. J Hosp Infect. 2004;57:175-8.
30. Johansen C, Falholt P, Gram L. Enzymatic removal and disinfection of bacterial biofilms. Appl Environ Microbiol. 1997;63:3724-8.
30a. Health and occupational safety. Disinfectants which should you choose. Accessed from https://www.uab.edu/ohs/images/docs/ss/ss_2009_05_disinfectants.pdf).
30b. MacCall RE, Tankersley CM. Phlebotomy essentials. 2011. Accessed from https://books.google.co.in/books?isbn=1608311198.
31. Scott EM, Gorman SP. Glutaraldehyde. In: Block SS, (Ed). Disinfection, sterilization, and preservation. Philadelphia: Lippincott Williams & Wilkins. 2001:361-81.
32. Scott EM, Gorman SP. Glutaraldehyde. In: Block SS (Ed). Disinfection, Sterilization, and Preservation. Philadelphia: Lea & Febiger; 1991:596.pp.616.
33. Babb JR, Bradley CR, Ayliffe GAJ. Sporicidal activity of glutaraldehydes and hypochlorites and other factors influencing their selection for the treatment of medical equipment. J Hosp Infect. 1980;1:63-75.
34. Scott EM, Gorman SP. Glutaraldehyde. In: Block SS (Ed). Disinfection, sterilization, and preservation. Philadelphia: Lippincott Williams & Wilkins; 2001.pp.361-81.
35. Hanson PJ, Bennett J, Jeffries DJ, Collins JV. Enteroviruses, endoscopy and infection control: An applied study. J Hosp Infect. 1994;27:61-7.
36. Wardle E, Jones D. Determination of rinsing volumes following manual endoscope disinfection with ortho-phthalaldehyde (OPA). J Gastroenterol Nurses College Australia. 2003:7-9.
37. Leaper S. Influence of temperature on the synergistic sporicidal effect of peracetic acid plus hydrogen peroxide in *Bacillus subtilis* SA22(NCA 72-52). Food Microbiol. 1984;1:199-203.
38. Rutala WA, Weber DJ. Disinfection of endoscopes: review of new chemical sterilants used for high-level disinfection. Infect Control Hosp Epidemiol. 1999;20:69-76.
39. Jonas G, Mahoney A, Murray J, Gertler S. Chemical colitis due to endoscope cleaning solutions: A mimic of pseudomembranous colitis. Gastroenterol. 1988;95:1403-8.
40. Crow S. Peracetic acid sterilization: A timely development for a busy healthcare industry. Infect Control Hosp Epidemiol. 1992;13:111-3.
41. Malchesky PS. Medical applications of peracetic acid. In: Block SS (Ed). Disinfection, sterilization, and preservation. Philadelphia: Lippincott Williams & Wilkins. 2001:979-96.
42. Mannion PT. The use of peracetic acid for the reprocessing of flexible endoscopes and rigid cystoscopes and laparoscopes. J Hosp Infect. 1995;29:313-5.
43. Alasri A, Roques C, Michel G, Cabassud C, Aptel P. Bactericidal properties of peracetic acid and hydrogen peroxide, alone and in combination, and chlorine and formaldehyde against bacterial water strains. Can J Microbiol. 1992;38:635-42.
44. Widmer AF, Frei R. Antimicrobial activity of glucoprotamin: A clinical study of a new disinfectant for instruments. Infect Control Hosp Epidemiol. 2003;24:762-4.
45. Health and Safety Executive (1999) Occupational exposure limits. EH 40/99 Norwich: HMSO.
46. Croshow B. Disinfectant testing with particular reference to the Rideal - Walker and Kelsey Syke test Chapter XVII. In: Collins

CH, Allwood MC, Bloomfield SF, Fox A (Eds). Disinfectants, their use and evaluation of effectiveness. 1981.pp.1-15.

47. Kelsey JC, Sykes G. A new test for the assessment of disinfectants with particular reference to their use in hospitals. Pharmaceutical Journal, 1969;202:607-9.
48. Kelsey JC, Maurer IM. Monthly bulletin of the Ministry of Health and Public Health Laboratory Service. 1966;25:180.
49. JG Collee, JP Duguid, AG Fraser, BP Marmion. In use Test. Testing Disinfectants. Chapter 4. Sterilization and disinfection in the laboratory. In: Mackie and McCartney (Eds). Practical Medical Microbiology,13th edition. Vol 2; 1989.p.84-5.
50. Rutala WA. APIC Guidelines for Selection and Use of Disinfectants. Guidelines for Infection Control Practice. American Journal of Infection Control. 1990;24(4):313-42. August 1996.
51. Shriniwas. Hospital-acquired infections: guideline for control. Government of India. Ministry of Health and Family Welfare; 1992
52. Cheesbrough M. Decontamination of infectious material and disposal of laboratory waste. District Laboratory Practice in Tropical Countries, 2nd edition, Part 1; 2009.p.69.
53. Molinari JA, Gleason MJ, Cottone JA, Barrett ED. Comparison of dental surface disinfectants. Gen Dent. 1987;35:171-5.
54. Rutala WA, Weber DJ. Surface disinfection: should we do it? J Hosp Infect. 2001;48 (supplement A):S64-S68.
55. Rutala WA, Weber DJ. Disinfection of endoscopes: review of new chemical sterilants used for high-level disinfection. Infect Control Hosp Epidemiol. 1999;20:69-76.

Chapter 9

Decontamination of the Environment, Equipment and the Skin

Chapter Outline

- Infection Risks to Patients from Equipment, Material and the Environment
- Hospital Environment
- Hospital Domestic Staff (Housekeeping Staff), their Duties and Responsibilities
- Decontamination
- Disinfection of Rooms
- Decontamination of Non-clinical Equipment
- Curtains
- Bed Cradles
- Decontamination of Instruments for Clinical Procedures
- Decontamination of Medical Equipment (High-risk Items)
- Intermediate High-risk Items
- Miscellaneous High-risk Items
- Decontamination of Respiratory Equipment
- Decontamination of Infant Incubators
- Decontamination of Vaginal Speculae and Sigmoidoscopes
- Decontamination of Tonometers
- Decontamination of Equipment Used on Patients with Creutzfeldt-Jacob Disease
- Cleaning and Disinfection of Skin and Mucous Membranes

INTRODUCTION

All medical devices, equipment, and the environment in healthcare settings may become contaminated with micro-organisms and thus can present a risk to patients, as well as to those subsequently handling or using equipment. Safe and effective decontamination of all re-useable equipment between uses is an essential part of routine infection prevention and control practice. Inadequate decontamination has been responsible for outbreaks of infection in healthcare establishments. Staff has a duty to ensure that all equipment they use in whatever setting is clean when used and effectively decontaminated between patients/clients.

Similarly skin may also be contaminated with microorganisms and can develop into a source of infection due to flora transfer both to the patient and others. It is therefore essential to practice and encourage standard principles of infection control (including hand hygiene) at all times and with all patients.

Prior to purchasing equipment staff **must** ensure that the item can be decontaminated effectively and that the company supplying the equipment offers clear instructions on suitable cleaning, disinfection and sterilization methods.

The choice of the method of decontamination (i.e. cleaning, disinfection or sterilization) depends on many factors, but the initial choice is made on the basis of risk to the patients.[1] These can be classified as high, intermediate, low and minimal risks.[2] However, there is an overlap between these categories and requirements for decontamination may vary within a category.

Guidance on the Use of Healthcare Devices

Single Use

The medical device is intended to be used once on an individual patient during a single procedure and then discarded. It is not intended to be re-processed or re-used on another patient. The re-use of single-use medical devices can affect their safety, performance and effectiveness, exposing patients and staff to unnecessary risk.

Single Patient Use

The medical device can be used more than once on **one patient only**. The device may need to be decontaminated between each use.

Reusable

The medical device can be used for repeated episodes on different patients, but requires appropriate decontamination between each use.

Why should single-use items not be reused?

Single use items should not be reused because of risk of:

- Cross-infection—because of inability to clean and decontaminate due to design
- Endotoxin reaction—due to excessive bacterial breakdown products, which cannot be removed adequately by cleaning
- Patient injury—because of device failure from reprocessing or reuse because of fatigue, material alteration and embrittlement
- Chemical burns or sensitization—due to residues from chemical decontamination agents on materials that can absorb/adsorb chemicals.

Also if you reuse a single-use device you may be legally liable for the safe performance of the device.

Decontamination

Decontamination is a process that removes or destroys contamination and thereby prevents microorganisms or other contaminants reaching a susceptible site in sufficient numbers to initiate infection or any other harmful response.

It includes the processes of:

- Cleaning
- Disinfection
- Sterilization.

INFECTION RISKS TO PATIENTS FROM EQUIPMENT, MATERIALS AND THE ENVIRONMENT

High Risk

The risk is said to be high due to invasive items, which come in close contact with a break in the skin or mucous membrane, or are introduced into sterile body area (e.g. surgical instruments, dressings, catheters, prosthetic devices). These items require sterilization. If sterilization is not practically achievable, high level disinfection, although not optimal may be adequate.

Intermediate Risk

The risk is intermediate for items, which come in contact with intact mucous membranes, body fluids, or contaminated with particularly virulent or readily transmissible organisms, or items to be used on highly susceptible patients or sites (e.g. gastrointestinal endoscopes, respiratory equipment) and for this disinfection is required.

Low Risk

The risk is low for items in contact with normal and intact skin (e.g. washing bowls, toilets and bedding) and for these cleaning and drying is usually adequate. Disinfection is needed only if there is a known risk of infection (e.g. bath of a MRSA patients).

Minimal Risk

The risk is minimal when the items are not in close contact with the patient or his/her immediate surroundings, for surfaces that are unlikely to be contaminated with a significant number of pathogens, or these transferred to a susceptible site (e.g. floors, walls and sinks), cleaning to remove organisms and drying is usually adequate.

Choosing the Appropriate Method of Decontamination

Risk	Indication	Recommendation
High	Items that penetrate skin/mucous membranes or enter sterile body areas	Cleaning followed by **sterilization**
Medium	Items in contact with intact mucous membranes, or contaminated with blood/body fluids	Cleaning followed by **disinfection** (Except for instruments used in the vagina or cervix, e.g. speculae which must be sterilized between each use)
Low	Items in contact with intact skin or not in direct patient contact	Cleaning

Environmental Cleaning Following Patient Discharge or Bed Movement or During an Outbreak

1. Patient bed areas (to include beds, table, locker, chair and all other equipment used in that area, e.g. drip stands) must be cleaned thoroughly with hot water and detergent following discharge before next patient can be admitted into the vacated bed space.
2. Areas occupied by patients with a known infection should be cleaned using hot water and detergent then disinfected using a chlorine releasing agent.
3. The Infection Prevention and Control team may be contacted for further advice regarding curtain changes and steam cleaning, etc.
4. Any contamination of the walls should be cleaned immediately therefore terminal wall washing is not required.

Cleaning of Skin Procedure

	Product
Skin Hand washing	For normal hand washing liquid soap is adequate. Patients at bed side must be offered hand wipes after using the commode and before meals if unable to access soap and water
Skin Hand rubs	Hand sanitizer should be used if hands visibly clean and no contact with patient suffering from diarrhea. This gel should be available at the point of use and be an approved brand
Skin Injection sites	• Clean with 70% isopropyl alcohol prior to injection unless otherwise contraindicated by the manufacturer
Venepuncture	• Swab the intended site with a swab containing 70% alcohol and allow to dry
Cannulation site	• Swab the intended site with a swab containing 70% isopropyl and 2% chlorhexidine gluconate and allow to dry

Contd...

Contd...

	Product
Wound cleaning	Wounds with minimal to moderate discharge can be cleaned with warm normal saline 0.9% sterile solution Tap water of drinking quality can be used to irrigate wounds and to soak leg ulcers prior to dressings. Surgical/acute wounds must be cleaned with a sterile solution

HOSPITAL ENVIRONMENT

Usually, the inanimate environment of the hospital is of little importance in the spread of endemic hospital infection, as it is unlikely to make contact with a susceptible site, but it may occasionally have a role in outbreaks.

Ward

If the environment in the ward is clean, and the surfaces of the floor, furniture, equipment or wall are physically clean and dry, there is very little risk of infection. A clean environment is necessary to provide good standards of hygiene and asepsis and to maintain the confidence of patients and the morals of the staff. Wet surfaces and equipment are more likely to encourage the growth of microorganisms and to spread potential pathogens. The equipment used for cleaning and the cleaning solutions may be heavily contaminated with bacteria, and therefore should be removed from the patients vicinity and food preparation areas as soon as cleaning is completed. Thorough cleaning will remove microorganisms and the organic material on which they thrive. This will render most items free of risk of infection and safe to handle. Though it was initially thought that disinfectants are usually not required, CDC guidelines 2008 suggests that there are five important reasons why a disinfectant should be used for non-critical surfaces, first is that soap and water was less effective in reducing the number of bacteria than was a phenolic disinfectant, second detergents become contaminated and result in seeding the patient's environment with bacteria, third the CDC Isolation guidelines recommends that noncritical equipment contaminated with blood, body fluids, secretions or excretions be cleaned and disinfected after use, forth OSHA requires that surfaces contaminated with blood and other potentially infectious materials be disinfected. Fifth using a single product throughout the facility can simplify both training and appropriate practice (for details see chapter of Disinfection).

HOSPITAL DOMESTIC STAFF (HOUSEKEEPING STAFF), THEIR DUTIES AND RESPONSIBILITIES

Ideally a special domestic staff under control of a domestic service manager should be appointed for routine cleaning of the environment including floors, toilets, baths, wash-basins, beds, furniture, etc. They should be specially trained and aware of possible infections hazards. They should be available to clean and if necessary disinfect the rooms occupied or vacated by infected patients. Nursing and other patient care staff, whenever possible should be relieved of cleaning tasks. If the specially trained domestic staffs are not available the nurses should clean and disinfect the surfaces or equipment contaminated with potentially infectious material. If there is an unusual risk of infection associated with the presence of particular patient (e.g. on cleaning blood spillage from an HBV- or HIV-infected patient, or on a high-risk department), the ward sister should ensure that the domestic staff is aware of that risk. This task if possible can be more safely performed by a trained nurse.

DECONTAMINATION

Decontamination of Floors

In the past, it was said the floors should be cleaned with a detergent rather than a disinfectant, because the advantage of using a disinfectant is very less. In a busy ward, recontamination from airborne settlement or transfer from shoes and trolley wheels is rapid. Levels of bacterial contamination on floors may be restored to their original values within 2 hours of cleaning, whether or not disinfectants are used.[3] Infection rates are not influenced by the use of disinfectant and a detergent will normally suffice.[4] But even then as mentioned above a disinfectant should be used to clean the floors rather than a detergent alone for the reasons mentioned above.

Dry Cleaning

Brooms should not be used in patient treatment areas or food preparation and service areas, as they redisperse dust and bacteria in its air. Use of vacuum cleaners is most suitable. The inner paper bag must be closed before and discarded if more than half full. Bags should be exchanged away from patient care area with minimal dispersal of dust. Filters should be inspected at regular scheduled intervals (e.g. monthly) and must be changed if they are dirty or blocked.

Dust attracting mops are also available and can be used as an alternative for vacuum cleaners though they are less efficient. These may be disposable or reprocessable. If they are used for an extensive period of time without replacement, they will fail to retain the dust and may disperse it and adherent bacteria into the air. So an acceptable period of use should be decided upon for each area. To avoid dispersal during use, the head should remain in contact with the floor during sweeping and should not be lifted at the end of each stroke.

However, it should be remembered that dry cleaning would remove the soil, but will not remove stains or scuff marks.

Wet Cleaning

Wet cleaning is essential to remove stains and scuff marks (marks made by shoes). Sluice rooms (where surplus water is drained), toilets and moist areas require cleaning at least once in a day. This can be done with a neutral detergent prepared freshly. Wet mops and cleaning cloths are used for cleaning, but these have been found to be heavily contaminated by microbes and therefore may spread such contamination. Therefore, effective policies must be formulated for decontamination and maintenance of reusable cleaning cloths or mops. Immersion in hypochlorite solution (4,000 ppm) for 2 minutes can be done. If reusable cleaning cloths or mops are used, they should be decontaminated regularly to prevent surface contamination during cleaning with subsequent transfer of organisms from these surfaces to patients or equipment by the hands of healthcare workers. Wetting the mops with disinfectant significantly removes microbes (95% v/s 68%).

Mops and equipment should be drained, cleaned and stored dry. Buckets should be rinsed and stored inverted to assist drying. Mops are difficult to dry completely and are therefore frequently contaminated with gram-negative bacilli.

All cleaning equipment must be examined at regular intervals and cleaned if soiled. In case the equipment is worn out or damaged, it should be repaired or replaced. Cleaning solutions should be changed frequently to prevent multiplication of bacteria and should be discarded as soon as cleaning is completed. During mopping a stand with two buckets is ideal, so that used water from the mop can be discarded in a separate bucket. Surfaces should be left dry after cleaning. The cleaning and maintenance of all new equipment should be agreed upon before putting it into use.

Decontamination of Carpets (or Other Soft Flooring Materials) in Hospital Wards

Although bacteria are present in large numbers and survive longer on carpets than hard floors, there is no evidence that carpets are associated with an increased risk[5] Nevertheless, it is still reasonable to minimize potential infection hazards by selecting carpets with specifically desirable properties. The carpets should have a waterproof backing and the joints should be sealed. The fibers should be non-absorbent and water repellent, so that they can be cleaned and dried easily. The carpet should be washable and not damaged by the commonly used disinfectants. Disinfection may be required, if there is spillage of blood from patients at high risk of blood-borne infections, where chlorine-releasing agents may have to be used. But as these damage the carpets, alternatives to chlorine-releasing compounds may be used (e.g. peroxygen powders), which cause less damage to the carpets. However, carpets with spillage can be cleaned by thorough washing with detergent solution, provided gloves are worn by the operator. Carpets should be vacuum cleaned daily and periodically wet cleaned with specially designated equipment (e.g. steam cleaners with vacuum extraction facility).

Decision to use carpets is based on the infection risk of that area with other factors (e.g. appearance, comfort, sound reduction, etc). Carpets should not be fitted in an area, with frequent or large volume spillage, which may be inadequately maintained. Other clinical areas like surgical and obstetric wards may also be frequently contaminated with blood and other body fluids, and routine cleaning may be inadequate. Problems of smell and staining have been responsible for removing carpets from these areas. Now, it is preferred not to have carpets in these areas, as attractive alternative flooring is available. Washable floors are advisable in isolation wards, as carpets may prolong the survival of organisms (e.g. multiresistant strains of *Staphylococcus aureus* such as MRSA).

Decontamination of Spillage

For most forms of spillage (e.g. food, urine, etc.), cleaning with a detergent and water may be adequate. But for a spillage containing potentially hazardous organisms, a disinfectant should be used. Disposable gloves should be worn, when known contaminated spillage is being cleaned. Granules or powder of chlorine-releasing agent may be sprinkled with a sprinkler to cover small amount of spillage. When the fluid is completely absorbed, a reabsorbable paper should be immediately used to remove the residue and discarded into a plastic bag. Finally, the surface should be washed using a disposable paper wipe. Powders or granules are to be used for wet spillage only. Liquid disinfectants (e.g. chlorine-releasing agents or clear soluble phenolics) can be used for large spillages (>30 mL). Chlorine-releasing powder, granules or fluids containing 10,000 ppm of available chlorine should be used for blood or body fluid spillage that is known or suspected to be contaminated with HIV or HBV. If chlorine-releasing agents are added to hot water, anionic detergents or acidic body fluids (e.g. urine), this may result in rapid release of toxic levels of chlorine. At such concentration these chlorine-releasing agents are toxic and corrosive and likely to damage or decolorize many surfaces.

For other spillages or previously cleaned surfaces, chlorine-releasing agents can be used at 1,000 ppm concentrates.

All wastes, wipes, disposable gloves, aprons should be discarded, sealed and disposed off as clinical waste.

Universal precautions assume that all blood and certain body fluids are potentially infectious and routine disinfection before cleaning is recommended. However, this would seem to be unnecessary in hospitals where the infection rate with HBV or HIV is low, provided that gloves and plastic apron are worn and hands are washed. Thorough cleaning alone is sufficient. Clear soluble phenolics (0.6–2%) are less likely to damage surfaces and are suitable for decontamination with enteric organisms or *Mycobacterium*, but they are poor virucidal agents.

Disinfectants should be prepared freshly and in accurate dilution for each task. Chlorine-releasing powders, granules and tablets, i.e. sodium dichloroisocyanurate

(NaDCC) are stable but solutions are not, and so should be discarded soon after the task is completed, or at the end of the day.

Decontamination of Walls and Ceilings

Usually, there are very few bacteria on walls, which are clean, smooth, dry and intact. Therefore, they are unlikely to pose an infection hazard. Ceilings have an even smaller number of bacteria. Cleaning of wall and ceilings should however be carried out at regular and frequent intervals say 12–24 months to prevent accumulation of visible dirt. In operation theaters, the cleaning should be done at 6 months interval.

Disinfection of walls is usually not required. However if splashes of blood occur, they should be removed promptly. After the cleaning is over, the walls should be left as dry as possible. If there are damaged areas of the wall and the plaster has come out, this area can be heavily colonized with bacteria especially if it becomes moist and cleaning and disinfection of this area would be difficult as such areas can not be cleaned effectively. Therefore, damaged surfaces should be repaired promptly especially in an operating theater. A moist surface may encourage the growth of *Aspergillus*.

Decontamination of Other Surfaces

Locker tops and furniture should be wiped daily with freshly prepared detergent/disinfectant solutions using disposable wipes. So also shelves and ledges should be damp-dusted weekly, or more often if dust accumulates. Disinfection is a must if the surface is contaminated with body fluids or other potentially infectious material.

Decontamination of Baths

Should be cleaned daily. Detergent is usually adequate for routine cleaning. A cream cleaner can be used to remove scum. Baths will have to be disinfected if used for infected patients, or those carrying multi-resistant or problematic strains (e.g. MRSA), or before use by patients with open wounds. A non-abrasive chlorine-releasing powder can be used for this purpose. Abrasive powders are effective, but they damage porcelain surfaces and must never be used on fiberglass.

Solutions or cream cleaners containing chlorine-releasing agents may also be used with a detergent, provided the detergent is known to be compatible.

Decontamination of Wash Basins

Washbasins should be solely used for washing hands and wrist/elbow operated taps are preferred. This can be cleaned with a suitable detergent, or if necessary with a chlorine-releasing agent or a phenolic.

Decontamination of Toilets and Drains

The toilet seats and handles should be cleaned at least once daily and also when they are visibly soiled. A detergent solution can be used for routine cleaning, but if the seat is obviously contaminated, or if a patient with gastrointestinal infection uses it, disinfection can be done with chlorine-releasing agent or a clear soluble phenolic. If a disinfectant is used, the seat should be rinsed with water and dried before use. Pouring disinfectant into lavatory pans or drains is unlikely to reduce infection risks.

Decontamination of Crockery and Cutlery

Food remnants should be scraped out or washed out first, and then crockery should be rinsed, and washed with hot water (at comfortable temperature) and detergent in one sink. In the next sink, the crockery should be immersed in hot water at 77–82°C for one minute and disinfected. It should be allowed to dry by itself, do not wipe.

A washing machine and a facility for drying all crockery and cutlery is preferable to individual washing in wards. A washing machine with a final rinse temperature of 80°C for one minute or other appropriate disinfection time/temperature combination (71°C for 3 minutes) can be used in ward kitchens.

Cleaning Material

Material used for cleaning surfaces (e.g. baths, sinks, mattresses, beds and furniture) must be disposable. If disposable single-use wipes are not available, nylon brush may be used, these can be dried quickly. Absorbent cotton mops or bristle brushes should not be used, as they get heavily contaminated, and are difficult to disinfect. In case non-disposable cloths are used, they should be washed after use (preferably in a washing machine with a disinfection stage in the cycle).

Separate cloths should be used in the kitchen, sluice and other wards areas. Color codes may be used to distinguish them.

Toilet brushes should be rinsed well in the flushing water of the lavatory pan. After excess water has been taken out, they should be stored dry.

Sponges dry slowly, are difficult to disinfect and should not be used.

DISINFECTION OF ROOMS

The Need for Terminal Room Cleaning and Disinfecting

For many years, experts believed that contaminated environmental surfaces in hospitals did not play a significant role in transmission of pathogens to patients. However, recent studies have provided increasing evidence that contaminated surfaces in hospitals may be a source of transmission of pathogens.

For such transmission to occur, the following factors are necessary:

- Relatively frequent contamination of environmental surfaces by pathogens;
- Pathogens that are able to survive in the environment; and
- Direct or indirect transmission of the pathogen to a susceptible patient.

Contaminated Surfaces as Sources of Nosocomial Transmission

Evidence that patients who are colonized or infected with such organisms as methicillin-resistant *Staphylococcus aureus* (MRSA), vancomycin-resistant enterococci (VRE), *Clostridium difficile* spores, *Acinetobacter* species, and Norovirus shed these organisms onto surfaces in their immediate environment in abundance. These pathogens can survive for days or weeks (even months for *C. difficile* spores) on various environmental surfaces. Numerous studies have shown that healthcare workers can contaminate their hands or gloves by touching contaminated surfaces in patient rooms, and it is likely that this could result in transmission to patients.

Monitoring Cleaning and Disinfecting Practices

Methods for assessing the adequacy of room cleaning and disinfecting practices in healthcare facilities is an important element of infection control programs. Numerous studies have established that previous room occupancy by patients with VRE or MRSA increases risk for acquiring these multidrug-resistant organisms in patients subsequently admitted to the same rooms.. On the basis of this, cleaning hospital rooms include the following:

- Have housekeeping managers conduct visual inspection: Although quick and easy, visual inspection does not give reliable information about the cleanliness of surfaces
- Marking high touch surfaces with a fluorescent solution and checking the surfaces with a black light after rooms have been cleaned can determine whether the surfaces have been wiped with a liquid

detergent or disinfectant well enough to remove the marker solution

- Count aerobic colonies of specimens obtained from high touch surfaces: Unfortunately, no standardized criteria for defining hospital surfaces as "clean" or "not clean" on the basis of aerobic colony counts currently exist
- Use adenosine triphosphate (ATP) bioluminescence assay to assess the cleanliness of surfaces: Because all organic material (including microorganisms, human secretions and excretions, and food particles) contains ATP, ATP bioluminescence assay has been used to assess the level of cleanliness of surfaces in hospitals to monitor the adequacy of cleaning practices. With this approach, surfaces are sampled with a specialized swab that is placed in a reaction tube that contains luciferase. The tube is then placed in a luminometer, which quickly yields a digital readout of the amount of generated light, expressed as the number of relative light units. Surfaces that remain contaminated with substantial organic material yield high relative light unit readings, whereas clean surfaces yield low readings.

In most instances, terminal cleaning of patient rooms can be performed using standard hospital-grade surface disinfectant solutions at the manufacturer's recommended concentration and contact times. Currently, in the United States quaternary ammonium compounds are the most commonly used for this purpose. Newer surface disinfectants, such as activated hydrogen peroxide liquid formulations, have recently gained popularity in Canada.

Because *C. difficile* spores are relatively resistant to standard surface disinfectants, current guidelines recommend that hospitals with highly endemic or epidemic *C. difficile*-associated diarrhea use dilute (10%) bleach solutions for terminal cleaning of environmental surfaces in the rooms of patients with *C. difficile*-associated diarrhea. Noroviruses, like *C. difficile* spores, are also relatively resistant to commonly used surface disinfectants. Facilities that are experiencing nosocomial transmission of noroviruses and viral hemorrhagic fever viruses should use dilute bleach solutions to disinfect surfaces following discharge of patients with infections caused by these organisms.

Newer Strategies for Terminal Room Decontamination

Area decontamination technologies that have been studied recently in hospital settings include micro-condensation hydrogen peroxide vapor, a hydrogen peroxide dry mist system, gaseous ozone, an alcohol/quaternary ammonium power sanitizing system, and ultraviolet light room decontamination. Hydrogen peroxide vapor technology has also been used to decontaminate rooms that were vacated by patients who had been infected with norovirus or multidrug-resistant organisms, such as MRSA, VRE, *Serratia,* or *Acinetobacter.* An alcohol/quaternary ammonium power sanitizing system was found to significantly reduce MRSA and VRE contamination on hospital surfaces, but was not consistently as effective as 10% bleach solution.

Ultraviolet (UV) light has been used for years to reduce microbial contamination of air-handling systems. UV-C, particularly in the 254-nm range, destroys microorganisms by creating thymine dimers and inhibiting replication. A recent study demonstrated that an automated mobile UV-C light unit reduced bacterial contamination of surfaces by 2–3 logs (99–99.9%). Because it has proven to be difficult for housekeepers to clean and disinfect environmental surfaces consistently according to hospital policies, these newer room decontamination technologies warrant further investigation to determine their cost-effectiveness and their role in terminal room disinfection.

Recommendations for Post-discharge Cleaning

1. Establish policies for which objects in patient rooms are to be cleaned/disinfected by housekeepers, and which (if any) should be cleaned by other personnel, such as nurses.
2. Educate housekeepers about the surfaces that should be cleaned, the appropriate concentration and contact times for each detergent/disinfectant solution in use, and the importance of room disinfection in reducing transmission of healthcare-associated pathogens.
3. Standard hospital-grade detergent/disinfectant solutions can be used for routine terminal room disinfection. If rates of transmission of *C. difficile* or norovirus are high, use of a dilute bleach solution for surface disinfection in rooms vacated by patients affected by these microorganisms is recommended.
4. Develop methods for periodically monitoring the practices of housekeepers who are responsible for terminal room cleaning/disinfection, and provide them with feedback on their performance.
5. Consider using a fluorescent marking solution to target surfaces, an ATP bioluminescence assay to monitor cleanliness, or aerobic colony counts to monitor cleaning/disinfection practices. Involve infection control personnel in determining which approach to use.
6. For situations in which routine terminal room disinfection practices continue to be problematic despite the above measures or fail to adequately reduce transmission of pathogens that survive well in the environment (e.g. VRE, *C. difficile*, MRSA, *Acinetobacter*, or norovirus), consider use of a newer area decontamination technology to supplement terminal room cleaning/disinfecting protocols.

DECONTAMINATION OF NON-CLINICAL EQUIPMENT

Washing and Shaving Equipment

Plastic Washing Bowls

In general wards—plastic bowls should be thoroughly washed with a detergent and hot water after each use. It should then be stored separately and kept inverted for drying.

In intensive care and high-risk units each patient should have his/her own washing bowl. The bowl should be heat sterilized or disinfected with chlorine-releasing agents or phenols, or alcohol or quaternary ammonium compound before it is used for another patient.

Nail Brushes

Their use should be avoided except for special procedures (e.g. first scrub of the day in operating theaters). This is because the brushes become frequently contaminated with gram-negative bacilli even when stored in a disinfectant solution.

Soap Dishes and Dispensers

Soap dishes are usually not necessary and may encourage growth unless they are washed daily and kept dry. The nozzles of liquid dispensers and the outside should be cleaned and dried. Disposable cartridge type refills with an integral nozzle are preferred, but they tend to be too expensive. If non-disposable reservoirs are used, topping-up should be avoided and the inside of containers cleaned and dried before refilling. Liquid soaps used in hospitals should contain a preservative, which should prevent growth during periods of use.

Razors

Razors are used for preoperative shaving. It should be disposable or autoclavable. If common razors are used, they should be wiped clean and disinfected after each shave using 70% alcohol. Electric razors should also be used after being immersed in alcohol for 5 minutes.

Beds and Beddings

Bed Frames

They should be cleaned weekly and as required and after discharge of patient with a disinfectant.

Of course in the cleaning schedules, they should be included and be wiped with a detergent-disinfectant solution and dried.

If bed belongs to an infected patient like MRSA, or in an outbreak situation, clean twice in a day.

If contaminated, chlorine-releasing agent (1,000 ppm of chlorine) or phenol can be used or a QAC can be used.

Mattresses and Pillows

Mattresses and pillows cannot be disinfected readily if they are contaminated. They should be enclosed in a waterproof cover and if possible a waterproof draw sheet especially if they are being used for patients where contamination with body fluids is likely.

Wiping the cover with a disinfectant solution and thorough drying is adequate. For disinfection chlorine-releasing agents should be used. Phenols should not be used as they may make the covers permeable. After disinfection with chlorine-releasing agents, they should be rinsed well.

Some pillows may be disinfected using hot water laundering at 71°C for 3 minutes or 65°C for 10 minutes, or by low temperature steam (73–80°C). Some mattress covers are often permeable to fluids and should be changed daily. All mattresses should be routinely inspected for damage.

Decontamination of pillows should be done weekly and following patient's discharge and immediately if soiled.

Bedding

Bedding can get heavily contaminated with colonized skin scales very rapidly; therefore frequent changing of bedding is not of much value in controlling the spread of infection. However bedding should be laundered, procedures for laundering are given in section of laundry.

Mattress must have plastic waterproof cover. In the event of the outer plastic cover becoming damaged (split), the item should be disposed of as clinical waste.

Cotton blankets should be used and they should be changed after discharge of patient or if they become soiled or contaminated with potentially infectious spillage.

Bed sheets should be changed twice a week at least, and at any other time when they are soiled or contaminated with potentially infectious material.

CURTAINS

The level of microbial contamination on the curtains will depend on the amount of dispersal by patients in the immediate vicinity. Even if they are changed frequently, they will regain that level. Therefore, they should be washed only when obviously soiled or after every 6 months.

The curtains in the vicinity of a patient who is a disperser of an epidemic strain of *Staphylococcus aureus*, may remain heavily contaminated for some hours, and should be changed if the same area is to be occupied by a susceptible patient within 24 hours.

The degree of microbial contamination is usually not related to the type of material used, or the time since the curtains were changed.

BED CRADLES

Cradles should be maintained and kept in a good condition. They should be disinfected only after use by an infected patient. The cradle should be wiped with chlorine-releasing agent or phenol, and rinsed.

DECONTAMINATION OF INSTRUMENTS FOR CLINICAL PROCEDURES

Dressing Trolley Tops

Washing with a detergent solution and then wiping with a disposable paper to keep it dry is enough. In case it is necessary to disinfect it, it should be wiped with 70% alcohol.

Instruments for Clinical Procedures

Usually all items required for clinical procedures are sterilized, packed and supplied by the SSD. But if this is required at the ward level, a bench top autoclave could be used. If this is not possible boiling water bath may be used rather than chemicals, as it is a more reliable method of disinfection than chemical agents. If there is an emergency, precleaned instruments can be disinfected (not sterilized) by boiling in water bath for 5–10 minutes. Immersion of clean instruments in 70% alcohol, or 2% glutaraldehyde for 10 minutes will disinfect but not as effectively as hot water or steam. Instruments immersed in glutaraldehyde should be thoroughly rinsed with distilled water so as to remove the irritant residues before use. Sterile water is used for invasive items. If glutaraldehyde is used in wards, adequate protection is given to prevent skin, eye and respiratory contact. Wiping with alcohol is not a very reliable method of disinfection of items like scissors though it is a rapid method, and therefore should be used for other items like electrical equipment, etc. that cannot be immersed. Cheatle forceps should preferably not be used for aseptic techniques. If they have to be used (e.g. in hospital without CSSD) the forceps, with its container should be cleaned autoclaved or boiled between use and stored dry.

Used instruments must be washed with water to remove blood or body fluids if soiled, disinfected and then transferred to a paper or plastic bag and sent for sterilization. Suitable protective clothing (e.g. gloves and apron) should be worn.

Thermometers

Oral Thermometers

Should be stored clean and dry. They should not be kept in a disinfectant as used to be done in the past, because, the solution may be contaminated and there may be growth of gram-negative bacilli. Thermometers should be disinfected by immersion in 70% alcohol or 1–2% clean phenolic solution for 10 minutes. If separate thermometers are used for each patient, they should be disinfected by wiping with alcohol and kept back in their respective holders. If not kept for individual patients, they may be wiped clean, and disinfected with alcohol at the end of the round and stored dry.

Rectal Thermometers

Usually, a lubricant is used for introducing the rectal thermometers. After recording the temperature, the thermometer is removed, all traces of the lubricant on the thermometer should be removed and then it should be disinfected as mentioned above. In the West, disposable sleeves are used, which reduce the risk of contamination. If used, the sleeve should be removed and its thermometer treated as for oral thermometers.

Bedpans

Reusable Bedpans

Simplest method is to empty the bedpan in the sluice, after using, washing it and allowing it to dry thoroughly before reuse. This is for the non-infected patients.

If they are used for infected patients bedpans may be boiled in boiling water for 5–10 minutes. Chemical disinfection is usually not practicable. Immersion tanks are not advocated, as they may be ineffective if not well maintained, and may encourage the growth of gram-negative bacilli. Wiping of the entire surface of a cleaned bedpan with a clear soluble phenolic or chlorine-releasing solution, rinsing it and allowing it to dry is an alternative, but this is not as effective as heat disinfection and should be used only when there is emergency especially in a country like ours.

Whenever bedpan washing machine with heat-disinfection cycle is available, that should be used, for washing and disinfection of the bedpans. The thermal disinfection should ensure that the surfaces reach 90°Cor are raised to 80°C and maintained at the temperature for at least one minutes.[6] The cycle should be checked regularly to ensure that the desired temperature is reached. Washing machines without heat disinfection cycles can be used for normal situations, but not in urological wards, infectious diseases wards or where enteric infections are likely to occur.

Disposable Bedpans

Are being used in other countries. They are made up of paper pulp and disposed off in a macerator. These may however cause blockage of pipes. In case, there is heavy contamination they should be washed and wiped with chlorine-releasing agent or a clean phenolic. This should be disinfected if soiled and also on discharge of the patient.

Commodes

If the seat of the commode is soiled, or a patient with enteric infection uses it; it should be disinfected with a clear soluble phenolic or chlorine-releasing agent and dried before use. Ideally, it should be cleaned with disposable wipes, wearing disposable gloves and apron, and then hands washed at the end of the task even if gloves were worn.

Urine Bottles

Recommendations are as suggested for bedpans.

DECONTAMINATION OF MEDICAL EQUIPMENT (HIGH-RISK ITEMS)

High-risk Items

Majority of the items, e.g. surgical instruments, prosthetic devices, and dressings, surgical drapes, gowns, parenteral fluids, etc. can be sterilized by moist heat at high temperature (autoclaving). For other instruments like some delicate sharp instruments used in ophthalmic and dental surgery, glass syringes, oils, powders can be sterilized by dry heat. Single use or disposable items (like catheters, plastic syringes, needles grafts and internal pacemakers) are usually sterilized by the manufacturer using ethylene oxide or irradiation.

Ideally, inexpensive items, especially those that are heat sensitive and difficult to clean, should not be reused. All reusable items should be cleaned thoroughly before sterilization prior to reuse. Manufacturers should state the methods of decontamination, which can be used, for any reusable item or equipment. Non-disposable items should be able to withstand autoclaving at 134°C or at least 80°C. If items are damaged at these temperatures or cannot easily be cleaned, then their use should be discouraged. There are some items which are expensive, and are heat sensitive, e.g. flexible endoscopes, for them decontamination can be done by using less effective methods like immersion in disinfectants.

Operative Endoscopes (Arthroscopes and Laparoscopes)

Use of various scopes is on an increase. Some of these are flexible and may be damaged by heat. So these should be cleaned thoroughly and if possible sterilized with ethylene oxide. If this is not available, then for the more rigid endoscopes low temperature steam and formaldehyde can be used (LTSF). As these methods may not be available or sometimes not practicable, immersion in 2% glutaraldehyde for 3–10 hours is acceptable, but this method is not very reliable due to possible presence of airbubbles and recontamination in subsequent rinsing. Many a-times short immersion times (10–20 minutes) are usually used because of the limited availability of instruments. The short contact time is effective against some pathogenic spores, e.g. *Clostridium difficile*.[7] This process is effective against vegetative bacteria including *Mycobacterium tuberculosis*, viruses and fungi, but usually not all bacterial spores or some atypical *Mycobacterium*.[8] If the endoscope is well cleaned, the risk of infection is small, but the remote risk of infection due to spore-forming organisms cannot be excluded. All invasive endoscopes immersed in glutaraldehyde should be thoroughly rinsed in sterile or bacteria free (filtered <0.45 M) water to remove toxic residues prior to reuse.

Cystoscopes

Autoclaving is widely preferred for rigid cystoscopes, but high level disinfection, i.e. immersion in 2% glutaraldehyde for 10 minutes is usually used.[9] The longer exposure of 20 minutes is required if an effect against *M. tuberculosis* is required.[10,11] Solutions should not be used beyond the manufacturers recommended post-activation use life (e.g. 14–28 days), or if reuse reduces the concentration to below 1.5%. If sufficient instruments are available, autoclaving at low temperature steam with or without formaldehyde may be used. Pasteurization in a water bath at 70–80°C for 10 minutes can be used as an alternative to disinfection, but the manufacturer should be consulted on heat tolerance if hot water or steam is used.

Thermal disinfection/sterlization is unsuitable for flexible cystoscopes. Another alternative is immersion in 70°C ethanol for 5 minutes, but this may damage the instrument if immersion is prolonged beyond the time limit indicated by the manufacturer.

INTERMEDIATE HIGH-RISK ITEMS

Noninvasive Endoscopes

These are now being routinely used by surgeons not being aware that infections are also very frequently transmitted by the use of these scopes. *Pseudomonas* and other gram-negative bacilli, including *Salmonella*, have been transferred from one patient to another on inadequately decontaminated flexible fiber optic endoscopes.[12] However, there have been no reports of transmission of *Mycobacterium*, very rarely of HBV, and no evidence of transfer of HIV. Nevertheless, it is essential to take care to avoid the spread of any infection due to ineffective decontamination.[13] Endoscopic retrograde cholangiopancreatography (ERCP) is a particularly vulnerable procedure, and severe gram-negative infections have been reported. Thorough cleaning and disinfection are important with this procedure.

Potential pathogens such as gram-negative bacilli can grow overnight in the channels of the endoscope, the water bottle and in its processing equipment, and disinfection is required at the beginning of the list as well as after each patient. The time available for processing between patients is often short (20–30 minutes). However, vegetative bacteria and most viruses are killed or inactivated by 1-2 minutes exposure to 2% glutaraldehyde.[14-16]

Having automated machines for cleaning and disinfection are always preferable, as it protects the user from toxic processing chemicals. But even then a preliminary brushing of the suction/biopsy channel and wiping of the insertion tube are still required. All channels should be cleaned and disinfected. In automated systems and otherwise too the concentration of glutaraldehyde is reduced due to repeated use and so the solution must be regularly changed. The rinse water should also be changed preferably after each instrument. Infection has been reported from gram-negative bacilli growing in the rinse water tank. This should be routinely disinfected.

Bacteria free or filtered (0.2–0.45 μ) or sterile water is recommended for invasive instruments and those for ERCP (endoscopic retrograde cholangiopancreatography) and bronchoscopy.

Before we change the method of decontamination, it is advisable to consult the manufacturer, giving them the details of the method to be used. It must be remembered that many of the disinfectants are corrosive and may damage the endoscope. So also low temperature steam may reach 80°C and ethylene oxide may reach 55°C with considerable variations in pressure. Furthermore not all endoscopes and accessories are totally submersible.

Flexible Gastrointestinal Endoscopes

Two percent glutaraldehyde is the disinfectant most widely used for endoscopes. Immersion for 10 minutes at the beginning of the test and in between pateints should be done for decontamination (It is important to clean all the channels and external surfaces of the endoscope before decontamination). This will destroy all the vegetative bacteria, viruses including HIV and HBV. If however the endoscope has been used for a patient suspected of having pulmonary tuberculosis, immersion in 2% glutaraldehyde should be done for 20 minutes. For patients of AIDS and other immunocmpromised patients, endoscope should be disinfected for 20 minutes before and after the procedure, to protect the patients from opportunistic pathogens, some of which are relatively resistant to glutaraldehyde. Similarly a 20 minutes immersion is recommended between cases for ERCP when high-level disinfection is required.

Cryptosporidia are resistant to glutaraldehyde but thorough cleaning of the endoscope will be adequate or though glutaraldehyde is recommended, an alternative agent may be used, e.g. 70% ethanol can be used for in-between patients. But immersion of endoscope in ethanol for longer than 5 minutes may damage the lens cements. Therefore, other agents like peracetic acid, chlorine dioxide and superoxidized water are being investigated. These agents are said to be more rapidly effective than 2% glutaraldehyde especially against *Mycobacterium* (5 minutes) and spores (10 minutes). However, they cause more damage to instruments and processing equipment, and their long-term toxicity is not known.

In view of the toxic, irritant and sensitizing properties of aldehyde, it is necessary to find an effective, non-damaging and less irritant alternative to glutaraldehyde.

Flexible Bronchoscopes

Bronchoscopes should be immersed in 2% glutaraldehyde for 20 minutes between patients—for one hour after being used for a patient, i.e. of pulmonary tuberculosis.

Since there is risk of contamination of instrument with environmental *Mycobacterium* (*Mycobacterium chelonae*), the instrument should be rinsed in sterile water, filtered water (0.2–0.45 μ) or tap water followed by 70% alcohol. This procedure must be followed especially, when the instrument has to be used in an immunocompromised patient.

Endoscope Accessories

There are two types—(1) autoclavable and (2) non-autoclavable. The ones which are autoclavable should be dismantled, cleaned thoroughly, dried, reassembled and autoclaved. Non-autoclavable items should be dismantled, cleaned and immersed in 2% glutaraldehyde or a suitable alternative.

Examples of endoscopic accessories are biopsy forceps, brushes, snares, water bottles, etc.).

Use of 2% Glutaraldehyde

As glutaraldehyde is irritant to the skin, eyes and respiratory tract (even though it is effective) certain precautions are to be taken.

1. Impermeable gloves and apron should always be worn as well as eye protection if splashing is likely.
2. It is important to rinse thoroughly all items immersed in glutaraldehyde.

All staff that comes into contact with glutaraldehyde should undergo health screening which includes a pre-employment enquiry regarding asthma, skin and mucosal symptoms (e.g. rhinitis and conjunctivitis). Lung function tests by spirometry and annual completion of a health questionnaire and immediate notification of skin rashes, chest and sinus problems are also recommended.

MISCELLANEOUS HIGH-RISK ITEMS

Catheters

Single use is preferred. However, there are some catheters (like cardiac catheters), which are too expensive for single use and reprocessing, may be necessary though not usually recommended. These may be sterilized with ethylene oxide provided proper cleaning has been done and its structure and function remains unimpaired. Single use items should be used only if it is cost-effective and safe to do so. Single use items must not be reused if suitable reusable items are available.

Grafts (Heart Valves, Arterial Grafts, Joints and Other Implants)

All these should be autoclaved if possible. In case, they are likely to be damaged by heat, use ethylene oxide. Usually, sterilization of these items in the hospital is not necessary, unless the package containing the device has been opened and the device has not been used immediately.

Cryoprobes

These should be autoclaved. But if it is not possible because they are heat sensitive, use ethylene oxide or LTSF. Immersion in 2% glutaraldehyde or 70% alcohol may be necessary if cryoprobes are heat sensitive and gaseous sterilization facilities are not available.

Transducers and Blood Monitoring Equipment

These may be a source of infection. Single use items are preferable, or else ethylene oxide of LTSF should be used. High-level disinfection (e.g. 2% glutaraldehyde or 70% alcohol) may sometimes be necessary.

Hemodialysis Equipment

For decontamination of hemodialysis equipment—see Chapter 12 (Dialysis).

DECONTAMINATION OF RESPIRATORY EQUIPMENT

Ventilators

There are many types of ventilators. Ventilators may have filters or may not have them. For ventilators, which have filters, the need to decontaminate is minimized. Some ventilators have internal air circuits, which are removable. These can be autoclaved or disinfected by low temperature steam. Sometimes, chemical disinfection may be required. Most of the methods of chemical disinfection are not practicable, as they do not work efficiently in the presence of organic matter, and none of the methods is entirely reliable.

Two methods have been used; one is nebulization with hydrogen peroxide[17] and the use of formaldehyde vapor. The hydrogen peroxide method is quick and the peroxide breaks down and is not toxic to pateints or the staff. If the ventilator is visibly contaminated, it must be striped down and cleaned prior to disinfection. An alternative method is use of formaldehyde vapour.[18]

This method can however be used only for machines with a closed circuit, besides great care has to be taken to remove residual formaldehyde and protect the staff from irritant vapor. Formaldehyde cabinets are also effective, provided that the ventilator is kept working during the cycle. If patient is known to be suffering from tuberculosis and the ventilator is not protected by filters, the use of formaldehyde is advisable. For machines with single circuits you can either use nebulized hydrogen peroxide, or since it can be dismantled easily, it can be washed and disinfected by heat. Smaller machines like infant ventilators can be sterilized by using ethylene oxide. If gaseous methods are used, care should be taken to ensure that all toxic products are removed by flushing with air or oxygen before the ventilator is reused.

Humidifiers

With this water vapor is blown towards the patient. These humidifiers should be changed together with the ventilator circuit, every 48 hours. The condensate may contaminate the hands of staff and humidifiers should be cleaned and disinfected, preferably by heat, before refilling with sterile water. It should be emptied daily and refilled with sterile water. Disinfect when contaminated with 1% hypochlorite for 20 minutes, wash and dry. Autoclave after each patient's use. Autoclave when respiratory circuit is changed. Alcohol (70%) may be used to disinfect evaporator type humidifiers in infant incubators. If antiseptics like chlorhexidine are added to the water, they are not only ineffective, but may select resistant organisms.

Sometimes nebulizers may be contaminated and produce aerosals, which may be responsible for lung infections, caused by gram-negative bacilli, especially *Pseudomonas aeruginosa*. Hence unless, it is possible to disinfect them daily, the nebulizers should not be used. The water in it should also be replaced and not just topped up. If the nebulizing part of the machine is likely to get damaged by heat, it should be flushed with water and dried. If drying is not possible, it should be rinsed in 70% alcohol and allowed to dry.

Oxygen Tents

These should be washed and dried after each patient. Oxygen masks and tubing should be disposable. There is no evidence that piped medical gases become contaminated with bacteria, provided that the lines remain dry.

Anesthetic Equipment

Normally, the anesthetic machines are unlikely to get significantly contaminated and therefore routine decontamination is rarely possible or necessary. However, if filters are not used, then decontamination may be required if it is used for a patient with a known or suspected communicable disease (e.g. pulmonary tuberculosis), when formaldehyde gas may be required. In this case, the machine should be sent to the SSD. The external surface should be kept clean and dry. Contamination is likely to occur in the facemask and tubing nearest to the patient. This equipment (i.e. the tubing, reservoir, ambu bags, face masks, endotracheal tubes and airways) if not meant for single use, should be cleaned and thermally disinfected. The medical equipment cleaning is most suitable for this. The items should be disinfected in a water disinfector (>80°C) or using low temperature steam (73°C) as frequent autoclaving at 121°C or 134°C may damage the equipment.

It is usually desirable to provide a decontaminated set of equipment for every patient, but this is usually not possible. Sessional or daily treatment of the tubing and reservoir bag is reasonable, unless patient has a respiratory infection or pulmonary tuberculosis is suspected.[19]

However, all patients should have a decontaminated facemask, airway and endotracheal tube. Disposable facemasks, tubing and reservoir bags are preferred on patients with known or suspected infections such as tuberculosis. If disposable items are not available, all items used on such patients should be autoclaved immediately or disinfected using hot water or subatmospheric steam.

Laryngoscope Blades

Cleaning and drying is usually sufficient. If disinfection is required, immersion in 70% alcohol for 10 minutes should be effective.

Scavenging Equipment

The tubing close to the patient should be autoclaved, or if it is heat labile, disinfection using LTS (low-temperature steam) or a washer/disinfector should be used. It should be changed regularly (e.g. weekly) and after use on an infected patient.

Suction Equipment

It is ideal to have a piped suction, but if this is not possible, a separate machine should be available for each patient requiring suction. After use the contents should be discarded and the bottle washed, dried, and fresh connection tube attached. If the aspirate in the bottle is allowed to stand for long, bacterial multiplication may occur in it. If there is aspirate in the bottle, this should be emptied in the sluice and the bottle washed with a detergent solution and dried. A washer/disinfector may be used as an alternative if available. The bottle should be emptied at least daily irrespective of the amount of fluid aspirated. This should be done using non-sterile gloves and hands washed after handling the bottle contents. A fresh catheter should be used; each time a patient undergoes suctions (e.g. bronchial aspiration). If detergents are used to clean the bottles, there may be excessive foaming of the bottle contents, which may then wet the filter and enter the pump mechanism. The filter will have to be changed if moist or discolored. To prevent foaming, an anti-foaming agent may be used. Disinfectants are usually not used during suction because many of them are toxic and ineffective. However if the contents are likely to be hazardous to the staffs or if the suction equipment has been used to irrigate instruments, then it should be disinfected. This is done by adding sufficient disinfectant (e.g. chlorine releasing agent) to give a final concentration suitable for dirty situation, which is drawn through the tubing and added to the bottle and left for at least 10 minutes. The tubing should then be flushed and the bottle washed and dried before re-use. The machine should periodically be returned to the SSD where the pumps can be checked, the filter changed, and the tubing lid, non-return valve and bottle autoclaved or processed in a washer/disinfector. If a patient requires suction for more than 24 hours, the bottle tubing should be changed. When the suction machine is not in use, the bottle should be kept dry and the catheter should not be connected until it is required. Now-a-days disposable suction bottles are available, but they are expensive. In this, the container itself is disposable or a disposable liner is fitted within a container.

DECONTAMINATION OF INFANT INCUBATORS

These are to be preferably cleaned in the SSD. After discharge of a patient, the inner surface of the incubator should be thoroughly cleaned with a moist paper wipe and detergent and dried. As cleaning and drying is usually effective, disinfection is rarely necessary. Even if disinfection becomes necessary, prior cleaning has to be done for proper disinfection. For disinfection, the cleaned surface can be wiped with a freshly prepared chlorine-releasing agent (e.g. 125 ppm available chloride) rinsed and dried. As an alternative 70% alcohol may be used. However care should be taken since alcohol is inflammable, and the incubator must be aired thoroughly before reuse.

Formaldehyde cabinets are occasionally used but these are expensive and involve the use of a hazardous chemical.

DECONTAMINATION OF VAGINAL AND OTHER SPECULA AND SIGMOIDOSCOPES

Such instruments should be thoroughly cleaned and autoclaved. Bench top autoclaves are now available and appropriate for use in clinics. Boiling water (for 5–10 minutes) is effective, but care is necessary to ensure that all items are thoroughly cleaned and completely immersed, and that the instrument is exposed to boiling water for the required time (i.e. at least 5 minutes). The boiling water bath preferably should have a timing mechanism. Use of chemical disinfectants should be avoided as far as possible especially for vaginal specula.[20] but immersion in 70% alcohol for 10 minutes should disinfect adequately. Immersion in 2% glutaraldehyde for 10 minutes is also effective, but is irritant and sensitizing, so its use should be avoided unless suitable controlled exhaust-vented processing equipment is available.

DECONTAMINATION OF TONOMETERS

These should be rinsed and immersed in a disinfectant solution for at least 5 minutes. The use of chlorine-releasing agents for 10 minutes (550 ppm of available chlorine) or 3–6% stabilized hydrogen peroxide is recommended by CDC (Center for Disease Control). Tonometers should be rinsed thoroughly and dried before use. Hydrogen peroxide in particular is irritant to the conjunctiva, and therefore thorough rinsing or neutralization is important. Wiping with 70% ethanol is probably effective, although the exposure time is short and alcohol can damage the conjunctiva if it is still present on the instrument when it is used. Immersion in 70% alcohol for 5–10 minutes should be effective, but care should be taken that this does not damage the instrument, and that the alcohol has completely evaporated before use.

DECONTAMINATION OF EQUIPMENT USED ON PATIENTS WITH CREUTZFELDT-JACOB DISEASE

Creutzfeldt-Jacob disease (CJD) is one of the rare transmissible degenerative diseases of human and animals with a long incubation period (10–20 years in humans) and is characterized by progressive dementia. The agent that causes this disease is referred to as prions that are a self-replicating protein without detectable RNA or DNA. It has not been grown in tissue cultures and is extremely resistant to disinfection and sterilization procedures. Transmission of CJD has occurred from contaminated human pituitary growth hormones, corneal transplants and surgical instruments. It is also likely that transmission of variant CJD (VCJD) to humans has occurred from cows with BSE (Bovine spongiform encephalopathy).

Usually, the main risk of spread of CJD is from the central nervous system (i.e. brain and spinal cord), although careful handling of blood is also advised. The Advisory Committee of Dangerous Pathogens (ACDP) and spongiform encephalopathies (SEAC) have jointly prepared guidelines.[21] These unconventional agents are extremely resistant to physical and chemical agents.[22] They are not significantly susceptible to the disinfectants normally used to disinfect instruments, environmental surfaces and skin. They are also resistant to gaseous sterilants, e.g. ethylene oxide and formaldehyde), ionizing radiation, UV light, microwaves and the conventional steam-sterilization cycles (i.e. 121°C for 15 minutes and 134°C for 3 minutes). It is advised that the instruments used on patients known to have, or suspected of having CJD or related disorders and at risk patients (i.e. those who are asymptomatic, but have a clinical or family history which places them in one of the risk groups), and which have been exposed to brain, spinal cord and eye tissue must be destroyed by incineration. If the instruments have been used on at-risk patient where there has been no involvement of brain, spinal cord or eye tissue should be thoroughly cleaned, and sterilized or disinfected using an appropriate physical or chemical process. The methods, which could be used, for sterilization are porous-load steam sterilization at 134°C to 137°C for a single cycle of 18 minutes or steam sterilization at 132°C for 30 minutes in a gravity displacement sterilizer, immersion in sodium hypochlorite (20,000 ppm available chlorine) for one hour, immersion in 1 N sodium hydroxide for one hour followed by steam sterilization at 121°C for 30 minutes and for histological specimens, immersion in 96% formic acid for one hour. These chemical agents, at the concentration and contact times described here, are likely to damage most instruments, therefore wherever possible single use items are advised. If it is not possible to avoid expensive reusable items, it is essential to confirm the process compatibility of the device with the manufacturers and to clean the item thoroughly first.

CLEANING AND DISINFECTION OF SKIN AND MUCOUS MEMBRANES

Principles

There are three principal reasons for removing or reducing the number of microorganisms present on the skin or mucous membranes:

1. To reduce the number of organisms present before any invasive procedure is carried out.
2. To remove or destroy potentially pathogenic organisms present on the hands of staff.
3. To treat a carrier or disperser of a resistant, virulent or highly communicable strain of bacteria.

The bacteria present on the healthy skin have been classified for practical purposes into two types:

1. Resident organisms that colonize the skin, i.e. survive and multiply in the superficial layers. For example, *Coagulase-negative Staphylococcus* and diphtheroids and occasionally *S. aureus*. Gram-negative bacilli (e.g. *Klebsiella* are usually transients, but may be temporary residents for periods ranging from several days to many weeks.). *Acinetobacter calcoaceticus var, anitratum* has many of the survival properties of staphylococci and may be considered a true resident.
2. Transient organisms—those that are recent contaminants, they are usually acquired from a colonized or infected patient or from inanimate hospital environment and deposited on the skin. They survive only for a limited period of time and do not multiply there. However, these include pathogens like GNB (*E. coli, Klebsiella*), *S. aureus*, etc., which may cause nosocomial infections.

Most of the transient flora can be removed with soap and water. This may be as effective as disinfection. However, the resident bacteria are mostly left on the skin after washing with soap and water, but these can be reduced by disinfection. Some bacteria are naturally acquired and present on the skin, but do not multiply on the skin (e.g. *Clostridium perfringens* present through fecal contamination) may be difficult to remove by washing with soap and water.

On the mucus membranes of mouth, nose and vagina also a large number of bacteria are found as residents, but different organisms predominate at different sites. The urethra normally has few commensal bacteria, but can become contaminated after passing a catheter or other instruments. Disinfection of urethra is one of the most important features of prophylaxis against infection of urinary tract. The conjunctiva also has a few bacteria, but these may include *Staphlococcus aureus.*

Cleaning and Disinfection of Hands

Handwashing plays a very important role in preventing the transmission of infection between the healthcare workers and patients in the hospital. Pathogenic organisms from infected patients or colonized patients are present on the hands of the staff and from an important mode of spread of infection in the hospital.

Hands should be washed between patient contacts and after contact with blood, body fluids, excretions, secretions and equipment or articles contaminated with these.

There are two types of flora on the skin as has been already mentioned, the resident flora and the transient flora. The transient flora can be easily removed by soap and water, but the resident flora has to be removed by disinfection.

There are various methods of decontamination of hands, depending on the purpose for which it is required.

Social Handwashing (10–15 Seconds)

Social handwashing (10-15 seconds) is washing with plain soap and water.

Aims: It is to remove transient microorganisms from the moderately soiled hands.

It is done:

a. Before handling food, eating or feeding the patient.
b. After—the toilet
c. Before and after nursing a patient (e.g. bathing and bed making)
d. Whenever hands are soiled.

Note: Handwashing is not needed for superficial contact with patient (e.g. taking blood pressure).

Method: This is done using only soap and water. It has to be done vigorously, applying mechanical friction to all surfaces of hands, for at least 10 seconds, using a defined technique. The hands are then rinsed under a stream of water and dried with paper towel. If there is no running water available, a clean bowl of water should be used for hand washing purposes. The bowl should be cleaned and water changed in between each use. Alternatively a drum with a tap could be elevated to serve as running water. Similarly in absence of paper/towels, a clean cloth should be used (measuring 12" × 12"), for individual drying of hands. This cloth/towel should not be used for common use and should be discarded after each use into a bag specifically meant for laundering and re-use. In places where there is frequent disruption of water supply, it is necessary to store water in large receptacles wherever a water supply is available. This can be used during periods of scarcity of water. The water should be free from pathogens such as cholera.

Hygienic Handwashing or Disinfection (30 Seconds to 1 Minute)

It is a procedure where an antiseptic detergent preparation is used for washing hands. A thorough hand wash may be appropriate if disinfectants are not available, but a single application of 60–70% ethanol or isopropanol with an emollient (e.g. 1% glycerol) with or without antiseptic (e.g. chlorhexidine or povidone-iodine) is significantly more effective against transients than soap and water wash.[23,24]

Aim: It is to remove and kill the transient flora and to decrease the resident organisms to prevent the risk of wound contamination (when gloves are not available or damaged).

Agents used are:[25]

Acqueous:

- 4% chlorhexidine gluconate/detergent solution
- 7.5% povidone—iodine/detergent solution containing 0.75% available iodine (e.g. betadine, videne).

Alcohol based: 0.5% chlorhexidine or povidone-iodine in 70% isopropanol or ethanol, 60% isopropanol or 70% ethanol with emollient (e.g. 0.5% glycerol).

Aim: It is done:

a. Before performing invasive procedure
b. Before caring for susceptible patient (immunocompromised)
c. Before and after use of gloves
d. After contact with blood secretions or following situations in which microbial contamination is likely to occur.
e. Before and between caring for high-risk patients
f. Upon leaving an isolation room.

Method: Wet hands with clean running water, if not available, from water in a bowl, apply cleanser (3–5 mL of 70% alcohol or an alcoholic antiseptic preparation with emollient to the hands and rub to dryness (i.e. at least for 30 seconds to 1 minute), applying friction over all hand surfaces. Alcohol-based antiseptic is more effective than acqueous antiseptic solution.

Alcohol is an effective alternative when there is no water or towels readily available and there is need for rapid hand disinfection.

If disinfectant is not available a thorough hand wash (using soap) may be appropriate.

Standard procedure of handwashing technique[26]

The hands are rubbed, with five strokes for each movement backwards and forwards, palm to palm, right palm over left dorsum, left palm over right dorsum, palm to palm with fingers interlaced, backs of fingers to opposing palm with the fingers interlaced, rotational rubbing of right thumb clasped in left palm and left thumb in right palm, rotational rubbing with clasped fingers of the right hand in the palm of left hand, and the left hand in the palm of the right hand, complete hands and wrists (Fig. 9.1).

If using antiseptic hand rub (e.g. alcoholic handrub)

- Apply product to palm of one hand and rub hands together, covering all surfaces of hands and fingers, take an adequate amount and rub on all surfaces for the recommended time

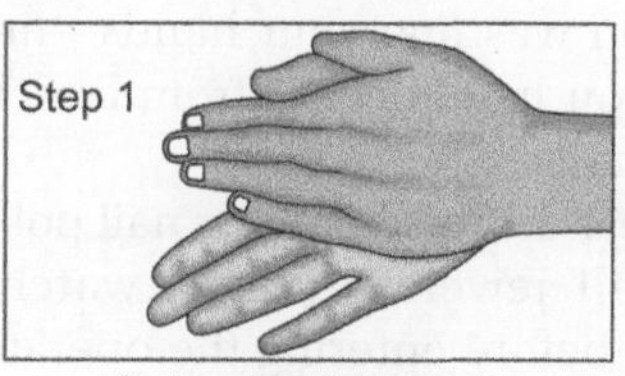

Rub palms together

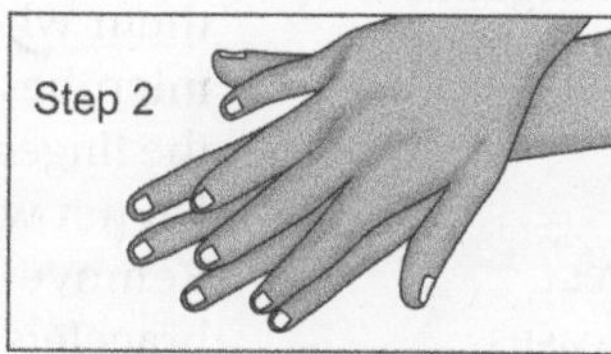

Rub the back of both hands

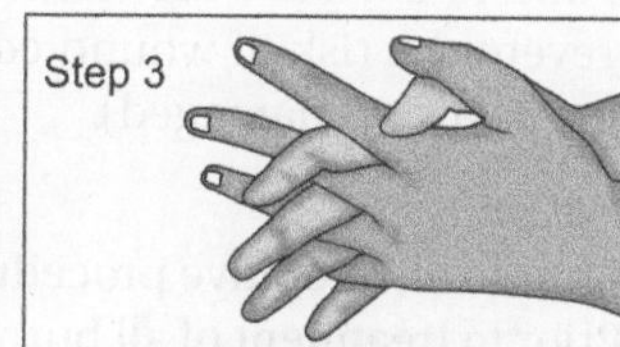

Interface fingers and rub hands together

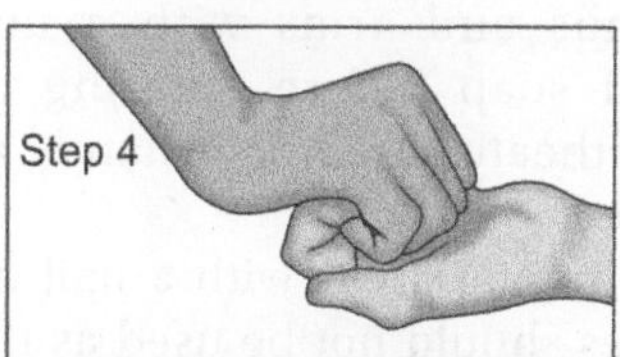

Interface fingers and rub the back of fingers of both hands

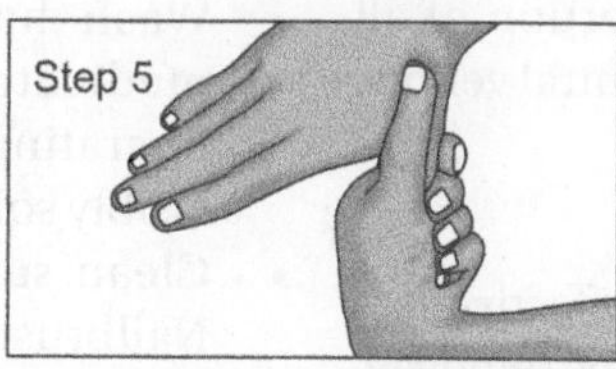

Rub thumb in a rotating manner followed by the area between index finger and thumb for both hands

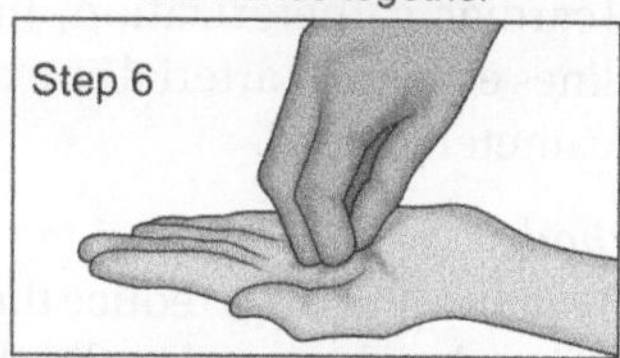

Rub fingertips on palm for both hands

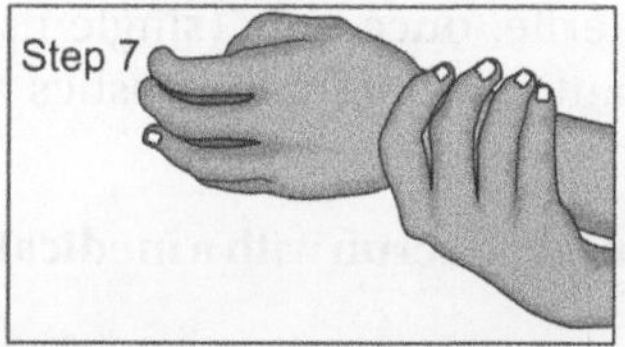

Rub both wrists in a rotating manner. Rinse and dry thoroughly

Fig. 9.1: Handwashing technique[26]

- Let the antiseptic dry on its own. Follow the manufacturer's recommendations regarding the volume of product to use (usually at least 3 mL is required).

The use of an alcohol-based handrub instead of washing with soap and water is preferable since, an alcohol-based handrub requires less time, is microbiologically more effective and is less irritating to skin than traditional hand washing with soap and water.[2]

Handrub: Alcohol-based handrub (ABHR) should be provided in all patient care areas. In case, there is an outbreak of MRSA or *Candida* infections a combination of alcohol with triclosan (anti-MRSA) and chlorhexidine should be used.

Surgical Handwashing

Aim: In this no disinfectant other than soap/ detergent is used, however defined technique for decontamination of hands is now important than the detergent used.

Aim is to remove and kill all transient flora and to decrease the resident organisms to prevent the risk of wound contamination (when gloves are damaged).

Indication:

- Prior to all operative procedures
- Prior to treatment of all burns cases
- Before insertion of all invasive devices (cardiac catheterization, Insertion of all lines especially arterial and central venous catheterization).

Method:

a. Watches and rings reduce the effectiveness of handwashing and so should be removed.
b. The time of scrub is increased to 2–3 minutes. The hands should be scrubbed at least twice using warm water and should include wrists and forearms (i.e. up to the elbow) besides palms and fingers.

After washing, the water should not drop down from unwashed area of arm to washed hands. To assure this, the hands are kept in upright position folded at elbow. After drying the surgeon must put on gown and gloves.

After washing hands with soap and water, a handrub with an alcoholic base formulation should be used if possible. This will not only remove the transient flora more effectively,[23] but also enhance the destruction or inhibition of resident skin flora.[25] Surgical scrubs and alcohol rub should preferably contain emollients and moisturizers to counter the drying/detrimental effects of repeated hand washing.

Sterile towels should be used to dry the hands thoroughly after washing and before alcohol is applied.

Alcohol alone may be used before subsequent operations during an operation session.

Sterile disposable or autoclavable nail brushes may be used to clean the fingernails only, but it should be used only during the first wash of the day or the first application of the antiseptic detergent during that day.

Steps before starting surgical hand preparation

Key steps:

- Keep nails short and pay attention to them when washing your hands—most microbes on hands come from beneath the fingernails
- Do not wear artificial nails or nail polish. Remove all jewelery (rings, watches, bracelets) before entering the operating theater
- Wash hands and arms with a non-medicated soap before entering the operating theater area or if hands are visibly soiled
- Clean subungual areas with a nail file. Nailbrushes should not be used as they may damage the skin and encourage shedding of cells. If used, nailbrushes must be sterile, once only (single use). Reusable autoclavable nail brushes are available.

Protocol for surgical scrub with a medicated soap

- Start timing. Scrub each side of each finger, between the fingers, and the back and front of the hand for 2 minutes

- Proceed to scrub the arms, keeping the hand higher than the arm at all times. This helps to avoid recontamination of the hands by water from the elbows and prevents bacteria-laden soap and water from contaminating the hands
- Wash each side of the arm from wrist to the elbow for 1 minute
- Repeat the process on the other hand and arm, keeping hands above elbows at all times. If the hand touches anything at any time, the scrub must be lengthened by 1 minute for the area that has been contaminated
- Rinse hands and arms by passing them through the water in one direction only, from fingertips to elbow. Do not move the arm back and forth through the water
- Proceed to the operating theater holding hands above elbows
- At all times during the scrub procedure, care should be taken not to splash water onto surgical attire
- Once in the operating theater, hands and arms should be dried using a sterile towel and aseptic technique before donning gown and gloves.

Surgical procedures may be carried out one after the other, without the need for handwashing, provided that the handrubbing technique for surgical hand preparation is followed (Fig. 9.2).

Note:

1. That alcoholic solutions may not be effective against some viruses (e.g. enteroviruses), due to the relatively short exposure time of the agent on the hands, and washing with soap and water prior to the use of alcohol is therefore preferable if contamination with these agents is likely.[27] However, 70% alcohol is effective against rotaviruses on the hands.[28]
2. Triclosan or hexachlorophene preparations are less frequently used, but they are useful if hypersensitivity develops to other agents.

For handwashing, the following facilities are required:

- Running water, large washbasins with hands free control, which requires less maintenance and anti-splash devices
- Products—dry soap or liquid antiseptic depending on procedure
- Suitable material for drying of hands, disposable towels, reusable sterile single use towels, or roller towels, which are suitably maintained (Automatic hand dryer).

Cleaning and Disinfection of Operation Site

For preoperative preparation of an operation site, a quick acting antiseptic is desirable. Alcoholic solutions containing chlorhoxidine, povidone-iodine or triclosan are preferable to aqueous solutions for intact skin.[29] The antiseptic should be applied with friction, on a sterile gauze swab. This should extend well beyond the operation site for 3–4 minutes. If a gloved hand is used to apply the antiseptic, a second glove should be worn by the surgeon over his or her operatory glove, and removed when the preparation of the operation site is complete.[30] Alcoholic solutions should be allowed to dry.

Before operations on hands with ingrained dirt (in gardeners), or on the legs of patients with a poor arterial supply (e.g. amputations for diabetic gangrene of the foot), the application of a compress soaked in povidone-iodine solution to the operation site for 30 minutes, will greatly reduce the numbers of spores of gas gangrene bacilli that present a special hazard in such patients. Ordinary methods of disinfection are ineffective against bacterial spores. However, some spores may remain and antibiotic prophylaxis is still required. Washing with detergents and grease solvent jellies helps to remove ingrained dirt and the dead skin scales in which organisms are carried.

- The handrubbing technique for surgical hand preparation must be performed on perfectly clean, dry hands
- On arrival in the operating theater and after having donned theater clothing (cap/hat/bonnet and mask), hands must be washed with soap and water
- After the operation when removing gloves, hands must be rubbed with an alcohol-based formulation or washed with soap and water if any residual talc or biological fluids are present (e.g. the glove is punctured)

Surgical procedures may be carried out one after the other without the need for handwashing, provided that the handrubbing technique for surgical hand preparation is followed (Steps 1 to 17).

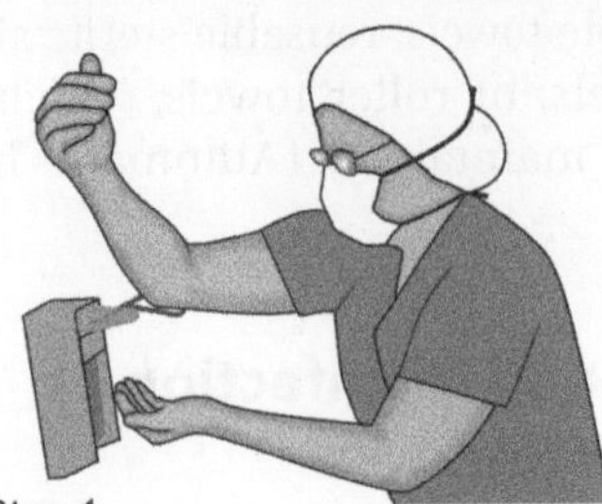

Step 1
Put approximately 5 mL (3 doses) of alcohol-based handrub in the palm of your left hand, using the elbow of your other arm to operate the dispenser

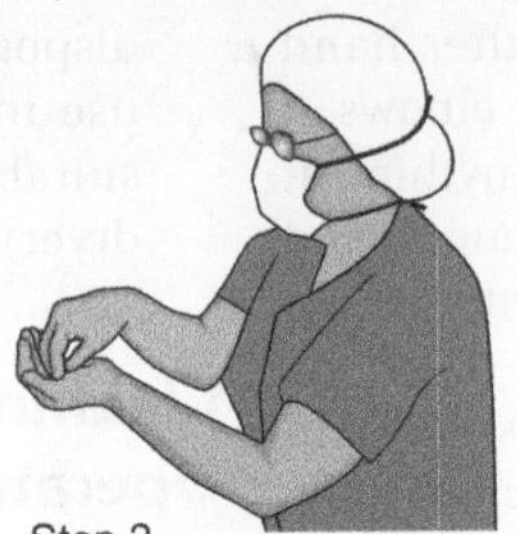

Step 2
Dip the fingertips of your right hand in the handrub to decontaminate under the nails (5 seconds)

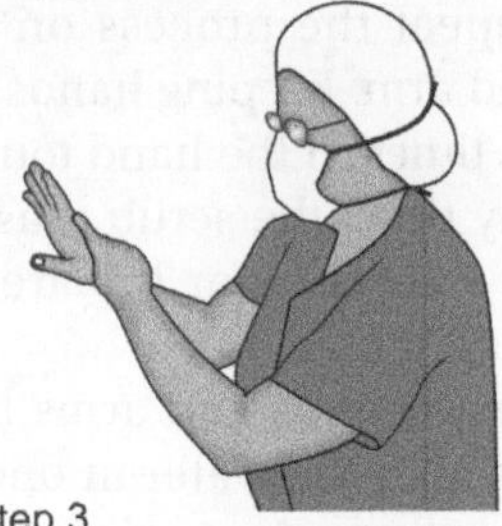

Step 3
Steps 3–7: Smear the handrub on the right forearm up to the elbow. Ensure that the whole skin area is covered by using circular movements around the forearm until the handrub has fully evaporated (10–15 seconds)

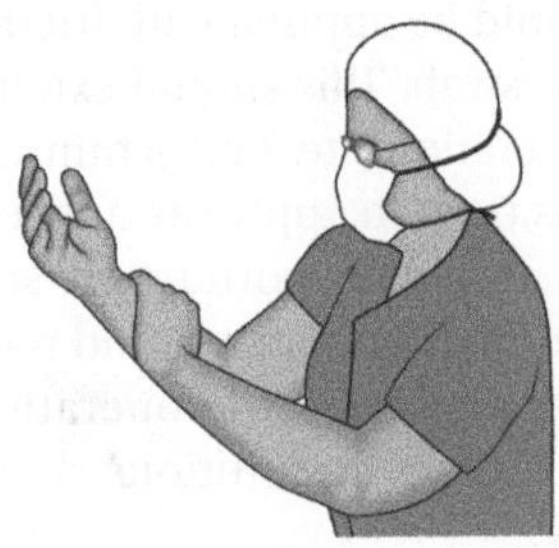

Step 4
See legend for Step 3

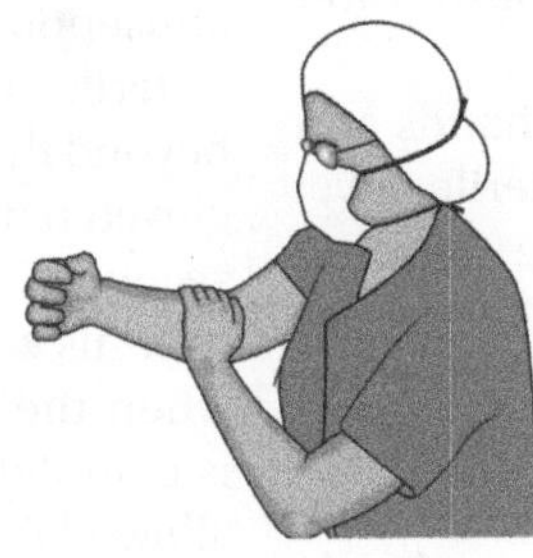

Step 5.
See legend for Step 3

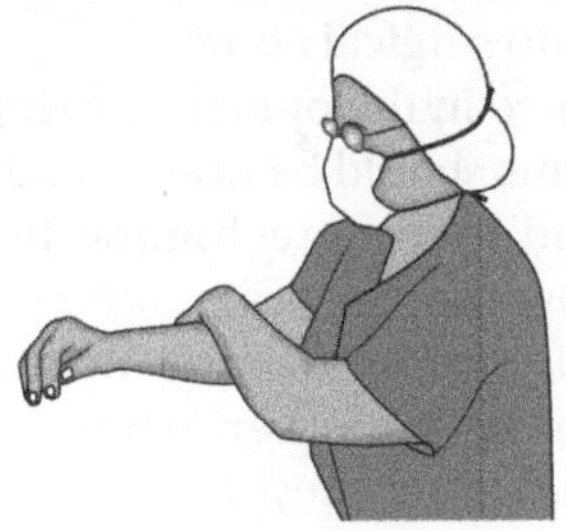

Step 6
Se legend for Step 3

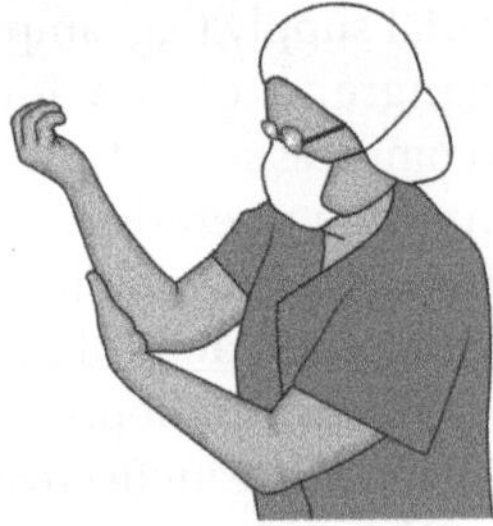

Step 7
See legend for Step 3

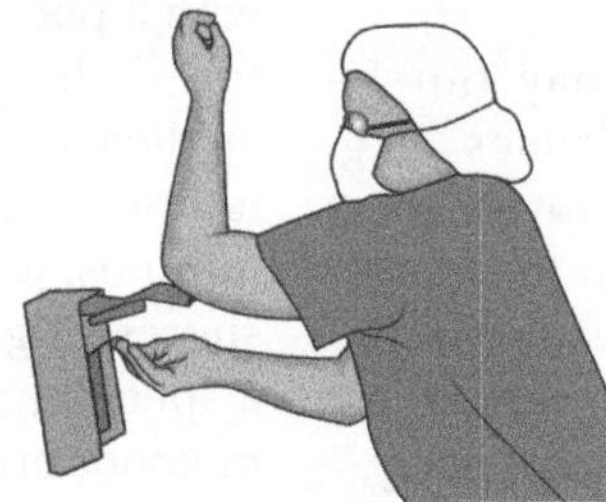

Step 8
Put approximately 5 mL (3 doses) of alcohol-based handrub in the palm of your right hand, using the elbow of your other arm to operate the dispenser

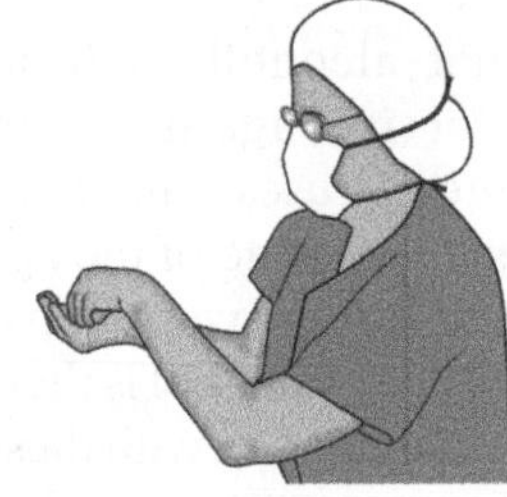

Step 9
Dip the fingertips of your left hand in the handrub to decontaminate under the nails (5 seconds)

Contd...

Contd...

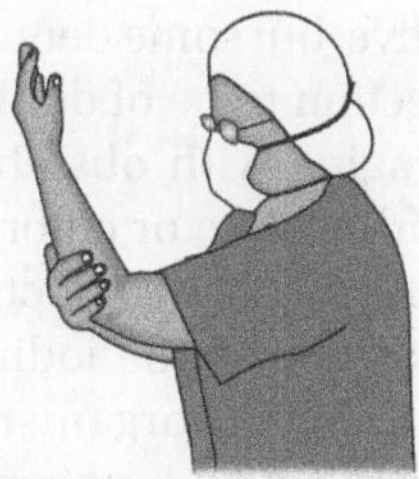

Step 10
Smear the handrub on the left forearm up to the elbow. Ensure that the whole skin area is covered by using circular movements around the forearm until the handrub has fully evaporated (10–15 seconds)

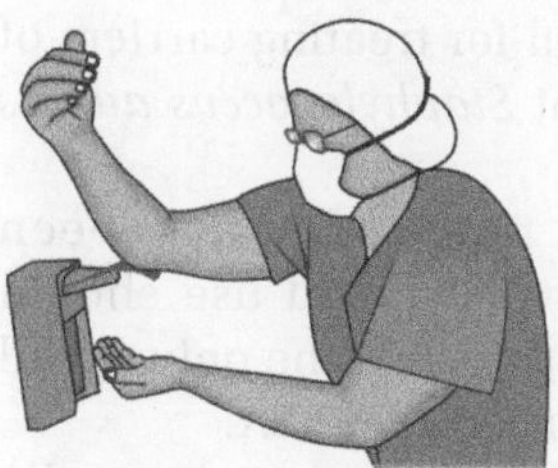

Step 11
Put approximately 5 mL (3 doses) of alcohl-based handrub in the palm of your left hand, using the elbow of your other arm to operate the distributor. Rub both hands at the same time up to the wrists, and ensure that all the steps represented in Steps 12–17 are followed (20–30 seconds)

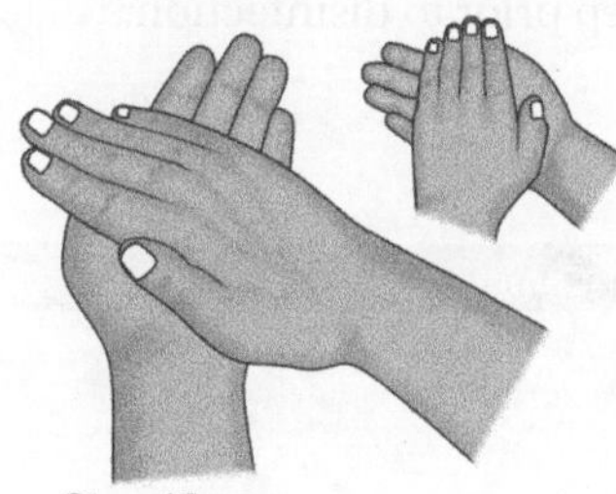

Step 12
Cover the whole surface of the hands up to the wrist with alcohol-based handrub, rubbing palm against palm with a rotating movement

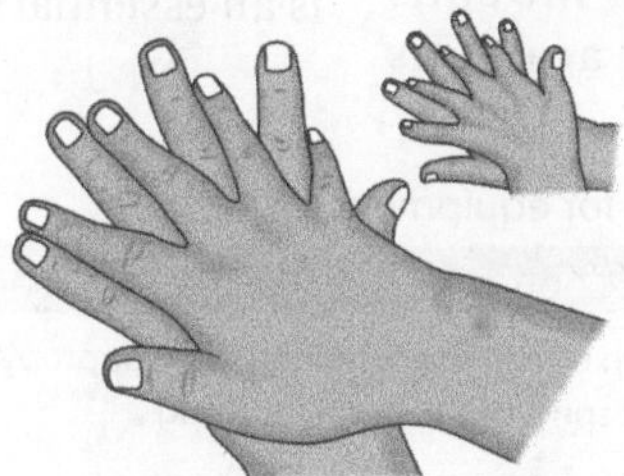

Step 13
Rub the back of the left hand, including the wrist, moving the right palm back and forth, and vice versa

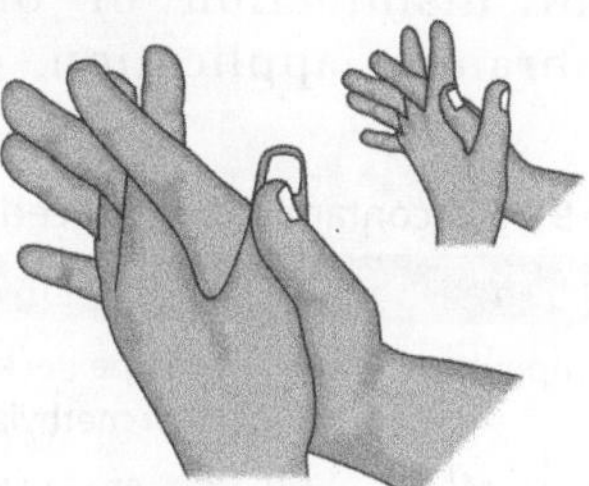

Step 14
Rub palm against palm back and forth with fingers interlinked

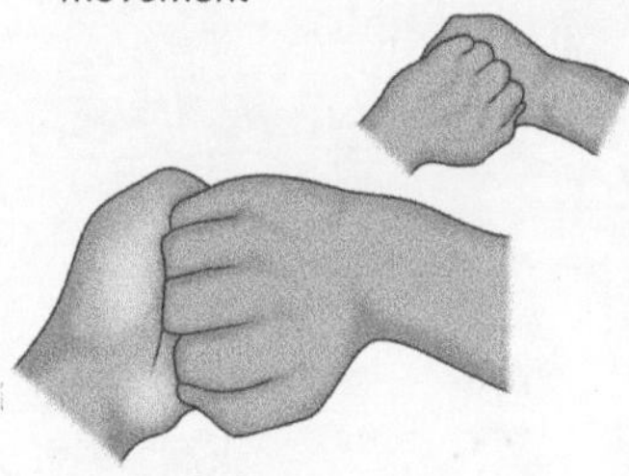

Step 15
Rub the back of the fingers by holding them in the palm of the other hand with a sideways back and forth movement

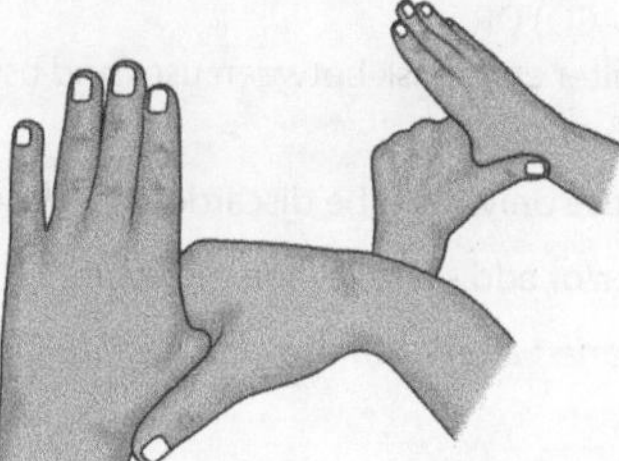

Step 16
Rub the thumb of the left hand by rotating it in the clasped palm of the right hand and vice versa

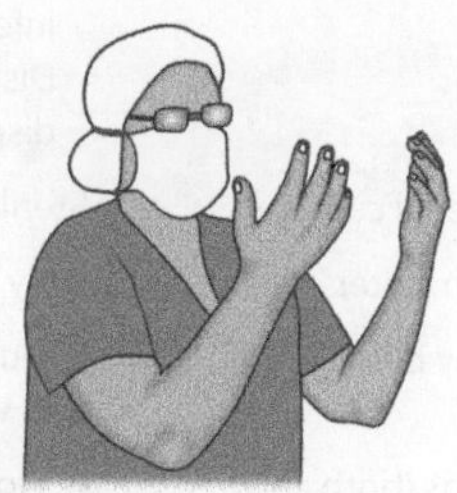

Step 17
When the hands are dry, sterile surgical clothing and gloves can be donned

Repeat the above-illustrated sequence (average duration, 60 seconds) according to the number of times corresponding to the total duration recommended by the manufacturer for surgical hand preparation with an alcohol-based handrub

Fig. 9.2: Surgical hand preparation technique with an alcohol-based handrub formulation

Cleaning and Disinfection of Mucous Membranes

Repeated applications (three to four times a day) of a cream containing 0.5% neomycin and 0.1% chlorhexidine, to the inside of nostrils has been shown to remove *Staphylococcus aureus* from a fairly large proportion of nasal carriers. Alternative for this could be neomycin-bacitracin ointment or 1% chlorhexidine cream.[31] Mupirocin cream is more rapidly effective and more likely to eliminate the

Staphylococcus than other preparations and is particularly useful for treating carriers of methicillin-resistant *Staphylococcus aureus* (MRSA).

Resistance to mupirocin has been described and its widespread use should therefore be avoided, as it is the only useful agent for treating carriers of MRSA.

Streptococcus pyogenes can usually be cleaned from the throat by a course of penicillin (injected or given by mouth, but not by local application). Erythromycin is effective and should be used in patients who are sensitive to penicillin.

For disinfection of oral mucous membranes, application of aqueous solutions of chlorhexidine or povidone-iodine are effective, but some dental surgeons consider disinfection to be of doubtful value. Treatment of vagina with obstetric creams containing chlorhexidine or chloroxylenol is considered to have little disinfectant action. An application of a povidone-iodine solution reduces the number of organisms, but its effect on clinical infection is uncertain.

Decontamination Procedure for Equipment (Table 9.1)

Note: Pre-cleaning of any item/medical device is an essential step prior to disinfection.

Table 9.1: Decontamination procedure for equipment

Article	Standard procedure	Comments
1. Ampoules	Wipe neck with 60–70% alcohol (ethyl or isopropyl) or methylated spirit or PVI before cutting	
2. Ambu bags	• Should be cleaned with detergent and water; dried and sterilized OR • Disinfect by heat or immerse in 2% glutaraldehyde and then wash with sterile distilled water to reduce the risk of chemical irritation which can precipitate respiratory infection (NACO) OR • Dispose of filter and mask between uses and use disposable Ambu bags	
3. Arterial catheters	Sterile single use only. Must be discarded after use	
4. Bath water	Only hot water/or add savlon when necessary	
5. Baby bath	Should be cleaned after each use with detergent and water	
6. Baths (both children and adults)	• Noninfected—wash with detergent and water, and let dry • If used for infected patients with open wounds—Disinfect with sodium hypochlorite solution 0.1% (1000 ppm) and 2 tsf soap	
7. Bedpans and urinals	Should be cleaned and disinfected with Saniquad' (Banzalkonium chloride) 2% for 30 minutes (If possible autoclave before reuse for bedpans) or disinfect with 0.5% sodium hypochlorite for 20–30 minutes	Heat disinfect if facility available at 80°C or 90°C for 1 minute or in boiling water for 5–10 minutes
8. Bowls a. Surgical bowls (for washing)	Wash with hot water and keep dry If used for infected patients—disinfect with alcohol 60–70%/saniquad 2%—30 minutes or 0.5% sodium hypochlorite for 20–30 minutes. Wash and autoclave before reuse	

Contd...

Contd...

Article	Standard procedure	Comments
9. Baby equipment (Feeding bottles and teats)	• Disposable—single use • Reusable - Feeds—pre-sterilized and heat disinfected - Use teats and bottles sterilized and packed by SSD Or - Disinfectant used (chlorine-releasing agent) in small units where other methods are unavailable	Rinse with sterile distilled water before use
10. Baby weighing scales	• A fresh liner should be used for each baby • Clean tray as necessary. Wash with detergent and water	If contaminated should be wiped with hypochlorite 1000 ppm (0.1%) after washing/wipe with 70% isopropyl alcohol
11. Beds and couches or frames	Damp dust with detergent and water between patients and as required	If contaminated wipe with phenol or lysol or saniquad or with sodium hypochlorite solution (if required). If used in isolation room, clean and then wipe with above said disinfectants
12. Breast pumps	Should be washed with detergent and water, immersed in sodium hypochlorite freshly made	
13. Brushes (nail, toilet)	• Disposable—single use • Re-usable—returned to CSSD after each use should be rinsed well in flush water and stored dry	Should not be left on sink after use
14. Crockery and cutlery	• Scoop or wipe the food remnants • Rinse and wash with detergent in one sink • In the second sink filled with water at 77–82°C, immerse the crockery for one minute, this will disinfect it, then let it dry spontaneously. Do not wipe	
15. Carpets	• Vacuum daily (Vacuum) • Carpets in clinical area require a 6 monthly carpet shampoo • Should be shampooed or steam cleaned in isolation room as part of terminal cleaning • For blood spills—sodium hypochlorite/ peroxygen and shampoo immediately	• Carpets are not recommened for clinical areas as they are impractical to clean • Alternative types of flooring must be considered when replacing
16. Commodes	Seat and arms should be cleaned with detergent and water and dried	If soiled or used in isolation, should be wiped with sodium hypochlorite 2% and dried after cleaning
17. Cradles	Should be cleaned with detergent and water, and dried	If used by infected patient—wipe with sodium hypochlorite or phenol
18. Curtains	Routine change every 6 months + immediately, if contaminated	• Should be changed as a part of terminal cleaning • Additional cleaning for some specific infections
19. Drainage bottles	Disposable—single use If reusable—rinse with hot water and detergent—disinfect with 2% lysol, phenol or saniquad/or 1% sodium hypochlorite according to requirement	Autoclave before reuse. To be stored clean and dry

Contd...

Contd...

Article	Standard procedure	Comments
20. Denture pots	Patients must have their own named denture pot to be cleaned by patients themselves with detergent and water Or use disposable single use pots Discard after patient discharge	
21. Drip stands	Should be cleaned with detergent and water, and dried	After use in isolation, should be wiped with sodium hypochlorite 2% and dried after cleaning
22. Endoscopes	• Clean and heat disinfect or sterilize • If heat sensitive, clean and disinfect with 2% glutaraldehyde	Cleaning with detergent and then with 70% ethanol however this is a less effective method (Immersion for >5 minutes can damage epoxy lens cement)
23. Ear pieces for auroscope	Should be cleaned with detergent and water, and dried	To be returned to CSSD after use in isolation
24. Earphone	Should be cleaned with detergent and water, and dried	Foam should be replaced after use in isolation
25. Eye testing glasses and vision eye patches	Wipe with a dilute detergent solution or detergent wipe between patients and store clean and dry	Eye patches should be made of a wipeable material
26. Floors	Should be vacuum cleaned daily. A damp mop with detergent and water should be used	For blood splashes blood spillage policy should be followed
27. Flower vases	Should be cleaned with detergent and water, and dried. Should be stored inverted	
28. Furniture	Should be damp dusted with detergent and water	Contaminated areas damp dust with phenol/saniquad/chlorine releasing agent
29. Humidifiers	Should be cleaned with detergent and water, and sterilized at low temperature	Empty daily, refill with sterile water. Disinfect when contaminated with 1% hypochlorite—20 minutes, wash and dry. Autoclave after each patient's use. Autoclave when respiratory circuit is changed.
30. Incubators	Should be cleaned with detergent and water and dried. Wipe with 70% isopropyl alcohol from inside	
31. Instruments	• Sterilize by heat • If heat sensitive chlorine releasing agents/2% glutaraldehyde/alcohol 60–70%	Contaminated surgical instruments should be cleaned before sterilization, preferably in a washer-disinfector
32. Intravenous monitoring pumps (and feed pumps)	Should be cleaned with detergent and water, and dried	After use in isolation or for infected patients wipe with 2% sodium hypochlorite and dry after cleaning
33. Linen Contaminated linen (especially if belonging to HIV infected patient	Wash with detergent and hot water and dry (Soak in hot water and send to laundry if available) Soak in sodium hypochlorite in a concentration achieving 150 ppm. Rinse in this at least for 5 minutes Boiling/autoclaving	

Contd...

Contd...

Article	Standard procedure	Comments
34. Mattresses/pillows a. With water impermeable cover	Wash with detergent solution and dry in between patients and as required	Disinfect with 1% sodium hypochlorite if contaminated. Do not disinfect unnecessarily as this may damage the mattress. Should not be used if cover is damaged. Contaminated pillows must be discarded. Torn mattress covers must be replaced before mattress is reused
35. Mops	Disposable—use for one day If reusable—rinse after each use, store dry, heat disinfect Laundry—laundered in washing machine	Mops must not be stored wet. If disinfection with chemicals is required soak in 0.1% (1000 ppm) sodium hypochlorite
36. Nebulizers	Cleaning and low temperature sterilization Single patient use—between uses wash chamber and mask thoroughly with hot water and detergent, rinse and dry thoroughly. Replace weekly or if heavily soiled. When patient discharged discard single patient use item	Clean the machine as per manufacturers instructions
37. Nail brushes	Use only if essential. A sterile or heat decontaminated brush should be used for all clinical procedures	
38. Proctoscopes	• Disposable—single use • Reusable—rinsed • Returned to CSSD	
39. Pressure relieving devices	Should be cleaned with detergent and water, and dried	
40. Razors	• Safety—single use disposable • Electric—detachable head, clean with 70% isopropyl alcohol	• Patients should use their own razors • Razors should not be shared
41. Rooms (terminal cleaning or disinfection)	**Non-infected patients** • Wash surfaces with detergent solution and allow to dry **Infected patients** • Wash with detergent solution, allow drying Disinfect with sodium hypochlorite 1% or 2% lysol Or saniquad (Benzalkonium chloride)•	
42. Shaving brushes	Should not be used unless supplied by the patients for their own use	
43. Sputum container	• Should be discarded into clinical waste for incineration • Use disposable only with closed lids • Reusable—should be emptied with care and heat disinfected or sterilized	Add 0.5% of sodium hypochlorite to the sputum
44. Suction bottles	Bottles: Disposable liners must be sealed when 75% full and placed in yellow plastic bag • If reusable—should be cleaned with sodium hypochlorite and dried or heat sterilized • All new suction machines purchased must be of a type with disposable collection bottle liners	• Must be changed daily and between each patient • To be stored dry when not in use

Contd...

Contd...

Article	Standard procedure	Comments
	At Hospital sites • Change liner daily when in use **Accessories** • *Suction catheters*—single use. Use once and discard • *Filters*—disposable—change every three months or when wet or visibly soiled or as otherwise instructed by manufacturers • *Tubing* must be single patient use • *Machines*—wipe weekly or when soiled with hot water and detergent/detergent wipes. Dry thoroughly **In patients own homes** • *Bottles*—if disposable available change liner daily. If non-disposable collection jars used, the contents should be emptied down a lavatory and then cleaned with hot water and detergent and dried thoroughly • *Suction catheters*—single use only • *Tubing*—single patient use, flush through after each use and change every seven days unless copious amounts of secretions are present—if this is the case change daily • *Machine*—it is the user's responsibility to keep equipment dust free. If visibly soiled clean with warm water and detergent	
45. Skin disinfection	Showers are preferred to bath	A particular site—tincture iodine/ alcohol
46. Soap dispensers	Should be cleaned weekly with detergent and water and dried	
47. Sphygmomanometer cuffs	• After use in isolation/infected patients, laundered in washing machine Or • Wipe with hot water and detergent at least weekly or sooner if visibly contaminated	
48. Spillages	• Should be cleaned with detergent • Spillages from known HIV-infected patient or hepatitis B patient—blood spillage policy should be followed	
49. Stethoscopes	• Should be cleaned with detergent and water and dried should be wiped with 70% alcohol OR • Wipe the bell and diaphragm (the ends) with (70% alcohol) between patient contacts • Earpieces should be removed and cleaned with detergent and hot water/detergent wipes	
50. Stretchers	• Wash with hot water and detergent—wipe with 0.5% sodium hypochlorite/phenol/— saniquad • If used for infected patient—wash as above and wipe with 1% sodium hypochlorite. If not available phenol/saniquad can also be used	
51. Telephones	To be wiped with 70% alcohol	

Contd...

Contd...

Article	Standard procedure	Comments
52. Thermometers	• To be covered with disposable sleeve (must for oral or rectal temperatures) before use, and stored dry in individual holder. In between patients, it should be cleaned with 70% isopropyl alcohol swab • If disposable sleeve is not used in between patients—wash in general purpose detergent and water, then wipe with 70% alcohol swab. To be stored in individual holder	Collect after round, and disinfect with 70% isopropyl alcohol for 10 minutes, store dry
53. Toilet seats	Washed with detergent and dried at least twice daily. If used by infected patient/grossly contaminated—disinfect with 1% sodium hypochlorite or 2% Lysol rinse and dry	
54. Tooth mugs	• Use disposable • If reusable—autoclave	
55. Toys	Toys—to be cleaned with detergent and water If contaminated: • Heat disinfect • Wipe surface with 70% isopropyl alcohol or 1% sodium hypochlorite	• For isolation patients—toys that cannot be decontaminated to be avoided • Heavily contaminated toys may have to be destroyed
56. Trolleys (Dressing, etc.)	To be cleaned daily with detergent and water. After each use should be wiped with 70% alcohol—If contaminated with blood or body fluids clean with detergent and water followed by disinfection using sodium hypochlorite 0.1%	
57. Tubings (Anesthetic/ ventilator)	• Use disposable tubing • If reusable—washer disinfector/low temperature steam sterilization/wash thoroughly and disinfect with 2% glutraraldehyde/or 1% sodium hypochlorite	For patients with tuberculosis—use disposable tubing and disinfect with 2% glutaraldehyde after use and then dispose
58. Scopes—arthroscope/ cystoscopes/ endoscopes/ bronchoscopes/ laparoscopes fibreoptic endoscopes, etc.	• 2% glutaraldehyde (alkaline) Cidex under controlled conditions—as per manufacturer's instructions • Ethylene oxide • Alcohol disinfection • Hydrogen peroxide/peracetic acid	• Permissible level is 0.2 ppm with 0.82 mg/cm^3 at 25°C for 8 hours for aldehyde • Use latex gloves, eye protection plastic covering mask while handling • Environment should be checked for aldehyde every 14 months by gas chromatography or methylene blue, tetrazolium hydrochloride or by colorimetric method
59. Endotracheal suction catheter	• Use disposable • If reusable—flush catheters with sterile distilled water after each use • If used for infected patient disinfect with 2% glutaraldehyde followed by proper rinsing with sterile distilled water to avoid chemical irritation • Bowl—must be washed clean after each suction disinfected/autoclaved if required	

Contd...

Contd...

Article	Standard procedure	Comments
60. Endotracheal tubes	Recycled after cleaning and autoclaving	
61. Oxygen delivery face mask	Wash and then dry. Wipe with 70% isopropyl alcohol to remove mucus	
62. Ventilatory circuits ***Note:*** Do not use these instruments for more than 72 hours without sterilization. If filters are installed on the expiratory and inspiratory ends of ventilation, the same circuit can be used for 4–5 days before sterilization becomes necessary	Heat disinfect at 80°C for 3 minutes or autoclave or ethylene oxide sterilization	Protect machine with filters. If machine is unprotected by filters, disinfect with hydrogen peroxide or formaldehyde (for tuberculosis)
63. Vomit bowls	Contents emptied into sluice—rinsed, washed with hot water with detergent	
64. Wash basins	Clean with detergent. Disinfection normally not required	If disinfection required—use 0.5% sodium hypochlorite
65. Walls	Should be cleaned with detergent and water	
66. Wheel chairs	Patients own—should be cleaned with detergent and water as necessary. Hospital—clean between patients with detergent and water	
67. Urinals	• Use—disposable • If reusable—use washer—disinfector or disinfect with 0.5–1.0% sodium hypochlorite or 2% lysol/2% Saniquad (Benzalkonium chloride)	
68. Urinary catheter	• Ideally—single use • Disposable	
69. X-ray equipment	Damp dust with detergent, switch off, do not overwet. Allow to dry before use, wipe with 70% alcohol	
70. Drinking water (contact time should be half an hour, and this concentration should be at end-use	0.2–0.4 ppm (1–2 liters of sodium hypochlorite to 250,000 liters of water)	
71. Food and dairy equipment	200–300 ppm of sodium hypochlorite (0.02–0.03%)	

Common Disinfectants (Table 9.2)[33]

Table 9.2: Common disinfectants

Disinfectants	Recommended use	Precautions
1. Sodium hypochlorite	Disinfection of material contaminated with blood and body fluids	• Should be used in well ventilated areas • Protective clothing required while handling and using undiluted • Not to be mixed with strong acids to avoid release of chlorine gas • Corrosive to metals

Contd...

Contd...

Disinfectants	Recommended use	Precautions
2. Bleaching powder 7 g/ liter with 70% available chlorine	Toilets, bathrooms, may be used in place of liquid bleach if liquid bleach is not available	• Some as above
3. Alcohol (70%), isopropyl, ethyl alcohol, methylated spirit	Smooth metal surfaces table tops and other surfaces on which bleach cannot be used	• Flammable, toxic, to be used in well-ventilated area, avoid inhalation • To be kept away from heat sources, electrical equipment, flames, hot surfaces • Should be allowed to dry completely—Particularly when using diathermy, as it can cause diathermy burns
4. Glutaraldehyde (2%)	For disinfection of endoscopes, respiratory therapy equipment, and for materials that are destroyed by heat can work as a sterilant if contact time is 6–8 hours and if used under strictly controlled condition	• Eye and nasal irritant, may cause asthma and skin allergies, hence should be used in well-ventilated area, keep covered with well-fitting lids • Eye protection, plastic apron and gloves should be worn while handling
5. Detergent with enzyme	Cleaning endoscopes surgical instruments before disinfection	
6. Chlorhexidine combined with alcohol or detergents	Antiseptic, for skin and mucous membranes, preoperative skin preparation, disinfection of hands	• Inactivated by soap, organic matter • Relatively non-toxic • Should not be allowed contact with eye or middle ear
7. Quarternary ammonium compounds (e.g. dettol may be combined with chlorhexidine	Antiseptic for cleaning dirty wounds (Low level disinfection only)	• Relatively non-toxic • Dilutions in use are likely to get contaminated and grow gram-negative bacteria • Should be used in correct dilution • Solution in use should be changed every 8 hours • Stock bottle should not be topped up

Universal Precautions[32]

These have become extremely important with the advent of the HIV pandemic. This implies regarding blood, body fluids and tissues of all persons and objects contaminated with them as potentially infected. With this in mind direct contact of skin and mucous membranes with blood and body fluids, tissues of persons and all objects likely to be contaminated with infected material should be avoided. This can be done using barrier precautions, and carrying out all the procedures safely, and avoiding accidental injuries with needles and sharps. Blood and body fluid precautions should be consistently used for all the patients. This approach is referred to a "Universal precautions".

The following barrier precautions are to be used (Fig. 9.3):

1. Gloves—to prevent exposure of skin when contact with body fluids is anticipated, e.g. when touching blood or other body fluids (amniotic fluid, pericardial fluid, peritoneal fluids, pleural fluid, synovial fluid, semen, vaginal secretions and any body fluid visibly contaminated with blood), mucous membranes or non-intact skin of all patients, for handling items or surfaces soiled with blood or body fluids and for performing venepuncture, vascular access or invasive procedures. Gloves should be changed after contact with each patient. Hands should be washed immediately after removing the gloves.

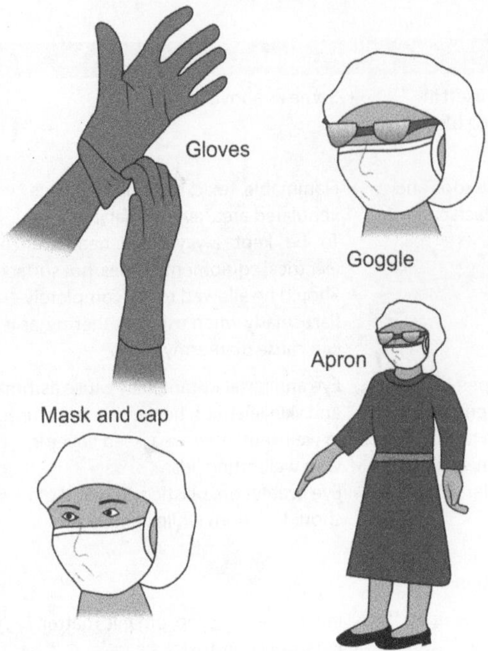

Fig. 9.3: Universal precautions

2. Masks and protective eye wear or face shields—should be worn during procedures which are likely to generate droplets of blood or other body fluids to prevent exposure of mucous membranes of the eyes, nose and mouth.
3. Gowns or aprons should be worn during procedures that are likely to generate splashes of blood or other body fluids.
4. Hands and other skin surfaces should be washed thoroughly if contaminated with blood or other body fluids.
5. Great care should be taken to prevent injuries caused by needles, scalpels or other sharp instruments, or devices during procedures and during handling, cleaning or disposal of these after the procedure is over.
   For avoiding needle stick injuries, needles should not be recapped, purposely bent or broken by hand, removed from disposable syringes or manipulated by hand. After use, the disposable syringes and needles, scalpel blades and other sharp items should be placed in puncture-resistant containers for disposal, these containers must be located as close as possible to the work area. The usable needles or other "sharps" should be placed in a puncture-resistant container containing appropriate disinfectant to render these safe for handling and reprocessing.
6. To minimize the need for emergency mouth-to-mouth resuscitation, mouth-pieces, resuscitation bags, or other ventilation devices should be available for use in areas in which the need for resuscitation is likely to occur.
7. HCW who have lesions on their skin, which are exudative, should be refrained from direct patient care and also from handling patient care equipment until the lesions are treated and resolved.
8. Healthcare workers (females) who are pregnant should adhere strictly to Universal precautions, so as to minimize the risk of acquiring HIV infection. Of course pregnant health care workers are not known to be at a greater risk of contracting HIV infection than HCW who are not pregnant. However, in case a pregnant HCW gets infected, her infant is also at risk of infection.
9. Linen and articles soiled with blood or body fluids should be placed in the appropriate bags and transported bagged so as to prevent leakage.

Gloves

Gloves are meant to supplement and not replace the hygienic practice of thorough hand washing with soap and water.

Gloves: Sterile surgical gloves of vinyl or latex should be used. Single use is better. General-purpose utility gloves should be used for instrument cleaning, decontamination.

- Gloves for reuse should be washed and sterilized before reuse. Gloves that are cracked, discolored, peeling or have visible tears or holes must be discarded. Most invisible holes can be detected by filling them with air and holding them under water. Bubbles will appear if holes are present

- HCWs with break in skin of hands should wear gloves in all situations
- When a series of venepuncture are to be done, and if the gloves are not soiled during venepuncture, the procedure may be carried out on several patients after washing the gloved hands after each venepuncture
- However, if gloves get soiled with blood, they should be changed. Before removal of gloves, the gloved hand should be washed with soap and water. Hands should again be washed after removing the gloves.

Gowns and aprons

- It prevents contact infection as long as it remains dry, when it is wet/soiled it must be changed
- Cotton gowns have pores in the fabric through which bacteria can escape (on the skin scales of wearer). Better types of gown are available (ventile, body exhaust ventilation) for 'high risk patients.' A gown or apron of plastic or water-resistant paper should be worn when splashes of blood or other body fluids are likely to occur e.g. during surgery, obstetric procedures, lifting a patient with bleeding wounds, invasive procedures, postmortem and embalming. In operating room instead of plastic apron, preferably apron made of antistatic rubber or synthetic material should be worn.

Masks and caps

- Deflector type of mask made of paper should be used
- It should be discarded after an hour at the end of a procedure if it lasts more than an hour
- These should be worn during all routine and emergency surgical and invasive procedures.

Eye covers: These should be worn when droplets or splashes of blood or other body fluids are expected, e.g. obstetric, dental, orthopedic (where motorized drills are used) procedures and during autopsy.

Shoe covers

- Linen overshoes prevent contamination of shoes if the floor is dry
- Better are overshoes made up of waterproof material or changing to footwear with impervious soles
- Shoe covers should be worn where shoes are likely to be soiled by body fluids, e.g. during vaginal delivery, urological procedures, emergency care or severe trauma, surgery in the perineal region, abdominothoracic surgery and during prolonged surgical procedures.

Syringes and needles: For collection of blood samples it is safer to use vacuum collection of blood than conventional syringe and needle.

Mouth-to-mouth resuscitation

- Although HIV has been isolated from saliva, there is no evidence that saliva is involved in transmission
- However, to reduce occupational exposure to HIV, mouthpieces, resuscitation bags, or other ventilation devices should be available and used
- Resuscitation should however, continue to be used when other methods are not available.

REFERENCES

1. Babb J. Decontamination of the environment, equipment and the skin. In Control of Hospital Infection—A Practical Handbook. 4th (Edn). Graham AJ Ayliffe, Adam P Fraise, Alasdair M, Geddes Edr. Oxford University Press Inc. New York, 2000.pp.92.
2. Ayliffe, GAJ, Coates D, Hoffman PN. Chemical disinfection in hospitals. 2nd Edn. Public Health Laboratory Service. London; 1993.
3. Ayliffee GAJ, Collins BJ, Lowbury EJL. Cleaning and disinfection of hospital floors. Br Med J. 1966;ii:442.
4. Donforth D, Nicolle LE, Hume K, et al. Nosocomial infections on nursing units with

floors cleaned with a disinfectant compared with detergent. J Hosp Infect. 1987;10:229.

5. Ayliffe GAJ, Babb JR, Collins BJ. Carpets in hospital wards. Health and Social Services Journal, 1974; 84:12. (Quoted by Ref.No. 1).
6. British Standards Institute (1993) BS 2745. Washer-disinfectors for medical purposes. Part 1.Specification for general requirements. Part 2. Specification for human-waste container washer-disinfectors Part 3 Specification for washer-disinfectors except those used for processing human waste and laundry. London. British Standard Institute. Quoted by Ref. No. 1.
7. Dyas A, Das BC . The activity of glutaraldehyde against Clostridium difficile. J Hosp Infect. 1985;6:41.
8. Rutala WA. APIC guidelines for selection and use of disinfectants. IS J Infect Control. 1990; 18:99.
9. Cook RPD, Feneley RCL, Ayliffe GAJ, et al. Decontamination of urological equipment: Interim report of working group of the Standing Committee on urological instruments of the British Association of Urological surgeons. Br J Urol. 1993;71:5 (Quoted by Ref.No.1).
10. Best M, Sattar SA, Springthorpe VS, et al. Efficacies of selected disinfectants against *Mycobacterium tuberculosis*. J Clin Microbiol. 1990; 28:10.
11. Griffiths PA, Babb JR, Fraise AP. Mycobacterial activity of selected disinfectants using a quantitative suspension test. J Hosp Infec. 1999;41:111.
12. Ayliffe GAJ. Nosocomial infections associated with endoscopy. In: Mayhall CG (Ed). Hosptial Epidemiology and Infection Control, 2nd Edn, Baltimore, MD: Williams and Williams; 1999.
13. Spach DH, Silverstein FE, Stamm WE. Transmission of infection by gastrointestinal endoscopy and bronchoscopy. Ann Int Med. 1993;118:117.
14. Hansen PJV, Gor D, Jeffries DJ, et al. Chemical inactivation of HIV on surfaces. Br Med J. 1989; 298:862.
15. Hansen PVJ, Gor D, Jeffries DJ, Collins JV. Elimination of high titre HIV from fibreoptic endoscopes. Gut. 1990;31:657.
16. Tyler R, Ayliffe GAJ, Bradley CR. Virucidal activity of disinfectants: studies with the poliovirus. J Hosp Infec. 1990;15:339.
17. Judd PA, Tomlin PJ, Whitby JL, et al. Disinfection of ventilators by ultrasonic nebulisation. Lancet. 1968;2:1019.
18. Benn RAV, Dulton AAC, Tully M. Disinfection of mechanical ventilators: an investigation using formaldehyde in a cape ventilator. Anaesthesiology. 1973;27:265.
19. Deverill CEA, Dutt KK. Methods of decontamination of anaesthetic equipment: daily sessional exchange of circuits. J Hosp Infec. 1980;1:165.
20. Royal College of Obstetricians and Gynaecologists. HIV infection in Maternity care and Gynaecology. Working Party Report, London RCOG Press; 1997.
21. Advisory Committees on Dangerous Pathogens and Spongiform Encephalopathies. Transmissible encephalopathy agents: Safe working and prevention of infection. London HMSO; 1998.
22. Taylor DM. Inactivation of unconventional agents of the transmissible degenerative encephalopathies. In: Russel AW, Huge WG, Ayliffe GAJ (Eds). Disinfection, preservation and sterilization, 3rd edition. Oxford Blackwell Scientific Publications; 1992.pp.222.
23. Ayliffe GAJ, Babb JR, Davier JG, Lily HA. Hand disinfection a comparison of various agents in laboratory and ward studies. J Hosp Infec. 1988;11:226.
24. Rotter M. Hand washing and hand disinfection. Hospital Epidemiology and Infection Control. 1996;79:1052.
25. Manual for Infection control LTMGH and LTMCC - Johnson and Johnson.
26. Ayliffe GAJ, Babb JR, Quoraishi AH. A test for hygienic hand disinfection. J Clin Pathol. 1978; 31:923.
27. Davies JG, Babb JR, Bradley CR, Ayliffe GAJ. Preliminary study of test methods to assess the virucidal activity of skin disinfectants using poliovirus and bacteriophages. J Hosp Infec. 1993;25:125.
28. Bellamy K, Alcock R, Babb JR, Davies JG, Ayliffe GAJ. A test for assessment of hygienic hand disinfection using rotovirus. J Hosp Infec. 1993; 24:201.
29. Davies JG, Babb JG, Ayliffe GAJ. Disinfection of skin of abdomen. Br J Surg. 1978;65:885.
30. Lowbury EJL, Lilly HA. Gloved hands as applicator of antiseptic to operation sites. Lancet. 1975;ii:153.

31. Williams JD, Waltho CA, Ayliffe GAJ, Lowbury EJL. Trials of five antibacterial creams in the control of nasal carriage of *Staphylococcus aureus*. Lancet. 1967;2:390.
32. Aggarwal DS. Microbiology Department University College of Medical Sciences and GTB University College of Medical Sciences and GTB Delhi, Universal Precautions in Guidelines for Nosocomial Infection—Surveillance and Control, Hospital, WHO South East Asia Regional Office, New Delhi. Pg 51-6.
33. WHO: Guidelines on prevention and control of hospital-associated infections; 2002.

Chapter 10

Surgical Site Infections

Chapter Outline

- Microbiology of Hospital-acquired Surgical Infection
- Classification of Surgical Site Infections
- Recording of Data
- Operations, and Likely Surgical Site Infection Pathogens
- Risk Factors
- Surveillance of Surgical Site Infection
- Special Problems of Infections due to *Clostridium perfringens* and Other Gas Gangrene Bacilli
- Microbiologic Sampling
- Disinfection of Operation Theater
- Fumigation/Fogging
- Conventional Sterilization of Surgical Instruments
- Flash Sterilization of Surgical Instruments

Practical Aspects

- Risk Factors of SSI and General Guidelines for Prevention of SSI
- Methods of Cleaning Operation Theater and Equipment Inside Operation Theater
- Fumigation of Operation Theaters
- Use of Machines for Fumigation/Fogging
- Cold Fogging of Operation Theaters
- Biological Test for Monitoring Autoclaves
- Recommendations for Prevention of Surgical Site Infection
- Summary of SSI Prevention (Including SSI Bundle)

INTRODUCTION

Surgical site infections comprise 17–18% of the nosocomial infections. The global data suggests the surgical site infection (SSI) incidence rate varies from 1.5 to 20%.[1ab] Recently CDC has found a prevalence rate for SSI to be 31%.[1c] In India six studies reported an overall incidence of 9–23% for all surgical procedures. However, the incidence varied between different surgical procedures, higher incidence was generally observed for gastrointestinal surgery (3–36%) and cardiothoracic surgery (5–19%). Incidence of SSI following neurological surgery appeared to be lower (0.5–2.5%), however, these studies considered only SSIs per-discharge. Other surgical procedures included breast surgery and genitourinary surgery, with incidences ranging from 4–18%.[1d]

Surgical site infection (SSI) can be defined as "Infection on the surgical site that occurs within 30 days of the surgical procedure or within one year if there is an implant or foreign body, such as prosthetic heart valve or joint prosthesis."[1e]

Surgical wound infections occur in up to 10% of patients undergoing clean surgery, with the incidence varying with complexity of surgery, intrinsic patient risk and surgical skills.[2] Most surgical wound infections result from contamination of the surgical wound with the patient's own flora, or that of operating room personnel or environment at the time of surgery. Postoperative hematogenous seeding of the wound site is uncommon.

Infection may present clinically during hospitalization. However, the current trend to shorter postoperative stays and day surgery result in more than 50% of surgical wound infection becoming apparent after discharge from hospital. Clinically infection may occur up to four weeks after deep surgery and up to 12 months after surgery involving an implanted prosthesis (e.g. joint replacement).

The common clinical features of surgical wound infection are localized pain, redness and discharge. Fever that occurs within 4 weeks of surgery, without other localizing features, is likely to be caused by infection at the surgical site. Superficial wound infection may resolve with or without antibiotics. Deeper or organ-space infection may require imaging for diagnosis, surgical drainage and antimicrobial therapy guided by culture of the purulent material.

The likely causative organisms depend on the location and type of surgery. Most common is *S. aureus* with MRSA common in some hospitals. For gastrointestinal or genitourinary tract surgery, gram-negative bacilli (e.g. *E. coli*) are more common causes of infection.

Advances in infection control practices include improved operating room ventilation, sterilization methods, barriers, surgical technique, and availability of antimicrobial prophylaxis. Despite these activities, SSIs remain a substantial cause of morbidity and mortality among hospitalized patients. This may be partially explained by the emergence of antimicrobial-resistant pathogens and the increased numbers of surgical patients who are elderly and/or have a wide variety of chronic, debilitating, or immunocompromising underlying diseases. There also are increased numbers of prosthetic implant and organ transplant operations performed. Thus, to reduce the risk of SSI, a systematic but realistic approach must be applied with the awareness that this risk is influenced by characteristics of the patient, operation, personnel, and hospital.[3]

MICROBIOLOGY OF HOSPITAL-ACQUIRED SURGICAL INFECTION[2,3]

In the past, infections due to streptococci were common, later they were replaced by *S. aureus*. Then there was a gradual shift towards gram-negative bacilli like *Escherichia. coli*, *Enterobacter*, *Proteus*, *Pseudomonas*, *Klebsiella*, etc.

The pathogens isolated from SSI have not changed markedly during the last decade.

Staphylococcus aureus, Coagulase-negative Staphylococci, Enterococcus species and *Escherichia coli* remain the most frequently isolated organisms. Increasing proportions of SSIs are caused by antimicrobial resistant pathogens, such as *Methicillin-resistant S. aureus* (MRSA) or by *Candida albicans.* The increased proportions of SSI, caused by resistant pathogens and *Candida* may reflect increasing numbers of severely ill and immunocompromised surgical patients, and the impact of wide spread use of broad spectrum antimicrobial agents.

Outbreaks or clusters of SSIs have also been caused by unusual pathogens, such as *Rhizopus oryzae, Clostridium perfringens, Rhodococcus bronchialis, Nocardia farcinica, Legionella pneumophila, Legionella dumoffi, and Pseudomonas multivorans.* These rare outbreaks have been traced to contaminated adhesive dressings; elastic bandages, colonized surgical personnel, tap water or contaminated disinfectant solutions. Where cluster of SSIs involves an unusual organism, an epidemiological investigation should be conducted.

CLASSIFICATION OF SURGICAL SITE INFECTIONS[3]

The CDC's NNIS (National Nosocomial Infection Surveillance) system had developed standardized surveillance criteria for defining SSIs (Fig. 10.1).

By these criteria's SSIs have been classified into three types:

1. Superficial incisional SSI
   Those involving only skin and subcutaneous lesions.
2. Deep incisional SSI
   These involving deeper soft tissues of the incision.
3. Organ or space SSI
   Those involving any part of the anatomy.

Organ/space SSIs involve any part of the anatomy (e.g. organ or space) other than incised body layers that was opened or manipulated during an operation. Organ/space SSIs have been classified according to specific site, e.g. in a patient who had an appendicectomy, and subsequently developed an intra-abdominal abscess, not draining through the incision, the infection would be reported as an organ/space SSI at the intra-abdominal site.

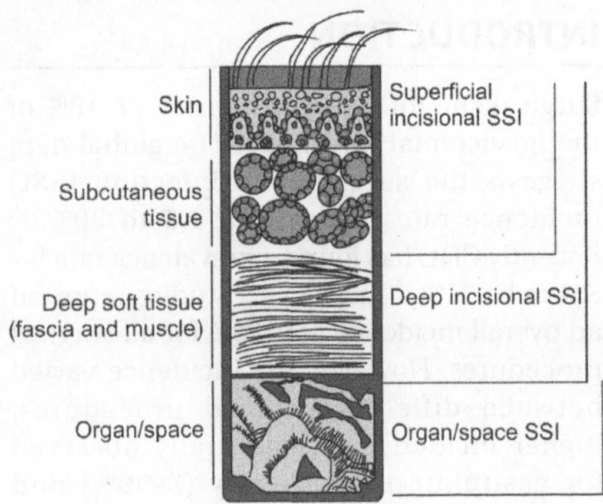

Fig. 10.1: Classification of surgical site infections

Among surgical patients, SSIs were the most common nosocomial infections accounting for 38% of all such infections. Of these SSI's two-thirds were confined to the incision and one-third involved organs or spaces accessed during the operation. When surgical patients with nosocomial SSI died, 77% of the deaths were reported to be related to the infection and the majority were serious infections involving organ or spaces accessed during the operation.

Record of wound infection should be kept. Wound infection rate must be defined if comparisons are to be made either within a hospital or between hospitals. For this obtain a list of all operations performed from the operating theater. They should be classified into clean, clean contaminated or contaminated, but even in these, there may be wide variation in infection rates for different types of operations. It is also useful to record the severity of each type of infection and whether the infection was drained or not. Accuracy may be further improved by comparing individual types of operation (e.g. hernia) and introducing risk factor into calculation).[4] The incidence or prevalence rate can be corrected for risk factors such as age, sex, type of operation (clean, clean contaminated or contaminated) preoperative stay, wound drainage and special factors such as diabetes. Infections that occur after discharge from hospital must also be included if accurate rates are to be obtained. Infection rate should be based on clinical and not bacteriological findings. Only operation in which there has been a breach in the skin should be included in the assessment. Non-operative endoscopies, manipulations and examinations under anesthesia, vaginal operations and also incision of abscess, should not be included in the total operations at risk for acquired infection. Ulcerations and pressure sores should also be excluded, but should be recorded separately.

Criteria for Defining a Surgical Site Infections[3,5]

Superficial Incisional SSI

Infection occurs within 30 days after the operation *and* infection involves only skin or subcutaneous tissue of the incision *and* at least *one* of the following:

1. Purulent drainage, with or without laboratory confirmation, from the superficial incision.
2. Organisms isolated from an aseptically obtained culture of fluid or tissue from the superficial incision.
3. At least one of the following signs or symptoms of infection: pain or tenderness, localized swelling, redness, or heat *and* superficial incision is deliberately opened by surgeon, *unless* incision is culture-negative.
4. Diagnosis of superficial incisional SSI by the surgeon or attending physician.

Do *not* report the following conditions as SSI:

1. Stitch abscess (minimal inflammation and discharge confined to the points of suture penetration).
2. Infection of an episiotomy or newborn circumcision site.
3. Infected burn wound.
4. Incisional SSI that extends into the fascial and muscle layers (see deep incisional SSI).

Note: Specific criteria are used for identifying infected episiotomy and circumcision sites and burn wounds.[6]

Deep Incisional SSI

Infection occurs within 30 days after the operation if no implant† is left in place or within 1 year if implant is in place and the infection appears to be related to the operation *and* infection involves deep soft tissues (e.g. fascial and muscle layers) of the incision *and* at least *one* of the following:

1. Purulent drainage from the deep incision but not from the organ/space component of the surgical site.
2. A deep incision spontaneously dehisces or is deliberately opened by a surgeon when the patient has at least one of the following signs or symptoms: fever (>38°C), localized pain, or tenderness, unless site is culture-negative.
3. An abscess or other evidence of infection involving the deep incision is found on direct examination, during reoperation, or by histopathologic or radiologic examination.
4. Diagnosis of a deep incisional SSI by a surgeon or attending physician.

Notes:

1. Report infection that involves both superficial and deep incision sites as deep incisional SSI.
2. Report an organ/space SSI that drains through the incision as a deep incisional SSI.

†National Nosocomial Infection Surveillance definition: a nonhuman-derived implantable foreign body (e.g. prosthetic heart valve, nonhuman vascular graft, mechanical heart, or hip prosthesis) that is permanently placed in a patient during surgery.

Organ/Space SSI

Infection occurs within 30 days after the operation if no implant is left in place or within 1 year if implant is in place and the infection appears to be related to the operation *and* infection involves any part of the anatomy (e.g. organs or spaces), other than the incision, which was opened or manipulated during an operation *and* at least *one* of the following:

1. Purulent drainage from a drain that is placed through a stab wound‡ into the organ/space.
2. Organisms isolated from an aseptically obtained culture of fluid or tissue in the organ/space.
3. An abscess or other evidence of infection involving the organ/space that is found on direct examination, during reoperation, or by histopathologic or radiologic examination.
4. Diagnosis of an organ/space SSI by a surgeon or attending physician.

RECORDING OF DATA[7]

Type of Operation

(Type of operation and whether the wound is drained or not)

Operations are classified as **(Surgical wound classification):**[8,9]

Class I/Clean: An uninfected operative wound in which no inflammation is encountered and the respiratory, alimentary, genital, or uninfected urinary tract is not entered. In addition, clean wounds are primarily closed and, if necessary, drained with closed drainage. Operative incisional wounds that follow nonpenetrating (blunt) trauma should be included in this category if they meet the criteria.

Class II/Clean-contaminated: An operative wound in which the respiratory, alimentary, genital, or urinary tracts are entered under controlled conditions and without unusual contamination. Specifically, operations involving the biliary tract, appendix, vagina, and oropharynx are included in this category, provided no evidence of infection or major break in technique is encountered.

Class III/Contaminated: Open, fresh, accidental wounds. In addition, operations with major breaks in sterile technique (e.g. open cardiac massage) or gross spillage from the gastrointestinal tract, and incisions in which acute, nonpurulent inflammation is encountered are included in this category.

Class IV/Dirty-infected: Old traumatic wounds with retained devitalized tissue and those that involve existing clinical infection or perforated viscera. This definition suggests that the organisms causing postoperative infection were present in the operative field before the operation.

Sepsis and Degree of Severity

- *Mild sepsis:* When there is a small or superficial area of inflammation with minimal discharge
- *Moderate sepsis:* When there is superficial inflammation of the whole wound (or over one-third of it) with a serous or small amount of purulent discharge, or a deeper infection involving a small area (one-third or less) usually with a purulent discharge.
- *Severe sepsis:* A deep purulent infection, with or without sinuses, or fistulae, or widespread cellulitis, or wound breakdown with an obvious inflammatory reaction and pus.

Severity may also be classified as major and minor infections:

- *Major:* When the purulent discharge is accompanied by complete dehiscence of the fascial layers of the wound; deep tissue destruction, or spreading cellulitis

‡ If the area around a stab wound becomes infected, it is not an SSI. It is considered a skin or soft tissue infection, depending on its depth.[6]

and lymphangitis that requires antibiotic therapy

- *Minor:* When there is discharge of pus without lymphangitis or tissue destruction.

Infections may also be classified into primary and secondary:

- *Primary:* When there is no predisposing condition.
- *Secondary:* When infection follows a complication, which results in discharge of bile, serum, gastric juice, intestinal contents, urine, CSF or a hematoma.

Probable Location of Wound Infection[7]

It is important to know where the infection was acquired. The following points will help in determining this.

Infection Acquired in Operating Theater

This may be indicated by:

- Deep infection in a clean, undrained wound at any time
- Infection occurring within 3 days of operation, or prior to first dressing in a clean wound.

Supporting evidence includes the following:

- Pyrexia
- *Staphylococcus* of the same type not isolated from any patients in the ward
- *Staphylococcus* of the same type isolated from a member of the operating staff and not present in the ward
- *Staphylococcus* of the same type in different wards from patients operated in the same operating theater.

Infection Acquired in the Ward

Indicated by:

- Superficial infection in a wound (usually drained)
- Occurring after first dressing
- Culture of discharge may initially be negative, and deep infection may develop later in a drained wound.

Supporting evidence includes: *Staphylococcus* of the same type isolated from other patient or members of staff in the ward.

Place of Acquisition of Infection Not Known

When there is superficial infection in any wound after first dressing, and no available evidence from bacteriology in support of theater or ward infection.

Infection Acquired from Patients' Own Bacterial Flora

These include infections due to *Staphylococcus epidermidis* or *Staphylococcus aureus* that was present in the patient's nose or on their skin prior to or at the time of surgery, however, resistant strains may have been acquired by the patient in the ward before operation.

Infections that are due to antibiotic sensitive gram-negative bacilli usually involve *E. coli* or *Bacteroides species.*

Post-discharge Infections

Nowadays, since most of the patients are discharged rapidly, many of the hospital-acquired infections manifest themselves after discharge of the patient. In case of surgical wound infections, 21–70% of surgical wound infections become apparent only after leaving the hospital. Detection of these infections is difficult and time consuming. Even though, it is true that infection rates would be less valuable without this information, but cost-effectiveness if considered, one should really think over it, as severe infections would be re-admitted to the hospital, and the minor infections are not worth considering.

OPERATIONS, AND LIKELY SURGICAL SITE INFECTION PATHOGENS[3]

Operations and Likely Pathogens

1. Placement of all grafts, prostheses, or implants: *Staphylococcus aureus;* coagulase-negative staphylococci.

2. Cardiac operations: *S. aureus;* coagulase-negative staphylococci.
3. Neurosurgery: *S. aureus;* coagulase-negative staphylococci.
4. Breast surgery: *S. aureus;* coagulase-negative staphylococci.
5. Ophthalmic surgery: Limited data; however, commonly used in procedures such as anterior segment resection, vitrectomy, and scleral buckles-S. *aureus;* coagulase-negative staphylococci; streptococci; gram-negative bacilli.
6. Orthopedic surgery:
   - Total joint replacement, closed fractures/use of nails, bone plates, other internal fixation devices, functional repair without implant/device, trauma
   - *S. aureus;* coagulase-negative staphylococci; gram negative bacilli.
7. Noncardiac thoracic surgery: *S. aureus;* coagulase-negative staphylococci.
8. Thoracic (lobectomy, pneumonectomy, wedge resection, other noncardiac mediastinal procedures), closed tube thoracostomy: *Streptococcus pneumoniae;* gram-negative bacilli.
9. Vascular surgery: *S. aureus;* coagulase-negative staphylococci.
10. Appendectomy: Gram-negative bacilli; anaerobes.
11. Biliary tract: Gram-negative bacilli; anaerobes.
12. Colorectal surgery: Gram-negative bacilli; anaerobes.
13. Gastroduodenal surgery: Gram-negative bacilli; streptococci; oropharyngeal anaerobes (e.g. peptostreptococci)
14. Head and neck (major procedures with incision through oropharyngeal mucosa) *S. aureus;* streptococci; oropharyngeal anaerobes (e.g. peptostreptococci).
15. Obstetric and gynecologic: Gram-negative bacilli; enterococci; group B streptococci; anaerobes.
16. Urologic: Gram-negative bacilli.

RISK FACTORS[1,3]

Risk Factors in Patients that May Influence the Risk of SSI

Age

Usually, operating in very old or very young poses a higher risk of developing infections.

Nutritional Status

Usually, poor nutrition may have a bad effect on the operated patient. Severe protein caloric malnutrition may be associated with postoperative nosocomial infections, impaired wound healing or death.

Diabetes

The contribution of diabetes to SSI risk is controversial, because the independent contribution of diabetes to SSI risk has not typically been assessed after controlling for potential confounding factors. Recent preliminary findings from a study of patients who underwent coronary artery bypass graft showed a significant relationship between increasing levels of HbA1c and SSI rates, but it has been shown that increased glucose level (>200 mg/dL) in the immediate postoperative period (<48 hours) was associated with increased risk of SSI.[3] However, more studies are needed to assess the efficacy of preoperative blood glucose control as prevention measure.

Smoking

Nicotine delays primary wound healing and may increase the risk of SSI. So smoking may be an independent risk factor for SSI.

Steroids

Patients who are receiving steroids or other immunosuppressive drugs preoperatively may be predisposed to developing SSI.

Obesity

It can increase risk of SSI.

Coexistent Infections in a Remote Body Site

Infection at any other site in the body may increase risk of SSI, so that has to be adequately treated.

Colonization of Carriers

Many persons may be carrying the organisms, so screening for carriers is a must (especially preoperative nares colonization with *S. aureus* has been associated with risk of SSI). In fact, it has been noted that such carriage was the most powerful independent factor for SSI following cardiothoracic operations.

Mupirocin ointment is effective as a topical agent for excluding *S. aureus* from the nares of colonized patients or healthcare workers.

Length of Preoperative Stay

Increased length of preoperative stay will lead to colonization with bacteria from infected patients. A study has shown that the longer the patient stays in the hospital; he is more likely to develop a SSI. They have found that one day preoperative stay is associated with an infection rate of 1.1%, 1 week with 2%, and over 2 weeks with 4.3%. This might suggest that the patient become colonized with a hospital strain for which they lack defense.

Risk Factors Related to Preoperative Issues (Preoperative Patient Related)

Preoperative Antiseptic Bath

Preoperative antiseptic bath or shower reduces the microbial load of the skin. Chlorhexidine gluconate reduces the bacterial colony counts by nine fold, whereas povidone-iodine achieves a reduction in colony count by 1–2 folds. In our country, where the standard of hygiene is poor, the practice of preoperative antiseptic bath/showers should be recommended and encouraged.

Preoperative Hair Removal

Shaving of the skin in the previous night, i.e. 24 hours before is a significant risk factor for SSI. The method recommended is shaving immediately before the operation or use of depilatories.

The increased risk of SSI associated with shaving has been attributed to microscopic cuts in the skin that later serve as foci for bacterial multiplication.

Preoperative Skin Preparation (Table 10.1)

Several antiseptic agents are available for preoperative preparation of skin at incision site. The most commonly used agents are:

1. Iodophors (povidone-iodine).
2. Alcohol containing products.
3. Chlorhexidine gluconate.

Alcohol is readily available and non-expensive and rapidly acting, but the disadvantage is it has no action on spores, and it is inflammable. Both chlorhexidine and iodophors have broad spectra of antimicrobial activity, but chlorhexidine gluconate is preferred, its advantage being its greater reduction in skin microflora and greater residual activity after a single application than povidone-iodine, and blood or serum proteins do not inactivate it.

Before the skin preparation of a patient is initiated, the skin should be free of gross contamination (i.e. dirt, soil, or any other debris). The patient's skin is prepared by applying an antiseptic in concentric circles, beginning in the area of the proposed incision. The prepared area should be large enough to extend the incision or create new incisions or drain sites, if necessary. The application of the skin preparation may need to be modified, depending on the condition of the skin (e.g. burns) or location of the incision site (e.g. face).

Preoperative Hand/Forearm Antisepsis (Table 10.1)

Members of the surgical team who have direct contact with the sterile operating field or sterile instruments or supplies used in the field, wash their hands and forearms by performing a traditional procedure known as scrubbing (or the surgical scrub) immediately before donning sterile gowns and gloves. Ideally, the optimum antiseptic used for the scrub should have a broad spectrum of activity, be fast acting, and have a persistent effect.

Alcohol is considered the gold standard for surgical hand preparation in several European countries. Alcohol containing products are used less frequently in the United States than in Europe, possibly because of concerns about flammability and skin irritation. Povidone-iodine and chlorhexidine gluconate are the current agents of choice for most US surgical team members. However, when 7.5% povidone-iodine or 4% chlorhexidine gluconate was compared to alcoholic chlorhexidine (60% isopropanol and 0.5% chlorhexidine gluconate in 70% isopropanol), alcoholic chlorhexidine was found to have greater residual antimicrobial activity.

Factors other than the choice of antiseptic agent influence the effectiveness of the surgical scrub. Scrubbing technique, the duration of the scrub, the condition of the hands, or the techniques used for drying and gloving are examples of such factors. Recent studies suggest that scrubbing for at least 2 minutes is as effective as the traditional 10-minute scrub in reducing hand bacterial colony counts, but the optimum duration of scrubbing is not known. The first scrub of the day should include a thorough cleaning underneath fingernails (usually with a brush). It is not clear that such cleaning is a necessary part of subsequent scrubs during the day. After performing the surgical scrub, hands should be kept up and away from the body (elbows in flexed position), so that water runs from the tips of the fingers toward the elbows. Sterile towels should be used for drying the hands and forearms before the donning of a sterile gown and gloves.

A surgical team member who wears artificial nails may have increased bacterial and fungal colonization of the hands despite performing an adequate hand scrub. Hand carriage of gram-negative organisms has been shown to be greater among wearers

Table 10.1: Mechanism and spectrum of activity of antiseptic agents commonly used for preoperative skin preparation and surgical scrub[3]

Agent	Mechanism of action	Gram-positive bacteria	Gram-negative bacteria	MTB	Fungi	Viruses	Rapidity of action	Residual activity	Toxicity	Uses
Alcohol	Denature proteins	Excellent	Excellent	Good	Good	Good	Most rapid	None	Drying, volatile	SP, SS
Chlorhexidine	Disrupt cell membranes	Excellent	Good	Poor	Fair	Good	Interme-diate	Excellent	Ototoxicity, keratitis	SP, SS
Iodine/ iodophors	Oxidation/ substitution by free iodine	Excellent	Good	Good	Good	Good	Interme-diate	Minimal	Absorption from skin with posssible toxicity, skin irritation	SP, SS
Triclosan	Disrupt cell wall	Good	Good	Good	Poor	Un-known	Interme-diate	Excellent	More data needed	SS

Abbreviations: MTB, *Mycobacterium tuberculosis,* SP, skin preparation; SS, surgical scrubs.

Source: Data from Larson E[10]

of artificial nails than among non-wearers. While the relationship between nail length and SSI risk is unknown, long nails—artificial or natural—may be associated with tears in surgical gloves. The relationship between the wearing of nail polish or jewelry by surgical team members and SSI risk has not been adequately studied.

Management of Infected or Colonized Surgical Personnel

Surgical personnel who have active infections or are colonized with certain microorganisms have been linked to outbreaks or clusters of SSIs. Thus, it is important that healthcare organizations implement policies to prevent transmission of microorganisms from personnel to patients. These policies should address management of job-related illnesses, provision of postexposure prophylaxis after job-related exposures and, when necessary, exclusion of ill personnel from work or patient contact. While work exclusion policies should be enforceable and include a statement of authority to exclude ill personnel, they should also be designed to encourage personnel to report their illnesses and exposures and not penalize personnel with loss of wages, benefits, or job status.

Antimicrobial Prophylaxis[3] (Table 10.2)

Surgical antimicrobial prophylaxis (AMP) refers to a very brief course of an antimicrobial agent initiated just before an operation begins.

This is a necessary step to be taken before operation. AMP is not an attempt to sterilize tissues, but a critically timed adjunct used to reduce the microbial burden of intra-operative contamination to a level that cannot overwhelm host defenses.

Four principles necessary for preoperative antibiotic prophylaxis:

i. Use an antibacterial agent which is safe, inexpensive and bactericidal, and covers most of the probable intraoperative contaminants for the operation.
ii. Time the initial dose, such that bactericidal concentration of the drug is established in serum and tissues by the time the skin is incised.
iii. Maintain therapeutic levels of the antimicrobial agent in both serum and tissues throughout the operation and until, at most, a few hours after the incision is closed in the operating room.
iv. A single dose with induction of anesthesia is recommended except in surgeries lasting for more than 3 hours, wherein a second dose is given. Exceptions to this rule are immunocompromised patients.

Table 10.2: Antimicrobial prophylaxis for surgery[22]

	Likely organisms	Suitable agent	
1. Gastrointestinal			
Esophageal, gastroduodenal	Enteric gram-negative bacilli, gram-positive cocci	High-risk[5] only: Cefazolin[6]	1–2 g IV[2]
Biliary tract	Enteric gram-negative bacilli, enterococci, *Clostridia*	High risk[7] only: Cefazolin[6,8]	1–2 g IV[2]
Colorectal	Enteric gram-negative bacilli, enterococci, anaerobes	Oral: Neomycin + erythromycin base[9] or metranidazole[9]	See footnote 9

Contd...

Contd...

	Likely organisms	Suitable agent	
		Parenteral: Cefoxitin[6] or cefotetan[6]	1–2 g IV
		OR Cefazolin + metronidazole or	1–2 g IV[2] 0.5 g IV
		ampicillin/sulbactam[6,10]	3 g IV
Appendicectomy, non-perforated	Same as colorectal	Cefoxitin[6] or Cefotetan [6] or cefazolin[6] + metronidazole	1–2 g IV 1–2 g IV[2] 0.5 g IV
2. Cardiac	*S. aureus* *S. epidermidis*	Cefazolin or cefuroxime or vancomycin[4]	1–2 g IV[2,3] 1.5 g IV[3] 1 g IV
3. Orthopedic surgery	*S. aureus* *S. epidermidis*	Cefazolin[16] or vancomycin[4,16]	1–2 g IV[2] 1 g IV
4. Genitourinary			
Cystoscopy alone	Enteric gram-negative bacilli, enterococci	High risk[12] only: Ciprofloxacin[10]	500 mg PO or 400 mg IV
		or trimethoprim-sulfamethoxazole	1 DS tablet
Cystoscopy with manipulation or upper tract instrumentation[13]	Enteric gram-negative bacilli, enterococci	Ciprofloxacin[10]	500 mg PO or 400 mg IV
		or trimethoprim-sulfamethoxazole	1 DS tablet
Open or laparoscopic surgery[14]	Enteric gram-negative bacilli, enterococci	Cefazolin[6]	1–2 g IV[2]
5. Gynecologic and obstetric			
Vaginal, abdominal or laparoscopic hysterectomy	Enteric gram-negative bacilli, anaerobes, Group B streptococci, enterococci	Cefazolin[6], Cefoxitin [6] or cefotetan[6] or ampicillin-sulbactam[6,10]	1–2 g IV[2] 3 g IV
Ceserian section	Same as for hysterectomy	Cefazolin[6]	1–2 g IV[2]
Abortion, surgical	Same as for hysterectomy	Doxycycline	300 mg PO[15]
6. Head and neck surgery			
Incisions through oral or pharyngeal mucosa	Anaerobes, enteric gram-negative bacilli, *S. aureus*	Clindamycin or cefazolin + metronidazole or ampicillin/sulbactam[10]	600–900 mg IV 1–2 g IV [2] 0.5 g IV 3 g IV
7. Neurosurgery	*S. aureus, S. epidermidis*	Cefazolin OR vancomycin[4]	1–2 g IV[2] 1 g IV

Contd...

Contd...

	Likely organisms	Suitable agent	
8. Ophthalmic	*S. aureus, S. epidermidis,* streptococci, enteric gram-negative bacilli, *Pseudomonas species.*	Gentamicin, tobramycin, ciprofloxacin, gatifloxacin, levofloxacin, moxifloxacin, ofloxacin or neomycin, gramicidin-polymyxin B or cefazolin	Multiple drops topically over 2–24 hours 100 mg subconjunctivally
9. Thoracic (non-cardiac)	*S. aureus, S. epidermidis* streptococci, enteric gram-negative bacilli,	Cefazolin or ampicillin/sulbactam[10] or vancomycin[4]	1–2 g IV[2] 3 g IV 1 g IV
10. Vascular			
Arterial surgery involving prosthesis, the abdominal aorta, or a groin incision	*S. aureus, S. epidermidis,* enteric gram-negative bacilli,	Cefazolin OR vancomycin[4]	1–2 g IV[2] 1 g IV
Lower extremity amputation for ischemia	*S. aureus, S. epidermidis,* enteric gram-negative bacilli, *Clostridia*	Cefazolin or vancomycin[4]	1–2 g IV[2] 1 g IV

[1]Parenteral prophylactic antimicrobials can be given as a single IV dose begun within 60 minutes before the procedure. For prolonged procedures (>3 hours) or those with major blood loss, or in patients with extensive burns, additional intraoperative doses should be given at intervals 1–2 times the half-life of the drug (ampicillin-sulbactam q2 hours, cefazolin q4 hours, cefuroxime q4 hours, cefoxitin q2 hours, clindamycin q6 hours, vancomycin q12 hours) for the duration of the procedure in patients with normal renal function. If vancomycin or a fluoroquinolone is used, the infusion should be started within 60 to 120 minutes before the initial incision to have adequate tissue levels at the time of incision and to minimize the possibility of an infusion reaction close to the time of induction of anesthesia.

[2]The recommended dose of cefazolin is 1 g for patients who weigh <80 kg and 2 g for those $\geq$ 80 kg. Morbidly obese patients may need higher doses.

[3]Some experts recommend an additional dose when patients are removed from bypass during open heart surgery.

[4]Vancomycin can be used in hospitals in which Methicillin-resistant *S. aureus* and *S. epidermidis* are a frequent cause of postoperative wound infection and also in patients previously colonized with MRSA, or those who are allergic to penicillins or cephalosporins. Rapid IV administration may cause hypotension, which could be especially dangerous during induction of anesthesia. Even when the drug is given over 60 minutes, hypotension may occur; treatment with diphenhydramine (Benadryl and others) and further slowing of the infusion rate may be helpful. Some experts would give 15 mg/kg of vancomycin to patients weighing more than 75 kg, up to a maximum of 1.5 g, with a slower infusion rate (90 minutes for 1.5 g). For procedures in which enteric gram-negative bacilli are common pathogens, many experts would add another drug such as an aminoglycoside (Gentamicin, tobramycin or amikacin), aztreonam or a fluoroquinolone.

[5]Morbid obesity, GI obstruction, decreased gastric acidity or GI motility, gastric bleeding, malignancy or perforation, or immunosuppression.

[6]For patients allergic to penicillin and cephalosporins, clindamycin or vancomycin with either gentamicin, ciprofloxacin levofloxacin or aztreonam is a reasonable alternative. Fluoroquinolones should not be used for prophylaxis in cesarean section.

[7]Age 70 years , acute cholecystitis, non-functioning gall bladder, obstructive jaundice, or common bile duct stones.

[8]Cefotetan, cefoxitin and ampicillin-sulbactam are reasonable alternatives.

[9]In addition to mechanical bowel preparation, 1 g of neomycin plus 1 g of erythromycin at 1 PM, 2 PM and 11 PM or 2 g of neomycin plus 2 g of Metranidazole at 7 PM and 11 PM the day before an 8 AM operation.

[10]Due to increasing resistance of *E. coli* to fluoroquinolones and ampicillin-sulbactam, local sensitivity profiles should be reviewed prior to use.

[11]For a ruptured viscus, therapy is often continued to five days.

[12]Urine culture positive or unavailable, preoperative catheter, transrectal prostatic biopsy or placement of prosthetic material.

[13]Shock wave lithotripsy, ureteroscopy.

[14]Including percutaneous renal surgery, procedures with entry into the urinary tract, and those involving implantation of a prosthesis. If manipulation of bowel is involved, prophylaxis is given according to colorectal guidelines.

[15]Divided into 100 mg before the procedure and 200 mg after.

[16]If a tourniquet is to be used in the procedure, the entire dose of antibiotic must be infused prior to its inflation.

(Also refer to Recommendations for Surgical Antimicrobial Prophylaxis in Chapter 25 on ,"Use of Antibiotics and Chemotherapeutic Agents)

Two well recognized exceptions of clean surgeries requiring prophylactic antimicrobials are:

- Insertion of intravascular prosthesis/joint prosthesis
- Any operation in which incisional or organ/space SSI would pose a catastrophic risk.

A simple way to organize AMP indications is based on using the surgical wound classification scheme. A surgeon makes the decision to use AMP by anticipating *preoperatively* the surgical wound class for a given operation.

AMP is indicated for all operations that entail entry into a hollow viscus under controlled conditions. Certain clean-contaminated operations, such as elective colon resection, low anterior resection of the rectum, and abdominoperineal resection of the rectum, also require an additional preoperative protective maneuver called "preparation of the colon," to empty the bowel of its contents and to reduce the levels of live microorganisms. This maneuver includes the administration of enemas and cathartic agents followed by the oral administration of nonabsorbable antimicrobial agents in divided doses the day before the operation.

By definition, AMP is not indicated for an operation classified as contaminated or dirty. In such operations, patients are frequently receiving therapeutic antimicrobial agents perioperatively for established infections.

The choice of antibiotic will depend on the endogenous flora likely to contaminate the site. Cephalosporins are the most widely studied agents for surgical prophylaxis. These drugs are effective against many gram-positive and gram-negative microorganisms. They also share the features of demonstrated safety, acceptable pharmacokinetics, and a reasonable cost per dose. In particular, cefazolin is widely used and generally viewed as the AMP agent of first choice for clean operations. If a patient is unable to receive a cephalosporin because of penicillin allergy, an alternative for gram-positive bacterial coverage is either clindamycin or vancomycin.

Cefazolin provides adequate coverage for most clean-contaminated operations. For operations on distal intestinal tract cefoxitin (or some other second generation cephalosporin) that provides anaerobic coverage will be necessary. If patient cannot safely receive a cephalosporin because of allergy, a reasonable alternative for gram- negative coverage is aztreonam. However an agent such as clindamycin or metronidazole should also be included to ensure anaerobic coverage.

Aminoglycosides are seldom recommended as first choice either alone or in combination. Similarly routine use of vancomycin is not recommended exception being a cluster of MRSA-related SSIs or MRSA mediastinitis.

Basic "rules of thumb" guide decisions about AMP dose sizes and timing. For example, it is believed that a full therapeutic dose of cefazolin (1–2 g) should be given to adult patients no more than 30 minutes before the skin is incised. There are a few exceptions to this basic guide. With respect to dosing, it has been demonstrated that larger doses of AMP agents are necessary to achieve optimum effect in morbidly obese patients. With respect to timing, an exception occurs for patients undergoing cesarean section in whom AMP is indicated: the initial dose is administered immediately after the umbilical cord is clamped. If vancomycin is used, an infusion period of approximately 1 hour is required for a typical dose.

Operation-related Issues: Intraoperative Environmental Issues[3,11,12]

Operating Room Environment

Airborne contamination is mainly derived from the personnel in the operation theater and their activities. Number of factors influences the bacterial count in the operation theater. They are:

A. Sources of microorganisms in the OR (operating room) environment:

They are: dust, lint, skin squames (epithelial cells) and respiratory droplets. These act as exogenous sources of infection. (They are mostly *Staphylococcus aureus* and *S. epidermidis* which are shed into the environment in skin scales)

- The microbial level in the OR is directly proportional to the number of people moving about in the room
- Movement of swinging doors also creates turbulence and adds to the microbial burden. Sliding doors are thus to be preferred.

B. Zones in OT: The theater should be segregated into different zones to achieve a high degree of asepsis in the OT. OT is divided into 4 zones. The aim of zoning is that when staff members, patients or supplies enter the OT suite, the risk factors of carrying the chances of infection with them get lesser and lesser, as they pass from the protective through clean to aseptic zone.

- Clean from dirty traffic-flow within the OT suite should be segregated as best as possible
- Spaces in the suite should be arranged in such a way that while moving from one space to another, there is continuous progression of cleanliness from entrance of OT suite to the operating room
- Staff working in the OT department should be able to move from one clean area to the other without having to pass through unprotected areas
- Soiled materials and waste should be removed from the operating rooms without passing through clean areas
- OT ventilation should be independent of the air movement of the rest of the hospital. Therefore, the direction of airflow within the OT suite should be from cleaner to less clean areas.

Zones[13,14]

- *Protective zone:* This is at the entrance of operating theater. The main facilities which lie in this area are:
  a. Patient's waiting area and reception
  b. Trolley bay
  c. Lifts
  d. Stairs
  e. Switch room
  f. Preanesthesia room, changing room, store room.
- *Clean zone:* Next zone is the clean zone. It provides:
  a. Preoperating room
  b. Recovery room
  c. Theater work room
  d. X-ray room, plaster room
  e. Sister's room, staff nurse room
  f. Storage space for clean surgical supplies
  g. Medical stores including parental solutions, and instruments
  h. Anesthesia induction rooms, anesthesia stores and anesthetist's room are located in this zone
  i. A frozen section laboratory, if provided and any darkroom facility should be located in the clean zone.
- *Sterile zone:* This zone will include:
  a. Operating suite in particular
  b. Scrub room
  c. Anesthesia room
  d. Instruments trolley area.
- *Disposal zone:* It will include dirty room, disposal corridor and janitors corridor. Disposal zone is the corridor from where used instruments and used linen and operating room debris is taken out. This zone must have an independent access to the outside corridor. Disposal zone has only one-way traffic, viz. from inside the operating room to the outside and never vice versa. This is achieved by a door or a hatch from operating room opening into the disposal corridor.

Following physical facilities must be provided in operating theater:

a. Reception and office
b. Transfer area
c. Entrance
d. Cloak room
e. Preoperative room
f. Staff changing room
g. Notice board
h. Holding bay

i. Anesthesia room
j. Scrub room
k. Operating room.

C. Ventilation and air flow: Proper design and ventilation of operation theaters is the most important means of controlling airborne contamination and thus preventing air borne infection in the operation theaters. The theater should be segregated into zones like aseptic, clean and less clean. It should have mechanical ventilation. Failure to provide proper operation theater ventilation is associated with risk of postoperative infection.[15]

Ventilation/heating ventilation air-conditioning (HVAC): HVAC system maintains indoor air temperature and humidity, control odors, remove contaminated air and minimize the risk of transmission of airborne organisms.

They consist of air inlets, filter beds, and humidity modification mechanisms, heating and cooling equipment, fans, ducts and air exhausts.

Decreased performance of HVAC systems can contribute to the transmission of air-borne infection in the OR.

Critical parameters of operating rooms

i. Operating rooms should be maintained at positive pressure with respect to corridors and adjacent areas. Positive pressure prevents airflow from less clean areas into more clean areas.
ii. All ventilation air conditioning system in hospitals including the operating rooms should have two filter beds in series, with the efficiency of the first filter bed being ≥30% and that of the second filter bed being ≥90%.
iii. There should be minimum of 15 to 20 air changes of filtered air per hour, three (20%) of which must be fresh air.[9] Air should be introduced at the ceiling and exhausted near the floor.
iv. An additional measure could be use of laminar airflow and use of UV radiations to reduce SSI risk for operations. Laminar flow is designed to move particle free air (called "ultra clean air") over the aseptic operating field at a uniform velocity (0.3 to 0.5 mm/sec) sweeping away particles in its path. Laminar flow can be directed vertically or horizontally, and recirculated air is usually passed through a high efficiency particulate air (HEPA) filter to remove particles >0.3 mm in diameter with an efficiency of 99.97%. Laminar flow is recommended for prosthetic and joint surgery. Laminar flow may provide over 400 air changes per hour.[2,9,16]

   The effects of ultraclean air alone, antimicrobial prophylaxis alone, and ultraclean air in combination with antimicrobial prophylaxis on the rate of deep SSIs were compared and it was found that the SSI rate following operations in which ultraclean air alone was used decreased from 3.4 to 1.6%, whereas the rate for those who received only antimicrobial prophylaxis decreased from 3.4 to 0.8%. When both interventions were used in combination, the SSI rate decreased from 3.4 to 0.7%.[17] These findings suggest that both ultraclean air and antimicrobial prophylaxis can reduce the incidence of SSI following orthopedic implant operations, but antimicrobial prophylaxis is more beneficial than ultraclean air. Intra-operative UV radiation has not been shown to decrease overall SSI risk.[18,19]
v. Temperature of 20–22°C is comfortable and inhibits bacterial growth (heating systems to raise the temperature whenever required need to be provided).
vi. Relative humidity 30–60% to slow down bacterial growth.
vii. Direction of air flow: In addition to bacterial load of air, the direction of air flow is also important and should be from clean to less clean area. Recommended airflow rates are 0.28–0.47 m^3/sec across an open door to

prevent back flow into cleaner areas. In ultraclean air enclosure, airflow should not be less than $0.2\ m^3/sec$ one meter above the door.[2]

In hospitals that lack HVAC systems the quality of air in the OR cannot be guaranted.

When a window air-conditioner is used, proper maintenance is required.

In a developing country like India, other innovative methods of providing clean air need to be investigated in clinical trials, particularly with reference to their influence on SSI rates.

The use of fans in operating rooms is not recommended, since this adds to turbulence and lifts dust particles.

D. Environmental surfaces: Environmental surfaces in operating rooms (e.g. tables, floors, walls, ceilings, lights) are rarely implicated as the sources of pathogens important in the development of SSIs. Nevertheless, it is important to perform routine cleaning of these surfaces to reestablish a clean environment after each operation. There are no data to support routine disinfecting of environmental surfaces or equipment between operations in the absence of contamination or visible soiling. When visible soiling of surfaces or equipment occurs during an operation, an hospital disinfectant should be used to decontaminate the affected areas before the next operation. This is in keeping with the Occupational Safety and Health Administration (OSHA) requirement that all equipment and environmental surfaces be cleaned and decontaminated after contact with blood or other potentially infectious materials. Wet-vacuuming of the floor with an hospital disinfectant is performed routinely after the last operation of the day or night. Care should be taken to ensure that medical equipment left in the operating room be covered, so that solutions used during cleaning and disinfecting do not contact sterile devices or equipment. There are no data to support special cleaning procedures or closing of an operating room after a contaminated or dirty operation has been performed.

Operation-related Issues: Other Issues

Surgical Attires

It is necessary to use barriers like scrub-suits, caps, mask, gloves to minimize the exposure of the patient to the skin, mucous membrane or hair of the surgical team members, and to protect the surgical team members from exposure to blood or bloodborne pathogens.

All personnel working in operating rooms must wear clean surgical attire in place of their ordinary clothes. Operation room clothes should not be worn outside this area.

Scrub suits: Must be designed for maximum skin coverage since skin squames are a potential source of microbial contamination.

Masks: Disposable deflector masks, which should be well fitting, must be worn, cloth masks are ineffective barriers for micro-organisms particularly once they get moistened during breathing. OSHA (Occupational Safety and Health Administration) has advised using a N95 mask (respirator) or higher when the patient has or is suspected of having infectious tuberculosis.

Caps: Caps must cover the head and hair falling on the forehead and face. They will reduce contamination of surgical field by organisms shed from the hair and scalp.

Shoes/shoe covers: Footwear should be worn in the operation rooms. They should be designed to protect the wearer from spills of blood and body fluids.

Sterile gloves: All scrubbed members of the surgical team wear sterile gloves. They help to minimize the transmission of microorganisms from the hands of the surgical team to the patient. They also protect the surgical team members from contamination with the patient's blood and body fluids.

Double gloving is recommended for protection during operations on patients infected with bloodborne pathogens viz. HBV, HCV and HIV. In fact, this can be recommended for all surgeries. (Reuse of surgical gloves is not recommended).

Gowns and drapes: Sterile surgical gown and drapes are used to create a barrier between the surgical operative field and potential sources of microorganisms. All surgical team members should wear gowns and drapes are placed over the patients.

The gowns and drapes should ideally be made of material that is impermeable to liquids. However such gowns are uncomfortable, they also inhibit heat loss, and the evaporation of sweat from the wearer's body. Hence, careful selection of gowns should be made.

It is a common practice to use cotton gowns and drapes. A plastic apron should be worn under the gown. The cotton gowns and drapes are laundered following use and steam sterilized for reuse.

Asepsis and Surgical Technique

All scrubbed personnel must strictly adhere to aseptic practice at all times. Members who work in close proximity to the sterile surgical field such as anesthesia personnel must also follow the same standards of asepsis. Invasive procedures like endotracheal intubation, intravascular devices have all been associated with outbreaks of postoperative infections including SSI.

Surgical technique: Excellent surgical skill reduces the risk of SSI. This includes:

- *Effective hemostasis:* While preserving adequate blood supply
- *Prevention of hypothermia:* Hypothermia in surgical patients, defined as a core body temperature below 36°C, may result from general anesthesia, exposure to cold, or intentional cooling such as is done to protect the myocardium and central nervous system during cardiac operations. In one study of hypothermia (temperature below 36°C) during a procedure (colorectal surgery) has been shown to be associated with an increased risk of postoperative SSI.[20] Hypothermia appears to increase incisional SSI, by causing vasoconstriction, decreased delivery of oxygen to the wound space and subsequent impairment of function of phagocytic leukocytes (e.g. neutrophils)
- Gentle handling of tissues during surgery
- Removal of devitalized (e.g. necrotic, charred) tissue, and avoiding inadvertent entries into a hollow viscus
- *Appropriate use of drains:* Drains placed through an operative incision increase incisional SSI. Drains should be placed through separate incisions distant from operative incisions. Closed suction drains are at less risk of SSI than open drain; as they are more effective in evacuating postoperative hematomas or seromas. Timing of removal of drain is important. Bacterial colonization of initially sterile drain tracts increases with duration of time the drain is left in place.
- *Use of appropriate suture material:* In general, monofilament sutures appear to have the lowest infection promoting effects.

Operative Characteristics and Postoperative Issues

Incision Care

A surgical incision that is closed primarily (i.e. the skin edges are re-approximated at the end of the operation) is usually covered with a sterile dressing for 48 hours. In case of delayed primary closure (surgical incision is left open at the skin level for a few days before it is closed) or healing by second intention, the incision is packed with a sterile dressing.

Discharge Planning

In current practice, many patients are discharged very soon after their operation, before surgical incisions have fully healed. The purpose of discharge planning is to maintain integrity of the healing incision, educate the patient about the signs and symptoms of infection and advise the patient about whom to contact to report any problems.

Additional Issues

Managing Clinical Wastes from OR

The waste emerging from the operation room would consist of the following:

- Patient contaminated wastes like disposable plastics, linen and gauze contaminated with blood and body fluids
- Sharps
- Gloves
- Anatomical body parts and tissues
- Wrapping paper and other wrappers:
  - All sharps including needles, IV cannulae, scalpels, blades, etc. should be segregated into puncture proof containers at source
  - Infectious waste requiring disposal like gloves, plastics, cotton, gauze, etc., should be segregated into color coded bags for transportation to the site of treatment
  - Non-infectious wraps should be collected in color-coded bags for disposal/recycling
  - Anatomical body parts should be transported in appropriately sealed containers/bags for pathological examination
  - Specimens fixed in formalin should be stored in closed containers. These are no longer considered as "infectious".

Laundry

- Contaminated linen may be a source of infection and should be placed in impervious bags for transportation
- Disinfection in a sluice area may be achieved using mechanical washers/ sluicing machines or hot water and or bleach
- Laundered linen should be autoclaved before being supplied to ORs.

Pest Control

It is essential to keep OR free from pests like flies, which can sometimes gain entry through open doors.

There has to be a regular schedule for pest control.

Water

This is an important reservoir of microorganisms like *Pseudomonas* species. Some water sources may also be responsible for outbreaks of legionellosis.

If the OR does not have a dedicated water tank, it is advisable to treat the water at the user end by means prior to its being used in the OR.

There are several commercial gadgets available for this purpose.

Water has been implicated as an important reservoir in outbreaks of postoperative infections.

SURVEILLANCE OF SURGICAL SITE INFECTION[3]

Surveillance of SSI with feedback to surgeons has been shown to be an important component of strategies to reduce risk of SSI. In Indian hospitals, little or no surveillance data exists. Now it has become important to concentrate on the SSIs' and acquire our own data.

Three categories of variables have proven to be reliable predictors of SSI risk.

1. Those that estimate the intrinsic degree of microbial contamination of the surgical site, i.e. the wound classification—as clean, clean-contaminated or dirty.
2. Those that measure the duration of operation, i.e. length of operation > T hours, where T is the approximate 75th percentile of the duration of the specific operation performed.
3. Physical status of the patient classification >2 for example.

Code Patient's preoperative physical status:

1. Normally healthy patient
2. Patient with mild systemic disease
3. Patient with severe systemic disease that is not incapacitating
4. Patient with an incapacitating system disease that is a constant threat to life
5. Moribund patient who is not expected to survive for 24 hours with or without operation.

Surveillance methods may be:

1. Inpatient surveillance.
2. Post discharge surveillance.
3. Outpatient surveillance.

Calculation of SSI rate:

Surgical site infection rate

$$= \frac{\text{No. of surgical site infections}}{\text{No. of patients operated on}} \times 100$$

SPECIAL PROBLEMS OF INFECTIONS DUE TO *CLOSTRIDIUM PERFRINGENS* AND OTHER GAS GANGRENE BACILLI[21]

Hospital-acquired infections due to *Clostridium perfringens* is almost always postoperative and derived from patient's own flora. Gas gangrene is rare but it occasionally follows orthopedic operations on the leg (especially above the knee) when the arterial blood supply is defective, and may occur after some abdominal operations.

Since *Clostridial perfringens,* which causes gas gangrene, are found in abundance in the bowel flora of healthy individuals and are also found commonly in the environmental air and dust, there is no reason to close the theater after the operation. Although for the same reason isolation of the patient to prevent cross infection with *Clostridial* species is unnecessary, patient with gas gangrene is isolated for proper nursing care since this patient is dangerously ill and requires special nursing.

MICROBIOLOGIC SAMPLING

Because there are no standardized parameters by which to compare microbial levels obtained from cultures of ambient air or environmental surfaces in the operating room, routine microbiologic sampling cannot be justified.

Such environmental sampling should only be performed as part of an epidemiologic investigation.

Environmental Sampling

Consists of:

1. *Air sampling:* Sampling of air in OT (OR).
2. *Surface sampling:* Sampling of surfaces in OT.

Air Sampling

Sampling of air in OR can be done by two methods:

i. Settle plate method.
ii. By using air sampler either a centrifugal sampler or a slit sampler. Slit sampler is in vogue at present.

Settle plate method: It relies on gravity. This reflects large particles and lacks sensitivity for respirable particles. It is commonly used for sampling air for bacteria and fungi. Settle plates may be useful to detect aerosols of fungi. Though commonly used in our country this method lacks sensitivity and also correlation with clinical isolates. This method has the advantage that it is very simple, but its disadvantage is that it measures only the rate of deposition of large particles from air and not the total number of large and small bacteria-carrying particles suspended in it (Bacteria-carrying particle may be a dust particle or droplet nuclei which may carry one to a hundred or more bacteria, but generally carry a few bacteria).

Air sampler: Air sampling is used to detect aerosols or particles of microorganisms. These may be respirable particles (25 μm) or larger particles. Slit samplers are in vogue. These are capable of collecting larger volumes of air in short period. This method helps to verify filter efficacy and is performed in undisturbed conditions when air is sampled during or after human activity, a higher number of airborne microorganisms is detected.

Particle counter is also required and is a practical method for evaluating the efficiency of filters.

The detection of pathogenic micro-organisms and/or fungi from the operating room environment should thus be an indicator of inadequacy of cleaning/air quality. Microbiologic sampling remains controversial since there are no standards for comparison. Both the methods should therefore be interpreted in the right context. Concentrating all efforts on microorganisms detected during sampling can often be misleading. The true factors for SSI may thereby be neglected.

Environmental Sampling or Sampling of Surfaces

Surface sampling is done with the assumption that inanimate sources are important causes of nosocomial infection. However, it must be kept in mind that for the inanimate environment to act as source of infection two factors are necessary (1) Inadequate cleaning and disinfection thereby increasing the bacterial load and (2) vehicle of transmission by which the environment is brought in contact with the patients' vulnerable areas through hands, inadequately disinfected or sterilized equipment like gloves, dressings and instruments. It has been said that surfaces not in contact with surgical wound are unlikely to pose a major infection risk.[7] The routine sampling of the inanimate environment particularly of surfaces does not contribute to the prevention of nosocomial infections or predict when postoperative infections are likely to occur.[12] Also rates of occurrence of nosocomial infections have not been correlated with levels of general environmental contamination, standards for acceptable levels of environmental contamination are arbitrary.

Surfaces are not uniformly contaminated like air and therefore the results of bacteriological tests on them are difficult to evaluate. Routine sampling of floors, wall, furniture and equipment not in direct patient contact are not recommended. A quantitative or semiquantitative test of a large area and search for specific pathogen can at best give an idea of a lapse of the cleaning and disinfection processes. However, the best of cleaning cannot totally eliminate organisms. Environmental swabs are an issue of the past and should be abondened. It has been recommended that surfaces should only be sampled when there is a clear epidemiological indication to do so.[7]

Environmental surface in operating rooms (e.g. tables, floor, walls, ceilings, lights) are rarely implicated as sources of pathogens important in the development of SSIs. However, it is important to perform routine cleaning of these surfaces to establish a clean environment after each operation.

DISINFECTION OF OPERATION THEATER

The choice of disinfectant is important for example; a routine use of quaternary ammonium compounds can lead to selection of gram-negative bacteria in the environment.

The ideal disinfectant should have a broad spectrum, be safe and economical. There is a wide choice available: commonly used agents include sodium hypochlorite, environmental iodophors, hydrogen peroxide (stabilized with silver), chlorhexidine gluconate combinations, etc. The disinfectant should be approved/selected by the hospital infection control committee taking into consideration all the above factors.

Rotation of disinfectant remains a controversial issue.

Schedule for cleaning of operation rooms:
- Beginning of the day, i.e. before the first surgery
- During a procedure
- Between procedures
- End of the day
- Weekly/monthly.

Beginning of the Day—Prior to the First Surgery

The furniture, equipments, lights are damp dusted with detergent germicide. Particular attention should be paid to horizontal surfaces because dust and lint transport microorganisms settled on them.

During the Procedure

Spills/blood splashes in the vicinity of the sterile area should be absorbed with a cloth and cleaned with a germicide. All instruments opened for a procedure whether used or not are treated as contaminated.

In Between Procedure (in Between Cases)

The furnitures, operating lights, suction canisters and other equipment used is wiped with a detergent germicide. Mattress is wiped and patient transport vehicles are wiped. Three to four feet area of the floor around the table should be cleaned. Wet mops, fresh for every patient is preferred or wet vacuum cleaner. Walls, doors, push plates and other areas that have come in contact with the patient's blood and body fluids are cleaned.

Days End

OR, scrub utility, corridor, furnishings and equipment to be cleaned.

FUMIGATION/FOGGING[11]

This ancient routine is still practiced. However, there is no substitute for vigorous washing of surfaces that come in contact with patients.

Fumigation traditionally consists of a mixture of formalin and potassium permanganate being placed in a bowl. The room is then sealed and opened after 12–24 hours. Alternatively formalin can be sprayed with humidification by a spraying device.

Fogging hastens the process of settling of airborne microorganisms. Mist, generated by a disinfectant or water would achieve the same process. This procedure is no longer recommended in the Western literature.

Since most of the ORs of hospitals in our country do not have the recent sophisticated ventilation system, fogging continues to be a primary method of decontamination in our country.

It is said that fogging gives a false sense of security, but as has been mentioned earlier, since majority of our ORs are without the modern ventilation system, therefore fogging will help maintain a continuous awareness regarding the cleanliness of ORs.

However, formalin should not be used for fumigation/fogging, as it is not only toxic, but also carcinogenic. If this procedure is to be continued, safer agents like hydrogen peroxide stabilized with a silver salt or any other disinfectant of proven efficacy should replace formalin.

It should be remembered that fogging has no role in ORs with modern day HVACS.

If surgeries are being performed with window air-conditioners, fogging should be performed on daily basis, not on weekends alone as is practiced.

CONVENTIONAL STERILIZATION OF SURGICAL INSTRUMENTS

Inadequate sterilization of surgical instruments has resulted in SSI outbreaks. Therefore, all surgical instruments should be soaked in a disinfectant—detergent and thoroughly washed prior to steam sterilization or use of other approved methods, i.e. dry heat, ethylene oxide, etc. Microbial monitoring of steam sterilizers is necessary and can be accomplished by use of biological indicators.

Short-cut method like boiling and chemical disinfection of surgical instruments should be avoided. Appropriate packing of surgical instruments also needs to be emphasized.

FLASH STERILIZATION OF SURGICAL INSTRUMENTS

The Association for the Advancement of Medical Instrumentation defines flash sterilization as "the process designated for the steam sterilization of patient care items for immediate use. During any operation, the need for emergency sterilization of equipment may arise (e.g. to reprocess an inadvertently dropped instrument). However, flash sterilization is not intended to be used for either reasons of convenience or as an alternative to purchasing additional instrument sets or to save time. Also, flash sterilization is not recommended for implantable devices because of the potential for serious infections.

Flash sterilization is not recommended as a routine sterilization method because of the lack of timely biologic indicators to monitor performance, absence of protective packaging following sterilization, possibility for contamination of processed items during transportation to operating rooms, and use of minimal sterilization cycle parameters (i.e. time, temperature, pressure). To address some of these concerns, many hospitals have placed equipment for flash sterilization in close proximity to operating rooms and new biologic indicators that provide results in 1 to 3 hours are now available for flash-sterilized items. Nevertheless, flash sterilization should be restricted to its intended purpose until studies are performed that can demonstrate comparability with conventional sterilization methods regarding risk of SSI.

PRACTICAL ASPECTS

RISK FACTORS FOR SSI AND GENERAL GUIDELINES FOR PREVENTION OF SSI

Definition

Infection in the surgical site that occurs within 30 days of the surgical procedure or within one year if there is an implant or foreign body such as prosthetic heart valve or joint prosthesis.

The key factors to be recorded clinically are:[1]

- Severity and extent of infection in the patient
- Type of operation
- Time period between the operation and the development of infection.

Factors, which influence the frequency of SSIs, include (Tables 10.3 to 10.6):

- Surgical technique
- Extent of endogenous contamination of the wound at surgery (clean, clean-contaminated)
- Duration of operation
- Underlying patient status
- Operating room environment
- The number of organisms shed from the skin of the operating room team and from the skin of the patient.

Do's and Don'ts for SSI[1]

Adapted from "Guidelines on prevention and control of hospital associated infections WHO Regional Office for South-East Asia, New Delhi, January 2002.

Table 10.3: Risk factors for SSI and prevention

Risk factors for SSI	Prevention
1. Patient age	Avoid operating on very old or very young as they are at higher risk for developing infections
2. Nutritional status	Build a good nutritional status
3. Diabetes	Control and maintain blood sugar levels
4. Smoking	Cessation of smoking at least one month prior to surgery
5. Obesity	Reduce weight prior to surgery
6. Co-existent infections in a remote body site	Treat adequately before operation
7. Colonization with microorganisms	Screen and treat carriers (avoid preoperative shaving)
8. Altered immune response	Boost immunity if possible
9. Length of preoperative stay	Avoid long stay in hospital
10. Prevention of SSI	Preoperative shower/bath with antiseptic on night before

Table 10.4: Operational procedures and guidelines

Operational procedures	Guidelines
1. Duration of surgical scrub	2 minutes as effective as 10 minutes
2. Skin antisepsis	Use povidone-iodine/ chlorhexidine gluconate (preferable)
3. Preoperative shaving	Avoid if possible or shave immediately prior to operation preferably with depilator
4. Preoperative skin preparation	Allow drying of antiseptic
5. Duration of operation	Keep procedures as short as possible

Table 10.5: General factors and guidelines

General factors	Guidelines
1. Antimicrobial prophylaxis	Give suitable antimicrobial cover
2. Operating room ventilation	Adhere to specifications
3. Inadequate sterilization of instruments	Monitor CSSD procedures
4. Foreign material in the operative site	Maintain high level of sepsis
5. Surgical drains	Avoid unless really necessary
6. Surgical technique - Poor hemostasis - Failure to obliterate dead space - Tissue trauma	Maintain good surgical technique and ensure minimal tissue trauma

Table 10.6: Measures for prevention of infection[2]

Infection	Proven effective	Proven not effective
Surgical site infection	1. Surgical technique 2. Clean operating environment 3. Staff attire (clothes) 4. Limiting preoperative hospital stay 5. Preoperative shower and local skin preparation of patient 6. Optimal antibiotic prophylaxis 7. Aseptic practice in operation room 8. Surgical wound surveillance	1. Fumigation 2. Preoperative shaving

Source: Adapted from Prevention of hospital-acquired infections. 2nd edition, WHO—A Practical Guide; 2002.

Microbiological Surveillance of OR/(OTs)

- Monitoring of bacterial load of OR surfaces
- Monitoring of bacterial load of OR air.

Microbiological Surveillance of the Operation Theaters[3] (Operation Rooms)

In hospital ORs where planar ventilation systems and infection control nurses monitoring infection control processes are available, surface swabs are often not indicated.

There are no standard parameters by which we can compare microbial levels from cultures of ambient air or environmental surfaces in the operating rooms, therefore, routine microbiologic sampling cannot be justified. Such environmental sampling should only be formed as part of epidemiological investigation.[3]

Operation theater infections with anaerobes like *Clostridium tetanii* are associated with bad surgical procedures with a lot of dead tissue in the surgical site at the end of the procedure and also with presence of heavy dust in the OT environment. Surveillance for clostridial spores is an age old concept and has lost importance with the available OT sterilization and disinfection programs and practices. Today we rarely encounter a infection with *Clostridium tetanii.*[23]

Thus aerobic cultures of OT swabs should be done only as a part of epidemiological investigation and routine testing for *Clostridium tetanii* is not mandatory and could be done in situations like new constructions or structural alterations made in the theater.

It is to be noted that environmental swabs are an issue of the past and should be abandoned.

A. Monitoring the bacterial load of surfaces: Swabs are usually taken from the OT table and its vicinity.

Sites from where samples are to be collected:

1. Boyle's apparatus (Anesthesia trolley)
2. OT table
3. Instrument trolley
4. Overhead lamp
5. Window sills
6. Floor near the OR table

(Sterile swabs soaked in sterile normal saline are streaked on the surface)

Processing of OR (OT) swabs:[3]

The swabs have to be processed aerobically and anaerobically

Routine screening for *Clostridium tetani* has lost its relevance and should be done only when suspected tetanus case is operated or whenever there is some renovation work done in the OT complex.[23-27]

Results of prefumigation/fogging microbiological monitoring indicates the prevalent bacterial load to which the patient could be exposed.

Results of postfumigation/fogging microbiological monitoring indicates the effectiveness of the fumigation procedure.

Anaerobic cultures: OT swabs are immersed in test tubes containing RCM (Robertson's cooked meat medium) and incubated for up to seven days. They are observed for turbidity, blackening of meat and a foul odor. Smears are made from the RCM if these changes are noted, and screened for *Clostridium tetani.*

Interpretation of anaerobic cultures: If no change in RCM is seen after seven days then the respective samples are reported as negative for *Clostridium tetani.* If in any smears showing the typical morphology of *Clostridium tetani* is noted then the sample from which that particular smear was made is reported as positive for *Clostridium tetani.*

Clostridia being the most difficult to eradicate, are used as indicators of efficacy of fumigation/fogging of OR surfaces.

Aerobic cultures: The swabs are immediately put into nutrient broth and incubated at 37°C for 48 hours. Subcultures are then done on blood agar and MacConkey agar plates and the plates are examined after overnight incubation at 37°C. Colonies are then identified by standard methods.

B. Monitoring bacterial load in OR air: Monitoring bacterial load of air can be done in different ways, the two methods used routinely are:

1. *Active air sampling:* By use of air samplers.
2. *Passive air sampling:* By use of settle plates.

Both methods are widely used and have their own set of advantages and disadvantages.

Air samplers have the advantage that the results are expressed as numbers of cfu per cubic meter (cfu/m^3) of air, which correlates well with most official guidelines. Drawback is that they are heavy, expensive and noisy, cause turbulance while sampling, need continuous calibration and are difficult to sterilize. So also each active sampler gives different results in the same place at the same time showing a high variability as well as different active samplers gives different results. Therefore, it is difficult to compare data collected using different samplers.[24,25]

Settle plate on the other hand is simple and inexpensive, economical readily available and most important are sterile. The chief advantage in context of operation theaters is that settle plates reflect the bacterial load nearest the operative site without creating any turbulence.[24,25] It is said to reproduce the circumstances of infection by dust particles sedimenting into the wound better than a slit sampler.[26] It predicts the likely contamination rate at the surgicak site, as it allows a direct measure of the number of organisms settling on surfaces.[27]

Unfortunately settle plates too are used in different ways. Petri dishes used for this are of different diameters, different exposure time, and different incubation temperatures used, making it difficult to compare data. It was first standardized by Fisher in 1970s,[28] and a schedule of 1/1/1 was devised as a standard for measuring the microbial air contamination in hospital environments at bio-risk. The petri

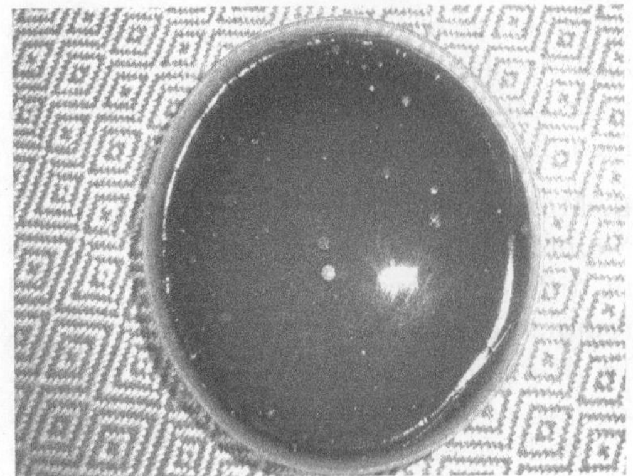

Fig. 10.2: Settle plate method

dish is left open to air for 1 hour, 1 m above the floor, 1 m from the wall or any obstacle.[24]

The data is now interpreted according to the scientifically determined baseline values initially suggested by Fisher in 1970s and now widely adopted by the European Cooperation for Accreditation of Laboratories.[29]

Since no Indian standard limits are provided by any Indian official documents the Swiss Hospital Official Standards could be followed as maximum levels in operation theaters, i.e. ≤5 CFU/9 cm[29] diameter plate in ultra-clean rooms like neurosurgery, cardiothoracic vascular surgeries (CTVS) and joint replacement theatres, ≤25 in other operation theaters.

i. *Settle plate method (Fig. 10.2 and Table 10.7):*[3,4,24]

1. Blood agar plate is exposed for 1 hour at various places in the OT (kept on a table one meter above the ground) and one meter away from walls or any obstacles.
2. Plate is then incubated at 37°C for 48 hours.
3. After incubation colonies are counted. Results are expressed in CFU/plate/hour.
4. Maximum acceptable level of contamination for ultra-clean ORs is up to 5 CFU/hour and up to 25 CFU/hour in other ORs.
5. Not a single colony of *Staphylococcus aureus, Pseudomonas* or fungus should be present.

In epidemiological situations other selective media for staphylococci or fungi or other pathogens could be used in addition.

The formula used is number of bacteria settling on 1 sq meter of medium per minute = number of such particles per 0.3 cubic meter of air. By using this formula settle plate counts can be converted into air counts.

Note: Many plates may have to be used to obtain an overall assessment of conditions

Table 10.7: Interpretation of settle plate culture results[24,30]

Sr. No.	Average colony count per plate/60 minutes	Interpretation	Action to be taken
1.	<25 bacterial colonies (for general OTs like ENT, gynecology, surgery, etc.) <5 bacterial colonies (for ultraclean OTs)	Acceptable	No special action Maintain regular fumigation/fogging and mopping
2.	>25 bacterial colonies (for general OTs like ENT, gynecology, surgery, etc.) >5 bacterial colonies for ultraclean OTs	Unacceptable	Repeat fumigation/fogging with microbiological monitoring
3.	Isolation of any number of *Staphylococcus aureus* and *Pseudomonas* species	Unacceptable	Repeat fumigation/fogging with microbiological monitoring and follow precautions to keep bacterial counts low in the OT *
4.	More than 2 fungal colonies	Unacceptable	Repeat fumigation/fogging and thorough cleaning of all objects intimate with the patient using 70% alcohol. See for any obvious fungal growth on walls and ceiling

*Interpretation of settle plate results and action to be taken:[30]

in the room, for the count on any one plate is subject to wide variation from the effects of air current and any temporary dust-raising disturbance in its vicinity.

ii. Air Sampler:[3,4]
According to British standards air sampling is recommended in plenum ventilated operation theaters at commissioning or after refurbishing (making clean again). In ultra clean theaters it is recommended on a regular basis several times a year and should be done inside and outside the enclosed area.[7]

The above protocol is recommended presuming that the theater has plenum ventilation and that ventilation standards are being met. However, in our country where many theaters do not have adequate ventilation and requisite number of air changes are not taking place, routine microbiological surveillance is being justified keeping in mind that factors like theater discipline, protective clothing, number of persons in the theater and their activity influence the level of bacterial contamination and sampling may serve educational and deterrent value to prevent the breach of theater discipline. However, it should not be treated as replacement for the lack of provision of proper ventilation. It should be the endeavor of every infection control officer (may be a microbiologist, administrator or clinician) to prevent the use of improperly ventilated rooms as operation theaters.[7]

Using a device called as air sampler one can carry out bacterial counts. There are two types of air samplers, centrifugal air sampler and slit sampler (Figs 10.3A and B). Both the air samplers can be used, the centrifugal air sampler though more convenient, all the calculations for laminar flow systems have been made on the slit sampler, which is now the gold standard.

The centrifugal sampler is a small portable device with a centrifugal fan, which draws in air and passes it over a strip of agar, which is placed facing the fan. This type of sampler is more convenient to transport and use, however it is less efficient than slit sampler in detecting particles below 5 μ in diameter and the size of the sample may not be accurately controlled. It is inadequate therefore for ultraclean areas.

The slit sampler is a large vacuum extractor with a nozzle, which is pointed to the area to be sampled. This air is passed directly over an

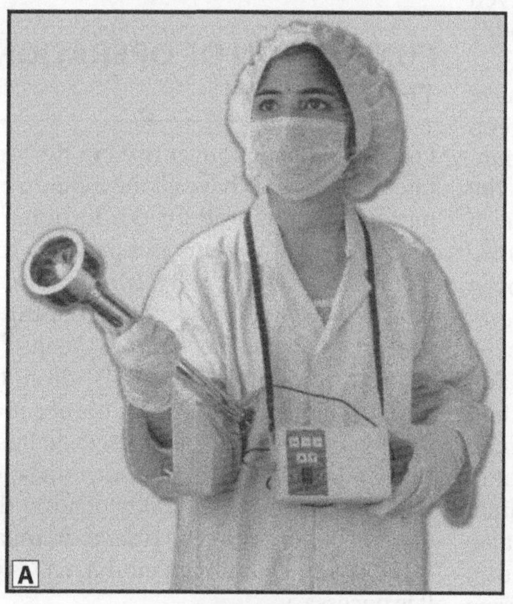

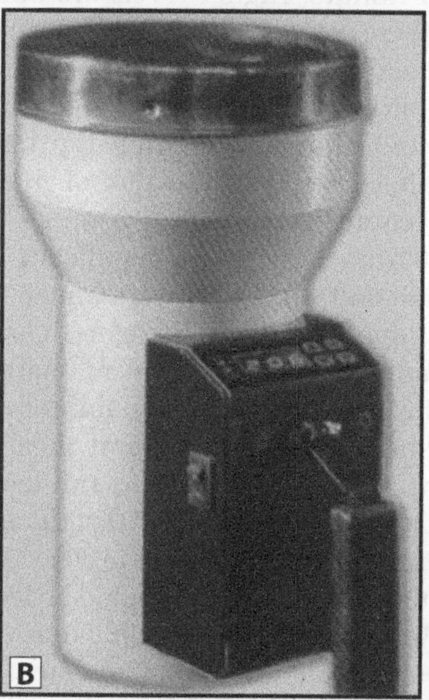

Figs 10.3A and B: (A) Centrifugal air sampler; (B) Petri air sampler

agar plate, which can then be incubated, and the counts calculated the next day.

The principle of an air sampler is that a known quantity of air (40 liters) is passed over the blood agar plates for a given time period (e.g. four or eight minutes and the number of bacteria carrying particles are calculated per cubic liter of air.

Air contamination standards: The level of bacterial contamination of air is usually expressed as the number of bacteria carrying particles per m^3 (bcp m^3) or the bioload B. B can be calculated from the formula:

$$B = \frac{1000\ N\ \text{bcp m}^3}{RT}$$

Where N is the number of colonies counted on the sample plate, T is the duration of time in minutes and R is the air sampling rate in liters/min. In studies concerned with airborne infection of man, the particles counted are those that carry bacteria capable of growth on blood agar during aerobic incubation for 24 or 48 hours at 37°C. Conventionally ventilated rooms commonly show contamination levels between 150/m^3 and 4000/m^3, and deposition on settle plates from values 10/m^2 to 1000/ m^2 per minute. Higher levels are observed when there are many occupants, more bodily movement or other dust raising activities.[31]

Studies in a number of theaters have suggested a general relationship between total air counts and the risk of infection. When counts were within a range of 700 to 1,800/m^3, there was a significant risk of infection and when they were under 180/m^3 the risk appeared slight. Therefore, it has been recommended that for conventional operation theater the bioload should not exceed 35/m^3 of air space in an empty theater and 180/m^3 during an operation, and less than one colony-forming unit (CFU) of *Clostridium perfringens* or *Staphylococcus* in 30 m.[3] In ultra clean theaters the bioload should be less than 1.0 CFU/m^3 in the center of an empty theater, and less than 10 CFU/m^3 at the center (and 20 cfu/m^3 at the periphery of the enclosure) during operation, and not more than one colony of *C. perfringens* or *S. aureus* should be found.[3,7]

METHODS OF CLEANING OPERATION THEATER AND EQUIPMENT INSIDE OPERATION THEATER[30]

Wash the operation theater with soap and water. See that all crevices and windowsills are also cleaned.

1. Mopping of the floors should be done using 10 g of bleaching powder per liter. Let the floor dry after the first mop. Second round of mopping is done using 2 to 5 % phenol (carbolic acid 20 to 50 mL per liter of water) or use a good quality disinfectant like Lysol as per manufacturer's instructions.
2. Clean the operation table, Mackintosh, instrument trolley and instruments coming in close contact with the patient and door handles with 70% alcohol.
3. Do not enter OT till completely dry.
4. After mopping, mops must be kept dry by exposure to sunlight. Continuous use of mops without intermittent drying leads to contamination more than disinfection.

FUMIGATION OF OPERATION THEATERS[3,7,11]

Fumigation is no longer used in the Western Literature as they have all the modern critical parameters required for OT. In India, there are extreme situations in operation theater (OT) facilities, ranging from rooms with fans, window air conditioning, to the more sophisticated laminar airflow systems.

More than 60–80% of OTs, do not have air handling unit (AHU) and other modern facilities with critical parameters. In hospitals that lack heat ventilation air conditioning (HVAC) systems, the quality of air in the OT cannot be guaranteed. Hence, fumigation/ fogging is still continued in Indian OTs where it is necessary.

However, formalin should not be used since it has been identified as a carcinogen.

Fumigation with formalin if used should be carried out by trained personnel under strictly defined conditions. All workers using formaldehyde must be aware of safe handling techniques. Formaldehyde is a Schedule 1 chemical under the Control of Substances Hazardous to Health (COSHH) and has a maximum exposure limit (MEL) of 2 ppm.[32]

Method I

Preparation

- Clean the floor, walls and all washable equipment thoroughly with soap and water. Close windows and ventilators tightly. Plug all other openings with cotton wool, sheets or tape
- Put off all the lights, fans, and air-conditioner, exhaust fans, other electrical and electronic devices and oxygen control
- Calculate the room size in cubic feet (L×B×H) and calculate the required amount of formaldehyde as given in the next step.

Precaution

1. Adequate care must be taken by wearing cap, mask, foot cover, spectacle, etc.
2. Formaldehyde is irritant to eye and nose; and it has been recognized as a potential carcinogen.
3. So the fumigating employee must be provided with the personal protective equipments (PPE).

Fumigation

Keep fumigation chamber on the floor in the center of the room (boil 500 mL of 40% formaldehyde + 1,000 mL of water per 1,000/ft^3 of air space) in an electric boiler. As soon as the formaldehyde is kept for boiling, leave the room quickly closing the door. Seal the door with gum paper or adhesive tape for 24 hours. After 45 minutes (time will vary according to volume used, should be switched off just before the evaporation is complete) switch off the boiler without entering the room. (Switch of boiler should be outside the OT).[24] Put label on the door "Room under fumigation". From (time and date) To (time and date).[32]

Next day: Keep a cloth soaked in ammonia solution (i.e. 250 mL of liquid ammonia per 1000 mL of formalin solution used).

Leave it in the room for 2 to 3 hours, to neutralize the formaldehyde. The room may then be used.

Method II

For 10 × 10 × 10 rooms – 250 g of potassium permanganate + 500 cc of formalin[33] (exact amount of potassium permanganate should be used, as excess amount may lead to explosion). Divide the formaldehyde solution into 6 to 8 heat resistant bowls and also divide the potassium permanganate into the same number of parts and add it to the bowls containing formaldehyde solution. This will lead to autoboiling and generation of fumes.

Neutralization

After the fumigation process neutralize the formaldehyde vapor with ammonia solution. On next day, enter the operation theater at 7 am with 250 mL of 10% ammonia (for 1000 mL of formaldehyde used).[34] Place the ammonia solution in the center of the room and leave it for 3 hours to neutralize the formalin vapor.

Example:

1. Operation Theater Volume = L × B × H = 20 × 15 × 10 = **3,000 cubic feet.**
2. Formaldehyde required for fumigation = 500 mL for 1000 cubic feet = So **1,500 mL of formaldehyde** required
3. Ammonia required for neutralization = 250 mL of 10% ammonia for 1000 mL of formaldehyde = So **375 mL of 10% ammonia** required.

a. Duration of fumigation: 48 hours in case done after any construction in the OT.
   Three swabs to be taken from walls, equipment at intervals:
   First swab—48 hours after fumigation
   Second swab—24 hours later, after first swab.
   Third swab—12 hours after second swab.
   All the three swabs should come negative and then OT can be used.
b. 24 hours fumigation in case infected cases were operated.
c. 12 hours fumigation for routine clean cases.

Swabs for monitoring the disinfection of OT to be collected after fumigation.

Note: Walls should be disinfected only once in 6 months and the ceiling disinfected only once a year unless obvious fungal growth/dampness is noted. In such case report immediately to the authorities.

USE OF MACHINES FOR FUMIGATION/FOGGING (FIG. 10.4)

Nowadays, machines are available in which you can put the required amount of formalin and water and start the machine. The disinfector splits the solution of formalin and water into microparticles. Due to high aerodynamic stability the formalin droplets remain suspended in the atmosphere for longer duration and is claimed to ensure 100% sterile germ free environment within six hours.

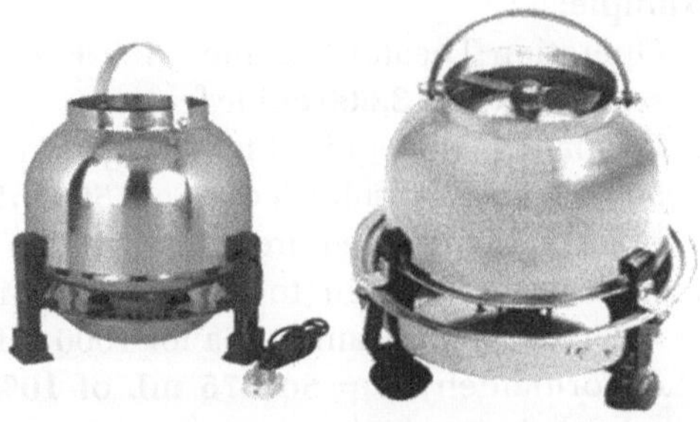

Fig. 10.4: Aerosol disinfector

COLD FOGGING OF OPERATION THEATERS

Operation theaters (OTs)/Operating rooms (ORs) are commonly disinfected by fumigation with formaldehyde. This is a toxic process, which causes eye irritation too. It is also said to be carcinogenic. Besides the OR has to be kept closed for nearly 10 hours after fumigation. Hospitals and surgeons therefore reluctantly sterilize the OR once a month, some weekly and do not carry out disinfection between operations.

Now newer products have been launched which contain hydrogen peroxide (5%) with colloidal silver (40 ppm).[15,16] The oxidizing agent and silver are capable of controlling microbes individually, but when combined exhibit tremendous synergy. Silver has a antimicrobial property and is potent in traces, which are harmless for human beings. It is effective against bacteria, virus, fungi, protozoa, mycobacteria, bacteriophages and biofilms.

Mechanism of Action

With the help of fogging machine, droplets of 7 to 20 microns are released (of H_2O_2 + Silver). It traps suspended particulate matters and kills the microorganisms.

Advantage

The OT (OR) can be used just after an hour after cold fogging.

So also other agents like quaternary ammonium compounds, chemically bound formaldehydes, etc. have been used as agents for fogging.

Table 10.8 shows the surgical protocol for microbiological surveillance of operation theater.

Table 10.8: Surgical protocol for microbiological surveillance of operation theater[7]

Procedure	When to do it	Method
1. Airflow check and ventilation (not truly a microbiological procedure, performed with the help of engineering dept)	1. At commissioning and refurbishing, after completion of a. All engineering work b. Vacuum cleaning of ducting c. Plant has been running at full power for 24 hours 2. Yearly thereafter	Direction of airflow by smoke test Air velocity by hot air anemometer
2. Air microbial sampling	1. At commissioning and refurbishing as above 2. Weekly	Settle plate using 5% sheep blood or slit sampler
3. Monitoring of sterilization A. Steam	1. With every cycle/load 2. Daily 3. Weekly	Physical (time and temperature record, manual or automatic Bowie-Dick *B. stearothermophilus* spores
B. Ethylene oxide gas (ETO)	Every cycle	Physical (time and temperature) Concentration of ETO moisture content *B. subtilis* spores
C. Equipment and instruments—sterilized/disinfected by liquid chemicals (e.g. glutaraldehyde	Weekly	Spot check for sterility by Swab rinse method/Glutaraldehyde testing strip
4. Testing of disinfectants and antiseptics	1. At introduction of disinfectant into hospital 2. Weekly	Use dilution Kelsey-Sykes test In-use test
5. Surface sampling	1. At commissioning and refurbishing 2. During outbreak if epidemiologically indicated	Rodac plate and swab rinse method
6. Testing for carriers among staff	1. At entry, employment 2. During outbreak	Nasal swab, throat swab, rectal swabs/ stool culture Routine culture techniques using selective media

Note: The laboratory should establish protocol for carrying out surveillance with consultation of HAICC. Interpretation and action there upon are critical factors for meaningful surveillance

BIOLOGICAL TEST FOR MONITORING AUTOCLAVES[3]

When microbiological tests are required for hospital sterile equipment, first ensure that there is a good and sufficient reason to justify their employment.

1. Ensure that the autoclave has passed its physical checks, including a Bowie-Dick test (Bowie et al., 1963)[35,36] to prove that air removal is effective.
2. Purchase paper disks or strips containing at least 10^6 spores of *Bacillus stearothermophilus* (NCTC 10,003, ATCC 7,953, CIP 52,181) with Z factor of 10–14. (The Z value is a measure of the thermal resistance of the spore to the particular process. It is the number of degree centigrade required to produce a 10-fold change in thermal death time).
3. Place the spore strip in the center of one or more packs in the coolest (lowest) part of the chamber.
4. After autoclaving, transfer the strips with aseptic precautions into tryptone soya broth pH 7.3.
5. Incubate aerobically at 56°C for 5 days. At the same time incubate a positive, nonautoclaved control disk.

After 5 days incubation, make smears if turbidity is seen and look for the presence of *Bacillus stearothermophilus*. Presence of the organisms suggests that sterilization was not proper. Absence of turbidity and *Bacillus stearothermophilus* indicates that sterilization was proper. If organisms other than gram-positive bacilli (*Bacillus stearothermophilus*) are seen, then the test must be repeated.

Nowadays, biological indicators are available in ampoules containing the liquid medium (trypticase soya broth), which is in the upper portion of the vial and the indicator strip (spore strip) at the bottom. After sterilization the ampoule is removed and the ampoule is crushed and then tapped on a hard surface, so that the medium goes down and wets the strip. Then this ampoule with the BI is incubated for 48 hours (or in a Rapid Incubator (results in one to three hours) and results read. If there is no color change the sterilization was effective. But if there is a color change the sterilization was not effective.

Autoclave tapes on the surface of the packs merely provide an indication that the process has been carried out. It does not indicate that the contents of the pack are sterile.

It is unwise to manufacture one's own test spores. Biological variability creates considerable difficulty in producing consistent spores with a defined D value, i.e. the number of minute's exposure to produce a log reduction in the number of viable spores at the temperature of the test.

(For details refer to chapter on Central Sterile Supply Department—CSSD).

RECOMMENDATIONS FOR PREVENTION OF SURGICAL SITE INFECTION

Rationale

The Guideline for Prevention of Surgical Site Infection, 1999, provides recommendations concerning reduction of surgical site infection risk. Each recommendation is categorized on the basis of existing scientific data, theoretical rationale, and applicability. However, the previous CDC system for categorizing recommendations has been modified slightly.

Category I recommendations, including IA and IB, are those recommendations that are viewed as effective by HICPAC and experts in the fields of surgery, infectious diseases, and infection control. Both Category IA and IB recommendations are applicable for, and should be adopted by, all healthcare facilities; IA and IB recommendations differ only in the strength of the supporting scientific evidence.

Category II recommendations are supported by less scientific data than Category I recommendations; such recommendations may be appropriate for addressing specific nosocomial problems or specific patient populations.

No recommendation is offered for some practices, either because there is a lack of consensus regarding their efficacy or because the available scientific evidence is insufficient to support their adoption. For such unresolved issues, practitioners should use judgment to determine a policy regarding these practices within their organization.

Recommendations that are based on federal regulation are denoted with an asterisk.

Rankings

Category IA: Strongly recommended for implementation and supported by well-designed experimental, clinical, or epidemiological studies.

Category IB: Strongly recommended for implementation and supported by some experimental, clinical, or epidemiological studies and strong theoretical rationale.

Category II: Suggested for implementation and supported by suggestive clinical or epidemiological studies or theoretical rationale.

No recommendation; unresolved issue: Practices for which insufficient evidence or no consensus regarding efficacy exists.

Practices required by federal regulation are denoted with an asterisk (*).

Recommendations

Preoperative

Preparation of the patient

1. Whenever possible, identify and treat all infections remote to the surgical site before elective operation and postpone elective operations on patients with remote site infections until the infection has resolved (*Category IA*).
2. Do not remove hair preoperatively unless the hair at or around the incision site will interfere with the operation (*Category IA*).
3. If hair is removed, remove immediately before the operation, preferably with electric clippers (*Category IA*).
4. Adequately control serum blood glucose levels in all diabetic patients and particularly avoid hyperglycemia perioperatively (*Category IB*).
5. Encourage tobacco cessation. At minimum, instruct patients to abstain for at least 30 days before elective operation from smoking cigarettes, cigars, pipes, or any other form of tobacco consumption (e.g. chewing/dipping) (*Category IB*).
6. Do not withhold necessary blood products from surgical patients as a means to prevent SSI (*Category IB*).
7. Require patients to shower or bathe with an antiseptic agent on at least the night before the operative day (*Category IB*).
8. Thoroughly wash and clean at and around the incision site to remove gross contamination before performing antiseptic skin preparation (*Category IB*).
9. Use an appropriate antiseptic agent for skin preparation (*Category IB*).
10. Apply preoperative antiseptic skin preparation in concentric circles moving toward the periphery. The prepared area must be large enough to extend the incision or create new incisions or drain sites, if necessary (*Category II*)
11. Keep preoperative hospital stay as short as possible while allowing for adequate preoperative preparation of the patient (*Category II*).
12. No recommendation to taper or discontinue systemic steroid use (when medically permissible) before elective operation (*Unresolved Issue*).
13. No recommendation to enhance nutritional support for surgical patients solely as a means to prevent SSI (*Unresolved Issue*).
14. No recommendation to preoperatively apply mupirocin to nares to prevent SSI (*Unresolved Issue*).
15. No recommendation to provide measures that enhance wound space oxygenation to prevent SSI (*Unresolved Issue*).

Hand/forearm antisepsis for surgical team members

1. Keep nails short and do not wear artificial nails (*Category IB*).
2. Perform a preoperative surgical scrub for at least 2 to 5 minutes using an appropriate antiseptic. Scrub the hands and forearms up to the elbows (*Category IB*).
3. After performing the surgical scrub, keep hands up and away from the body (elbows in flexed position) so that water runs from the tips of the fingers toward the elbows. Dry hands with a sterile towel and don a sterile gown and gloves (*Category IB*).
4. Clean underneath each fingernail prior to performing the first surgical scrub of the day (*Category II*).
5. Do not wear hand or arm jewelry (*Category II*).
6. No recommendation on wearing nail polish (*Unresolved Issue*).

Management of infected or colonized surgical personnel

1. Educate and encourage surgical personnel who have signs and symptoms of a transmissible infectious illness to report conditions promptly to their supervisory and occupational health service personnel (*Category IB*).
2. Develop well-defined policies concerning patient care responsibilities when

personnel have potentially transmissible infectious conditions. These policies should govern (a) personnel responsibility in using the health service and reporting illness, (b) work restrictions, and (c) clearance to resume work after an illness that required work restriction. The policies also should identify persons who have the authority to remove personnel from duty (*Category IB*).

3. Obtain appropriate cultures from, and exclude from duty, surgical personnel who have draining skin lesions until infection has been ruled out or personnel have received adequate therapy and infection has resolved (*Category IB*).
4. Do not routinely exclude surgical personnel who are colonized with organisms such as *S. aureus* (nose, hands, or other body site) or group A *Streptococcus,* unless such personnel have been linked epidemiologically to dissemination of the organism in the healthcare setting (*Category IB*).

Antimicrobial prophylaxis

1. Administer a prophylactic antimicrobial agent only when indicated, and select it based on its efficacy against the most common pathogens causing SSI for a specific operation and published recommendations (*Category IA*).
2. Administer by the intravenous route, the initial dose of prophylactic antimicrobial agent, timed such that a bactericidal concentration of the drug is established in serum and tissues when the incision is made. Maintain therapeutic levels of the agent in serum and tissues throughout the operation and until, at most, a few hours after the incision is closed in the operating room (*Category IA*).
3. Before elective colorectal operations in addition to above, mechanically prepare the colon by use of enemas and cathartic agents. Administer nonabsorbable oral antimicrobial agents in divided doses on the day before the operation (*Category IA*).
4. For high-risk cesarean section, administer the prophylactic antimicrobial agent immediately after the umbilical cord is clamped (*Category IA*).
5. Do not routinely use vancomycin for antimicrobial prophylaxis (*Category IB*).

Intraoperative

Ventilation

1. Maintain positive-pressure ventilation in the operating room with respect to the corridors and adjacent areas (*Category IB*).
2. Maintain a minimum of 15 air changes per hour, of which at least 3 should be fresh air (*Category IB*).
3. Filter all air, recirculated and fresh, through the appropriate filters (*Category IB*).
4. Introduce all air at the ceiling, and exhaust near the floor (*Category IB*).
5. Do not use UV radiation in the operating room to prevent SSI (*Category IB*).
6. Keep operating room doors closed except as needed for passage of equipment, personnel, and the patient (*Category IB*).
7. Consider performing orthopedic implant operations in operating rooms supplied with ultraclean air (*Category II*).
8. Limit the number of personnel entering the operating room to necessary personnel (*Category II*).

Cleaning and disinfection of environmental surfaces

1. When visible soiling or contamination with blood or other body fluids of surfaces or equipment occurs during an operation, use an EPA-approved hospital disinfectant to clean the affected areas before the next operation (*Category IB**).
2. Do not perform special cleaning or closing of operating rooms after contaminated or dirty operations (*Category IB*).
3. Do not use tacky mats at the entrance to the operating room suite or individual

operating rooms for infection control (*Category IB*).

4. Wet vacuum the operating room floor after the last operation of the day or night with an EPA-approved hospital disinfectant (*Category II*).
5. No recommendation on disinfecting environmental surfaces or equipment used in operating rooms between operations in the absence of visible soiling (*Unresolved Issue* 1).

Microbiologic sampling: Do not perform routine environmental sampling of the operating room. Perform microbiologic sampling of operating room environmental surfaces or air only as part of an epidemiologic investigation (*Category IB*).

Sterilization of surgical instruments

1. Sterilize all surgical instruments according to published guidelines (*Category IB*).
2. Perform flash sterilization only for patient care items that will be used immediately (e.g. to reprocess an inadvertently dropped instrument). Do not use flash sterilization for reasons of convenience, as an alternative to purchasing additional instrument sets, or to save time (*Category IB*).

Surgical attire and drapes

1. Wear a surgical mask that fully covers the mouth and nose when entering the operating room if an operation is about to begin or already under way, or if sterile instruments are exposed. Wear the mask throughout the operation (*Category IB**).
2. Wear a cap or hood to fully cover hair on the head and face when entering the operating room (*Category IB**).
3. Do not wear shoe covers for the prevention of SSI (*Category IB**).
4. Wear sterile gloves if one is a scrubbed surgical team member. Put on gloves after donning a sterile gown (*Category IB**).
5. Use surgical gowns and drapes that are effective barriers when wet (i.e. materials that resist liquid penetration) (*Category IB*).
6. Change scrub suits that are visibly soiled, contaminated, and/or penetrated by blood or other potentially infectious materials (*Category IB**).
7. No recommendations on how or where to launder scrub suits, on restricting use of scrub suits to the operating suite, or for covering scrub suits when out of the operating suite (*Unresolved Issue*).

Asepsis and surgical technique

1. Adhere to principles of asepsis when placing intravascular devices (e.g. central venous catheters), spinal or epidural anesthesia catheters, or when dispensing and administering intravenous drugs (*Category IA*).
2. Assemble sterile equipment and solutions immediately prior to use (*Category II*).
3. Handle tissue gently, maintain effective hemostasis , minimize devitalized tissue and foreign bodies (i.e. sutures, charred tissues, necrotic debris), and eradicate dead space at the surgical site (*Category IB*).
4. Use delayed primary skin closure or leave an incision open to heal by second intention if the surgeon considers the surgical site to be heavily contaminated (e.g. Class III and Class IV) (*Category IB*).
5. If drainage is necessary, use a closed suction drain. Place a drain through a separate incision distant from the operative incision. Remove the drain as soon as possible (*Category IB*).

Postoperative Incision Care

a. Protect with a sterile dressing for 24 to 48 hours postoperatively an incision that has been closed primarily (*Category IB*).
b. Wash hands before and after dressing changes and any contact with the surgical site (*Category IB*).
c. When an incision dressing must be changed, use sterile technique (*Category II*).
d. Educate the patient and family regarding proper incision care, symptoms of SSI,

and the need to report such symptoms (*Category II*).

e. No recommendation to cover an incision closed primarily beyond 48 hours, nor on the appropriate time to shower or bathe with an uncovered incision (*Unresolved Issue*).

Surveillance

a. Use CDC definitions of SSI without modification for identifying SSI among surgical inpatients and outpatients (*Category IB*).
b. For inpatient case-finding (including readmissions), use direct prospective observation, indirect prospective detection, or a combination of both direct and indirect methods for the duration of the patient's hospitalization (*Category IB*).
c. When post-discharge surveillance is performed for detecting SSI following certain operations (e.g. coronary artery bypass graft), use a method that accommodates available resources and data needs (*Category II*).
d. For outpatient case-finding, use a method that accommodates available resources and data needs (*Category IB*).
e. Assign the surgical wound classification upon completion of an operation. A surgical team member should make the assignment (*Category II*).
f. For each patient undergoing an operation chosen for surveillance, record those variables shown to be associated with increased SSI risk (e.g. surgical wound class, ASA (American Society of Anesthesiologists) class, and duration of operation) (*Category IB*).
g. Periodically calculate operation-specific SSI rates stratified by variables shown to be associated with increased SSI risk (e.g. NNIS risk index) (*Category IB*).
h. Report appropriately stratified, operation-specific SSI rates to surgical team members. The optimum frequency and format for such rate computations will be determined by stratified case-load sizes (denominators) and the objectives of local, continuous quality improvement initiatives (*Category IB*).
i. No recommendation to make available to the infection control committee coded surgeon-specific data (*Unresolved issue*).

SUMMARY OF SSI PREVENTION (INCLUDING SSI BUNDLE)[27,28]

Definition

Surgical site infection (SSI) can be defined as "Infection on the surgical site that occurs within 30 days of the surgical procedure or within one year if there is an implant or foreign body, such as prosthetic heart valve or joint prosthesis."[1]

Signs and Symptoms

- The common clinical features of surgical wound infection are localized pain, redness and discharge.
- Fever that occurs within 4 weeks of surgery, without other localizing features, is likely to be caused by infection at the surgical site.
- Deeper or organ-space infection may require imaging for diagnosis, surgical drainage and antimicrobial therapy guided by culture of the purulent material.

Classification of Surgical Site Infections

Surgical site infections (SSIs) have been classified into three types:

1. Superficial incisional SSI
   - Those involving only skin and subcutaneous lesions
2. Deep incisional SSI.
   - These involving deeper soft tissues of the incision
3. Organ or space SSI
   - Those involving any part of the anatomy.

- Organ/space SSIs involve any part of the anatomy (e.g. organ or space) other than incised body layers that was opened or manipulated during an operation.
- Organ/space SSIs have been classified according to specific site, e.g. in a patient who had an appendicectomy, and subsequently developed an intra-abdominal abscess, not draining through the incision the infection would be reported as an organ/ space SSI at the intra-abdominal site.

Prevention of Surgical Site Infections[27,28]

There are two types of strategies:

1. Core strategies:
   - High levels of scientific evidence demonstrated
   - Demonstrated feasibility.
2. Supplemental strategies:
   - Some scientific evidence
   - Variable levels of feasibility.

Prevention Strategies

Core Strategies

Preoperative measures

1. Administer antimicrobial prophylaxis in accordance with evidence-based standards and guidelines
   - Administer within 1 hour prior to incision
     - 2 hours for vancomycin and fluoroquinolones
   - Select appropriate agents on basis of:
     - Surgical procedure
     - Most common SSI pathogens for the procedure
     - Published recommendations.
2. Remote infections-whenever possible:
   - Identify and treat before elective operation
   - Postpone operation until infection has resolved.
3. Do not remove hair at the operative site unless it will interfere with the operation; do not use razors:
   - If necessary, remove by clipping or by use of a depilatory agent.
4. Skin preparatons:
   - Use appropriate antiseptic agent and technique for skin preparation
5. Maintain immediate postoperative normothermia.
6. Colorectal surgery patients:
   - Mechanically prepare the colon (Enemas, cathartic agents)
   - Administer non-absorbable oral antimicrobial agents in divided doses on the day before the operation.

Core Intraoperative Measures

1. Operating room (or) traffic
   - Keep OR doors closed during surgery except as needed for passage of equipment, personnel, and the patient.

Core Postoperative Measures

1. Surgical wound dressing
   - Protect primary closure incisions with sterile dressing for 24–48 hours postoperatively.
2. Control blood glucose level during the immediate postoperative period (cardiac)
   - Measure blood glucose level at 6 AM on POD#1 and #2 with procedure day = POD#0 (POD = postoperative day).
   - Maintain postoperative blood glucose level at <200 mg/dL.
3. Discontinue antibiotics within 24 hours after surgery end time (48 hours for cardiac).

Supplemental Strategies

Supplemental Preoperative Measures

- Nasal screen and decolonize only *Staphylococcus aureus* carriers undergoing elective cardiac and other procedures

(i.e. orthopedic, neurosurgery procedures with implants) with preoperative mupirocin therapy.
- Screen preoperative blood glucose levels and maintain tight glucose control POD#1 and POD#2 in patients undergoing select elective procedures (e.g. arthroplasties, spinal fusions).

Supplemental Perioperative Measures

- Redose antibiotic at the 3 hours interval in procedures with duration >3 hours or major blood loss.
- Adjust antimicrobial prophylaxis dose for obese patients (body mass index >30).
- Use at least 50% fraction of inspired oxygen intraoperatively and immediately postoperatively in select procedure(s).

Supplemental Postoperative Measures

- Do not tamper or remove the wound dressing for 48 hours postoperative unless clinically indicated
- Use aseptic technique for wound inspection and/or wound dressing changes
- Hand hygiene is mandatory before and after every time the wound is inspected or dressing changed.
- Feedback of surgeon specific infection rates.

REFERENCES

1a. Leper DJ, Van Goor H, Reilly J, Petrosillo N, Geiss HK, Torres AJ, et al. Surgical site infection—a European perspective of incidence and economic burden. Int Wound J. 2004;1(4):247-73.

1b. Hospital-acquired infection. From Wikipedia. Available at www.en.wikipedia.org/wiki/hospital-acquired-infection. Accessed on 9th July 2016.

1c. In surgical site infection (SSI) event—Centers for disease Control. Available at www.cdc.gov/nhsn/pdfs/pscmanual/9pscssicurrent.pdf. Jan 2016 (9-29).

1d. Tan JT, Coleman K, Norris S, Mapari J, Shastri S, Metz L. Health Technology Analysts Pty Ltd, Sydney, Australia,J ohnson and Johnson Asia-Pacific. Surgical site infection in India: A systematic review of the incidence and economic burden. Available at wwwaspjj.com/us/sites/www.aspjj.com.us/files/pdf/surgical-site-infection-in-india-pdf.

1e. WHO Guidelines for prevention and control of hospital-associated infections. Regional office for South-East Asia. WHO; 2002.

2. Speiman DW. Hospital-acquired infections. The Medical Journal of Australia. 2002;176(6):286-91. Available at the Med J Aust 2002 ISSH 0025-729X. www.mja.com.au. Accessed in Feb. 2004.

3. Mangram AJ, Horan TC, Pearson ML, Silver LC, Jarvis WR. Guideline for Prevention of Surgical Site Infection, 1999. The Hospital Infection Control Practices Advisory Committee. Accessed from www.md.ucl.ac.be/didac/hosp/ssi.pdf on 20/2 2015.

4. Cruse PJE, Ford R. A five-year prospective study of 23649 surgical wounds. Arch Surg. 1973;107:206.

5. Horan TC, Gaynes RP, Martone WJ, Jarvis WR, Emori TG. CDC definitions of nosocomial surgical site infections,1992: a modification of CDC definitions of surgical wound infections. Infect Control Hosp Epidemiol. 1992;13(10):606-8. Quoted in Ref No. 3.

6. Gaynes RP, Horan TC. Surveillance of nosocomial infections. In: Mayhall CG (Ed). Hospital Epidemiology and Infection Control. Baltimore: Williams & Wilkins; 1996.p.1017-31. Quoted in Ref No. 3.

7. Aggarwal DS. Microbiology Department, University College of Medical Sciences, a GTB University College of Medical Sciences. GTB, Delhi. Guidelines for Nosocomial Infection Surveillance and Control, WHO. South East Asia Regional Office, New Delhi, 21-5.

8. Garner JS. CDC guideline for prevention of surgical wound infections,1985. Supercedes guideline for prevention of surgical wound infections published in 1982. (Originally published in 1995). Revised Infect Control. 1986;7(3):193-200. Quoted in Ref No. 3.

9. Simmons BP. Guideline for prevention of surgical wound infections. Infect Control. 1982;3:185-96. Quaoted in Ref No. 3.

10. Larson E. Guideline for use of topical antimicrobial agents. Am J Infect Control. 1988;16:253-66. Quoted in Ref No. 3.
11. Consensus Guidelines for the Prevention of Infections in Operating Room-Hospital Infection Society, Mumbai Forum.
12. Mehta G. Microbiological surveillance of operation theatres. In: Issue special. Data available at http://www.orthoteers.co.uk/nrujp/ij331/orththeatresterile2.htm. Accessed on 26th June, 2004.
13. Teachers handbook hss404 - nq2014 operation theatre PSS Central Institute of Vocation Education, Shyamla Hills, Bhopal. Accessed from www.cive.org/nsqf/Healthcare/hc_IvI4/HSS-404-Thbk-GDA%2007.10.2014-pdf. On July 17th 2015.
14. Sapna, Majumdar S, Venkatesh P. The operation theatre: Basic architecture (Dr Rajendra Prasad Centre for Ophthalmic Sciences, AIIMS, New Delhi). Delhi Journal of Ophthalmology. 2011;21:3. Accessed from www.dja.org.in/pdfs/jan--march-2011.pdf on July 17 2015.
15. WHO Guidelines for Prevention and Control of Hospital-associated Infections—Regional Office for South East Asia, WHO; 2002.
16. Ducel G, Fabry J, Nicolle L. Prevention of Hospital-associated Infections—A Practical Guide. 2nd edition. WHO; 2002.
17. Lidwell OM, Elson RA, Lowbury EJ, Whyte W, Blowers R, Stanley SJ, et al. Ultraclean air and antibiotics for prevention of postoperative infection. A multicenter study of 8,052 joint replacement operations. Acta Orthop Scand. 1987:58:4-13. Quoted in Ref No. 3.
18. B'erard F, Gandon J. Postoperative wound infections; the influence of ultraviolet irradiation of the operating room and of various other factors. Ann Surg. 1964;160(suppl 1):1-192. Quoted in Ref No. 3.
19. Taylor GJ, Bannister GC, Leeming JP. Wound disinfection with ultraviolet radiation. J Hosp Infect. 1995;30(2):85-93. Quoted in Ref No. 3.
20. Kurz A, Sessler DI, Lenhardt R. Perioperative normothermia to reduce the incidence of surgical wound infection and shorten hospitalization. Study of Wound Infection and Temperature Group. New Engl J Med. 1996;334(19):1209-15.
21. Dani S, Kagal A, Kelkar R. Recommendations and guidelines for control of hospital-acquired infections in operation theatres. Vol 1. State level infection control committee. Government of Maharashtra.
22. Antimicrobial prophylaxis for surgery. Treatment Guidelines from the Medical Letter. 2012;10(122). Accessed from www.medicalletter.org. on 27th July 2015.
23. Rao TV. Operation Theatre Surveillance: Air sampling or Conventional Methods. Accessed on 26/8/2016. from www.sldeshare.net/doctorrao/operation-theatre-surveillance-air-sampling-or-conventional-methods.
24. Pasquarella C, Pitzurra O, Savino A. The index of microbial air contamination. J Hosp Inf. 2016;46(40):241-56. Accessed from www.ncbi.nim.nih.gov>pubmed on 29th August 2016.
25. Sabharwal ER, Sharma R. Estimation of microbial air contamination by settle plate method: are we within acceptable limit? Accessed from www.saspublisher.com. On 29th August 2016.
26. Charnley J, Eftekhar M. Postoperative infection in total prosthetic arthroplasty of the hip-joint with special reference to the bacterial content of air in the operating room. Br J Surg. 1969;56:641-64. Available at www.online library.wiley.com>doi >pdf on 39th August 2016.
27. Napoli C, Marcotrigiano V, Montagna MT. Research Article. Air sampling procedures to evaluate microbial contamination: a comparison between active and passive methods in operating theatres. Available at www.biomedcentral.com/1471-2458/12/594 on 30 th August 2016.
28. Fisher G, Fodre S, Nehez M. Versuche zur Festellung von Gesamtkeimzahl-Grenzwerten in der Raumluft von Gesundheitseinrichtungen. Z Ges Hyg. 1971:17:576-9. Quoted in Ref No. 25.
29. EAL-G18. Accreditation for Laboratories Performing Microbiological Testing Guidance on Interpretation of the EN 45 000 Series of Standards and ISO/IEC. Guide 25. EAL European Cooperation for Accreditation of Laboratories. EAL/EURACHEM Working Group 1995. Quoted in Ref No. 24 (CR 72).
30. Deep care Pest Control services, Mumbai. Ot Fumigation. Available at http://deepcareservices.com/o-t-fumigation-control-services.html.
31. Collee JG, Duguid JP, Fraser AG, Marmion BP. Mackie and McCartney Practical Medical Microbiology. 13th edition, Vol 2. Churchhill Livingstone; 1989.p.228.

32. Rao TV. Operation theatre sterilization by fumigation. Accessed from www.themicrobiologyblog.com.2009/08.
33. Chakraborty P. A Textbook of Microbiology. Second edition. New Central Book Agency; 2003.
34. Collee JG, Duguid JP, Fraser AG, Marmion BP. Mackie and McCartney Practical Medical Microbiology. 13th edition, Vol 2. Churchhill Livingstone; 1989.p.87.
35. Bowie Dick Test. Technical Bulettin. Accessed from www.steritecproducts.com/-assets/TB%20Bowie-Dick%20Testing.pdf.
36. Collee JG, Duguid JP, Fraser AG, Marmion BP. Mackie and McCartney Practical Medical Microbiology. 13th edition.Vol 2. Churchhill Livingstone; 1989.p.78.

Chapter 11

Urinary Tract Infections (Catheter-associated Urinary Tract Infections)

Chapter Outline

- Definitions
- Criteria for CAUTI
- Specific Problems
- Pathogens Associated with UTI
- Diagnosis of UTI
- Epidemiology of UTI
- Mechanism of Infection
- Control Measures
- Recommendations
- Practical Approach to Prevention of Urinary Tract Infection
- Summary of CAUTI Prevention (Including CAUTI Bundle)

INTRODUCTION

Urinary tract infections remain the most common hospital-associated infection despite the increasing awareness of the dangers of urethral catheterization. It is estimated that as many as 2% of hospital admissions acquire nosocomial urinary tract infections. These represent more than 30–40% of all reported hospital-acquired infections.[1,2] The patient who develops a nosocomial urinary tract infection is at a significant risk for developing bacteremia due to gram-negative bacilli or sepsis and are even at risk of death. Although only 5% of catheter-associated infections (UTIs) result in bacteremia, 15% of nosocomial bacteremias are attributable to nosocomial UTIs.

This high incidence of urinary tract infections is directly related to instrumentation of the genitourinary tract, and the use of urethral catheter. It was found that 66–86% of patients had undergone genitourinary instrumentation or catheterization.[2]

Virtually all healthcare-associated UTIs are caused by instrumentation of the urinary tract. Catheter-associated urinary tract infection (CAUTI) has been associated with increased morbidity, mortality, hospital cost, and length of stay.[3] In addition, bacteriuria commonly leads to unnecessary antimicrobial use, and urinary drainage systems are often reservoirs for multidrug-resistant bacteria and a source of transmission to other patients.[3]

Decrease in the incidence of nosocomial urinary tract infections depends on better understanding of the specific indications for urethral catheterization and a continued attempt to maintain and prolong a sterile catheter environment.

DEFINITIONS

An indwelling urinary catheter is a drainage tube that is inserted into the urinary bladder through the urethra, is left in place, and is connected to a closed collection system. Alternative methods of urinary drainage may be employed in some patients.

Intermittent ("in-and-out") catheterization involves brief insertion of a catheter into the bladder through the urethra to drain urine at intervals.

An external catheter is a urine containment device that fits over or adheres to the genitalia and is attached to a urinary drainage bag. The most commonly used external catheter is a soft flexible sheath that fits over the penis ("condom" catheter).

A suprapubic catheter is surgically inserted into the bladder through an incision above the pubis.

Although UTIs associated with alternative urinary drainage systems are considered device-associated, CAUTI rates reported to the National Healthcare Safety Network (NHSN) only refer to those associated with indwelling urinary catheters.

NHSN has recently revised the UTI surveillance definition criteria. Among the changes are removal of the asymptomatic bacteriuria (ASB) criterion and refinement of the criteria for defining symptomatic UTI (SUTI). However, asymptomatic bacteremic UTI (ABUTI) has been included in the surveillance. The time period for follow-up surveillance after catheter removal also has been shortened from 7 days to 48 hours to align with other device-associated infections. The new UTI criteria, which took effect in January 2009, can be found in the NHSN Patient Safety Manual (http://www.cdc.gov/nhsn/library.html).

The clinical significance of ASB (asymptomatic bacteriuria) in catheterized patients is undefined. Approximately, 75–90% of patients with ASB do not develop a systemic inflammatory response or other signs or symptoms to suggest infection. Monitoring and treatment of ASB is also not an effective prevention measure for SUTI (symptomatic urinary tract infection), as most cases of SUTI are not preceded by bacteriuria for more than a day. Treatment of ASB has not been shown to be clinically beneficial and is associated with the selection of antimicrobial-resistant organisms.

CRITERIA FOR CAUTI[3a,3b,3c]

There are two criteria that can be applied for identifying a CAUTI:

- Symptomatic UTI (SUTI)
- Asymptomatic bacteremic UTI (ABUTI).

Criteria for Symptomatic CAUTI (SCAUTI)

1. A UTI where an indwelling catheter was in place for >2 calendar days on the date of event*, with day of device placement being Day 1.

   and

   An indwelling urinary catheter was in place on the date of event or the day before. If an indwelling urinary catheter was in place for >2 calendar days and then removed, the date of event for the UTI must be the day of discontinuation or the next day for the UTI to be catheter associated.

*Date of event (DOE): For UTI, the date of event is the date the signs or symptoms appeared or the date the diagnosing urine specimen was collected, whichever comes first.

2. Accompanied by the relevant **signs and symptoms** and laboratory findings.

   Signs and symptoms:
   - At least 1 of the following signs or symptoms: **Fever (>38°C); suprapubic tenderness; costovertebral angle pain or tenderness** (if catheter is in place)
   and
   - At least 1 of the following signs or symptoms: **Fever (>38°C); urgency frequency; dysuria; suprapubic tenderness; costovertebral angle pain or tenderness** (if catheter is removed)

   If patient ≤1 year of age and at least one of the following signs and symptoms with no other recognized cause: **Fever (>38°C), hypothermia (<36°C), apnea, bradycardia, dysuria, lethargy or vomiting.** And an indwelling urethral urinary catheter in place within the 48-hour period before the onset of UTI or had the catheter removed 48 hours prior to specimen collection.
3. Accompanied by the **relevant laboratory findings.**

   Laboratory findings:
   - A positive urine culture with no more than 2 species of microorganisms identified, at least one of which is a bacterium of ≥ 10^5 CFU/mL
   or
   - At least 1 of the following findings (urine analysis):
     a. Positive dipstick for leukocyte esterase and/or nitrite.
     b. Pyuria [urine specimen with ≥10 white blood cells (WBC)/mm^3 of unspun urine or >5 WBC/high power field of spun urine].
     c. Microorganisms seen on Gram's stain of unspun urine.
   and
   - A positive urine culture of ≥10^3 and <10^5 CFU/mL with no more than 2 species of microorganisms.

Asymptomatic Bacteremic CAUTI (ABCAUTI)

1. Patient with an indwelling urinary catheter.
2. Has no signs or symptoms (i.e. for any age patient, no fever (>38°C), urgency, frequency, dysuria, suprapubic tenderness, or costovertebral angle pain or tenderness, OR for a patient ≤1 year of age, no fever (>38°C core), hypothermia (<36°C) core, apnea, bradycardia, dysuria, lethargy or vomiting)
   and
3. A positive urine culture with no more than 2 species of organisms identified, at least one of which is a bacterium ≥10^5 CFU/mL.
   and
   A positive blood culture with at least 1 matching uropathogen microorganism to the urine culture, or at least 2 matching blood cultures drawn on separate occasions if the matching pathogen is a skin contaminant (Antibiograms of the isolates do not have to match).

All ABUTIs will have a secondary bloodstream infection—secondary BSI.

SPECIFIC PROBLEMS

Predisposing Factors

Procedures and Manipulations

Urinary tract infections result from introduction of bacteria into the bladder, usually accompanied by some factor, which alters the normal protective mechanisms in the host. With simple urethral catheterization, bacteriuria results from introduction of organisms from the distal urethra into the bladder. In healthy outpatients, the risk of catheter-induced infection is only 1-2%.[4,5]

In the hospital setting however, and especially in patients who often have underlying abnormalities of the urinary tract, the risk is much higher. Severely ill patients and obstetrical and gynecologic patients, and patient over 50 years of age have up to a 20% risk of bacteriuria after a single catheterization.[6,7] Cystoscopy and surgical manipulations carries a similar high risk of infection. The incidence of infection ranges from 2–10% with the highest rate of infection occurring in patients who require retrograde pyelograms.

Indwelling Urethral Catheters

The indwelling Foley's catheter presents the greatest risk of all urinary manipulations for the development of urinary tract infection. With the open drainage system (i.e. no attempts to keep the catheter, tubing and bag connected and sterile) virtually all patients are bacteriuric within 4 days of introduction of the catheter. With the development of the closed system of urinary drainage (i.e. strict maintenance of a connected and sterile catheter, tubing and bag) the incidence of acquired bacteriuria has markedly diminished. Using this system, up to 50% of patients with an indwelling Foley's catheter have sterile urines even after 2 weeks of catheterization. Most patients who require short-term Foley's catheterization will never develop bacteriuria.

Method and Duration of Catheterization[2]

The risk of acquiring a urinary tract infection depends on the method and duration of catheterization, the quality of catheter care, and host susceptibility. Reported infection rates vary widely, ranging from 1–5% after a single brief catheterization to virtually 100% for patients with indwelling catheters draining into an open system for longer than 4 days. Adoption of the closed method of urinary drainage has markedly reduced the risk of acquiring a catheter-associated infection, but the risk is still substantial. Host factors, which appear to increase the risk of acquiring catheter-associated urinary tract infections include advanced age, debilitation and the postpartum state.

Catheter-associated urinary tract infections are generally assumed to be benign. Such infection in otherwise healthy patients is often asymptomatic and is likely to resolve spontaneously with the removal of the catheter. Occasionally infection persists and leads to such complications as prostatitis, epididymitis, cystitis, pyelonephritis, and gram-negative bacteremia, particularly in high-risk patients.

There is a greater risk for nosocomial urinary tract infection with increased duration of catheterization. The prevalence of asymptomatic bacteriuria is 15% in patients catheterized less than 30 days and 90% for patient catheterized more than 30 days.[8]

Risk Factors Associated with Nosocomial UTI

Risk factors associated with nosocomial UTIs are of two types:[9]

1. Those that are not alterable
2. Those that are alterable.

Those that are Not Alterable

a. Female gender
b. Postpartum status
c. Old age
d. Severe underlying illness
e. High blood creatinine levels.

Factors that are Alterable

a. The wrong reason for catheterization
b. Contamination during insertion
c. Errors in catheter care
d. Use of antibiotics.

PATHOGENS ASSOCIATED WITH UTI

The source of microorganisms causing CAUTI can be endogenous, typically via meatal, rectal, or vaginal colonization, or exogenous, such as via contaminated hands of healthcare personnel or equipment. Microbial pathogens can enter the urinary tract either by the extraluminal route, via migration along the outside of the catheter in the periurethral mucous sheath, or by the intraluminal route, via movement along the internal lumen of the catheter from a contaminated collection bag or catheter-drainage tube junction. The relative contribution of each route in the pathogenesis of CAUTI is not well known. The marked reduction in risk of bacteriuria with the introduction of the sterile, closed urinary drainage system in the1960's[3] suggests the importance of the intraluminal route. However, even with the closed drainage system, bacteriuria inevitably occurs over time either via breaks in the sterile system or via the extraluminal route.[3] The daily risk of bacteriuria with catheterization is 3–10%,[3] approaching 100% after 30 days, which is considered the delineation between short and long-term catheterization. Formation of biofilms by urinary pathogens on the surface of the catheter and drainage system occurs universally with prolonged duration of catheterization.[3] Over time, the urinary catheter becomes colonized with microorganisms living in a sessile state within the biofilm, rendering them resistant to antimicrobials and host defenses and virtually impossible to eradicate without removing the catheter. The role of bacteria within biofilms in the pathogenesis of CAUTI is unknown and is an area requiring further research.

The most frequent pathogens-associated with CAUTI (combining both ASB and SUTI) in hospitals reporting to NHSN between 2006–2007 were *Escherichia coli* (21.4%) and *Candida* species (21.0%), followed by *Enterococcus* species (14.9%), *Pseudomonas aeruginosa* (10.0%), *Klebsiella pneumoniae* (7.7%), and *Enterobacter* species (4.1%). A smaller proportion was caused by other gram-negative bacteria and *Staphylococcus* species.[6]

Antimicrobial resistance among urinary pathogens is an ever increasing problem. About a quarter of *E. coli* isolates and one-third of *P. aeruginosa* isolates from CAUTI cases were fluoroquinolone-resistant. Resistance of gram-negative pathogens to other agents, including third-generation cephalosporins and carbapenems, was also substantial.[6] The proportion of organisms that were multidrug-resistant, defined by non-susceptibility to all agents in 4 classes, was 4% of *P. aeruginosa*, 9% of *K. pneumoniae*, and 21% of *Acinetobacter baumannii*.[3]

Nonetheless, most complications of urinary catheterization remain a direct result of the patient's own bacteria which colonize the external and internal surfaces of the indwelling catheter.[10]

DIAGNOSIS OF UTI

Clinical

- Most episodes of short-term catheter-associated bacteriuria are asymptomatic, however, some patients present with symptoms of fever, dysuria, urgency and pain
- In addition to experiencing the same symptoms as short-term catheterized patients, long-term-catheterized patients may experience obstruction, urinary tract stones, local periurinary infections, chronic renal inflammation, renal failure and bladder cancer
- In upper UTIs (Pyelonephritis), flank pain, fever, blood in the urine (hematuria) and other physical findings may be present. In frail elderly patients, however, typical signs and symptoms of UTI may be absent.

Laboratory

- The CDC[11] and NNIS define UTI as $>10^5$ colony-forming units (CFU) with one or 2 organisms
- The Maki[12] definition of UTI is $>10^3$ CFU with 1 or 2 organisms.

EPIDEMIOLOGY OF UTI[2]

Most of the bacterial organisms responsible for urinary tract infections, including *E. coli,*

Enterococcus, Kelbsiella and Enterobacter species and *Proteus mirabilis* are part of normal colonic flora. With alterations in the normal barriers to infection, including the presence of a foreign body such as the urethral catheter, these strains may colonize and infect the urinary tract.

A number of other potential urinary pathogens are not part of the normal colonic flora, however, and are acquired by the patients from the hospital and environmental sources or other colonized patients. Strains of multiple-drug resistant *Klebsiella* are almost exclusively hospital-associated organisms, which may colonize the gastrointestinal tract after admission to the hospital. Patients carrying *Klebsiella* in the gastrointestinal tract may then become important reservoirs of subsequent nosocomial urinary tract infections. *Acinetobacter* species and *Pseudomonas aeruginosa* are frequently isolated from hospital environment sources. *Pseudomonas cepacia* has also been responsible for catheter-associated UTI—its acquisition is from an exogenous source.

With the use of closed sterile systems the hands of hospital personnel have become an increasingly important source of these infections. Maki et al. found that an endemic strain of *Serratia* was present on the hands of nursing personnel 50% of the time in random surveys and was not isolated from hospital equipment.[12]

Reported rates of UTI among patients with urinary catheters vary substantially. National data from NHSN acute care hospitals in 2006 showed a range of pooled mean CAUTI rates of 3.1–7.5 infections per 1000 catheter-days. Although morbidity and mortality from CAUTI is considered to be relatively low compared to other HAIs, the high prevalence of urinary catheter use leads to a large cumulative burden of infections with resulting infectious complications and deaths. While fewer than 5% of bacteriuric cases develop bacteremia,[7] CAUTI is the leading cause of secondary nosocomial bloodstream infections; about 17% of hospital-acquired bacteremias are from a urinary source, with an associated mortality of approximately 10%.[3] An estimated 17–69% of CAUTI may be preventable with recommended infection control measures,

MECHANISM OF INFECTION (FIGS 11.1 AND 11.2)[2]

Whether from exogenous or endogenous sources, infecting microorganisms gain access to the urinary tract by several routes.

The first mechanism involves the direct introduction of organisms into the bladder with the catheter. The distal one-third of the urethra and the perineum (and the meatus) are usually colonized by bacteria. With catheterization, a sufficient number of organisms can be introduced directly into the bladder and produce infection. Generally, however, low rates of infection have been reported after single brief catheterization suggesting that microorganisms introduced by this method are usually removed from healthy individuals by voiding or by antibacterial mechanisms of the bladder mucosa.

The second mechanism by which bacteria can reach the bladder is by migrating along the out side of the catheter in the periurethral mucous sheath. This may be an important mechanism of infection in patients with long-term indwelling catheters.

With an indwelling catheter the third method by which microorganisms reach the bladder is along the internal lumen of the catheter after the collection bag or catheter drainage tube junction has been contaminated. The importance of intraluminal introduction is suggested by the substantial reduction in infection that has been achieved through the use of closed urinary drainage system. However if closed sterile drainage can be maintained, extraluminal migration of microorganisms in the periurethral space becomes a relatively more important pathway of entry into the bladder.

Microorganisms reaching by migrating along the outside of catheter lumen are more common in women, because of their shorter

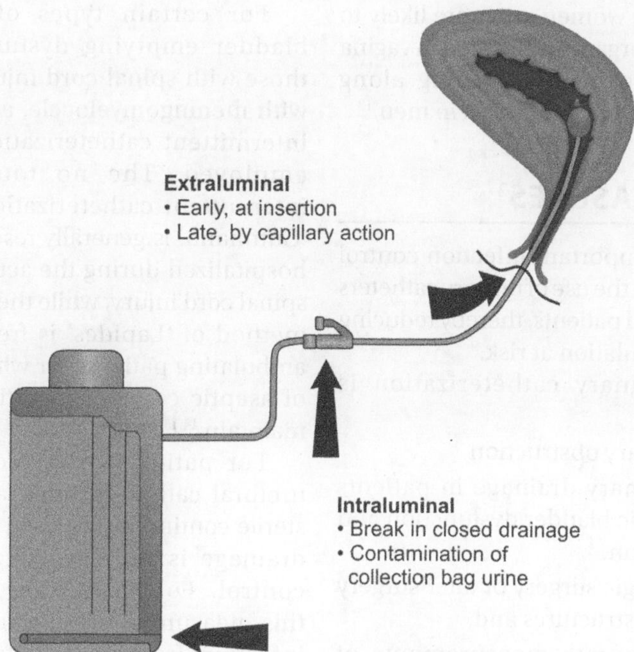

Fig. 11.1: Migration of urinary pathogens

Source of microorganisms may be endogenous (meatal, rectal, or vaginal colonization) or exogenous, usually via contaminated hands of healthcare personnel during catheter insertion or manipulation of the collecting system.

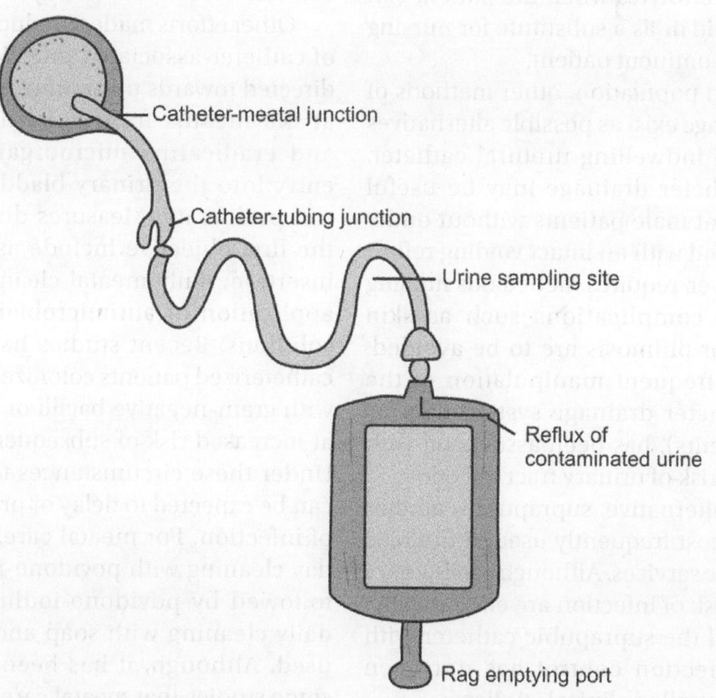

Fig. 11.2: Indwelling catheterization of urinary tract. Site of possible contamination

urethra. Therefore, women are more likely to develop UTI from organisms located in vagina whereas microorganisms reaching along internal lumen are more common in men.[13]

CONTROL MEASURES[2]

One of the most important infection control measures is to limit the use of urinary catheters to carefully selected patients, thereby reducing the size of the population at risk.

Generally urinary catheterization is indicated:

1. To relieve urinary obstruction
2. To permit urinary drainage in patients with neurogenic bladder dysfunction and urinary retention.
3. To aid in urologic surgery or after surgery on contiguous structures and
4. To obtain accurate measurements of urinary output in critically ill patients.

Specially, urinary catheterization should be discouraged as a means of obtaining urine for culture or certain diagnostic tests such as urinary electrolytes when the patient can voluntarily void or as a substitute for nursing care in the incontinent patient.

In selected population, other methods of urinary drainage exist as possible alternatives to the use of indwelling urethral catheter. Condom catheter drainage may be useful for incontinent male patients without outlet obstruction and with an intact voiding reflex. Its use, however, requires meticulous nursing care if local complications such as skin maceration or phimosis are to be avoided. In addition, frequent manipulation of the condom catheter drainage system (e.g. by agitated patients), has been associated with an increased risk of urinary tract infection.

Another alternative, suprapubic catheter drainage is most frequently used in urologic or gynecologic services. Although preliminary data on the risk of infection are encouraging, the benefit of the suprapubic catheter with regard to infection control has not been proven by controlled clinical studies.

For certain types of patients with bladder emptying dysfunction, such as those with spinal cord injuries, or children with meningomyelocele, a third alternative intermittent catheterization is commonly employed. The no touch method of intermittent catheterization advocated by 'Guttmann' is generally reserved for patients hospitalized during the acute phase of their spinal cord injury, while the clean non-sterile method of 'Lapides' is frequently used by ambulating patients for whom the practices of aseptic catheter insertion is difficult to maintain.[14,15]

For patients, who require indwelling urethral catheterization, adherence to the sterile continuously closed system of urinary drainage is the cornerstone of infection control. For short-term catheterization, this measure alone can reduce the rate of infection from an inevitable 100% when open drainage is employed to less than 25%. All other interventions can be viewed as additional measures since none have proven to be as effective in reducing the frequency of catheter-associated urinary tract infections.

Other efforts made to reduce the incidence of catheter-associated infections have been directed towards preventing microorganisms at the meatus from entering the bladder and eradicating microorganisms gaining entry into the urinary bladder before they can proliferate. Measures directed towards the first objective include aseptic catheter insertion, daily meatal cleansing and daily application of antimicrobial ointments or solutions. Recent studies have shown that catheterized patients colonized at the meatus with gram-negative bacilli or *enterococci* are at increased risk of subsequent infection.[16,17] Under these circumstances these measures can be expected to delay or prevent the onset of infection. For meatal care, either twice a day cleaning with povidone-iodine solution followed by povidone-iodine ointment or daily cleaning with soap and water can be used. Although, it has been mentioned in some studies that meatal care was ineffective in reducing the frequency of catheter-associated infections in patients on closed urinary drainage system, meatal care can definitely reduce the risk of infection.

Infection control measures for purposes of eradicating microorganisms in the urinary tract before they can proliferate and cause infection include irrigation of the bladder and the use of prophylactic systemic antibiotics. Though prophylactic systemic antibiotics delay the immergence of catheter-related infection,[18,19] but this protective effect is transient and is found to be associated with selection of antibiotic resistant microorganisms.

Sometimes, cross-infection is likely to be responsible for the spread of catheter-associated infection for which additional measures have been proposed. Catheterized patients with asymptomatic infection may serve as unrecognized reserviors of infecting organism. The mechanism of transmission is carriage of microorganisms in the hands of patient care personnel.[20,21] In these outbreaks, the implementation of control measures to prevent cross-infection, include renewing the emphasis on handwashing and spatial separation of catheterized patients, particularly infected from uninfected cases. Spatial separation of catheterized patients is effective in controlling catheter-associated infection only if there is an epidemic spread or frequent cross-infection.

Regular bacteriologic monitoring of catheterized patients has been advocated to ensure early diagnosis and treatment of urinary tract infection. Its possible value as an infection control measure lies in the potential usefulness in detecting and initiating treatment of clinically inapparent infection, which may serve as reservoirs of hospital pathogens, and thus reducing the likelihood of cross-infection.

RECOMMENDATIONS[3]

The new Healthcare Infection Contral Practices Advisory Committee (HICPAC) categorization scheme for recommendations is provided in Table 11.1.

Personnel

a. Only persons (e.g. hospital personnel, family members, or patients themselves) who know the correct technique of aseptic insertion and maintenance of catheter should handle catheters.
b. Hospital personnel and others who take care of catheter should be given periodic in-service training, stressing the correct techniques and potential complication of urinary catheterization.

Appropriate Catheter Use

Insert catheters only for appropriate indications (see Table 11.2 for guidance), and leave in place only as long as needed (*Category IB*). They should not be used solely for the convenience of patient care personnel.

Table 11.1: Modified HICPAC categorization scheme for recommendations

Category IA	A strong recommendation supported by high to moderate quality evidence suggesting net clinical benefits or harms
Category IB	A strong recommendation supported by low quality evidence suggesting net clinical benefits or harms or an accepted practice (e.g. aseptic technique) supported by low to very low quality evidence
Category IC	A strong recommendation required by state or federal regulation
Category II	A weak recommendation supported by any quality evidence suggesting a trade-off between clinical benefits and harms
No recommendation/ unresolved issue	Unresolved issue for which there is low to very low quality evidence with uncertain trade-offs between benefits and harms

Table 11.2: Uses of appropriate and inappropriate indications for indwelling catheters

A. Examples of appropriate indications for indwelling urethral catheter use[3]
- Patient has acute urinary retention or bladder outlet obstruction
- Need for measurements of urinary output in critically ill patients
- Perioperative use for perioperative use for selected surgical procedures: Patients undergoing urologic surgery or other surgery on contiguous structures of the genitourinary tract
  - Anticipated prolonged duration of surgery (catheters inserted for this reason should be removed in PACU)
  - Patients anticipated to receive large-volume infusions or diuretics during surgery
  - Need for intraoperative monitoring of urinary output
- To assist in healing of open sacral or perineal wounds in incontinent patients
- Patient requires prolonged immobilization (e.g. potentially unstable thoracic or lumbar spine, multiple traumatic injuries such as pelvic fractures)
- To improve comfort for end of life care if needed

B. Examples of *inappropriate* uses of indwelling catheters
- As a substitute for nursing care of the patient or resident with incontinence
- As a means of obtaining urine for culture or other diagnostic tests when the patient can voluntarily void
- For prolonged postoperative duration without appropriate indications (e.g. structural repair of urethra or contiguous structures, prolonged effect of epidural anesthesia, etc.)

Note: These indications are based primarily on expert consensus.

1. Minimize urinary catheter use and duration of use in all patients, particularly those at higher risk for CAUTI or mortality from catheterization such as women, the elderly, and patients with impaired immunity (*Category IB*).
2. Avoid use of urinary catheters in patients and nursing home residents for management of incontinence (*Category IB*).
   Further research is needed on periodic (e.g. night time) use of external catheters (e.g. condom catheters) in incontinent patients or residents and the use of catheters to prevent skin breakdown (*No Recommendation/Unresolved Issue*).
3. Use urinary catheters in operative patients only as necessary, rather than routinely.
4. For operative patients who have an indication for an indwelling catheter, remove the catheter as soon as possible postoperatively, preferably within 24 hours, unless there are appropriate indications for continued use.

Alternatives to Indwelling Catheter

For selected patients other methods of urinary drainage such as condom catheter drainage, suprapubic catheterization and intermittent urethral catheterization can be useful alternatives to indwelling catheters when appropriate.

Following are CDC Recommendations.

i. Consider using external catheters as an alternative to indwelling urethral catheters in cooperative male patients without urinary retention or bladder outlet obstruction (*Category II*).
ii. Consider alternatives to chronic indwelling catheters, such as intermittent catheterization, in spinal cord injury patients (*Category II*).
iii. Intermittent catheterization is preferable to indwelling urethral or suprapubic catheters in patients with bladder emptying dysfunction (*Category II*).
iv. Consider intermittent catheterization in children with myelomeningocele and neurogenic bladder to reduce the risk of urinary tract deterioration (*Category II*).
v. Further research is needed on the benefit of using a urethral stent as an alternative to an indwelling catheter in selected patients with bladder outlet obstruction (No *Recommendation/Unresolved Issue*).
vi. Further research is needed on the risks and benefits of suprapubic catheters as an alternative to indwelling urethral catheters in selected patients requiring

short- or long-term catheterization, particularly with respect to complications related to catheter insertion or the catheter site (*No Recommendation/ Unresolved Issue*).

Handwashing

Handwashing should be done immediately before and after any manipulation of the catheter site or apparatus.

Proper Techniques of Catheter Insertion

A. Perform hand hygiene immediately before and after insertion or any manipulation of the catheter device or site (*Category IB*).
B. In the acute care hospital setting, insert urinary catheters using aseptic technique and sterile equipment (*Category IB*).
   a. Catheters should be inserted using aseptic technique and sterile equipment (*Category IB*).
   b. Gloves, drapes, sponges, an appropriate antiseptic solution for periurethral cleaning and a single use packet of lubricant jelly should be used for insertion (*Category IB*).
   c. Routine use of antiseptic lubricants is not necessary (*Category II*).
   d. Further research is needed on the use of antiseptic solutions vs. sterile water or saline for periurethral cleaning prior to catheter insertion (*No Recommendation/Unresolved Issue*).
C. In the non-acute care setting, clean (i.e., non-sterile) technique for intermittent catheterization is an acceptable and more practical alternative to sterile technique for patients requiring chronic intermittent catheterization (*Category IA*).
D. Further research is needed on optimal cleaning and storage methods for catheters used for clean intermittent catheterization (*No Recommendation/Unresolved Issue*).
E. Properly secure indwelling catheters after insertion to prevent movement and urethral traction (*Category IB*).
F. Unless otherwise clinically indicated, consider using the smallest bore catheter possible, consistent with good drainage, to minimize bladder neck and urethral trauma (*Category II*).
G. If intermittent catheterization is used, perform it at regular intervals to prevent bladder overdistension (*Category IB*).
H. Consider using a portable ultrasound device to assess urine volume in patients undergoing intermittent catheterization to assess urine volume and reduce unnecessary catheter insertions (*Category II*).
   a. If ultrasound bladder scanners are used, ensure that indications for use are clearly stated, nursing staff are trained in their use, and equipment is adequately cleaned and disinfected in between patients (*Category IB*).

Proper Techniques for Urinary Catheter Maintenance

A. Following aseptic insertion of the urinary catheter, maintain a closed drainage system (*Category IB*):
   a. If breaks in aseptic technique, disconnection, or leakage occur, replace the catheter and collecting system using aseptic technique and sterile equipment (*Category IB*).
   b. Consider using urinary catheter systems with preconnected, sealed catheter-tubing junctions (*Category II*).
B. Maintain unobstructed urine flow (*Category IB*).
   a. Keep the catheter and collecting tube free from kinking (*Category IB*).
   b. Keep the collecting bag below the level of the bladder at all times. Do not rest the bag on the floor (*Category IB*).
   c. Empty the collecting bag regularly using a separate, clean collecting container for each patient; avoid splashing, and prevent contact of the drainage spigot with the nonsterile collecting container (*Category IB*).

C. Use standard precautions, including the use of gloves and gown as appropriate, during any manipulation of the catheter or collecting system (*Category IB*).
D. Complex urinary drainage systems (utilizing mechanisms for reducing bacterial entry such as antiseptic-release cartridges in the drain port) are not necessary for routine use (*Category II*).
E. Changing indwelling catheters or drainage bags at routine, fixed intervals is not recommended. Rather, it is suggested to change catheters and drainage bags based on clinical indications such as infection, obstruction, or when the closed system is compromised (*Category II*).
F. Unless clinical indications exist (e.g. in patients with bacteriuria upon catheter removal posturologic surgery), do not use systemic antimicrobials routinely to prevent CAUTI in patients requiring either short- or long-term catheterization (*Category IB*).
    a. Further research is needed on the use of urinary antiseptics (e.g. methenamine) to prevent UTI in patients requiring short-term catheterization (*No Recommendation/Unresolved Issue*).
G. Do not clean the periurethral area with antiseptics to prevent CAUTI while the catheter is in place. Routine hygiene (e.g. cleansing of the meatal surface during daily bathing or showering) is appropriate (*Category IB*).

Irrigation of Bladder

A. Unless obstruction is anticipated (e.g. as might occur with bleeding after prostatic or bladder surgery) bladder irrigation is not recommended (*Category II*).
    a. If obstruction is anticipated, closed continuous irrigation is suggested to prevent obstruction (*Category II*).
B. Routine irrigation of the bladder with antimicrobials is not recommended (*Category II*).
C. Routine instillation of antiseptic or antimicrobial solutions into urinary drainage bags is not recommended (*Category II*).
D. Clamping indwelling catheters prior to removal is not necessary (*Category II*).
E. Further research is needed on the use of bacterial interference (i.e. bladder inoculation with a nonpathogenic bacterial strain) to prevent UTI in patients requiring chronic urinary catheterization (*No Recommendation/Unresolved Issue*).

Catheter Materials

A. If the CAUTI rate is not decreasing after implementing a comprehensive strategy to reduce rates of CAUTI, consider using antimicrobial/antiseptic-impregnated catheters. The comprehensive strategy should include, at a minimum, the high priority recommendations for urinary catheter use, aseptic insertion, and maintenance (*Category IB*).
B. Further research is needed on the effect of antimicrobial/antiseptic-impregnated catheters in reducing the risk of symptomatic UTI, their inclusion among the primary interventions, and the patient populations most likely to benefit from these catheters (*No Recommendation/Unresolved Issue*).
C. Hydrophilic catheters might be preferable to standard catheters for patients requiring intermittent catheterization (*Category II*).
D. Silicone might be preferable to other catheter materials to reduce the risk of encrustation in long-term catheterized patients who have frequent obstruction (*Category II*).
E. Further research is needed to clarify the benefit of catheter valves in reducing the risk of CAUTI and other urinary complications (*No Recommendation/Unresolved Issue*).

Management of Obstruction

A. If obstruction occurs and it is likely that the catheter material is contributing to obstruction, change the catheter (*Category IB*).

B. Further research is needed on the benefit of irrigating the catheter with acidifying solutions or use of oral urease inhibitors in long-term catheterized patients who have frequent catheter obstruction (*No Recommendation/Unresolved Issue*).
C. Further research is needed on the use of a portable ultrasound device to evaluate for obstruction in patients with indwelling catheters and low urine output (*No Recommendation/Unresolved Issue*).
D. Further research is needed on the use of methenamine to prevent encrustation in patients requiring chronic indwelling catheters who are at high risk for obstruction (*No Recommendation/Unresolved Issue*).

Specimen Collection

Obtain urine samples aseptically (*Category IB*):

1. If a small volume of fresh urine is needed for examination (i.e. urinalysis or culture), aspirate the urine from the needleless sampling port with a sterile syringe/cannula adapter after cleansing the port with a disinfectant (*Category IB*).
2. Obtain large volumes of urine for special analyses (not culture) aseptically from the drainage bag (*Category IB*).

Spatial Separation of Catheterized Patients

Further research is needed on the benefit of spatial separation of patients with urinary catheters to prevent transmission of pathogens colonizing urinary drainage systems (*No Recommendation/Unresolved Issue*).

Quality Improvement Programs

Implement quality improvement (QI) programs or strategies to enhance appropriate use of indwelling catheters and to reduce the risk of CAUTI based on a facility risk assessment (*Category IB*).

The purposes of QI programs should be: (1) to assure appropriate utilization of catheters, (2) to identify and remove catheters that are no longer needed (e.g. daily review of their continued need), and (3) to ensure adherence to hand hygiene and proper care of catheters. Examples of programs that have been demonstrated to be effective include:

1. A system of alerts or reminders to identify all patients with urinary catheters and assess the need for continued catheterization.
2. Guidelines and protocols for nurse-directed removal of unnecessary urinary catheters.
3. Education and performance feedback regarding appropriate use, hand hygiene, and catheter care.
4. Guidelines and algorithms for appropriate perioperative catheter management, such as:
   a. Procedure-specific guidelines for catheter placement and postoperative catheter removal.
   b. Protocols for management of postoperative urinary retention, such as nurse-directed use of intermittent catheterization and use of bladder ultrasound scanners.

Administrative Infrastructure

Provision of Guidelines

1. Provide and implement evidence-based guidelines that address catheter use, insertion, and maintenance (*Category IB*).
   a. Consider monitoring adherence to facility-based criteria for acceptable indications for indwelling urinary catheter use (*Category II*).

Education and Training

1. Ensure that healthcare personnel and others who take care of catheters are given periodic in-service training regarding techniques and procedures for urinary catheter insertion, maintenance,

and removal. Provide education about CAUTI, other complications of urinary catheterization, and alternatives to indwelling catheters (*Category IB*).

2. When feasible, consider providing performance feedback to these personnel on what proportion of catheters they have placed meet facility-based criteria and other aspects related to catheter care and maintenance (*Category II*).

Supplies

1. Ensure that supplies necessary for aseptic technique for catheter insertion are readily available (*Category IB*).

System of Documentation

1. Consider implementing a system for documenting the following in the patient record: indications for catheter insertion, date and time of catheter insertion, individual who inserted catheter, and date and time of catheter removal (*Category II*).
   a. Ensuring that documentation is accessible in the patient record and recorded in a standard format for data collection and quality improvement purposes is suggested. Electronic documentation that is searchable is preferable (*Category II*).

Surveillance Resources

If surveillance for CAUTI is performed, ensure that there are sufficient trained personnel and technology resources to support surveillance for urinary catheter use and outcomes (*Category IB*).

Surveillance

A. Consider surveillance for CAUTI when indicated by facility-based risk assessment (*Category II*).
   a. Identify the patient groups or units on which to conduct surveillance based on frequency of catheter use and potential risk of CAUTI.

B. Use standardized methodology for performing CAUTI surveillance (*Category IB*).
   a. Examples of metrics that should be used for CAUTI surveillance include:
      i. Number of CAUTI per 1000 catheter-days.
      ii. Number of bloodstream infections secondary to CAUTI per 1000 catheter-days.
      iii. Catheter utilization ratio: (urinary catheter days/patient days) × 100.
   b. Use CDC/NHSN criteria for identifying patients who have symptomatic UTI (SUTI) (numerator data) (see NHSN Patient Safety Manual: http://www.cdc.gov/nhsn/library.html).
   c. For more information on metrics, please see the US. Department of Health and Human Services (HHS) Action Plan to Prevent Healthcare-associated Infections: http://www.hhs.gov/ophs/initiatives/hai/infection.html.

C. Routine screening of catheterized patients for asymptomatic bacteriuria (ASB) is not recommended (*Category II*).

D. When performing surveillance for CAUTI, consider providing regular (e.g. quarterly) feedback of unit-specific CAUTI rates to nursing staff and other appropriate clinical care staff (*Category II*).

USE OF NEW TYPES OF CATHETERS

Because of the substantial complications and costs associated with the use of urinary catheters, a number of practices have been evaluated in an effort to reduce the incidence of urinary catheter-related infections.

Evidences had been coming up recently supporting the use of silver alloy coated urinary catheters and urinary catheters impregnated with the antibiotics.

Such recommendations were based mostly on studies in relatively small populations or studies using methodologies other than randomized control trial.[22] It was found that silver alloy catheters are more effective in preventing urinary tract infections than are silver oxide catheters[23] and that the risk of infection declined by 32% among patients in whom silver coated catheters were used on the wards and that use of the more expensive silver coated catheter appeared to offer cost savings by preventing excess hospital costs from nosocomial UTI-associated with catheter use.[24,25]

However, there is a considerable controversy and doubt as to whether silver coated (or antimicrobial-coated) catheters reduce CAUTI rates. In the March 2009 guidelines by IDSA (Infectious Disease Society of America guidelines on CAUTI, they concluded that the evidence was insufficient to make a recommendation as to whether silver-coated or antibiotic-coated urinary catheters were effective in reducing catheter-related bacteriuria or CAUTI's. These guidelines were developed in collaboration with multiple other specialty societies.[26]

Also a large randomized trial published in The Lancet by Pickard and colleagues concluded that silver-alloy catheters were not effective for reduction of incidence of symptomatic CAUTI and that reduction in CAUTI with nitrofural-impregnated catheters was less than regarded as clinically important. Therefore, routine use of antimicrobial-impregnated catheters is not supported.[26,27] In the recommendations on the use of silver alloy coated catheters, the following recommendation was made by CDC—If the CAUTI rate is not decreasing after implementing a comprehensive strategy to reduce rates of CAUTI, consider using antimicrobial/antiseptic impregnated catheters. The comprehensive strategy should include, at a minimum, the high priority recommendations for urinary catheter use, aseptic insertion, and maintenance (*Category B*).[28]

In the recommendations on the use of antimicrobial-coated catheters by IDSA—Infectious Disease Society of America-In patients with short-term indwelling urethral catheterization, antimicrobial (silver alloy or antibiotic)-coated urinary catheters may be considered to reduce or delay the onset of CA-bacteriuria (*Category B, II*).[29]

PRACTICAL APPROACH TO PREVENTION OF URINARY TRACT INFECTION[30-32]

- UTI is one of the most frequent nosocomial infections[1] (40% of all reported nosocomial infections are UTI). 80% of these are due to indwelling urethral catheters
- UTIs can be prevented by reducing the unnecessary and inappropriately prolonged use of drainage devices, by a simple technique of handwashing, by the use of standard aseptic technique, and the use of closed drainage system
- Urinary catheterization is an aseptic procedure but is a common cause of bacteremia due to micro- or macro-trauma caused at the time of insertion or removal.
- Always think twice before using a urinary catheter.

Collection of Sample from a Catheterized Patient

- Inform the patient of the reasons for catheterization and explain the details of the procedures
- Collect all the requisite equipment and material required
- Wash and dry hands thoroughly (hygenic handwash)
- Wear sterile gloves for insertion
- Select a catheter of the right size, which fits the urethra without traumatizing the patient
- If the patient is male, foreskin is withdrawn and secretions are cleaned with sterile water (antiseptic solutions like povidone-

iodine solution or cetremide can be used for cleansing)

- If female patient labia separated and part cleaned with sterile water/antiseptic solution
- Xylocaine jelly is squeezed into the urethra. Do not contaminate the main tube during this procedure
- Advance the catheter by gripping through minor plastic sleeve of covering. Do not directly touch the catheter
- Collect the urine in a suitable container
- Fill the balloon with 5–10 mL of sterile water
- Connect up the urine drainage bag and hang it below the level of the bed to stop reflux
- Wash and dry hands
- It is important to use the correct urinary catheter as per the conditions. Foley's catheter requires no more than 5–10 mL of water, while hemostasis catheter requires 30 mL. The balloon can cause obstruction and stasis of urine if it is too large, thus increasing the risk of infection
- Emptying the drainage bag: This should be done wearing non-sterile gloves and via the drainage tap at the bottom of the bag. If the bag does not have a tap, replace it when full
- Do not disconnect the bag to empty and then reconnect
- If for financial reasons, drainage system have to be recycled, heat disinfection cannot be considered, and re-use is generally not recommended.

With proper handling, drainage bags with taps can be left in site for long periods and are more cost-effective in the long run.

For patients with a neurogenic bladder:

- Avoid an indwelling catheter if possible
- If assisted bladder drainage is necessary clean intermittent urinary catheterization should be used.

Prevention of UTI (Table 11.3)

Table 11.3: Prevention of UTI

Infection	Proven effective	Proven not effective
Urinary tract infection	1. Limit duration of catheter 2. Aseptic technique of insertion 2. Maintain closed drainage	1. Systemic antibiotic prophylaxis 2. Bladder irrigation or instillation of normal saline, antiseptic or antibiotics 3. Antiseptic added to drainage bag 4. Antimicrobial coated catheter 5. Daily antiseptic perineal cleaning

Measures for Prevention of Infection (Table 11.4)[2]

Table 11.4: Measures for prevention of infection

Hospital-associated UTI	Prevention[3]
Risk factors	
Invasive urological procedures	Aseptic technique should be maintained
Urinary catheter	Catheterization should be avoided unless absolutely necessary
Duration of catheterization	Prolonged catheterization should be avoided
Catheter care	
Selection of catheter size	The smallest size of catheter, which fits, should be used to avoid urethral trauma
Insertion technique of catheter	Aseptic "No touch" technique, use sterile gloves, hygienic hand and perineal disinfection prior to insertion
Drainage system	Closed system of drainage prevents infection. Hygienic hand disinfection prior to manipulation of drainage system
Training of HCW	Education and training helps to avoid infections
Traumatic insertion of catheter	Recommended technique should be followed

SUMMARY OF CAUTI PREVENTION (INCLUDING CAUTI BUNDLE)[33-39]

Definition: CAUTI

- UTI that occurs in a patient who had an indwelling urethral urinary catheter in place within the 48-hour period before the onset of UTI or had the catheter removed 48 hours prior to specimen collection
- Accompanied by the relevant signs and symptoms and laboratory findings.

Definition: Indwelling Catheter

- A drainage tube that is inserted into the urinary bladder through the urethra, is left in place and is connected to a closed collection system
- Also called as a Foley catheter
- Does not include straight in and out catheters or urinary catheters that are not placed in the urethra (e.g. suprapubic catheter) nor nephrostomy tubes, however, indwelling catheters used for intermittent or continuous irrigation are included in CAUTI surveillance.

Signs and Symptoms to be Looked for

- At least 1 of the following signs or symptoms: **Fever (>38°C); suprapubic tenderness; costovertebral angle pain or tenderness** (if catheter is in place)

and

- At least 1 of the following signs or symptoms: **Fever (>38°C); urgency; frequency; dysuria; suprapubic tenderness; costovertebral angle pain or tenderness** (if catheter is removed)

If patient ≤1 year of age and at least one of the following signs and symptoms with no other recognized cause: **fever (>38°C), hypothermia (<36°C), apnea, bradycardia, dysuria, lethargy or vomiting.**

Culture Report

- A positive urine culture with no more than 2 species of microorganisms identified, with at least one of which is a bacterium of $\geq 10^5$ CFU/mL

or

- At least 1 of the following findings:
  a. Positive dipstick for leukocyte esterase and/or nitrite.
  b. Pyuria (urine specimen with ≥10 white blood cells [WBC]/mm^3 of unspun urine or >5 WBC/high power field of spun urine).
  c. Microorganisms seen on Gram's stain of unspun urine.

and

- A positive urine culture of $\geq 10^3$ and $<10^5$ CFU/mL with no more than 2 species of microorganisms. Elements of the criterion must occur within a timeframe.

Collection of Sample from Catheterized Patient

- Explain procedure to patient
- Wash hands, put on disposable gloves
- Position the patient, so that catheter is accessible
- Clean the aspiration port of the drainage tubing with swabs and disinfectant
- Allow urine to collect in tubing by clamping or bending tubing
- Insert needle into aspiration port, draw urine sample by gentle aspiration, remove needle
- Transfer urine from syringe into sterile specimen container.

Risk Factors for CAUTI (Table 11.5)

Table 11.5: Risk factors for CAUTI

Symptomatic UTI	Bacteriuria
Prolonged catheterization	Disconnection of drainage system
Female sex	Lower professional training of inserter
Older age	Placement of catheter outside of OR
Impaired immunity	Incontinence
	Diabetes
	Meatal colonization
	Renal dysfunction
	Orthopedic/neurology services

Summary of Prevention Measures (Table 11.6)

Table 11.6: Summary of prevention of measures

Core measures	Supplemental measures
• Insert catheters only for appropriate indications • Leave catheters in place only as long as needed • Only properly trained persons insert and maintain catheters • Insert catheters using aseptic technique and sterile equipment • Maintain a closed drainage system • Hand hygiene and standard (or appropriate isolation) precautions	• Alternatives to indwelling urinary catheterization • Portable ultrasound devices to reduce unnecessary catheterizations • Antimicrobial/antiseptic impregnated chateters

Strategies not Recommended for CAUTI Prevention

- Complex urinary drainage systems (e.g. antiseptic-releasing cartridges in drain port)
- Changing catheters or drainage bags at routine, fixed intervals (clinical indications include infection, obstruction, or compromise of closed system)
- Routine antimicrobial prophylaxis
- Cleaning of periurethral area with antiseptics while catheter is in place (use routine hygiene)
- Irrigation of bladder with antimicrobials
- Instillation of antiseptic or antimicrobial solutions into drainage bags
- Routine screening for asymptomatic bacteriuria (ASB).

REFERENCES

1. Wallace RJ, Martin RR. Urinary tract infections. In: Groschel D (Ed). Hospital associated infections in the general hospital population and specific measures of control (Handbook on hospital associated infections, 3rd edition. Marcel Dekker INC, New York, US; 1979.p.89.
2. Wong ES, Hooton TM. Guideline for prevention of catheter associated urinary tract infections. CDC's issues in health care settings. 2002;15:36. Available at file //macintosh%20HDuritract.htm.
3. Gould CV, Craig A, Agarwal RK, Kuntz G, Pegues DA and the Health Care Infection Control Practices Advisory Committee (HICPAC). Guideline for prevention of catheter associated Urinary Tract Infections. Accessed from www.cdc.gov/hicpac/pdf/CAUTI guidelines on 27/9/2014.

3a. CDC/NHSN Surveillance Definition of Healthcare-associated Infection and Criteria for specific type of infections in the acute care setting. Accessed from www.cdph.ca.gov.on 28/9/2015.

3b. CDC. Device Associated module. Urinary Tract Infection (UTI), Catheter-associated Urinary Tract Infection (CAUTI) and Noncatheter-associated Urinary Tract Infection (NCAUTI) and other Urinary System Infection (USI) Events. Accessed from www.CDC.gov/nhsn/pdfsmanual/psicauticurrent.pdf.Accessed on 7th Sept 2016.

3c. NHSN CAUTI Definitions. Accessed from https//healthinsight.org/Internal/assets/hospital/resources/NHSN_CAUTI_12_16_11.pdf.

4. Kass EH. Bacteriuria and the diagnosis of infections of the urinary tract. Arch Int Med. 1957;100:709.

5. Turck M, Petersdorf RG. The role of antibiotics in the prevention of urinary tract infections. J Chronic Dis. 1962;15:683.
6. Marple CD. The frequency and character of urinary tract infections in an unselected group of women. Ann Intern Med. 1941;14:2220.
7. Kaye M, Vries J de, MacFarland KT. The initiation of urinary tract infection following a single bladder catheterisation. Can Med Assoc J. 1962;86:9.
8. Warren JW. Nosocomial urinary tract infections. In: Mandell GL, Bennet JE, Dolin R (Eds). Principles and practices of infectious diseases. 5th edition. App 328-339, Philadelphia. PA: Churchill Livingstone. Quoted in Timothy Decapite and Ann Richard: Nosocomial urinary tract infections. (Infectious Diseases) JHH (John Hopkin's Hospital, HEIC). Available at http:/hopkins-heic.org/infectious_diseases/urinary_tract.htm. 3/7/96. Accessed in March 2004.
9. Preventing urinary tract infections: Infection prevention guidelines. Chapter 22 Pp 22-1 to 22-10. Available at http://www.reproline.jhu.edu/english/4morerh/4ip/IP_manual/22_urinaryinfection.pdf.
10. Iannini PB. Hospital acquired urinary tract infections. Implications for treatment and prevention In: Current treatment options in infectious diseases. 2002;4:15-20. Available at search pubmed for: Iannini PB. Accessed in March 2004.
11. Garner JS, Jarvis WR, Emori TG, Horan TC, Hughes JM. CDC definitions for nosocomial infections. Am J Infec Control. 1988;16:128-40.
12. Maki DG, Hannekens CH, Bennet JV. Prevention of catheter-associated urinary tract infection. J Am Med Assoc. 1972;221:1270.
13. Garibaldi RA, et al. Medical colonization and catheter-associated bacteriuria. N Eng J Med. 1980;303(6):316-8.
14. Guttman L, Frankel H. The value of intermittent catheterization in the early management of traumatic paraplegia and tetraplegia. Paraplegia. 1966(4):63-83.
15. Lapides J, Dickno AC, Gould FR, Lowe BS. Further observation on self catheterization. J Urol. 1976;116:169-71.
16. Garibaldi RA, Burke JP, Britt MR, Miller WA, Smith CB. Meatal colonization and catheter-associated bacteriuria. New Engl J Med. 1980;303:316-8.
17. Garibaldi RA, Britt MR, Miller WA, Steinmuller P, Burke JP. Evaluation of periurethral colonization as a risk factor for catheter-associated bacteriuria. In: Proceedings of the 16th Interscience Conference on Antimicrobial agents and chemotherapy; 1976.p.142.
18. Garibaldi RA, Burke JP, Dickman ML, Smith CB. Factors predisposing to bacteriuria during indwelling urethral catheterization. N Eng J Med. 1974;291:215-8.
19. Britt MR, Garibaldi RA, Miller WA, Herbertson RM, Burke JP. Antimicrobial prophylaxis for catheter-associated bacteriuria—Antimicrob Agents Chemother. 1977;11:240-3.
20. Maki DG, Hennekens CH, Bennet JV, et al. Nosocomial urinary tract infection with *Serratia marcesens*: An epidemiologic study. J Infect Dis. 1973;128:579-87.
21. Kaslow RA, Lindsey JO, Bisno AL, Price A. Nosocomial infection with highly resistant *Proteus rettgeri*. Report of an epidemic. Am J Epidemiol. 1976;104:278-8.
22. Liedberg H, Lundeberg T. Silver Alloy Coated Catheters Reduce Catheter-associated Bacteriuria. British Journal of Urology. 1990;65(4):379-381. http://onlinelibrary.wiley.com/doi/10.1111/j.1464-410x.1990.tb14760.x/abstract. Accessed on 28/9/2014 from http://www.patientsafetysolutions.com/docs/january_2013_silver_coated_urinary_catheters_Dont_Reduce_CAUTIis.htm. in What's New in the Patient Safety World. January 2013 Silver Coated Urinary Catheters Don't reduce CAUTI's.
23. Saint S, Elmore JG, Sullivan SD, Emerson SS, Koepsell TD. The efficacy of silver alloy-coated urinary catheters in preventing urinary tract infection: a meta-analysis. Am J Med. 1998;105(3):236-41. Available at http://www.amjmed.com/article/S0002-9343%2898%2900240-X/abstract. Accessed on 28/9/2014 from http://www.patientsafetysolutions.com/docs/january_2013_silver_coated_urinary_catheters_Dont_Reduce_CAUTIis.htm. in What's New in the Patient Safety World. January 2013 Silver Coated Urinary Catheters Don't reduce CAUTI's.
24. Karchmer TB, Gianetta ET, Muto CA, et al. A Randomized Crossover Study of silver-Coated Urinary Catheters in Hospitalized Patients. Arch Intern Med. 2000;160(21):3294-8.

Available at http://archinte.jamanetwork.com/article.aspx?articleid=485555(Karchmer2000). Accessed on 28/9/2014 from http://www.patientsafetysolutions.com/docs/january_2013_silver_coated_urinary_catheters_Dont_Reduce_CAUTIis.htm. in What's New in the Patient Safety World. January 2013 Silver Coated Urinary Catheters Don't reduce CAUTI's.

25. Rupp ME, Fitzgerald T, Marion N, et al. Effect of silver-coated urinary catheters: efficacy, cost-effectiveness, and antimicrobial resistance. American Journal of Infection Control. 2004;32(8):445-50. Available at http://europepmc.org/abstract/MED/15573050/reload=0;jsessionid=iw2CF0dN1E2U8qDb2wdU.12. Accessed on 28/9/2014 from http://www.patientsafetysolutions.com/docs/january_2013_silver_coated_urinary_catheters_Dont_Reduce_CAUTIis.htm. in What's New in the Patient Safety World. January 2013 Silver Coated Urinary Catheters Don't reduce CAUTI's25.
26. What's New in the Patient Safety World. January 2013 Silver Coated Urinary Catheters Don't reduce CAUTI's. Accessed on 28/9/2014 from http://www.patientsafetysolutions.com/docs/january_2013_silver_coated_urinary_catheters_Dont_Reduce_CAUTIis.htm.in.
27. Pickard R, Lam T, MacLennan G, et al. Antimicrobial Catheters for Reduction of Symptomatic Urinary Tract Infection in adults Requiring Short-term Catheterization in Hospital. In: Gupta K, Bhadelia N (Eds). A Multicentre Randomised Controlled Trial Lancet. 2012;380:1927-35. Quoted in Preventing CAUTIs with Coated Catheters: Is the Jury Still Out? Feb 19, 2013.
28. Gould CV, Umscheid CA, Agarwal RK, Kuntz G, Pegues DA, and the Healthcare Infection Control Practices Advisory Committee (HICPAC). Guideline for prevention of catheter-associated urinary tract infections 2009. Available at www.cdc.gov/ncidod/dhqp/pdf/guidelines/CAUTI_Guideline 2009final.pdf).
29. Recommendation:Antimicrobial-Coated Catheters. IDSA http://www.journals.uchicago.Accessed on edu/doi/pdf/10.1086/650482?cookieSet=1). Quoted in BARDEX I.C. recommendations on the use of Silver Alloy Coated Catheters.http://www.bardmedical.com/Resources/Productes/Documents/Brochures/Urology/IC-CDC-Cathterisation Recommendations. Practical Approach to Prevention of UTI- References.
30. Manual for Hospital Infection Control: Compiled by Hospital Infection Control Committee. LTMGH and LTMMC. p 21.
31. Ducel G, Fabry J, Nicolle L. Prevention of hospital acquired infections—a practical guide. WHO, 2nd edition; 2002.p.38.
32. Guidelines on Prevention and Control of Hospital-associated infections WHO Regional Office for South-East Asia, New Delhi; 2002. p. 32.
33. Gould C. CAUTI Toolkit CDC Activity C: ELC Prevention Colloboratives. Accessed on 21 /1/ 2015. Available at www.cdc.gov/HAI/pdfs/toolkits/CAUTItoolkit_3_10.pdf.
34. CAUTI Bundle. Health protection, Scotland. Accessed on 21/1/2015. Available at www.hpsc.ie/A-Z/Microbiology/Antimicrobial Resistance/Infection Control and HAI/Urinary Catheters/Care Bundle/Fi Available at +www,hpsc.i.e/A-Z/Microbiology/Antimicrobial resistance/Infection Control and HAI/Urinary Catheters/Core Bundle/Fi.
35. CAUTI Toolkit CDC Activity (ELC Prevention Colloboratives). By Carolyn Gould MD MSCR. Available at www.cdc.gov/HAI/pdfs/toolkits/CAUTItoolkit-3-10.pdf.
36. Gould CV, Umscheid CA, Agarwal RK, Kuntz G, Pegues DA, and HICPAC. Guideline for Prevention of Catheter-associated Urinary Tract Infections 2009 Available at .http://www.cdc.gov/hicpac/cauti/001_cauti.html.
37. APIC CAUTI Elimination Guide: Available at http://www.apic.org.
38. IDSA Guidelines. Clin Infect Dis. 2010;50:625-63.
39. CDC/Medscape collaboration: Available at http://www.cdc.gov/hicpac.

Chapter 12

Dialysis Unit

Chapter Outline

- Methods of Dialysis
- Special Hazards in Dialysis Unit
- Prevention of Infections
- Subcutaneous Arteriovenous Fistula
- External Arteriovenous Fistula
- Routine Care of Access Site
- Training for Home Dialysis
- Infection in the Access Site
- Acute and Intermittent Dialysis: Precautions
- Continuous Ambulatory Peritoneal Dialysis
- Disinfection
- Infection Control Precautions for Outpatient Hemodialysis Settings Compared with Inpatient Hospital Settings
- Hepatitis B Infection
- Hepatitis C Infection
- Hepatitis Delta Virus Infection
- Human Immunodeficiencey Virus Infection
- Bacterial Infections
- Recommendations
- Practical Approach to Control of HAI in Dialysis Unit
- Microbial Testing of Dialysate

INTRODUCTION

Dialysis is a common procedure carried out in many hospitals. The general consideration with regard to hospital infection applies to dialysis, but there are special hazards. The number of patients with end-stage renal disease treated by maintenance hemodialysis in the United States has increased sharply during the past 30 years. Chronic hemodialysis patients are at high risk for infection because the process of hemodialysis requires vascular access for prolonged periods. In an environment where multiple patients receive dialysis concurrently, repeated opportunities exist for person-to-person transmission of infectious agents, directly or indirectly via contaminated devices, equipment and supplies, environmental surfaces, or hands of personnel. Furthermore, hemodialysis patients are immunosuppressed which increases their susceptibility to infection, and they require frequent hospitalizations and surgery, which increases their opportunities for exposure to nosocomial infections.[1]

Historically, surveillance for infections associated with chronic hemodialysis focused on viral hepatitis, particularly hepatitis B virus (HBV) infection. CDC began conducting national surveillance for hemodialysis-associated hepatitis in 1972. Other hemodialysis-associated diseases and practices not related to hepatitis have been included over the years (e.g. pyrogenic reactions, dialysis dementia, vascular access infections, reuse practices, vancomycin use), and the system is continually updated to collect data regarding hemodialysis-associated practices and diseases of current interest and importance.[1]

Recommendations for the control of hepatitis B in hemodialysis centers were first published in 1977 and by 1980, their widespread implementation was associated with a sharp reduction in incidence of HBV infection among both patients and staff members. In 1982, hepatitis B vaccination was recommended for all susceptible patients and staff members. However, outbreaks of both HBV and hepatitis C virus (HCV) infections continue to occur among chronic hemodialysis patients. Epidemiologic investigations have indicated substantial deficiencies in recommended infection control practices, as well as a failure to vaccinate hemodialysis patients against hepatitis B. These practices apparently are not being fully implemented because staff members (a) are not aware of the practices and their importance, (b) are confused regarding the differences between standard (i.e. universal) precautions recommended for all health-care settings and the additional precautions necessary in the hemodialysis setting, and (c) believe that hepatitis B vaccine is ineffective for preventing HBV infection in chronic hemodialysis patients.[1]

Bacterial infections, especially those involving vascular access, are the most frequent infectious complication of hemodialysis and a major cause of morbidity and mortality among hemodialysis patients. During the 1990s, the prevalence of antimicrobial-resistant bacteria [e.g. methicillin-resistant *Staphylococcus aureus* (MRSA) and vancomycin-resistant enterococci (VRE)] increased rapidly in health-care settings, including hemodialysis units. Although numerous outbreaks of bacterial infections in the hemodialysis setting have been reported, few studies exist regarding the epidemiology and prevention of endemically occurring bacterial infections in hemodialysis patients, and formal recommendations to prevent such infections have not been published previously. In 1999, CDC initiated a surveillance system for bloodstream and vascular access infections in outpatient hemodialysis centers to determine the frequency of and risk factors for these complications in order to formulate and evaluate strategies for control.[1]

The recommendations contained in this report were developed by reviewing available data and are based on consultations with specialists in the field. These recommendations provide guidelines for infection control strategies, unique to the hemodialysis setting, that should be used to prevent patient-to-patient transmission of blood-borne viruses and pathogenic bacteria.[1]

These recommendations do not address sources of bacterial and chemical contaminants in dialysis systems, water treatment or distribution, specific procedures for reprocessing dialyzers, clinical practice methods to prevent bacterial infections (e.g. techniques for skin preparation and access), or comprehensive strategies for preventing infections among healthcare workers.[1]

METHODS OF DIALYSIS

One is hemodialysis and the other one is peritoneal dialysis.

Hemodialysis System[2]

This consists of a water supply, a system for mixing water and concentrated dialysis fluid, and a machine to pump the dialysis fluid through the artificial kidney (dialyzer), the latter is connected to the patient's' circulatory system.

The supplied water is subjected to prefilters (if necessary), softener, carbon filters, and a particulate filter and is then passed through first a reverse osmosis unit and a deionization unit. Through, these phases the water becomes progressively chemically pure, but level of bacterial contamination increases. To compensate, an ultrafilter is included in the final step of the system to remove bacteria and bacterial endotoxins.

In the dialysis centers, the treated water is mixed with a dialysate concentrate and distributed through pipes.

Peritoneal Dialysis[2]

Peritoneal dialysis may be used for the treatment of acute renal failure, usually via a semi-rigid catheter inserted percutaneously into the abdomen followed by fairly rapid exchanges of dialysis fluid, often with automated control of inflow and outflow using a suitable design of peritoneal dialysis machine. Such a procedure can also be applied intermittently to patients with chronic renal failure, using a more permanent form of peritoneal access.

SPECIAL HAZARDS IN DIALYSIS UNIT[3]

Blood-borne Viruses (HBV, HCV, HIV)

Patients suffering from chronic renal failure may show few physical signs when infected with HBV, but become long-term carriers. This virus is often present in high titer, and transfer of infection to staff and other patients is a particular hazard. Blood transfusion is now a rare source of infection of HBV in most countries as transfusion blood is usually screened. Blood is also screened for HIV and HCV, but is more variable in countries with limited resources. Spread of HIV has not been reported in renal units. Spread of blood-borne viruses can also occur through stored and inadequately decontaminated equipment.

Risk Associated with Dialysis Machines

The dialysis fluid used for hemodialysis need not be sterile, but a heavy growth of bacteria leads to risk both of infection and of changes in the chemical composition of the fluid, which may be associated with endotoxins crossing the machine. Gram-negative bacilli (e.g. *Pseudomonas, Acinetobacter, Aeromonas* and *Serratia* species) and non-tuberculous *Mycobacterium* (e.g. *Mycobacterium chelonae*) can grow in dialysis machines and cause septicemia and pyrogenic reactions. Both these groups of bacteria multiply early in water.

Risk Associated with Vascular Access Site, Catheter Exit Site and Peritoneal Infections

Staphylococcus aureus and *Staphylococcus epidermidis* are the commonest cause of infection, but gram-negative bacilli (e.g. *E. coli, Pseudomonas aeruginosa*) can cause peritonitis. In addition to local sepsis and peritonitis, bacteremia and endocarditis are also possible complications.

PREVENTION OF INFECTIONS

Viral Infections

Patient should be screened for HBV (and possible HCV) on admission to the dialysis program. Screening for HIV remains controversial, as it is not essential as an infection control measure. Patients and staff should be immunized against hepatitis B if they are not already immune. Routine surveillance for HBV is important for susceptible patients (e.g. 3 monthly) and staff (6 monthly), but it is not necessary for HIV and HCV.[4]

Bacterial Infections

Meticulous attention should be paid to all aspects of environmental hygiene and to aseptic techniques. There are evidences that staphylococcal carriers are more likely to acquire clinical infections than non-carriers. Treatment of nasal carriers with mupirocin in varying regimens has been shown to reduce nasal carriage considerably, and to reduce infection rates significantly, including bacteraemias.[5] Continuous treatment with mupirocin appears to be more effective than an initial course plus a repeat course if a recurrence of carriage occurs.[6] However, resistance to mupirocin has emerged,[7] and many chronic staphylococcal carriers do not develop sepsis. It may be preferable to restrict nasal prophylaxis to those who develop repeated infections. The use of other less effective agents (e.g. neomycin, bacitracin, chlorhexidine) may be preferred for long-term prophylaxis.

SUBCUTANEOUS ARTERIOVENOUS FISTULA

The subcutaneous fistula has a great advantage over the external shunt in that there is no open wound once postoperative healing has occurred. The technique for management is as follows:

1. A wide area of arm is cleaned with 0.5% chlorhexidine in 70% ethyl alcohol. It is essential that this preliminary skin preparation should be very thorough, in order to avoid the introduction of bacteria directly into the bloodstream.
2. Local anesthesia is usually necessary in view of the wide bore of the needle to be inserted. Lignocaine (2%) in 2 mL ampoules is recommended for this purpose.
3. It is desirable to avoid inserting the needle through the same point of insertion made during the preceding dialysis, where a small-infected clot or scab may have formed.
4. The fistula needle is strapped into position after reinsertion into the fistula site, but no dressing is necessary.
5. Hemorrhage after withdrawal of the needle can occur and severe blood loss can be troublesome if adequate steps are not taken. To prevent this a protamine soaked or other hemostatic swab is placed over the site and held in place firmly for 10 minutes. This is replaced by a sterile gauze square, and firmly bandaged for 2 hours.

EXTERNAL ARTERIOVENOUS FISTULA

This is an external access device, and in this, the bacteriological problem is that, it is difficult to avoid infection in a permanently open wound containing a foreign body. This obviously presents considerable difficulties. However, prevention of infection at the access site is of major importance if suppuration is to be avoided. This may lead to destruction and abandonment of an important site, when the number of sites is strictly limited, and to the risk of septic emboli and fatal septicemia.

In view of these considerations, the care of the access site must begin with the general hygiene and ward cleanliness, and the measures used to control cross infection in the general hospital wards, should be applied more rigorously to the renal unit.

ROUTINE CARE OF ACCESS SITE

The main object is to prevent introduction of pathogens. This is achieved by observation of strict aseptic principles in the dressing and handling of the access site, by an occlusive dressing, and by keeping the site dry at all times as far as possible.

TRAINING FOR HOME DIALYSIS

It is important to train the patient for home dialysis to be self-sufficient, but it is equally important to train the spouse, relative or friend who may help the patient. They should be fully instructed in both the principles and practice of access site care. At the same time, the dangers of autogenous infection must be stressed in order to encourage the highest standards of personal hygiene.

INFECTION IN THE ACCESS SITE

If there is clinical evidence of infection at the site, a swab is taken for bacteriological examination and swabs of nose, throat, axilla and groin are also taken. If the clinical condition warrants antibiotic therapy pending the bacteriological report, antistaphylococcal drugs (e.g. flucloxocillin or an initial dose of vancomycin) are started. Treatment is reviewed and altered if necessary on receipt of the bacteriological report. If possible antibiotics that accumulate to toxic level in renal failure should be avoided.

Treatment is continued until there is bacteriological evidence of clearance. Carrier sites are treated as outlined above if they are found to carry pathogens.

The maintenance of infection control of access site depends on rigorous attention to basic aseptic principles, keeping the site dry, prevention of colonization of carrier sites by pathogens, and a high level of perineal and environmental hygiene.

ACUTE AND INTERMITTENT DIALYSIS: PRECAUTIONS

Peritoneal dialysis is used for treatment of acute renal failure and may sometimes be applied to patients with chronic renal failure; in which case, a more permanent form of peritoneal access is used. In such cases, sterile pyrogen free solutions and sterile cannulae and tubing are required. Abdominal drainage should be through a closed system.

Adequate skin preparation and stringent aseptic techniques are required for insertion of the peritoneal cannula. A suture should be placed around the catheter and tied, so that the latter cannot be pushed freely in and out by the staff attendant, and a simple gauze dressing should cover the site.

Manual methods often use a water bath or sink for warming the bottles of dialysate before use. This water is likely to be contaminated with gram-negative bacilli, including *Pseudomonas species*; the water should be changed frequently.

Automated systems for peritoneal dialysis include adequate instructions for sterilization.

Parts of the system that are likely to be in contact with dialysate must either be presterlized disposable items or be autoclaved.

Routine addition of prophylactic antibiotics to peritoneal dialysis fluid is not recommended. It is desirable to send samples to the laboratory every 24 hours for culture.

Peritoneal dialysis for chronic renal failure requires the use of a permanent indwelling silicone rubber peritoneal catheter. Such a catheter is plugged between uses except when continuous dialysis is practiced. The insertion and care of these catheters closely resemble to care of external arteriovenous shunts or cannulae. Whenever connections or disconnections are made, rigorous aseptic or no-touch techniques must be used. Peritonitis remains a common and serious complication of peritoneal dialysis.

CONTINUOUS AMBULATORY PERITONEAL DIALYSIS

The technique of continuous ambulatory peritoneal dialysis (CAPD) uses plastic bags of dialysate, which are changed by the patient several times daily. Patients must be taught to avoid contaminating the connections during these changes. Several types of connecting systems for CAPD are in use, and the manufacturer's instructions for each pattern should be followed. Various methods are available to reduce contamination of the line (e.g. flushing with hypochlorites and use of disinfectant impregnated cuffs), as well as systems using UV light and local heat application; spraying with 70% ethanol is also effective. The catheter connection is usually changed periodically by the staff of the parent unit using full aseptic precautions.

The major hazard of peritoneal dialysis is peritonitis. Infection in CAPD is most common by skin organisms, particularly *Staphylococcus epidermidis*. Meticulous attention to the details, like catheter care, and avoidance of wetting the exit site, greatly reduces the incidence of infection. Peritonitis, often indicated by cloudy dialysis effluent and abdominal pain requires antibiotic therapy, which is often added to the peritoneal dialysis fluid while awaiting for positive cultures, a broad spectrum antibiotic regime, including drugs active against *Staphylococcus epidermidis* is usually instituted. Gram negative and particularly fungal infections usually require temporary removal of the peritoneal catheter.

DISINFECTION[1]

Equipment, Supplies, and Environmental Surfaces

The hemodialysis machine and its components also can be vehicles for patient-to-patient transmission of blood-borne viruses and pathogenic bacteria. The external surfaces of the machine are the most likely sources for contamination. These include not only frequently touched surfaces (e.g. the control panel), but also attached waste containers used during the priming of the dialyzers, blood tubing draped or clipped to waste containers, and items placed on tops of machines for convenience (e.g. dialyzer caps and medication vials).

Internal Pathways of Hemodialysis Machines

In single-pass hemodialysis machines, the internal fluid pathways are not subject to contamination with blood. If a dialyzer leak occurs, dialysis fluid might become contaminated with blood, but this contaminated fluid is discarded through a drain and does not return to the dialysis machine to contaminate predialyzer surfaces. For dialysis machines that use a dialysate recirculating system (e.g. some ultrafiltration control machines and those that regenerate the dialysate), a blood leak in a dialyzer could contaminate the internal pathways of the machine, which could in turn contaminate the dialysis fluid of subsequent patients. However, procedures normally practiced after each use (i.e. draining the dialysis fluid and rinsing and disinfecting the machine) will reduce the level of contamination to below infectious levels. In addition, an intact dialyzer membrane will not allow passage of bacteria or viruses.

Pressure transducer filter protectors are used primarily to prevent contamination and preserve the functioning of the pressure monitoring (i.e. arterial, venous, or both) components of the hemodialysis machine. Hemodialysis machines usually have both external (typically supplied with the blood tubing set) and internal protectors, with the internal protector serving as a backup in case the external transducer protector fails. Failure to use an external protector or to replace the protector when it becomes contaminated (i.e. wetted with saline or blood) can result in contamination of the internal transducer protector, which in turn could allow transmission of blood-borne pathogens. However, no epidemiologic evidence exists that contamination of the internal transducer protector caused by failure of the external transducer protector has led to either mixing of blood or the transmission of blood-borne agents.

Dialyzer Reprocessing

Approximately, 80% of US chronic hemodialysis centers reprocess (i.e. reuse) dialyzers for the same patient. Although outbreaks of bacterial infections and pyrogenic reactions have occurred because of inadequate reprocessing procedures and failure to maintain standards for water quality, reuse has not been associated with transmission of blood-borne viruses. Any theoretical risk for HBV transmission from reuse of dialyzers would primarily affect staff members who handle these dialyzers. Although no increase in HBV (or HCV) infection among staff members who work in such centers has been reported, many centers do not reuse dialyzers from HBsAg-positive patients.

INFECTION CONTROL PRECAUTIONS FOR OUTPATIENT HEMODIALYSIS SETTINGS COMPARED WITH INPATIENT HOSPITAL SETTINGS[1]

Contact transmission is the most important route by which pathogens are transmitted in healthcare settings, including hemodialysis units. Contact transmission occurs most commonly when microorganisms from a patient are transferred to the hands of a healthcare worker who does not comply with infection control precautions, then touches another patient. Less commonly, environmental surfaces (e.g. bed rails, countertops) become contaminated and serve as an intermediate reservoir for pathogens; transmission can occur when a worker touches the surface then touches a patient or when a patient touches the surface.

In the hemodialysis setting, contact transmission plays a major role in transmission of blood-borne pathogens. If a healthcare worker's hands become contaminated with virus-infected blood from one patient, the worker can transfer the virus to a second patient's skin or blood line access port, and the virus can be inoculated into that patient when the skin or access port is punctured with a needle.

Contact transmission can be prevented by hand hygiene (i.e. hand washing or use of a waterless hand rub), glove use, and disinfection of environmental surfaces. Of these, hand hygiene is the most important. In addition, nonsterile disposable gloves provide a protective barrier for workers' hands, preventing them from becoming soiled or contaminated, and reduce the likelihood that microorganisms present on the hands of personnel will be transmitted to patients. However, even with glove use, hand washing is needed because pathogens deposited on the outer surface of gloves can be detected on hands after glove removal, possibly because of holes or defects in the gloves, leakage at the wrist, or contamination of hands during glove removal.

Standard precautions are the system of infection control precautions recommended for the inpatient hospital setting. Standard precautions are used on all patients and include use of gloves, gown, or mask whenever needed to prevent contact of the healthcare worker with blood, secretions, excretions, or contaminated items.

In addition to standard precautions, more stringent precautions are recommended for hemodialysis units because of the increased potential for contamination with blood and pathogenic microorganisms. For example, infection control practices for hemodialysis units restrict the use of common supplies, instruments, medications, and medication trays and prohibit the use of a common medication cart.

For certain patients, including those infected or colonized with MRSA or VRE, contact precautions are used in the inpatient hospital setting. Contact precautions include (a) placing the patient in a single room or with another patient infected or colonized with the same organism; (b) using gloves whenever entering the patient's room; and (c) using a gown when entering the patient's room if the potential exists for the worker's clothing to have substantial contact with the patient, environmental surfaces, or items in the patient's room. Workers also should wear a gown if the patient has diarrhea, an ileostomy, a colostomy, or wound drainage not contained by a dressing.

However, contact precautions are not recommended in hemodialysis units for patients infected or colonized with pathogenic bacteria for several reasons. First, although contact transmission of pathogenic bacteria is well-documented in hospitals, similar transmission has not been well-documented in hemodialysis centers. Transmission might not be apparent in dialysis centers, possibly because it occurs less frequently than in acute-care hospitals or results in undetected colonization rather than overt infection. Also, because dialysis patients are frequently hospitalized, determining whether transmission occurred in the inpatient or outpatient setting is difficult. Second, contamination of the patient's skin, bedclothes, and environmental surfaces with pathogenic bacteria is likely to be more common in hospital settings (where patients spend 24 hours a day) than in outpatient hemodialysis centers (where patients spend approximately 10 hours a week). Third, the routine use of infection control practices recommended for hemodialysis units, which are more stringent than the standard precautions routinely used in hospitals, should prevent transmission by the contact route.

HEPATITIS B INFECTION[1]

Epidemiology

Incidence and Prevalence

In 1974, the incidence of newly acquired (i.e. acute) HBV infection among chronic hemodialysis patients in the United States was 6.2%, and selected hemodialysis centers reported rates as high as 30%. By 1980, nationwide incidence among patients had decreased to 1%, and by 1999, to 0.06% (CDC, unpublished data, 2001), with only 3.5% of all centers reporting newly acquired infections. Prevalence of chronic HBV infection (i.e. hepatitis B surface antigen [HBsAg] positivity) among hemodialysis patients declined from 7.8% in 1976 to 3.8% in 1980 and to 0.9% by 1999 (CDC, unpublished data, 2001). In 1999, a total of 27.7% of 3,483 centers provided dialysis to ≥1 patient with either acute or chronic HBV infection (CDC, unpublished data, 2001).

Transmission

HBV is transmitted by percutaneous (i.e. puncture through the skin) or permucosal (i.e. direct contact with mucous membranes) exposure to infectious blood or to body fluids that contain blood, and the chronically infected person is central to the epidemiology of HBV transmission. All HBsAg-positive persons are infectious, but those who are also positive for hepatitis Be antigen (HBeAg) circulate HBV at high titers in their blood ($10^{8,9}$ virions/mL). With virus titers in blood this high, body fluids containing serum or blood also can contain high levels of HBV and are potentially infectious. Furthermore, HBV at titers of $10^{2,3}$ virions/mL can be present on environmental surfaces in the absence of any visible blood and still result in transmission.

HBV is relatively stable in the environment and remains viable for at least 7 days on environmental surfaces at room temperature. HBsAg has been detected in dialysis centers on clamps, scissors, dialysis machine control knobs, and doorknobs. Thus, blood-contaminated surfaces that are not routinely cleaned and disinfected represent a reservoir for HBV transmission. Dialysis staff members can transfer virus to patients from contaminated surfaces by their hands or gloves or through use of contaminated equipment and supplies.

Most HBV infection outbreaks among hemodialysis patients were caused by cross-contamination to patients via (a) environmental surfaces, supplies (e.g. hemostats, clamps), or equipment that were not routinely disinfected after each use; (b) multiple dose medication vials and intravenous solutions that were not used exclusively for one patient; (c) medications for injection that were prepared in areas adjacent to areas where blood samples were handled; and (d) staff members who simultaneously cared for both HBV-infected and susceptible patients. Once the factors that promote HBV transmission among hemodialysis patients were identified, recommendations for control were published in 1977. These recommendations included (a) serologic surveillance of patients (and staff members) for HBV infection, including monthly testing of all susceptible patients for HBsAg; (b) isolation of HBsAg-positive patients in a separate room; (c) assignment of staff members to HBsAg-positive patients and not to HBV-susceptible patients during the same shift; (d) assignment of dialysis equipment to HBsAg-positive patients that is not shared by HBV-susceptible patients; (e) assignment of a supply tray to each patient (regardless of serologic status); (f) cleaning and disinfection of nondisposable items (e.g. clamps, scissors) before use on another patient; (g) glove use whenever any patient or hemodialysis equipment is touched and glove changes between each patient (and station); and (h) routine cleaning and disinfection of equipment and environmental surfaces.

The segregation of HBsAg-positive patients and their equipment from HBV-susceptible patients resulted in 70–80% reductions in incidence of HBV infection among hemodialysis patients. National surveillance data for 1976–1989 indicated that incidence of HBV infection was substantially lower in hemodialysis units that isolated HBsAg-positive patients, compared with those that did not. The success of isolation practices in preventing transmission of HBV infection is linked to other infection control practices, including routine serological surveillance and routine cleaning and disinfection. Frequent serologic testing for HBsAg detects patients recently infected with HBV quickly so isolation procedures can be implemented before cross-contamination can occur. Environmental control by routine cleaning and disinfection procedures reduces the opportunity for cross-contamination, either directly from environmental surfaces or indirectly by hands of personnel.

Despite the current low incidence of HBV infection among hemodialysis patients, outbreaks continue to occur in chronic hemodialysis centers. Investigations of these outbreaks have documented that HBV transmission resulted from failure to use recommended infection control practices, including (a) failure to routinely screen patients for HBsAg or routinely review results of testing to identify infected patients; (b) assignment of staff members to the simultaneous care of infected and susceptible patients; and (c) sharing of supplies, particularly multiple dose medication vials, among patients. In addition, few patients had received hepatitis B vaccine. National surveillance data have demonstrated that independent risk factors among chronic hemodialysis patients for acquiring HBV infection include the presence of $\geq$1 HBV-infected patient in the hemodialysis center who is not isolated, as well as a <50% hepatitis B vaccination rate among patients.

HBV infection among chronic hemodialysis patients also has been associated with hemodialysis provided in the acute-care setting. Transmission appeared to stem from chronically-infected HBV patients who shared staff members, multiple dose medication vials, and other supplies and equipment with susceptible patients. These episodes were recognized when patients returned to their chronic hemodialysis units, and routine HBsAg testing was resumed. Transmission from HBV-infected chronic hemodialysis patients to patients undergoing hemodialysis for acute renal failure has not been documented, possibly because these patients are dialyzed for short durations and have limited exposure. However, such transmission could go unrecognized because acute renal failure patients are unlikely to be tested for HBV infection.

Clinical Features and Natural History

HBV causes both acute and chronic hepatitis. The incubation period ranges from 45–160 days (mean: 120 days), and the onset of acute disease is usually insidious. Infants, young children (aged <10 years), and immunosuppressed adults with newly acquired HBV infection are usually asymptomatic. When present, clinical symptoms and signs might include anorexia, malaise, nausea, vomiting, abdominal pain, and jaundice. Extrahepatic manifestations of disease (e.g. skin rashes, arthralgias, and arthritis) can also occur. The case fatality rate after acute hepatitis B is 0.5–1%.

In adults with normal immune status, most (94–98%) recover completely from newly acquired HBV infections, eliminating virus from the blood and producing neutralizing antibody that creates immunity from future infection. In immunosuppressed persons (including hemodialysis patients), infants, and young children, most newly acquired HBV infections result in chronic infection. Although the consequences of acute hepatitis B can be severe, most of the serious sequelae associated with the disease occur in persons in whom chronic infection develops. Although persons with chronic HBV infection are often asymptomatic, chronic liver disease develops in two-thirds of these persons, and approximately 15–25% die prematurely from cirrhosis or liver cancer.

Subtypes of HBV exist, and infection or immunization with one subtype confers immunity to all subtypes. However, reinfection or reactivation of latent HBV infection has been reported among certain groups of immunosuppressed patients, including those who have undergone renal transplant and those infected with human immunodeficiency virus (HIV). These patients were positive for antibody to hepatitis B core antigen (anti-HBc), with or without antibody to HBsAg (anti-HBs), and subsequently developed detectable levels of HBsAg. The frequency with which this occurs is unknown.

Monotherapy with alpha interferon or lamivudine is approved by the US Food and Drug Administration (FDA) to treat patients with chronic hepatitis B. Although the dosage of lamivudine should be modified based on creatinine clearance in patients with renal impairment, no additional dose modification is necessary after routine hemodialysis. The emergence of lamivudine-resistant variants has caused concern regarding long-term use of this drug.

Screening and Diagnostic Tests

Serologic Assays

Several well-defined antigen-antibody systems are associated with HBV infection, including HBsAg and anti-HBs; hepatitis B core antigen (HBcAg) and anti-HBc; and HBeAg and antibody to HBeAg (anti-HBe). Serologic assays are commercially available for all of these except HBcAg because no free HBcAg circulates in blood. One or more of these serologic markers are present during different phases of HBV infection (Table 12.1).

The presence of HBsAg is indicative of ongoing HBV infection and potential infectiousness. In newly infected persons, HBsAg is present in serum 30–60 days after exposure to HBV and persists for variable periods. Transient HBsAg positivity (lasting ≤18 days) can be detected in some patients during vaccination. Anti-HBc develops in all HBV infections, appearing at onset of symptoms or liver test abnormalities in acute HBV infection, rising rapidly to high levels, and persisting for life. Acute or recently acquired infection can be distinguished by presence of the immunoglobulin M (IgM) class of anti-HBc, which persists for approximately 6 months.

Table 12.1: Interpretation of serologic test results for hepatitis B virus infection

Serologic markers				Interpretation
HBsAg*	Total anti-HBc†	IgM§ anti-HBC	Anti-HBs¶	
–	–	–	–	Susceptible, never infected
+	–	–	–	Acute infection, early incubation**
+	+	+	–	Acute infection
–	+	+	–	Acute resolving infection
–	+	–	+	Past infection, recovered and immune
+	+	–	–	Chronic infection
–	+	–	–	False positive (i.e. susceptible), past infection, or "low-level" chronic infection
–	–	–	+	Immune if titer is ≥10 mIU/mL

*Hepatitis B surface antigen
†Antibody to hepatitis B core antigen
§Immunoglobulin M
¶Antibody to hepatitis B surface antigen
**Transient HBsAg positivity (lasting ≤18 days) might be detected in some patients during vaccination

In persons who recover from HBV infection, HBsAg is eliminated from the blood, usually in 2–3 months, and anti-HBs develops during convalescence. The presence of anti-HBs indicates immunity from HBV infection. After recovery from natural infection, most persons will be positive for both anti-HBs and anti-HBc, whereas only anti-HBs develops in persons who are successfully vaccinated against hepatitis B. Persons who do not recover from HBV infection and become chronically infected remain positive for HBsAg (and anti-HBc), although a small proportion (0.3% per year) eventually clear HBsAg and might develop anti-HBs.

In some persons, the only HBV serologic marker detected is anti-HBc (i.e. isolated anti-HBc). Among most asymptomatic persons in the United States tested for HBV infection, an average of 2% (range: <0.1–6%) test positive for isolated anti-HBc; among injecting-drug users, however, the rate is 24% . In general, the frequency of isolated anti-HBc is directly related to the frequency of previous HBV infection in the population and can have several explanations. This pattern can occur after HBV infection among persons who have recovered but whose anti-HBs levels have waned or among persons who failed to develop anti-HBs. Persons in the latter category include those who circulate HBsAg at levels not detectable by current commercial assays. However, HBV DNA has been detected in <10% of persons with isolated anti-HBc, and these persons are unlikely to be infectious to others except under unusual circumstances involving direct percutaneous exposure to large quantities of blood (e.g. transfusion). In most persons with isolated anti-HBc, the result appears to be a false positive. Data from several studies have demonstrated that a primary anti-HBs response develops in most of these persons after a three-dose series of hepatitis B vaccine. No data exist on response to vaccination among hemodialysis patients with this serologic pattern.

A third antigen, HBeAg, can be detected in serum of persons with acute or chronic HBV infection. The presence of HBeAg correlates with viral replication and high levels of virus (i.e. high infectivity). Anti-HBe correlates with the loss of replicating virus and with lower levels of virus. However, all HBsAg-positive persons should be considered potentially infectious, regardless of their HBeAg or anti-HBe status.

Nucleic Acid Detection

HBV infection can be detected using qualitative or quantitative tests for HBV DNA. These tests are not FDA-approved and are most commonly used for patients being managed with antiviral therapy.

Hepatitis B Vaccine

Hepatitis B vaccine has been recommended for both hemodialysis patients and staff members since the vaccine became available in 1982. By 1999, a total of 55% of patients and 88% of staff members had been vaccinated (CDC, unpublished data, 2001). Two types of vaccine have been licensed and used in the United States: plasma-derived and recombinant. Plasma-derived vaccine is no longer available in the United States, but is produced in several countries and used in many immunization programs worldwide. Recombinant vaccines available in the United States are Recombivax HB™ (Merck and Company, Inc., West Point, Pennsylvania) and Engerix-B® (SmithKline Beecham Biologicals, Philadelphia, Pennsylvania). Recombivax HB™ contains 10–40 μg of HBsAg protein per mL, whereas Engerix-B® contains 20 μg/mL.

Primary vaccination comprises three intramuscular doses of vaccine, with the second and third doses given 1 and 6 months, respectively, after the first. An alternative schedule of four doses given at 0, 1, 2, and 12 months to persons with normal immune status or at 0, 1, 2, and 6 months to hemodialysis patients has been approved for Engerix-B®.

Immunogenicity

The recommended primary series of hepatitis B vaccine induces a protective anti-HBs response [defined as ≥10 milli-International Units (mIU)/mL] in 90–95% of adults with normal immune status. The major determinant of vaccine response is age, with the proportion of persons developing a protective antibody response declining to 84% among adults aged >40 years and to 75% by age 60 years. Other host factors that contribute to decreased immunogenicity include smoking, obesity, and immune suppression. Compared with adults with normal immune status, the proportion of hemodialysis patients who develop a protective antibody response after vaccination (with higher dosages) is lower. For those who receive the three-dose schedule, the median is 64% (range: 34–88%), and for those who receive the four-dose schedule, the median is 86% (range: 40–98%).

Limited data indicate that concurrent infection with HCV does not interfere with development of protective levels of antibody after vaccination, although lower titers of anti-HBs have been reported after vaccination of HCV-positive patients compared with HCV-negative patients.

Vaccine Efficacy

For persons with normal immune status, controlled clinical trials have demonstrated that protection from acute and chronic HBV infection is virtually complete among those who develop a protective antibody response after vaccination. Among hemodialysis patients, controlled clinical trials conducted in other countries demonstrated efficacy of 53–78% after preexposure immunization.

Since the hepatitis B vaccine became available, no HBV infections have been reported among vaccinated hemodialysis patients who maintained protective levels of anti-HBs. This observation has been particularly striking during HBV infection outbreaks in this setting. In addition, a case-control study indicated that the risk for HBV infection was 70% lower among hemodialysis patients who had been vaccinated .Thus, most hemodialysis patients can be protected from hepatitis B by vaccination, and maintaining immunity among these patients reduces the frequency and costs of serologic screening.

Revaccination of Nonresponders

Among persons who do not respond to the primary three-dose series of hepatitis

B vaccine, 25–50% of those with normal immune status respond to one additional vaccine dose, and 50–75% respond to three additional doses. A revaccination regimen that includes serologic testing after one or two additional doses of vaccine appears to be no more cost-effective than serologic testing performed after all three additional doses. For persons found to be nonresponders after six doses of vaccine, no data exist to indicate that additional doses would induce an antibody response.

Few studies have been conducted of the effect of revaccination among hemodialysis patients who do not respond to the primary vaccine series. Response rates to revaccination varied from 40–50% after two or three additional 40 µg intramuscular doses to 64% after four additional 10 µg intramuscular doses.

Antibody Persistence

Among adults with normal immune status who responded to a primary vaccine series with a protective antibody level, antibody remained above protective levels in 40–87% of persons after 9–15 years. Only short-term data are available for hemodialysis patients. Among adults who responded to the primary vaccination series, antibody remained detectable for 6 months in 80–100% (median: 100%) of persons and for 12 months in 58–100% (median: 70%). Among successfully immunized hemodialysis patients whose antibody titers subsequently declined below protective levels, limited data indicate that virtually all respond to a booster dose.

Duration of Vaccine-induced Immunity

Among persons with normal immune status who respond to the primary series of hepatitis B vaccine, protection against hepatitis B persists even when antibody titers become undetectable. However, among hemodialysis patients who respond to the vaccine, protection against hepatitis B is not maintained when antibody titers fall below protective levels.

HEPATITIS C INFECTION[1]

Epidemiology

Incidence and Prevalence

Since 1990, limited data from US studies using testing for antibody to HCV (anti-HCV) to evaluate the incidence of HCV infection have reported annual rates of 0.73–3% among hemodialysis patients. None of the patients who seroconverted had received transfusions in the interim or were injecting-drug users.

During 1992–1999, national surveillance data indicated that the proportion of centers that tested patients for anti-HCV increased from 22–56% (CDC, unpublished data, 2001). In 1999, nationwide prevalence of anti-HCV was 8.9%, with some centers reporting prevalences >40% (CDC, unpublished data, 2001). Other studies of hemodialysis patients in the United States have reported anti-HCV prevalences of 10–36% among adults and 18.5% among children.

Transmission

HCV is most efficiently transmitted by direct percutaneous exposure to infectious blood, and like HBV, the chronically infected person is central to the epidemiology of HCV transmission. Risk factors associated with HCV infection among hemodialysis patients include history of blood transfusions, the volume of blood transfused, and years on dialysis. The number of years on dialysis is the major risk factor independently associated with higher rates of HCV infection. As the time patients spent on dialysis increased, their prevalence of HCV infection increased from an average of 12% for patients receiving dialysis <5 years to an average of 37% for patients receiving dialysis ≥5 years.

These studies, as well as investigations of dialysis-associated outbreaks of hepatitis C, indicate that HCV transmission most likely occurs because of inadequate infection control practices. During 1999–2000, CDC investigated three outbreaks of HCV infection among patients in chronic hemodialysis centers (CDC, unpublished data, 1999 and 2000). In two of the outbreaks, multiple transmissions of HCV occurred during periods of 16–24 months (attack rates: 6.6–17.5%), and seroconversions were associated with receiving dialysis immediately after a chronically infected patient. Multiple opportunities for cross-contamination among patients were observed, including (a) equipment and supplies that were not disinfected between patient use; (b) use of common medication carts to prepare and distribute medications at patients' stations; (c) sharing of multiple dose medication vials, which were placed at patients' stations on top of hemodialysis machines; (d) contaminated priming buckets that were not routinely changed or cleaned and disinfected between patients; (e) machine surfaces that were not routinely cleaned and disinfected between patients; and (f) blood spills that were not cleaned up promptly. In the third outbreak, multiple new infections clustered at one point in time (attack rate: 27%), suggesting a common exposure event. Although, the specific results of this investigation are pending, multiple opportunities for cross-contamination from chronically infected patients also were observed in this unit. In particular, supply carts were moved from one station to another and contained both clean supplies and blood-contaminated items, including small biohazard containers, sharps disposal boxes, and used vacutainers containing patients' blood.

Clinical Features and Natural History

HCV causes both acute and chronic hepatitis. The incubation period ranges from 14–180 days (average: 6–7 weeks). Persons with newly acquired (acute) HCV infection typically are either asymptomatic or have a mild clinical illness. The course of acute hepatitis C is variable, although elevations in serum alanine aminotransferase (ALT) levels, often in a fluctuating pattern, are the most characteristic feature. Fulminant hepatic failure after acute hepatitis C is rare.

Most (average: 94%) hemodialysis patients with newly acquired HCV infection have elevated serum ALT levels. Elevations in serum ALT levels often precede anti-HCV seroconversion. Among prospectively followed transfusion recipients who developed acute HCV infection, elevated ALT levels preceded anti-HCV seroconversion (as measured by second generation assays) in 59%, and anti-HCV was detectable in most patients (78%) within 5 weeks after their first ALT elevation. However, elevations in ALT or aspartate aminotransferase (AST) levels can occur that are not related to viral hepatitis, and compared with ALT, AST is a less specific indicator of HCV-related liver disease among hemodialysis patients. In a recent outbreak investigation, only 28% of 25 hemodialysis patients with newly observed elevations in AST levels tested anti-HCV positive (CDC, unpublished data, 1999).

After acute HCV infection, 15–25% of persons with normal immune status appear to resolve their infection without sequelae as defined by sustained absence of HCV RNA in serum and normalization of ALT. In some persons, ALT levels normalize, suggesting full recovery, but this is frequently followed by ALT elevations that indicate progression to chronic disease. Chronic HCV infection develops in most infected persons (75–85%). Of persons with chronic HCV infection, 60–70% have persistent or fluctuating ALT elevations, indicating active liver disease. Although similar rates of chronic liver disease have been observed among HCV-infected chronic hemodialysis patients (based on liver biopsy results), these patients might be less likely to have biochemical evidence of active liver disease. In seroprevalence studies of chronic hemodialysis patients, ALT elevations were reported in a median of 33.9% (range: 6–73%) of patients who tested positive for anti-HCV.

No clinical or epidemiologic features among patients with acute infection have been reported to be predictive of either persistent infection or chronic liver disease. Most studies have reported that cirrhosis develops in 10–20% of persons who have had chronic hepatitis C for 20–30 years, and hepatocellular carcinoma in 1–5%. Extrahepatic manifestations of chronic HCV infection are considered to be of immunologic origin and include cryoglobulinemia, membranoproliferative glomerulonephritis, and porphyria cutanea tarda.

At least six different genotypes and >90 subtypes of HCV exist. Unlike HBV, infection with one HCV genotype or subtype does not protect against reinfection or superinfection with other HCV strains.

Alpha interferon alone or in combination with ribavirin is FDA-approved for the treatment of chronic hepatitis C. Combination therapy should be used with caution in patients with creatinine clearance <50 mL/minute and generally is contraindicated in patients with renal failure. Interferon monotherapy results in low sustained virologic response rates.

Screening and Diagnostic Tests

Serologic Assays

The only FDA-approved tests for diagnosis of HCV infection are those that measure anti-HCV and include enzyme immunoassays (EIAs) and a supplemental recombinant immunoblot assay (RIBA™). These tests detect anti-HCV in ≥97% of infected persons, but do not distinguish between acute, chronic, or resolved infection. The average time from exposure to seroconversion is 8–9 weeks. Anti-HCV can be detected in 80% of patients within 15 weeks after exposure, in ≥90% within 5 months, and in ≥97% within 6 months. In rare instances, seroconversion can be delayed until 9 months after exposure. Anti-HCV persists indefinitely in most persons, but does not protect against reinfection.

As with any screening test, the positive predictive value of EIAs for anti-HCV is directly related to the prevalence of infection in the population and is low in populations with an HCV-infection prevalence <10%. Supplemental testing with a more specific assay (i.e. RIBA™) of a specimen with a positive anti-HCV result by EIA prevents reporting of false-positive results, particularly in settings where asymptomatic persons are being tested. Results of seroprevalence studies among chronic hemodialysis patients have indicated that 57–100% of EIA positive results were RIBA™ positive, and 53–100% were HCV RNA positive by reverse transcriptase polymerase chain reaction (RT-PCR) testing.

Nucleic Acid Detection

The diagnosis of HCV infection also can be made by qualitatively detecting HCV RNA using gene amplification techniques (e.g. RT-PCR). HCV RNA can be detected in serum or plasma within 1–2 weeks after exposure and weeks before onset of ALT elevations or the appearance of anti-HCV. In rare instances, detection of HCV RNA might be the only evidence of HCV infection. Although a median of 3.4% (range: 0–28%) of chronic hemodialysis patients who tested anti-HCV negative were HCV RNA positive, this might be an overestimate because follow-up samples to detect possible antibody seroconversions were not obtained on these patients.

Although not FDA-approved, RT-PCR assays for HCV infection are used commonly in clinical practice and are commercially available. Most RT-PCR assays have a lower limit of detection of 100–1,000 viral genome copies per mL. With adequate optimization of RT-PCR assays, 75–85% of persons who are positive for anti-HCV and >95% of persons with acute or chronic hepatitis C will test positive for HCV RNA. Some HCV-infected persons might be only intermittently HCV RNA positive, particularly those with acute hepatitis C or with end-stage liver disease caused by hepatitis C. To minimize false-negative results, blood samples collected for RT-PCR should not contain heparin, and serum must be separated from cellular components within 2–4 hours after collection and preferably stored frozen at –20°C or

-70°C. If shipping is required, frozen samples should be protected from thawing. Because of assay variability, rigorous quality assurance and control should be in place in clinical laboratories performing this assay, and proficiency testing is recommended.

Quantitative assays for measuring the concentration (i.e. titer) of HCV RNA have been developed and are available from commercial laboratories. These assays also are not FDA-approved and are less sensitive than qualitative RT-PCR assays. Quantitative assays should not be used as a primary test to confirm or exclude the diagnosis of HCV infection or to monitor the endpoint of treatment, and sequential measurement of HCV RNA levels has not proven useful in managing patients with hepatitis C.

HEPATITIS DELTA VIRUS INFECTION[1]

Delta hepatitis is caused by the hepatitis delta virus (HDV), a defective virus that causes infection only in persons with active HBV infection. The prevalence of HDV infection is low in the United States, with rates of <1% among HBsAg-positive persons in the general population and ≥10% among HBsAg-positive persons with repeated percutaneous exposures (e.g. injecting-drug users, persons with hemophilia). Areas of the world with high endemic rates of HDV infection include southern Italy, parts of Africa, and the Amazon Basin.

Few data exist on the prevalence of HDV infection among chronic hemodialysis patients, and only one transmission of HDV between such patients has been reported in the United States. In this episode, transmission occurred from a patient who was chronically infected with HBV and HDV to an HBsAg-positive patient after a massive bleeding incident; both patients received dialysis at the same station.

HDV infection occurs either as a co-infection with HBV or as a superinfection in a person with chronic HBV infection. Co-infection usually resolves, but superinfection frequently results in chronic HDV infection and severe disease. High mortality rates are associated with both types of infection. A serologic test that measures total antibody to HDV (anti-HDV) is commercially available.

HUMAN IMMUNODEFICIENCY VIRUS INFECTION[1]

During 1985–1999, the percentage of US hemodialysis centers that reported providing chronic hemodialysis for patients with HIV infection increased from 11–39%, and the proportion of hemodialysis patients with known HIV infection increased from 0.3–1.4% (CDC, unpublished data, 2001).

HIV is transmitted by blood and other body fluids that contain blood. No patient-to-patient transmission of HIV has been reported in US hemodialysis centers. However, such transmission has been reported in other countries; in one case, HIV transmission was attributed to mixing of reused access needles and inadequate disinfection of equipment.

HIV infection is usually diagnosed with assays that measure antibody to HIV, and a repeatedly positive EIA test should be confirmed by Western blot or another confirmatory test. Antiretroviral therapies for HIV-infected hemodialysis patients are commonly used and appear to be improving survival rates among this population. However, hepatotoxicity associated with certain protease inhibitors might limit the use of these drugs, especially in patients with underlying liver dysfunction.

BACTERIAL INFECTIONS[1]

Epidemiology

Disease Burden

The annual mortality rate among hemodialysis patients is 23%, and infections are the second most common cause, accounting for 15% of deaths. Septicemia (10.9% of all deaths) is the most common infectious cause of mortality. In various studies evaluating rates of bacterial infections in hemodialysis outpatients, bacteremia occurred in 0.63–1.7% of patients per month and vascular access infections (with or without bacteremia) in 1.3–7.2% of patients per month.

Infection Sites

Common sites involved in hemodialysis patients are vascular access, lungs, the urinary tract, skin and soft tissues, and other or unknown sites. The vascular access site is the most common site for infection. However, access site infections are particularly important because they can cause disseminated bacteremia or loss of the vascular access.

Vascular Access Infections

Vascular access infections are caused (in descending order of frequency) by *S. aureus,* coagulase-negative staphylococci (CNS), gram-negative bacilli, nonstaphylococcal gram-positive cocci (including enterococci), and fungi. The proportion of infections caused by CNS is higher among patients dialyzed through catheters than among patients dialyzed through fistulas or grafts.

The primary risk factor for access infection is access type, with catheters having the highest risk for infection, grafts intermediate, and native arteriovenous (AV) fistulas the lowest. Other potential risk factors for vascular access infections include (a) location of the access in the lower extremity; (b) recent access surgery; (c) trauma, hematoma, dermatitis, or scratching over the access site; (d) poor patient hygiene; (e) poor needle insertion technique; (f) older age; (g) diabetes; (h) immunosuppression; and (i) iron overload.

Transmission

Bacterial pathogens causing infection can be either exogenous (i.e. acquired from contaminated dialysis fluids or equipment) or endogenous (i.e. caused by invasion of bacteria present in or on the patient). Exogenous pathogens have caused numerous outbreaks, most of which resulted from inadequate dialyzer reprocessing procedures (e.g. contaminated water or inadequate disinfectant) or inadequate treatment of municipal water for use in dialysis.

Contaminated medication vials also are a potential source of bacterial infection for patients. In 1999, an outbreak of *Serratia liquefaciens* bloodstream infections and pyrogenic reactions among hemodialysis patients was traced to contamination of vials of erythropoietin. These vials, which were intended for single use, were contaminated by repeated puncture to obtain additional doses and by pooling of residual medication into a common vial.

Endogenous pathogens first colonize the patient and later cause infection. Colonization means that microorganisms have become resident in or on the body (e.g. in the nares or stool); a culture from the site is positive, but no symptoms or signs of infection exist. Colonization with potentially pathogenic microorganisms, often unknown to staff members, is common in patients with frequent exposure to hospitals and other healthcare settings. Colonization most often occurs when microorganisms are transmitted from a colonized or infected source patient to another patient on the hands of healthcare workers who do not comply with infection control precautions. Less commonly, contamination of environmental surfaces (e.g. bed rails, countertops) plays a role.

Infection occurs when microorganisms invade the body, damaging tissue and causing signs or symptoms of infection, and is aided by invasive devices (e.g. the hemodialysis vascular access). Evidence exists that when prevalence of colonization in a population is less frequent, infection in that population will also be less frequent, and infection control recommendations for hemodialysis units are designed to prevent colonization.

Antimicrobial Resistance[1]

Antimicrobial-resistant bacteria are more common in patients with severe illness, who often have had multiple hospitalizations or surgical procedures, and in those who have received prolonged courses of antimicrobial agents. In healthcare settings, including hemodialysis centers, such patients can serve as a source for transmission.

Clinically important drug-resistant bacteria that commonly cause healthcare-associated infections include MRSA, methicillin-resistant CNS, VRE, and multidrug-resistant gram-negative rods, including strains of *Pseudomonas aeruginosa*, *Stenotrophomonas maltophilia*, and *Acinetobacter* species, some of which are resistant to all available antimicrobials. In addition, strains of *S. aureus* with intermediate resistance to vancomycin and other glycopeptide antibiotics have recently been reported; these strains are called vancomycin-intermediate *S. aureus* (VISA) or glycopeptide-intermediate *S. aureus* (GISA). Intermediate resistance to vancomycin is reported even more frequently among CNS.

Prevalence of VRE has increased rapidly at US hospitals; among intensive care unit patients with nosocomial infections reported to the National Nosocomial Infections Surveillance (NNIS) system, the percentage of enterococcal isolates resistant to vancomycin increased from 0.5% in 1989 to 25.2% in 1999. (CDC, unpublished data, 2000). This increase is attributable to patient-to-patient transmission in healthcare settings and transmission of resistant genes among previously susceptible enterococci. Once vancomycin resistance has been transferred to a patient, antimicrobials select for resistant organisms, causing them to increase in number relative to susceptible organisms.

Vancomycin Use

Dialysis patients have played a prominent role in the epidemic of vancomycin resistance because this drug is used commonly in these patients, in part because vancomycin can be conveniently administered to patients when they come in for hemodialysis treatments. However, two studies indicate that cefazolin, a first-generation cephalosporin, could be substituted for vancomycin in many patients.[8,9] One of these studies reported that many pathogens causing infections in hemodialysis patients are susceptible to cefazolin,[7] and both studies reported therapeutic cefazolin blood levels 48–72 hours after dosing, making in-center administration three times a week after dialysis feasible.

RECOMMENDATIONS[1]

Rationale

Preventing transmission among chronic hemodialysis patients of blood-borne viruses and pathogenic bacteria from both recognized and unrecognized sources of infection requires implementation of a comprehensive infection control program. The components of such a program include infection control practices specifically designed for the hemodialysis setting, including routine serologic testing and immunization, surveillance, and training and education (Box 12.1).

The infection control practices recommended for hemodialysis units will reduce opportunities for patient-to-patient transmission of infectious agents, directly or indirectly via contaminated devices, equipment and supplies, environmental surfaces, or hands of personnel. These practices should be carried out routinely for all patients in the chronic hemodialysis setting because of the increased potential for blood contamination during hemodialysis and because many patients are colonized or infected with pathogenic bacteria. Such practices include additional measures to prevent HBV transmission because of the high titer of HBV and its ability to survive on environmental surfaces. For patients at increased risk for transmission of pathogenic bacteria, including antimicrobial-resistant strains, additional precautions also might be necessary in some circumstances.

Box 12.1: Components of a comprehensive infection control program to prevent transmission of infections among chronic hemodialysis patients

- Infection control practices for hemodialysis units.
  - Infection control precautions specifically designed to prevent transmission of blood-borne viruses and pathogenic bacteria among patients
  - Routine serologic testing for hepatitis B virus and hepatitis C virus infections
  - Vaccination of susceptible patients against hepatitis B
  - Isolation of patients who test positive for hepatitis B surface antigen
- Surveillance for infections and other adverse events
- Infection control training and education

Furthermore, surveillance for infections and other adverse events is required to monitor the effectiveness of infection control practices, as well as training and education of both staff members and patients to ensure that appropriate infection control behaviors and techniques are carried out.

Infection Control Practices for Hemodialysis Units

In each chronic hemodialysis unit, policies and practices should be reviewed and updated to ensure that infection control practices recommended for hemodialysis units are implemented and rigorously followed. Intensive efforts must be made to educate new staff members and reeducate existing staff members regarding these practices.

Infection Control Precautions for All Patients

During the process of hemodialysis, exposure to blood and potentially contaminated items can be routinely anticipated; thus, gloves are required whenever caring for a patient or touching the patient's equipment. To facilitate glove use, a supply of clean nonsterile gloves and a glove discard container should be placed near each dialysis station. Hands always should be washed after gloves are removed and between patient contacts, as well as after touching blood, body fluids, secretions, excretions, and contaminated items. A sufficient number of sinks with warm water and soap should be available to facilitate hand washing. If hands are not visibly soiled, use of a waterless antiseptic hand rub can be substituted for hand washing.

Any item taken to a patient's dialysis station could become contaminated with blood and other body fluids and serve as a vehicle of transmission to other patients either directly or by contamination of the hands of personnel. Therefore, items taken to a patient's dialysis station, including those placed on top of dialysis machines, should either be disposed of, dedicated for use only on a single patient, or cleaned and disinfected before being returned to a common clean area or used for other patients. Unused medications or supplies (e.g. syringes, alcohol swabs) taken to the patient's station should not be returned to a common clean area or used on other patients.

Additional measures to prevent contamination of clean or sterile items include (a) preparing medications in a room or area separated from the patient treatment area and designated only for medications; (b) not handling or storing contaminated (i.e. used) supplies, equipment, blood samples, or biohazard containers in areas where medications and clean (i.e. unused) equipment and supplies are handled; and (c) delivering medications separately to each patient. Common carts should not be used within the patient treatment area to prepare or distribute medications. If trays are used to distribute medications, clean them before using for a different patient.

Intravenous medication vials labeled for single use, including erythropoietin, should not be punctured more than once.[10,11] Once a needle has entered a vial labeled for single use, the sterility of the product can no longer be guaranteed. Residual medication from two or more vials should not be pooled into a single vial.

If a common supply cart is used to store clean supplies in the patient treatment area, this cart should remain in a designated area at a sufficient distance from patient stations to avoid contamination with blood. Such carts should not be moved between stations to distribute supplies.

Staff members should wear gowns, face shields, eye wear, or masks to protect themselves and prevent soiling of clothing when performing procedures during which spurting or spattering of blood might occur (e.g. during initiation and termination of dialysis, cleaning of dialyzers, and centrifugation of blood). Such protective clothing or gear should be changed if it becomes soiled with blood, body fluids, secretions, or excretions. Staff members should not eat, drink, or smoke in the dialysis treatment area or in the laboratory. However, patients can be served meals or eat food brought from home at their dialysis station. The glasses, dishes, and other utensils should be cleaned in the usual manner; no special care of these items is needed.

Cleaning and Disinfection

Establish written protocols for cleaning and disinfecting surfaces and equipment in the dialysis unit, including careful mechanical cleaning before any disinfection process (Table 12.2). If the manufacturer has provided instructions on sterilization or disinfection of the item, these instructions should be followed. For each chemical sterilant and disinfectant, follow the manufacturer's instructions regarding use, including appropriate dilution and contact time.

After each patient treatment, clean environmental surfaces at the dialysis station, including the dialysis bed or chair, countertops, and external surfaces of the dialysis machine, including containers associated with the prime waste. Use any soap, detergent, or detergent germicide. Between uses of medical equipment (e.g. scissors, hemostats, clamps, stethoscopes, blood pressure cuffs), clean and apply a hospital disinfectant (i.e. low-level disinfection); if the item is visibly contaminated with blood, use a tuberculocidal disinfectant (i.e. intermediate-level disinfection).

For a blood spill, immediately clean the area with a cloth soaked with a tuberculocidal disinfectant or a 1:100 dilution of household bleach (300–600 mg/L free chlorine) (i.e. intermediate-level disinfection). The staff member doing the cleaning should wear gloves, and the cloth should be placed in a bucket or other leak-proof container. After all visible blood is cleaned, use a new cloth or towel to apply disinfectant a second time.

Table 12.2: Disinfection procedures recommended for commonly used items or surfaces in hemodialysis units

Item or surface	Low-level disinfection*	Intermediate-level disinfection*
Gross blood spills or items contaminated with visible blood		×
Hemodialyzer port caps		×
Interior pathways of dialysis machine		×
Water treatment of distribution system	×	×†
Scissors, hemostats, clamps, blood pressure cuffs, stethoscopes	×	×§
Environmental surfaces, including exterior surfaces of hemodialysis machines	×	

*Careful mechanical cleaning to remove debris should always be done before disinfection

†Water treatment and distribution systems of dialysis fluid concentrates require more extensive disinfection if significant biofilm is present within the system.

§If item is visibly contaminated with blood, use a tuberculocidal disinfectant.

Published methods should be used to clean and disinfect the water treatment and distribution system and the internal circuits of the dialysis machine, as well as to reprocess dialyzers for reuse. These methods are designed to control bacterial contamination, but will also eliminate blood-borne viruses. For single-pass machines, perform rinsing and disinfection procedures at the beginning or end of the day. For batch recirculating machines, drain, rinse, and disinfect after each use. Follow the same methods for cleaning and disinfection if a blood leak has occurred, regardless of the type of dialysis machine used. Routine bacteriologic assays of water and dialysis fluids should be performed according to the recommendations of the Association for the Advancement of Medical Instrumentation.

Venous pressure transducer protectors should be used to cover pressure monitors and should be changed between patients, not reused. If the external transducer protector becomes wet, replace immediately and inspect the protector. If fluid is visible on the side of the transducer protector that faces the machine, have qualified personnel open the machine after the treatment is completed and check for contamination. This includes inspection for possible blood contamination of the internal pressure tubing set and pressure sensing port. If contamination has occurred, the machine must be taken out of service and disinfected using either 1:100 dilution of bleach (300–600 mg/L free chlorine) or a commercially available, EPA-registered tuberculocidal germicide before reuse. Frequent blood line pressure alarms or frequent adjusting of blood drip chamber levels can be an indicator of this problem. Taken separately, these incidents could be characterized as isolated malfunctions. However, the potential public health significance of the total number of incidents nationwide make it imperative that all incidents of equipment contamination be reported immediately to the FDA.

Housekeeping staff members in the dialysis facility should promptly remove soil and potentially infectious waste and maintain an environment that enhances patient care. All disposable items should be placed in bags thick enough to prevent leakage. Wastes generated by the hemodialysis facility might be contaminated with blood and should be considered infectious and handled accordingly. These solid medical wastes should be disposed of properly in an incinerator or sanitary landfill, according to local and state regulations governing medical waste disposal.

Hemodialysis in Acute-care Settings

For patients with acute renal failure who receive hemodialysis in acute-care settings, standard precautions as applied in all healthcare settings are sufficient to prevent transmission of blood-borne viruses. However, when chronic hemodialysis patients receive maintenance hemodialysis while hospitalized, infection control precautions specifically designed for chronic hemodialysis units should be applied to these patients. If both acute and chronic renal failure patients receive hemodialysis in the same unit, these infection control precautions should be applied to all patients.

Regardless of where in the acute-care setting chronic hemodialysis patients receive dialysis, the HBsAg status of all such patients should be ascertained at the time of admission to the hospital, by either a written report from the referring center (including the most recent date testing was performed) or by a serologic test. The HBV serologic status should be prominently placed in patients' hospital records, and all healthcare personnel assigned to these patients, as well as the infection control practitioner, should be aware of the patients' serologic status. While hospitalized, HBsAg-positive chronic hemodialysis patients should undergo dialysis in a separate room and use separate machines, equipment, instruments, supplies, and medications designated only for HBsAg-positive patients. While HBsAg-positive patients are receiving dialysis, staff members who are caring for them should not care for susceptible patients.

Routine Serologic Testing

Chronic Hemodialysis Patients

Routinely test all chronic hemodialysis patients for HBV and HCV infection, promptly review results, and ensure that patients are managed appropriately based on their testing results (see later recommendations for each virus). Communicate test results (positive and negative) to other units or hospitals when patients are transferred for care. Routine testing for HDV or HIV infection for purposes of infection control is not recommended.

The HBV serologic status (i.e. HBsAg, total anti-HBc, and anti-HBs) of all patients should be known before admission to the hemodialysis unit. For patients transferred from another unit, test results should be obtained before the patients' transfer. If a patient's HBV serologic status is not known at the time of admission, testing should be completed within 7 days. The hemodialysis unit should ensure that the laboratory performing the testing for anti-HBs can define a 10 mIU/mL concentration to determine protective levels of antibody.

Routine HCV testing should include use of both an EIA to test for anti-HCV and supplemental or confirmatory testing with an additional, more specific assay (Fig. 12.1). Use of RT-PCR for HCV RNA as the primary test for routine screening is not recommended because few HCV infections will be identified in anti-HCV negative patients. However, if ALT levels are persistently abnormal in patients who are anti-HCV negative in the absence of another etiology, testing for HCV RNA should be considered.

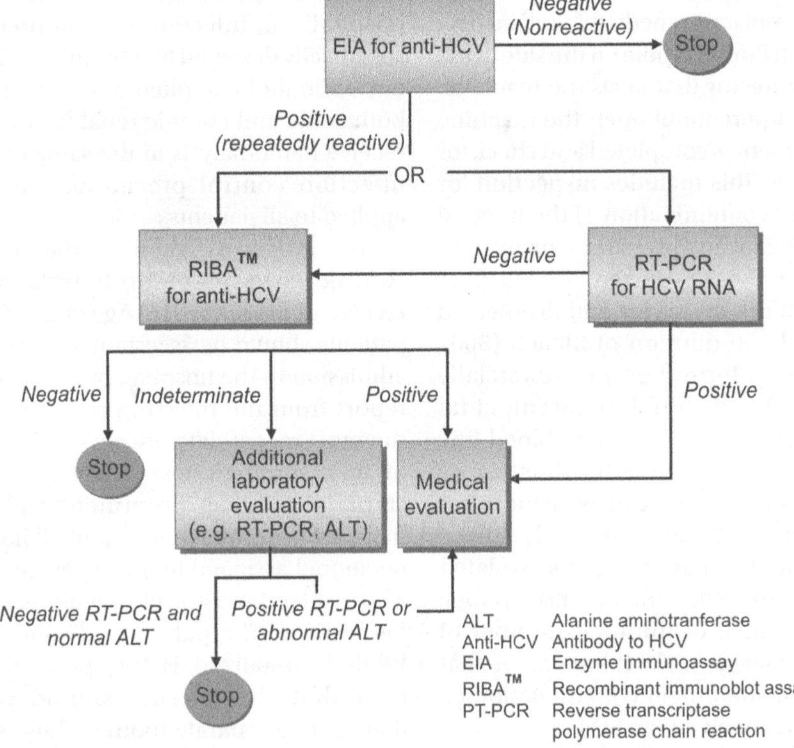

Fig. 12.1: Algorithm for hepatitis C virus (HCV) infection testing among persons who are asymptomatic
Source: CDC, Recommendations for prevention and control of hepatitis C virus (HCV) infection and HCV-related chronic disease. MMWR: 1998;47(No. RR-19):27.

Hemodialysis Staff Members

Previously, testing for HBV infection was recommended for all staff members at the time of employment and for susceptible staff members at routine intervals thereafter; however, such testing is no longer considered necessary. The risk for HBV infection among hemodialysis staff members is no greater than that for other healthcare workers. Thus, routine testing of staff members is not recommended except when required to document response to hepatitis B vaccination (see Postvaccination Testing and Revaccination of Nonresponders). Routine testing of staff members for HCV, HDV, or HIV infection is not recommended.

Hepatitis B Vaccination

Vaccine Schedule and Dose

Hepatitis B vaccination is recommended for all susceptible chronic hemodialysis patients and for all staff members (Table 12.3). Vaccination is recommended for pre-end-stage renal disease patients before they become dialysis dependent and for peritoneal and home dialysis patients because they might require in-center hemodialysis. Hepatitis B vaccine should be administered by the intramuscular route and only in the deltoid muscle for adults and children. Intradermal or subcutaneous administration of hepatitis B vaccine is not recommended.

If an adult patient begins the vaccine series with a standard dose before beginning hemodialysis treatment, then moves to hemodialysis treatment before completing the series, complete the series using the higher dose recommended for hemodialysis patients (Table 12.3). No specific recommendations have been made for higher doses for pediatric hemodialysis patients. If a lower than recommended vaccine dose is administered to either adults or children, the dose should be repeated.

If the vaccination series is interrupted after the first dose, the second dose should be administered as soon as possible. For the three-dose primary vaccine series, the second and third doses should be separated by an interval of at least 2 months; if only the third dose is delayed, that dose should be administered when convenient. When hepatitis B vaccine has been administered at the same time as other vaccines, no interference with the antibody response of the other vaccines has been demonstrated.

Table 12.3: Doses and schedules of licensed hepatitis B vaccines hemodialysis patients and staff members

Group	Recombivax HG™*			Engerix-B†		
	Dose	Volume	Schedule	Dose	Volume	Schedule
Patients aged ≥ 20 years						
Predialysis§	10 µg	1.0 mL	0, 1, and 6 months	20 µg	1.0 mL	0, 1, and 6 months
Dialysis-dependent	40 µg	1.0 mL¶	0, 1, and 6 months	40 µg	2–1.0 mL doses at one site	0, 1, 2, and 6 months
Patients aged <20 years**	5 µg	0.5 mL	0, 1, and 6 months	10 µg	0.5 mL	0, 1, and 6 months
Staff members aged ≥20 years	10 µg	1.0 mL	0, 1, and 6 months	20 µg	1.0 mL	0, 1, and 6 months

*Merck and Company, Inc., West Point, Pennsylvania.
†SmithKline Beecham Biologicals, Philadelphia, Pennsylvania.
§Immunogenicity might depend on degree or renal insufficiency.
¶Special formulation.
**Does for all persons aged <20 years approved by the US Food and Drug Administration; for hemodialysis patients, higher does might be more immunogenic.
Note: All does should be administered in the deltoid by the intramuscular route.

Postvaccination Testing and Revaccination of Nonresponders

Test all vaccinees for anti-HBs 1-2 months after the last primary vaccine dose, to determine their response to the vaccine (adequate response is defined as ≥10 mIU/mL). Patients and staff members who do not respond to the primary vaccine series should be revaccinated with three additional doses and retested for response. No additional doses of vaccine are warranted for those who do not respond to the second series.

Evaluate staff members who do not respond to revaccination to determine if they are HBsAg positive. Persons who are HBsAg positive should be counseled accordingly (e.g. need for medical evaluation, vaccination of sexual and household contacts). Primary nonresponders to vaccination who are HBsAg negative should be considered susceptible to HBV infection and counseled regarding precautions to prevent HBV infection and the need to obtain postexposure prophylaxis with hepatitis B immune globulin for any known or probable percutaneous or mucosal exposure to HBsAg-positive blood.

Follow-up of Vaccine Responders

Retest patients who respond to the vaccine annually for anti-HBs. If anti-HBs declines to <10 mIU/mL, administer a booster dose of hepatitis B vaccine and continue to retest annually. Retesting immediately after the booster dose is not necessary. For staff members who respond to the vaccine, booster doses of vaccine are not necessary, and periodic serologic testing to monitor antibody concentrations is not recommended.

Patients with a History of Vaccination

Routine childhood vaccination against hepatitis B has been recommended since 1991 and routine adolescent vaccination since 1995. Thus, many persons who develop end-stage renal failure will have a history of vaccination against hepatitis B. These persons should have responded to the vaccine when their immune status was normal, but if their anti-HBs levels are <10 mIU/mL when they begin dialysis, they should be revaccinated with a complete primary series.

Prevention and Management of HBV Infection

Preventing HBV transmission among chronic hemodialysis patients requires (a) infection control precautions recommended for all hemodialysis patients; (b) routine serologic testing for markers of HBV infection and prompt review of results; (c) isolation of HBsAg-positive patients with dedicated room, machine, other equipment, supplies, and staff members; and (d) vaccination. Additional infection control practices are needed because of the potential for environmentally mediated transmission of HBV, rather than internal contamination of dialysis machines. The need for routine follow-up testing, vaccination, or isolation is based on patients' serologic status (Table 12.1).

HBV-susceptible Patients

Vaccinate all susceptible patients (see hepatitis B vaccination). Test susceptible patients monthly for HBsAg, including those who (a) have not yet received hepatitis B vaccine, (b) are in the process of being vaccinated, or (c) have not adequately responded to vaccination. Although, the incidence of HBV infection is low among chronic hemodialysis patients, preventing transmission depends on timely detection of patients converting from HBsAg negative to HBsAg positive and rapid implementation of isolation procedures before cross-contamination can occur.

HBsAg Seroconversions

When a seroconversion occurs, review all patients' routine laboratory test results to identify additional cases. Perform additional testing as indicated later in this section. Investigate potential sources for infection to determine if transmission might have occurred within the dialysis unit, including review of newly infected patients' recent medical history (e.g. blood transfusion, hospitalization), history of high-risk behavior (e.g. injecting-drug use, sexual activity), and unit practices and procedures.

In patients newly infected with HBV, HBsAg often is the only serologic marker initially detected; repeat HBsAg testing and test for anti-HBc (including IgM anti-HBc) 1–2 months later. Six months later, repeat HBsAg testing and test for anti-HBs to determine clinical outcome and need for counseling, medical evaluation, and vaccination of contacts. Patients who become HBsAg negative are no longer infectious and can be removed from isolation.

HBV-infected Patients

To isolate HBsAg-positive patients, designate a separate room for their treatment and dedicate machines, equipment, instruments, supplies, and medications that will not be used by HBV-susceptible patients. Most importantly, staff members who are caring for HBsAg-positive patients should not care for susceptible patients at the same time, including during the period when dialysis is terminated on one patient and initiated on another.

Newly opened units should have isolation rooms for the dialysis of HBsAg-positive patients. For existing units in which a separate room is not possible, HBsAg-positive patients should be separated from HBV-susceptible patients in an area removed from the mainstream of activity and should undergo dialysis on dedicated machines. If a machine that has been used on an HBsAg-positive patient is needed for an HBV-susceptible patient, internal pathways of the machine can be disinfected using conventional protocols and external surfaces cleaned using soap and water or a detergent germicide.

Dialyzers should not be reused on HBsAg-positive patients. Because HBV is efficiently transmitted through occupational exposure to blood, reprocessing dialyzers from HBsAg-positive patients might place HBV-susceptible staff members at increased risk for infection.

Chronically infected patients (i.e. those who are HBsAg positive, total anti-HBc positive, and IgM anti-HBc negative) are infectious to others and are at risk for chronic liver disease. They should be counseled regarding preventing transmission to others, their household and sexual partners should receive hepatitis B vaccine, and they should be evaluated (by consultation or referral, if appropriate) for the presence or development of chronic liver disease according to current medical practice guidelines. Persons with chronic liver disease should be vaccinated against hepatitis A, if susceptible.

Chronically infected patients do not require any routine follow-up testing for purposes of infection control. However, annual testing for HBsAg is reasonable to detect the small percentage of HBV-infected patients who might lose their HBsAg.

HBV-immune Patients

Annual anti-HBs testing of patients who are positive for anti-HBs (≥10 mIU/mL) and negative for anti-HBc determines the need for booster doses of vaccine to ensure that protective levels of antibody are maintained. No routine follow-up testing is necessary for patients who are positive for both anti-HBs and anti-HBc.

HBV-immune patients can undergo dialysis in the same area as HBsAg-positive patients, or they can serve as a geographic buffer between HBsAg-positive and HBV-susceptible patients. Staff members can be assigned to care for both infected and immune patients on the same shift.

Isolated Anti-HBc-positive Patients

Patients who test positive for isolated anti-HBc (i.e. those who are anti-HBc positive, HBsAg negative, and anti-HBs negative) should be retested on a separate serum sample for total anti-HBc, and if positive, for IgM anti-HBc.

The following guidelines should be used for interpretation and follow-up:

- If total anti-HBc is negative, consider patient susceptible, and follow recommendations for vaccination.
- If total anti-HBc is positive and IgM anti-HBc is negative, follow recommendations for vaccination.
  - If anti-HBs is <10 mIU/mL even after revaccination, test for HBV DNA
  - If HBV DNA is negative, consider patient susceptible (i.e. the anti-HBc result is a false positive), and test monthly for HBsAg
  - If HBV DNA is positive, consider patient as having past infection or "low-level" chronic infection (i.e. the anti-HBc result is a true positive); no further testing is necessary.
  - Isolation is not necessary because HBsAg is not detectable.
- If both total and IgM anti-HBc are positive, consider patient recently infected and test for anti-HBs in 4–6 months; no further routine testing is necessary.
  - Isolation is not necessary because HBsAg is not detectable.

Prevention and Management of HCV Infection

HCV transmission within the dialysis environment can be prevented by strict adherence to infection control precautions recommended for all hemodialysis patients. Although isolation of HCV-infected patients is not recommended, routine testing for ALT and anti-HCV is important for monitoring transmission within centers and ensuring that appropriate precautions are being properly and consistently used.

HCV-negative Patients

Monthly ALT testing will facilitate timely detection of new infections and provide a pattern from which to determine when exposure or infection might have occurred. In the absence of unexplained ALT elevations, testing for anti-HCV every 6 months should be sufficient to monitor the occurrence of new HCV infections. If unexplained ALT elevations are observed in patients who are anti-HCV negative, repeat anti-HCV testing is warranted. If unexplained ALT elevations persist in patients who repeatedly test anti-HCV negative, testing for HCV RNA should be considered.

Anti-HCV Seroconversions

When a seroconversion occurs, review all other patients' routine laboratory test results to identify additional cases. Perform additional testing as indicated later in this section. Investigate potential sources for infection to determine if transmission might have occurred within the dialysis unit, including review of newly infected patients' recent medical history (e.g. blood transfusion, hospitalization), history of high-risk behavior (e.g. injecting-drug use, sexual activity), and unit practices and procedures.

If ≥1 patient seroconverts from anti-HCV negative to positive during a 6-month period, more frequent (e.g. every 1–3 months) anti-HCV testing of HCV-negative patients could be warranted for a limited time (e.g. 3–6 months) to detect additional infections. If no additional newly infected patients are identified, resume semiannual testing. If ongoing HCV transmission among patients is identified, implement control measures based on results of investigation of potential sources for transmission and monitor their effectiveness (e.g. perform more frequent anti-HCV testing of HCV-negative patients for 6–12 months before resuming semiannual testing).

HCV-positive Patients

Patients who are anti-HCV positive (or HCV RNA positive) do not have to be isolated from other patients or dialyzed separately on dedicated machines. Furthermore, they can participate in dialyzer reuse programs.

Unlike HBV, HCV is not transmitted efficiently through occupational exposures. Thus, reprocessing dialyzers from HCV-positive patients should not place staff members at increased risk for infection.

HCV-positive persons should be evaluated for the presence or development of chronic liver disease according to current medical practice guidelines. They also should receive information concerning how they can prevent further harm to their liver and prevent transmitting HCV to others. Persons with chronic liver disease should be vaccinated against hepatitis A, if susceptible.

Prevention and Management of HDV Infection

Because of the low prevalence of HDV infection, routine testing of hemodialysis patients is not necessary or recommended. However, if a patient is known to be infected with HDV, or if evidence exists of transmission of HDV in a dialysis center, screening for delta antibody is warranted. Because HDV depends on an HBV-infected host for replication, prevention of HBV infection will prevent HDV infection in a person susceptible to HBV. Patients who are known to be infected with HDV should be isolated from all other dialysis patients, especially those who are HBsAg-positive.

Prevention and Management of HIV Infection

Routine testing of hemodialysis patients for HIV infection for infection control purposes is not necessary or recommended. However, patients with risk factors for HIV infection should be tested so that, if infected, they can receive proper medical care and counseling regarding preventing transmission of the virus.

Infection control precautions recommended for all hemodialysis patients are sufficient to prevent HIV transmission between patients. HIV-infected patients do not have to be isolated from other patients or dialyzed separately on dedicated machines. In addition, they can participate in dialyzer reuse programs. Because HIV is not transmitted efficiently through occupational exposures, reprocessing dialyzers from HIV-positive patients should not place staff members at increased risk for infection.

Prevention and Management of Bacterial Infections

Follow published guidelines for judicious use of antimicrobials, particularly vancomycin, to reduce selection for antimicrobial-resistant pathogens. Infection control precautions recommended for all hemodialysis patients are adequate to prevent transmission for most patients infected or colonized with pathogenic bacteria, including antimicrobial-resistant strains. However, additional infection control precautions should be considered for treatment of patients who might be at increased risk for transmitting pathogenic bacteria. Such patients include those with either (a) an infected skin wound with drainage that is not contained by dressings (the drainage does not have to be culture positive for VRE, MRSA, or any specific pathogen) or (b) fecal incontinence or diarrhea uncontrolled with personal hygiene measures. For these patients, consider using the following additional precautions: (a) staff members treating the patient should wear a separate gown over their usual clothing and remove the gown when finished caring for the patient and (b) dialyze the patient at a station with as few adjacent stations as possible (e.g. at the end or corner of the unit).

Surveillance for Infections and Other Adverse Events

Develop and maintain a separate centralized record-keeping system (e.g. log book or electronic file) to record the results of patients' vaccination status, serologic testing results for viral hepatitis (including ALT), episodes of bacteremia or loss of the vascular access caused by infection (including date of onset, site of infection, genus and species of the infecting organism, and selected antimicrobial susceptibility results), and adverse events (e.g. blood leaks and spills, dialysis machine malfunctions). Designate a staff person to promptly review the results of routine testing each time such testing is performed and periodically review recorded episodes of bacteremia or vascular access infections. Specify a procedure for actions required when changes occur in test results or in the frequency of episodes of bacteremias or vascular access loss because of infection. Maintain records for each patient that include the location of the dialysis station and machine number used for each dialysis session and the names of staff members who connect and disconnect the patient to and from a machine.

Infection Control Training and Education

Training and education is recommended for both staff members and patients (or their family care givers). Training should be appropriate to the cognitive level of the staff member, patient, or family member, and rationales should be provided for appropriate infection control behaviors and techniques to increase compliance. The following recommendations are to be followed.

- Training and education for all employees at risk for occupational exposure to blood should be provided at least annually, given to new employees before they begin working in the unit, and documented. At a minimum, they should include information on the following topics:
  - Proper hand hygiene technique;
  - Proper use of protective equipment;
  - Modes of transmission for blood-borne viruses, pathogenic bacteria, and other microorganisms as appropriate;
  - Infection control practices recommended for hemodialysis units and how they differ from standard precautions recommended for other healthcare settings;
  - Proper handling and delivery of patient medications;
  - Rationale for segregating HBsAg-positive patients with a separate room, machine, instruments, supplies, medications, and staff members (Box 12.2);
  - Proper infection control techniques for initiation, care, and maintenance of access sites;
  - Housekeeping to minimize transmission of microorganisms, including proper methods to clean and disinfect equipment and environmental surfaces; and
  - Centralized record keeping to monitor and prevent complications,

Box 12.2: Management of HBsAg-positive patients

- Follow infection control practices for hemodialysis units for all patients
- Dialyze HBsAg-positive patients in a separate room using separate machines, equipment, instruments, and supplies
- Staff members caring for HBsAg-positive patients should not care for HBV-susceptible patients at the same time (e.g. during the same shift or during patient changeover)

Box 12.3: Hepatitis B vaccination

- Vaccinate all susceptible patients against hepatitis B
- Test for anti-HBs 1–2 months after last dose
  - If anti-HBs is <10 mIU/mL, consider patient susceptible, revaccinate with an additional three doses, and retest for anti-HBs
  - If anti-HBs is ≥10 mIU/mL, consider patient immune and retest annually
  - Give booster dose of vaccine if anti-HBs declines to <10 mIU/mL and continue to retest annually

  including routine serologic testing results for HBV and HCV, hepatitis B vaccine status (Box 12.3), episodes of bacteremia and loss of access caused by infection, and other adverse events.
  - Records of surveillance for water and dialysate quality should also be maintained.
- Training and education of patients (or family members for patients unable to be responsible for their own care) regarding infection control practices should be given on admission to dialysis and at least annually thereafter and should address the following topics:
  - Personal hygiene and hand washing technique;
  - Patient responsibility for proper care of the access and recognition of signs of infection, which should be reviewed each time the patient has a change in access type; and recommended vaccinations.

PRACTICAL APPROACH TO CONTROL OF HAI IN THE DIALYSIS UNIT[12]

1. In the dialysis centers, the treated water is mixed with a dialysis concentrate and distributed through pipes. It is essential to disinfect distribution pipe system at least weekly.
2. Storage tanks should not be used in dialysis system, unless they are frequently drained, and adequately disinfected, including scrubbing of the sides of the tank to remove bacterial biofilm. It is also recommended that an ultrafilter be used distal to the storage tank.
3. Types of dialysis system: Single pass dialysis machines tend to respond to adequate cleaning and disinfection procedures, and in general have lower levels of bacterial contamination in their dialysis fluid than the re-circulating machines. Hallow-fiber dialyzers are better than plate (Parallel-flow) dialyzers or coil dialyzers as the latter tend to amplify bacterial contamination in the dialysis system.
4. Simultaneous disinfection of the total dialysis system should be carried out (water treatment system, distribution system and dialysis machine) rather than of isolated components.
5. Chlorine based disinfectants are used just before the startup of the dialysis systems and formaldehyde, peroxyacetic acid or glutaraldehyde at the end of the day. Some dialysis systems use hot water (more than 80°C) disinfection and are found to be excellent.
6. The most common complications of dialysis are pyrogenic reactions and gram-negative sepsis. Peritonitis is a common problem after peritoneal dialysis. Patient's monitoring is therefore essential.
7. At least monthly bacteriological assays of water and dialysis fluid are done. The counts should not exceed the prescribed limits (200 and 2000 CFU/mL in water and dialysis fluid respectively).
8. Special problems in the control are viral hepatitis and HIV infection. Hepatitis B virus (HBV) is a risk for dialysis patients as well as HCWs in the unit. Other agents are the other hepatitis viruses like hepatitis C virus (HCV), delta virus (HDV) and rarely hepatitis A virus (HAV). Elaborate precautions have been recommended for control of HBV in dialysis unit. In contrast, control strategies for HCV and HIV include essentially universal precautions only.

HBV Control Strategy (Flowchart 12.1)

1. Dialysis patients and staff members to be screened for HbsAg and anti-HBs when they enter the center for treatment or employment respectively. They are identified as infected (HbsAg positive), immune (anti-HBs positive) or susceptible (negative for HbsAg or anti-HBs). Susceptible patients should

be tested monthly for HbsAg, but for anti-HBs testing every 6 months due to availability of effective hepatitis B vaccine. Susceptible HCWs should be tested for HbsAg and anti-HBs every 6 months.

2. All susceptible patients and HCW's in the unit should receive hepatitis B vaccine. HCWs who have anti-HBs on two consecutive tests at a level of at least 10.0 ml U/mL are considered immune and need no further routine testing for anti-HBs.
3. Patients who are HbsAg positive should be dialyzed in a separate room with the use of separate dedicated dialysis machines and these patients are not included in dialyzer reuse programs.
4. At the end of dialysis, non-disposable equipment should be cleaned and disinfected or sterilized. Special attention to be given to control knobs on the machine and the other external surfaces that are frequently contaminated. Storing

Flowchart 12.1: Evaluation and management of HBV infection in dialysis patient

Patient has come for dialysis

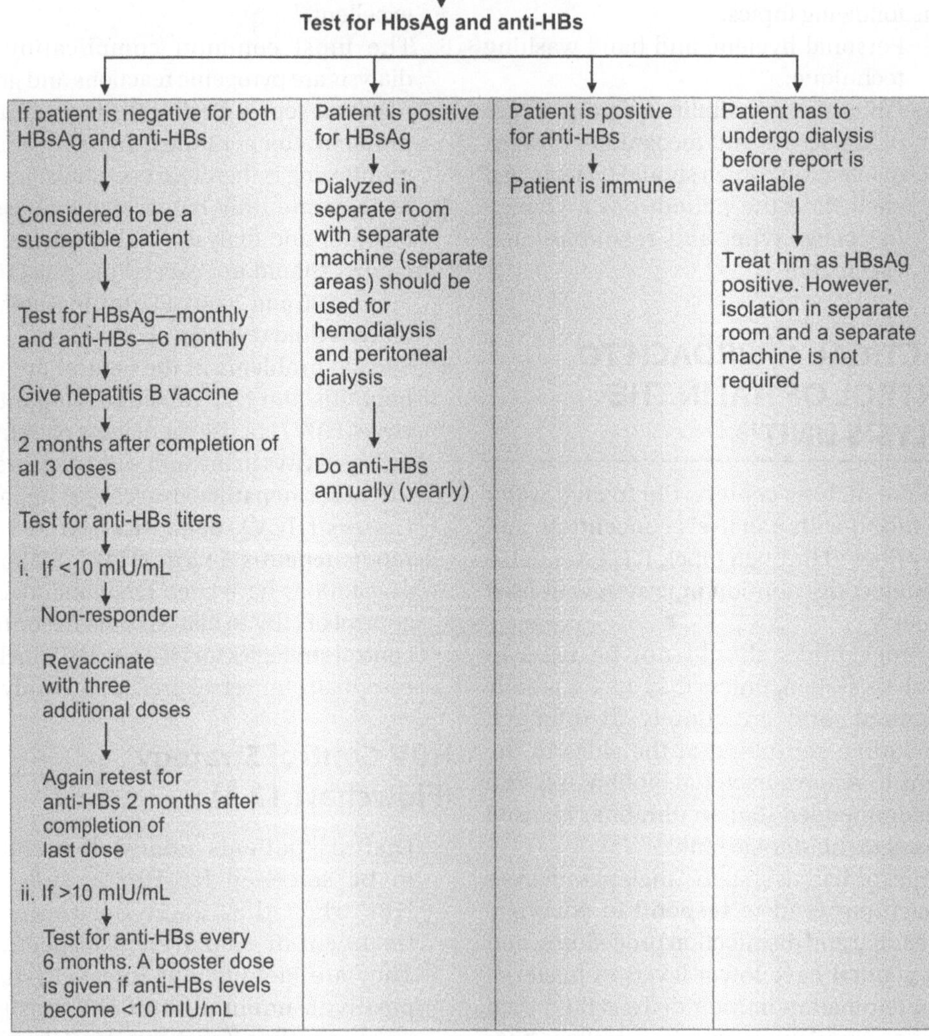

- If HBsAg is positive for > 6 months and anti-HBc is also positive-patient has chronic HBV infection and so medical expert team and microbiology team should discuss appropriate testing and time frames and treatment
- If anti-HBs and anti-HBc positive suggests past infection. Patient is immune. Nothing to be done

of ancillary supply equipment such as trays, blood pressure cuffs, clamps and scissors and other non-disposable items should be avoided. Chairs and beds should be cleaned after each use.

5. Dialysis staff should not attend to both HbsAg positive and seronegative patients during the same shift. They must wear disposable gloves for work and wash their hands after each patient. They should wear protective eyeglasses and masks for procedures in which spurting or spattering of blood may occur. They should also wear gowns while working in the unit. Staff in the unit should not eat, drink or smoke in the treatment area or laboratory.
6. Same precautions are taken for peritoneal dialysis.
7. Housekeeping should be of high order. It should be of a level similar to a surgical suite. Good cleaning and disinfection are essential. All disposables placed in sturdy bags for incineration. Needles and syringes put into a puncture-proof container for incineration/autoclaving. Linen is to be considered potentially infectious and bagged, sealed and treated with hot wash before laundering. Blood spills are to be decontaminated with standard procedure using hypochlorite.

For HCV (Flowchart 12.2)

1. Routine screening of patients and staff for anti-HCV is not necessary for control.
2. Diagnosis of HCV infection includes serologic exclusion of HBV, HAV, delta hepatitis, Epstein-Barr virus and now test for anti-HCV.
3. These patients need not be isolated from other patients or dialyzed separately on dedicated machines.
4. Infection control strategy is essentially strict observance of universal precautions.
5. Patients should be monitored for elevations in alanine-amino transferase and aspartate aminotransferase monthly.

For HDV

1. HDV infection may occur as coinfection with HBV or superinfection of an HBV carrier. Prevention of HBV by prophylaxis will prevent HDV infection for a person susceptible to hepatitis B.
2. If a patient is known to be infected with HDV or there appears to be evidence of transmission of HDV in a dialysis center, screening for delta antigen and its antibody should be done.
3. Patients who are infected with HDV should be separated from all other dialysis patients, including those who are HbsAg positive. They should be dialyzed in separate areas on dedicated machines.

HIV Infection

1. The mode of transmission of HIV in a dialysis unit is similar to HBV, but the

Flowchart 12.2: Evaluation and management of HCV infection in dialysis patient

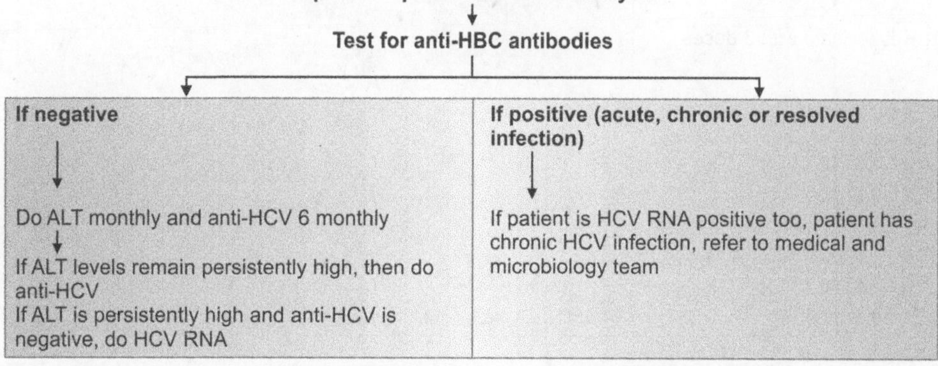

efficiency of transmission is significantly less.

2. The strategy for control is strict observance of universal precautions. Patients with HIV infection need not be isolated from other patients either in separate room or by using dedicated machine.
3. Routine testing of patients or HCWs in the unit for anti-HIV for infection control is not recommended. Although such testing may be required for patient management and treatment.
4. Disinfection and sterlization strategies as described for control of HBV should be used and consistently followed.

Hemodialysis Staff Members (Flowchart 12.3)

Previously, testing for HBV infection was recommended for all staff members at the time of employment and for susceptible staff members at routine intervals thereafter; however, such testing is no longer considered

Flowchart 12.3: Employees

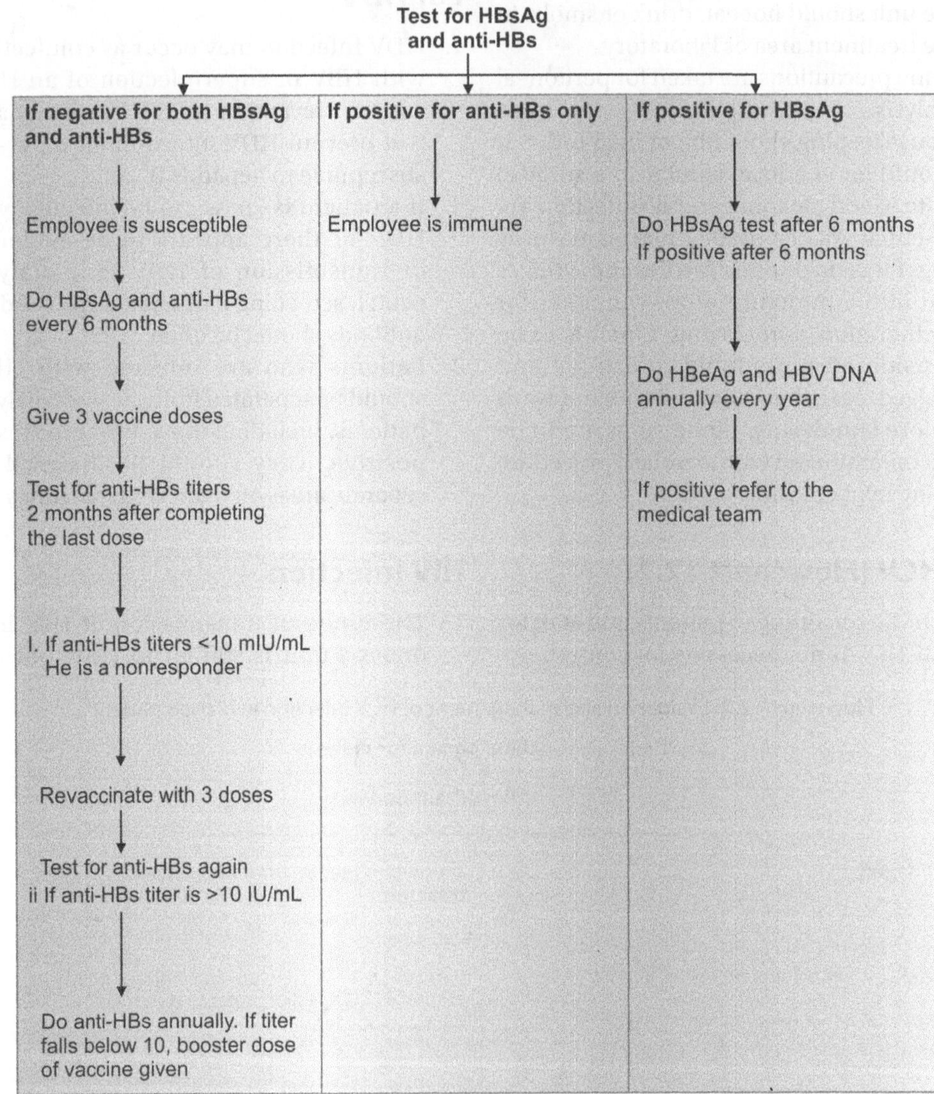

necessary. The risk for HBV infection among hemodialysis staff members is no greater than that for other healthcare workers. Thus, routine testing of staff members is not recommended except when required to document response to hepatitis B.

If done the following protocol can be followed:

- Staff members who are anti-HBs negative will not attend to a patient who is HbsAg positive
- Staff members attending to HbsAg positive should not attend to HBV susceptible patients at the same time (e.g. during the same shift or during patient change over).

MICROBIAL TESTING OF DIALYSATE[13]

The renal dialysis technician, the biomedical technologist or renal nurse who is trained and has demonstrated competency in dialysis water practices will use this procedure outlined below to collect dialysate samples for microbial testing.

Standards (Based on CSA-ISO)

Dialysate must not contain microbial contaminants at concentrations in excess of those specified in Table 12.4.

Table 12.4: Standard and ultrapure dialysates of microbial contaminants

	Standard dialysate	Ultrapure dialysate
Total viable microbial count	<100 CFU/mL	<0.1 CFU/mL
Action level	50 CFU/mL	–

The laboratory assaying technique used for testing microbial growth must be as follows (Table 12.5).

The calibrated loop technique is not an acceptable assay procedure, and blood agar and chocolate agar must not be used as culture media. For ultrapure dialysate, follow the requirements and instructions of the manufacturer of the dialysis machine.

Dialysate must be cultured weekly for new systems for a minimum of one month or until a pattern has been established (i.e. two consecutive tests have met the standards). Dialysate must also be cultured weekly if the acceptable limits are exceeded. For established systems, monitoring and testing the microbiology of dialysate must be performed at least monthly.

Definitions and Abbreviations

Action Level

Concentration of a contaminant at which steps should be taken to interrupt the trend toward higher, unacceptable levels.

Colony-forming Unit (CFU)

Measure of bacterial or fungal cell numbers that theoretically arise from a single cell or group of cells when grown on solid media; a cell or group of cells capable of replicating to form a distinct, visible colony on a culture plate.

Dialysate (Standard)

Aqueous fluid containing electrolytes and usually buffer and glucose, which is intended to exchange solutes with blood during

Table 12.5: The laboratory assaying technique used for testing microbial growth

	Standard Dialysate	Ultrapure Dialysate	
Acceptable test methods	Spread plate, pour plate, membrane filter techniques		
Preferred test method	Spread plate	Pour plate	Membrane filtration
Preferred sample volume	0.1–0.3 mL	0.1-1.0 mL	10–1,000 mL
Assaying time	Within 4 hours of collection or 24 hours if immediately refrigerated		
Culture media	TGEA (tryptone glucose extract agar) or R2A (Reasoners 2A)		
Incubation temperature	17 to 23°C		
Incubation time	168 hours (7 days)		

hemodialysis; also known as *dialysis fluid, dialyzing fluid,* or *dialysis solution.*

Dialysis Water

Water that has been treated to meet the requirements of the CSA-ISO standards and which is suitable for use in hemodialysis applications, including the preparation of dialysis fluid, reprocessing of dialysate, preparation of concentrates and preparation of substitution fluid for online convective therapies.

Hemodialysis

Form of renal replacement therapy in which waste solutes are removed primarily by diffusion from blood flowing on one side of a membrane into dialysis fluid flowing on the other side.

HPC

Heterotrophic plate count.

Microbial

Referring to microscopic organisms, such as bacteria, fungi, and algae.

Microbial Contamination

Contamination with any form of microorganism (e.g. bacteria, yeast, fungi and algae) or with the by-products of living or dead organisms such as endotoxins, exotoxins and cyanobacterial toxins (derived from blue-green algae).

R2A

Reasoners 2A.

RO

Reverse osmosis.

TGEA

Tryptone glucose extract agar.

Ultrapure Dialysate

Highly purified dialysis fluid that can be used in place of conventional dialysis fluid or as feed solution for possible further processing to create fluid intended for infusion directly into the blood.

Equipment

- 20 mL syringes
- HPC total count samplers
- Alcohol swabs
- Gloves
- Microbial testing of dialysate log sheet.

Procedure

Dialysate Sample Collection

1. Select the dialysis machines to be tested.
2. Record the machine IDs, date, time, and initials of the designated tester on the microbial testing of dialysate log sheet.
3. Draw the dialysate sample from the **inlet to the dialyzer** from each machine being tested.
4. Get a syringe, two alcohol swabs, and a HPC total count sampler.
5. Label the sampler with the machine ID, date, and time.
6. Put on a pair of gloves.
7. Open the alcohol swab and use it to clean the sample port at the inlet to the dialyzer. Make sure the alcohol swab is fully swabbed over the injection site. ***Be sure to use a new alcohol swab for each machine.***
8. Discard the alcohol swab after use and give the alcohol time to evaporate.
9. Using a new alcohol swab, fold the swab into a triangular shape and use the pointed end to clean the inside of the sample port.
10. Discard the swab and let the alcohol evaporate.
11. Using a syringe, aspirate dialysate out of and into the port before filling the syringe. Discard the filled syringe.

12. Use another new and sterile syringe to collect a fresh sample of dialysate.
13. Inject the dialysate sample into the HPC total count sampler. ***Be careful to not touch any inside part of the sampler.*** If the inside of the sampler comes into contact with anything, including the syringe or gloves, discard it and use a new one.
14. Collect 17 mL of fluid, or the volume specified by the laboratory performing the testing, in the HPC total count sampler.
15. Firmly seal the sampler. Discard the syringe.
16. Alternatively, if the hemodialysis machine permits, the dialysate sample can be drawn from the **outlet of the dialyzer**. This should be done aseptically by collecting a "free/clean" catch sample after allowing dialysis fluid to run for 30 to 60 seconds.
17. Send the samples to the microbiology laboratory for testing.
18. Fill out a lab requisition for each sample.
19. Attach the laboratory requisitions to the respective samples.
20. Submit the samples to the microbiology laboratory.
21. Upon receiving the results from the microbiology laboratory, record the results and the date the results are received on the microbial testing of dialysate log sheet.
22. Review the laboratory results.
    - If the microbial count does not exceed the action level of 50 CFU/mL (0.1 CFU/mL for ultrapure dialysate), resume routine microbial testing of dialysate the following month (i.e. on other machines).

      Otherwise, take corrective measures (go to step 23).
23. Perform corrective action (refer to the steps below):
    - If this is the 1st sample, retest the offending machine immediately (repeat steps from 2 to 22).

      Note: If the microbial count is 100 CFU/mL or greater (0.1 CFU/mL or greater for ultrapure dialysate), the offending machine must also be reselected for microbial testing the following month.
    - If this is the 2nd (or more) sample:
        - Remove the offending machine from service and immediately disinfect machine using peracetic acid
        - Notify the Area Renal Manager, the Biomed Lead Technician, Biomed Risk and Quality, and the Nephrologist.
    - If the microbial count exceeds 100 CFU/mL (0.1 CFU/mL for ultrapure dialysate), retest the offending machine after disinfection with peracetic acid and *do not* return the machine to service until after the lab results of this retest are returned.

      Otherwise, retest the offending machine after disinfection with peracetic acid and, if necessary, the machine *may* be returned to service before the lab results of this retest are returned.
24. Perform troubleshooting:

    Collect and test samples from other parts of the dialysis system.

    Evaluate/correct sample collection technique.

    Evaluate/correct compliance with disinfection procedure (refer to *Cleaning and Disinfection of Dialysis Water Equipment* clinical standard).

    Evaluate microbial data for previous 3 months to look for trends.
25. Record the corrective measure taken on the microbial testing of dialysate log sheet.

Documentation Considerations

All microbial test results for dialysate must be recorded on the microbial testing of dialysate log sheet. These results must be reviewed by the Area Renal Manager and Infection

Control, and reviewed and signed off by the Nephrologist every month.

REFERENCES

1. CDC Recommendations for Preventing Transmission of Infections among Chronic Haemodialysis Patients. MMWR. 2001;50(RR05):1-43.
2. Carpenter CB, Lazarus JM. Dialysis and transplantation in the treatment of renal failure. In: Isselbacher KJ, Eugene B, Wilson JD, Martin JB, Anthony S, Kasper DL (Eds). Chapter 238. In Harrison's Principles of Internal Medicine. 13th edition, Mc-Graw Hill. 1996;2:1281-4.
3. GAJ A, Fraise AP, Geddes AM. Control of hospital infection. A practical Hand Book. 4th edition. Oxford University Press Inc, New York; 2000.p.348.
4. Favero MS, Alter MJ, Bland LA. Control of infections associated with haemodialysis. In: Mayhall GI (Ed). Hospital epidemiology and infection control. Williams and Wilkins, Baltimore; 1996.p.693.
5. Hudson IRB. The efficacy of intranasal mupirocin in the prevention of staphylococcal infections: A review of recent experience. J Hosp Infec. 1994;27:81.
6. Boelaert JR, De Smedt RA, De Baere YA, et al. The influence of calcium mupirocin ointment on the incidence of *Staphylococcus aureus* infections in haemodialysis nephrology, dialysis and transplantation; 1989.
7. Eltringham I. Mupirocin resistance and methicillin-resistant *Staphylococcus aureus* (MRSA). J Hosp Infec. 1997;35:1.
8. Fogel MA, Nussbaum PB, Feintzeig ID, Hunt WA, Gavin JR, Kim RC. Cefazolin in chronic hemodialysis patients: a safe, effective alternative to vancomycin. Am J Kidney Dis. 1998;32:401-9.
9. Brady JP, Snyder JW, Hasbargen JA. Vancomycin-resistant *Enterococcus* in end-stage renal disease. Am J Kidney Dis. 1998; 32:415-8.
10. American Society of Health-System Pharmacists. AHFS Drug Information; 1999. In: Bethesda MD: American Society of Health-System Pharmacists; 1999.pp.1298-9.
11. US Food and Drug Administration. Medwatch: the FDA medical products reporting program. 2000. Available on the Internet at <http://www.fda.gov/medwatch/safety/2000/safety00.htm#epogen>.
12. *Aggarwal DS. Guidelines for nosocomial infection—surveillance and control. Lancet. 2008;371:126-34.
13. Clinical practice standards and procedures for dialysis. Water Quality: 1a: Microbial Testing of Dialysate. Section HD. Accessed from www.bcrenalagency/sites/default/filter/documents/files/1-a-Microbial-Testing-of-Dialysate-Final-2013pdf. on 23/4/2015.

Chapter **13**

Infections in Obstetrics and Gynecology

Chapter Outline

- Common Infections in Obstetrics and Gynecology
- Neonatal Infections
- Control Measures
- Preparation of Infant Feeds and Use of Milk Kitchens
- Practical Procedures for Prevention of HAI in Gynecology and Obstetrics

INTRODUCTION

Patients in the obstetrics and gynecology departments undergoing genital tract surgery are at a high risk of infection as most of these procedures involve the vagina, which has a contaminated field with an endogenous flora similar to that of large bowel. In addition tissue necrosis, hematoma and foreign bodies accompany these procedures making an environment, which is ideal for bacterial proliferation. However, most of the infections are endogenous (arising from patients lower genital tract) rather than from the hospital environment.

COMMON INFECTION IN OBSTETRICS AND GYNECOLOGY

Postoperative Infections in Gynecology

Most infections in gynecology occur after hysterectomy because of surgical entry into vagina. Other major gynecological surgery, such as removal of tube or ovary is "clean" surgery and has a much lower infection rate. Minor procedures, like dilatation and curettage are rarely followed by infection unless there is perforation or antecedent unrecognized infection.

For hysterectomy certain groups are predisposed to infection. Women with lower socioeconomic status have higher infection rates following this procedure as well as following all types of pelvic surgery. This observation has been made repeatedly and may be due to difference in flora, hygiene, nutrition or host defenses.

Other groups at risk for post-hysterectomy infection include women with acute pelvic inflammatory disease. Also premenopausal women are likely to develop postoperative infection (especially after vaginal hysterectomy because of increased vascularity of the pelvis with an increased likelihood of hematoma development.

Nowadays, because of advent of minimal invasive surgical techniques (laparoscopic operations) the risk of postoperative infections are likely to decrease.

Postpartum Infection

Incidence varies from 3 to 8%.[1] after delivery; bacteria from lower genital tract rapidly ascend into the uterine cavity. Here in the presence of blood and sloughing, endometrial infection may develop.

Patients predisposed to postpartum infection are those delivered by cesarean section (especially when it is performed after rupture of membranes in labor-incidence is 30–50%) and those with vaginal delivery complicated by early rupture of membranes, retained placental fragments or major trauma.

Postabortion Infection

The liberalization of abortion laws brought pregnancy termination under the medical supervision, and sharply decreased the number of septic abortions. But even though abortions have been legalized, infection still remains a leading cause (40%) of abortion deaths. The risk of death depends upon the type of abortion procedure performed. For example:

First trimester of pregnancy: Abortion is performed by dilatation of cervix and removal of products of conception by suction or curettage. With these procedures the reported infection rate varies from 0.2 to 5.0%.[1] Factors, which predispose to infection are incomplete abortion with retained placenta, which is an ideal environment for bacterial proliferation. Uncommon complications are uterine perforation, leading to peritonitis, injury to the bowel. Complications increase with duration of gestation and dilatation and curettage are generally contraindicated after first trimester.

Patients undergoing second trimester abortions are at a far greater risk for complications. Methods of second trimester abortions include intra-amniotic injections (of hypertonic saline, hypertonic urea or prostaglandins) hysterotomy and hysterectomy. Incidence of infection with IAS is 2 to 18%.[1]

Hysterotomy (a transabdominal incision into the uterus to remove pregnancy) is associated with so many complications that it has been abandoned.

Hysterectomy too is accompanied by a high complication rate and is reserved as an abortion technique in patients with other gynecological diseases such as severe cervical dysplasia or uterine leiomyomata.

Oncologic Patients and Pelvic Infection

Gynecologic patients who have received treatment for malignancy in the form of chemotherapy and radiation or radical surgery are compromised hosts, responding to infections less effectively, hence are prone to severe infections. In addition these patients may have been hospitalized for some time prior to treatment for evaluation and are likely to become colonized with organisms causing nosocomial infections. Thus, in these patients resistant gram-negative aerobes (such as *Pseudomonas*) and *Staphylococcus aureus* may become common pathogens. Antibiotic strategies, which may be used confidently in other gynecologic patients, must be altered accordingly.

Oncology patients may also be predisposed to more severe infections because of obstruction at various sites, e.g. patients with uterine cancer may obstruct the cervical canal and develop pyometra. Urinary tract injury by direct surgical trauma or by scarring from irradiation may lead to obstruction with subsequent severe pyelonephritis.

Diagnostic Problems in Pelvic Infections

Usually, there is no difficulty in diagnosing urinary or pulmonary infections, but diagnosis of postoperative pelvic infection may be difficult as localizing signs and symptoms are few and laboratory tests are often non-specific. Initial symptoms are often malaise, chills, abdominal pain and perhaps vaginal discharge. Early in the course of infection, physical examination may reveal fever, tachycardia and lower abdominal pain only. Hematomas and abscesses are not palpable for a few days. Furthermore, after hysterectomy, the vaginal apex is indurated and tender in nearly all patients.

Appropriate laboratory investigations should include blood count, a gram stain and culture of the infected site (endometrium, endocervix or vaginal apex) and blood culture.

Investigations of the flora of genital tract have shown that properly performed culture will be positive for variety of pathogens in 95% of asymptomatic postoperative[2] or postpartum[3] women. Therefore, caution must be used when interpreting culture reports from these patients, as isolation of the pathogen is not pathognomonic of an infection.

Clearly anaerobic organisms play a major role in pelvic infection, but it is impractical to perform anaerobic cultures in every infected patient. Anaerobic cultures are expensive and time consuming. Reports are available only after 48–72 hours and there is a major problem of avoiding contamination with vaginal and cervical organisms in transvaginal cultures.

Therefore, it is best to use anaerobic culture selectively such as: (1) when there is frank pus from a pelvic, vaginal or wound abscess, (2) when an intra-abdominal culture is taken during surgery, and (3) when there is a major infection characterized by a foul odor.

A suitable collection and transport system would be a syringe into which the pus or infected fluid may be aspirated. The air should be expressed and specimen should be capped tightly. If there is some delay in transport, the specimen may be injected into a commercially available transport vial or a swab may be placed in an oxygen free tube, agar or broth. The best results for quantitation of bacteria are obtained by direct plating of the specimen.

Gram stain is important to determine the predominant organism in the specimen. Also if organisms are seen on the stain but do not grow in culture; it may be presumed that these missing organisms are anaerobes.

Blood cultures are positive in only 10% pelvic infections, but it is still important to obtain them, to help detect the major pathogens. It is essential to recognize that the isolation of an organism from the blood stream does not mean that the organism is solely responsible for the infection, for example *Escherichia coli* may be recovered in the blood but other organisms, especially anaerobes, may also be involved at the operation site.

Special radiologic tests such as ultrasonography or intravenous pyelogram may be useful in localizing a pelvic abscess.

NEONATAL INFECTIONS

Postpartum and neonatal infections have been recognized as often being hospital associated. The introduction of handwashing procedures by Semmelweis led to a dramatic decrease in the incidence of these infections.

Though hospital-associated postpartum and neonatal infections have decreased since then, they still remain a problem. In United States infection rate of 1 to 1.5% was reported in 1976.[4] In 1998, the overall rates of nosocomial infections per patient (total number of infections per 100 patients) at US neonatal units ranged from 1.8 to 15.3.[5]

Though all infections acquired by babies born in hospital can be considered nosocomial infections, infections that become overt early (during the first week of life) are frequently caused by microorganisms transmitted by the mother to the newborn. These infections present a characteristic epidemiology, different from that of hospital infections acquired later in the neonatal period. Usually, neonatal infections are divided into early-onset (less than 3 to 7 days of life), originated by the mother, and late-onset (greater than 3 to 7 days of life), which are those acquired after birth and thus not originated by the mother.[6]

The Center for Disease Control and Prevention (CDC) considers that hospital infections includes those acquired intrapartum, during hospitalization, or up to 48 hours after hospital discharge. The exception includes transplacental infections (syphilis, toxoplasmosis, rubella, cytomegalovirus infection, hepatitis B, herpes simplex, HIV infection, and so on). Infections that occur up to 48 hours of life are considered hospital infections originated by the mother and those that occur after 48 hours of life are considered hospital infections originated by the environment.[6]

Specific Problems

Colonization vs Clinical Infections

The fetus is normally sterile. During birth and after birth, the child is quickly colonized with microorganisms from the mother and the hospital environment. The virulence of these colonizing microorganisms and the child defense mechanisms will determine whether a clinical infection will occur or not.

During delivery the child's upper respiratory tract is colonized with *Diphtheroids*, streptococci, staphylococci, *Candida species.* and other microorganisms from the vagina and vulva of the mother. In some 15% of the healthy mothers, the vagina and vulva are colonized by *Group B* streptococci, in these cases; the child may also be colonized with these microorganisms at delivery. Colonization with *Listeria species*, in the mother and subsequently the child is less common.

The gastrointestinal tract of the child is colonized with anaerobes, which will dominate the gastrointestinal flora (more than 99%) with *Escherichia coli* and other gram-negative rods. In breastfed children, the anaerobic fecal flora consists predominantly by *Bifidobacterium.*

The child skin, umbilicus, axilla, groin and nostrils are rapidly colonized, mainly with *Staphylococcus aureus* and *Staphylococcus epidermidis*. After a couple of weeks some 90% of children are colonized with *Staphylococcus aureus, Streptococci groups A, B, C and G* as well as *E. coli* and other gram-negative bacilli may also be found. The source for the colonization is mainly the mother and the nursery staff. Staff members with a paronychia constitute a special risk as sources of staphylococcal infection.

Some knowledge is necessary of the epidemiologic and clinical features of infection caused by the most important pathogens in order to prevent hospital associated infections.

Modes of Transmission

Babies can acquire infectious agents from fomites, by airborne transmission, from hands or bodies of personnel or from invasive procedures. Equipment, such as incubators, and humidifiers may also be an infection hazard. So also physical transmission from transducers, thermometers, stethoscopes, manometer, suction catheters and water may occur. Contaminated fluids, IV solutions, milk and blood derivatives may also be responsible for transmission of infection. Compared with these sources, others such as dust or healthy visitors play a minor role.[6]

Instances of nosocomial infections in newborn nurseries and NICUs are numerous. Some examples are:

1. Endotracheal suctioning—associated with transmission of HSV infection from a physician to a neonate.
2. Eye wash—contaminated with *P. aeruginosa* and other non-fermenting bacteria.
3. Hand carriage by personnel
4. Scrub brushes—contaminated with *Serratia marcescens.*
5. Contaminated hand lotions, topical ointments, phenolic disinfectants, intravenous fluids and total parenteral nutrition fluids, etc.

Although fomites and contaminated liquids carry a potential risk for spreading infection in nurseries, outbreaks are more often traced to personnel and poor aseptic techniques. Transmission of pathogen on hands of nursery personnel is the most common cause of outbreaks of infections in neonates.

Infection Sites[6]

Infections of term newborns and at normal nurseries are primarily cutaneous and of soft tissues, including omphalitis, pocks, abscess, and bullous impetigo. Outbreaks of conjunctivitis and bacterial or viral gastroenteritis can spread very rapidly in these nurseries. In the case of neonatal ICUs, bacteremia and sepsis are the most frequent infections and account for 30 to 50% of hospital infections; these infections are followed by pneumonia; eye, ear, nose, and throat infections; skin and soft tissue infections; and gastrointestinal and surgical site infections. There are variations in these sites of infection according to weight at birth and to the characteristics of the unit.

Causative Organisms

Bacteria

The microorganisms that cause hospital infections include bacteria, fungi, and virus; it is also possible to include all commensal pathogens and organisms of humans. In normal nurseries, the *Staphylococcus aureus*, the enteropathogens, and the respiratory virus are the main infection agents. At high-risk nurseries, there is a broad spectrum of infection agents that includes microorganisms normally nonpathogenic for term newborns, such as coagulase-negative staphylococci and *Candida*. In the assessment of the etiology of neonatal hospital infections, it is important to consider that it also depends on birth weight; on characteristics of the unit; on use of invasive procedures; on maternal or nonmaternal origin of the infection; and on evolution of etiological agents in the unit. It is fundamental that each institution register the microbiological ecology of its units through epidemiological surveillance.

Streptococci: Group A and Group B streptococci are to a large extent responsible for neonatal hospital-associated infections. The carrier rate for *Group A* streptococci in mothers and in hospital staff varies seasonally and may rise to 15% or more. Dispersers of these microorganisms are mainly throat carriers with symptoms of upper respiratory tract infection. If established in the skin or umbilicus of newborns, the microorganisms can spread from one baby to the other with the nurse's hands. Sometimes the baby may be colonized with Group A streptococci in the nursery, without signs of infection during the stay in the hospital. After discharge clinical infection may develop in their families in the form of omphalitis, paronychia, purulent skin infections and/or septicemia in newborns, mastitis and/or tonsillitis in the mother or scarlet fever.

Infection with Group B streptococci is also a common cause of septic infections in neonates. Approximately 15% of mothers carry these microorganisms in the vagina and vulva, and the child will be infected during delivery.[7] Normally, however, there will be no clinical symptoms of infection. It is said that only few babies get colonized from their mother and less than 1% of these develop overt infection[8] Group B streptococcal infection, must however be borne in mind in any sick neonate, particularly low birth weight or premature infant, and in those with respiratory distress.

Staphylococcus aureus: Approximately 50% of mothers and hospital staff are healthy skin carriers of *S. aureus*, in majority of cases intermittently, some permanently. Through the nursing routines, most infants are colonized with *S. aureus* during their first week of life, primarily in the umbilicus, skin and nostrils, but sometimes also in the gastrointestinal tract.

These *S. aureus* strains may then be responsible for hospital-associated infections, which may be caused by particular phage types. These days methicillin-resistant *S. aureus* has become common.

Most nursery infection in mothers and babies are caused by *S. aureus.* The infection rate varies in different reports from 1 to 2% or more than 15%. Difference may be due to different epidemiological situations of different hospitals at different times or due to variation in surveillance systems. So also as has been mentioned earlier, the incubation period is often so long, that patient has been discharged from hospital before the onset of clinical symptoms.

The clinical spectrum of staphylococcal infection is broad. It may lead to mild infections such as conjunctivitis, paronychia, pemphigus and umbilical infections or they may lead to more severe infection like sepsis and osteomyelitis. Severe forms of skin infection such as bullous impetigo or "Staphylococcal scalded skin syndrome" sometimes occurs when strains of *Staphylococcus,* which produce exfoliation spread within the hospital. Breast abscess may occur in mother, sometimes weeks after she has been discharged.

The *Staphylococcus aureus* is a concern for most nurseries around the world. Cutaneous lesions and invasive procedures are predisposing factors for occurrence of focal lesions, bacteremia, meningitis, or pneumonia. The main reservoir of this bacterium is the hospital staff and contamination usually occurs through the hands.[6]

Nowadays, the *Staphylococcus* is the main gram-positive infection agent of hospital infections of the newborn; the most important being coagulase-negative staphylococci such as *Staphylococcus epidermidis,* which frequently affects low-birth weight newborns with prolonged hospital stay, venous catheter, and administration of parenteral lipids. Bloodstream is the most frequent pathway of infection, presenting nonspecific and difficult to diagnose signs. This type of infection can, also, cause focal infections. Considering that the referred agents are a part of the normal cutaneous flora, they can also contaminate blood cultures.

Thus, the diagnosis after isolation of the agents becomes more difficult. Confirmed diagnosis of bloodstream infection follows criteria of resistance to at least six antimicrobial agents, since most strains are resistant to oxacillin.[6]

Enterococcus: The *Enterococcus* species can be acquired by the mother, but it is turning into a prevalent agent in nosocomial infections. The most common source of infection is the gastrointestinal tract of the newborn. There is also possibility of colonization of the mouth, respiratory tract, cutaneous lesions, and of contamination by objects and surfaces of the environment. Preterm newborns who remain hospitalized for more than 30–60 days, with prolonged use of venous catheters and exposed to multiple antimicrobials, are especially predisposed to infections by *Enterococcus.* These infections can be severe and include: necrotizing enterocolitis, sepsis, pneumonia, meningitis, and endocarditis.[6]

Gram-negative bacteria: Gram-negative bacteria are the cause of approximately 19% of cases of nosocomial sepsis, and of over 30% of pneumonias. These infections are severe and present high lethality rates (40–90%).[6]

Colonization with *E. coli* occurs early in life as mentioned earlier and mainly in the gastrointestinal tract. They are usually of little or no virulence, but may sometimes cause enteritis in infants. Non-maternal strains of *Escherichia coli* (other patients or environment) can cause invasive diseases.[6]

These microorganisms are mainly spread by contact, mostly with hands or gowns of staff. They are only to a small extent air borne.

The main reservoir of *Klebsiella* and *Enterobacter* are the gastrointestinal tract of the patient, invasive procedures, and catheters. Several gram-negative bacillus have been associated with outbreaks of hospital infections at neonatal units, especially those associated with environmental contamination, such as: *Pseudomonas aeruginosa*, *Serratia marcescens*, *Acinetobacter* species, *Stenotrophomonas maltophilia*, among others.[6]

Gram-negative bacteria, such as *Klebsiella* strains or *Pseudomonas* species may cause severe infections in severely ill premature babies. Incubators may be a source and spread the microorganisms between infants. They should be regularly and thoroughly cleaned. Breast milk stored in milk banks may become contaminated during collection or storage with *Salmonella* and *Klebsiella* leading to infections in preterm infants. *Clostridium difficile* infections are spread by fecal-oral route.

Viruses

Despite the fact that they are usually not identified, viral nosocomial infections are very common. Hospital staff, family members, and other infected patients represent the main conveyors of viral infections in neonatal units. The most frequent viral nosocomial infections are caused by respiratory syncytial virus and by rotavirus.[6]

Rotavirus is known to cause enteritis in children. A nosocomial spread of gastroenteritis in connection with Rotavirus excretion is common. The mode of spread is not known. Healthy adults rarely excrete Rotavirus. An environmental spread seems probable. Herpes simplex virus is also an important nosocomial pathogen.

Other viruses, which may cause nosocomial infections are, echovirus, coxsackievirus, respiratory syncitial virus. Echovirus and respiratory syncitial virus are spread both by droplets and by the hands of personnel touching contaminated objects since the virus survive well on hard surfaces in the nursery environment.

Nosocomial transmission of respiratory syncytial virus can result in increased morbidity and mortality for all infected newborns, but especially for premature newborns, with congenital cardiac disease or associated pulmonary conditions, and for post-surgical patients.[6]

Coxsackievirus is spread by fecal-oral route as with rotavirus. Neonatal outbreaks of rotavirus can be a result of transmission by contaminated hands. Both symptomatic and asymptomatic children can excrete the virus in feces. There are reports of viral excretion in feces of premature newborn infants for periods as long as 6 or more weeks.[6]

Fungi

Similarly to infections by gram-negative bacteria, those by fungi are increasingly prevalent in neonatal units. These infections are associated with prolonged exposure to antibiotics, with parenteral hyperalimentation, with tracheal intubation, and with IV infusion of lipids. *Candida* strains (albicans, tropicalis, parapsilosis) account for most hospital infections. The most common presentation is fungemia. However, the fungi can spread and cause meningitis, spleen or kidney abscess, endophthalmitis, osteomyelitis, or invasive dermatitis with mortality rates as high as 25–50%.[6]

Central venous catheters used for administering parenteral nutrition are a serious infection risk from preparation of the fluid, contamination when connections in the line are violated and entry wound infections are common. Frequency of infection (bacteremias) range from 3 to 8% due to CVC. Candidemia was a serious problem in approximately 10% of cases overall.

The infant may also be infected with organisms derived from mother either in utero (rubella, syphilis, tuberculosis, HBV, HIV) or during delivery (gonococcal ophthalmia, salmonellosis, Group B *Streptococcus*).

CONTROL MEASURES

Surveillance

Epidemiological surveillance is a set of activities aimed at active, systematic and continuous observation of collection, analysis and assessment of data regarding infection. The main objectives of surveillance of neonatal hospital infections, which is fundamental for prevention, are:[6]

1. To determine the epidemiological profile of hospital infections evaluating etiological agents, microbial sensitivity, and affected sites.
2. To observe the endemic levels of infection and early detection of outbreaks.
3. To define risk factors according to type of patient and procedures used.
4. To prioritize control and prevention measures, as well as the evaluation of necessary strategies of intervention.

Hence, the development of a surveillance program involves choosing a surveillance method, establishing uniform criteria for hospital infections, for identification of types of infection, and rationalizing control and use of antimicrobials.

Cases of hospital-associated infection should be registered, so that outbreaks may be discovered and preventive measures taken early. It is important to register not only infections that occur in hospital, but also during the first week after discharge.

There are several methods of epidemiological surveillance of hospital infections. The method of choice will depend on the characteristics of the hospital, on the available resources, on the type of patient, and on the most frequently identified infections. In epidemiological surveillance, it is possible to collect data passively, actively, or by review of medical records. In any of these methods, following the isolation of the etiological agent, it is necessary to characterize the susceptibility to antimicrobials.[6]

Routine bacteriological cultures from mother and child, especially from child's umbilicus 3-5 days after delivery can give valuable information on the epidimeologic situation in the maternity wards. If the colonization rate for *Staphylococcus* or Group A *Streptococcus* increases or if one phage pattern dominates among the staphylococcal strains, a common source should be suspected among the staff or it may be due to a decline in the discipline and investigative steps should be taken.

Investigation and Control of Hospital Infection Outbreaks in Nurseries[6]

Hospital infection outbreaks occur in cases of significant increase of infections (above the upper endemic limit of the neonatal unit). The increase in infection rates in specific sites or by a specific microorganism calls for measures aimed at identifying the agent, the reservoir, and the risk factors for transmission of the infection. Moreover, the occurrence of infections caused by unusual pathogens that are associated with high morbidity and/or mortality rates in newborns call for special concern with, and investigation of the matter.[6]

In cases of suspected outbreaks, all infection control measures should be reviewed. Special attention should be given to the washing of the hands of the staff between handling of newborn infants, to the sterilization and disinfecting routine procedures, to the preparation of formulas, and to the asepsis techniques for invasive procedures. The origin of cases of outbreak due to unusual microorganisms is probably on the nonobservance of infection control measures, such as overcrowding, understaffing, hygiene, and so on.[6]

If only one microorganism is responsible for the outbreak, infected or colonized patients, as well as the staff should be located in a cohort. The cohort can be located in a separate or marked area inside the neonatal unit with newborn infants isolated inside incubators. The collection of cultures for identification of reservoirs in staff or equipment is indicated only in cases in which preliminary epidemiological investigation is suggestive of association with the outbreak. One of the typical examples is that of outbreaks caused by *S. aureus* resistant to oxacillin and in which culture from the nasal mucosa indicates colonization of the staff. The topic use of mupirocin to the anterior nares is indicated.[6]

Use of Antimicrobials and Hospital Infection: The Need for Rationalization and Control[6]

Antimicrobials can save lives in the treatment of infected children; whereas in the case of newborns, there are substantial risks, such as: superinfection and infection by microorganisms resistant to drugs. That is because antimicrobials interfere in both the endogenous and pathogenic microbes.

The use of antibacterials is frequent in newborns, especially in those admitted to ICUs. The reported data indicates that the use of these drugs varies from 4.4 to 10.5% for all newborns, and from 42 to 60.4% for all preterm newborns. At ICUs, at least 75% of all newborns are administered antibacterials for at least 40 hours, with rates of use as high as 92% for preterm newborns with less than 1,500 g. In general, the frequent use of antibacterials is justifiable by the risks and high mortality rates of bacterial infections in newborns. However, it has not been demonstrated that the prophylactic use of antibiotics prevents nosocomial infections. Moreover, newborns whose normal flora is still not established and who are treated with antibiotics can develop colonization of microorganisms not detected in normal children. It has been reported that these microorganisms include those that are resistant to antibiotics. These microorganisms were selected from numerous patients on antibacterials and are part of the flora of the unit. In this sense, bacterial invasions are generally resistant to antibacterials used in the specific unit.

Multiresistance to antibacterial drugs has been identified with frequency. In this sense, over 80% of *Staphylococcus epidermidis* strains and at least 60% of *Staphylococcus aureus* strains that cause nosocomial infections in neonatal units are methicillin/oxacillin resistant.

The appearance of strains of *Enterococcus* resistant to vancomycin has been reported in ICUs. This could be a problem since these bacteria are resistant to all available antibiotics and have the potential of being reservoirs for glycopeptide-resistant genes that can be transferred to other more virulent pathogens.

As to the gram-negative bacteria, studies have reported that the appearance of resistance strains of *Klebsiella* and *Enterobacter* have caused problems and nosocomial outbreaks. The resistance, which is mediated by plasmid, induces extended-spectrum beta-lactamases (ESBLs) protection providing resistance to penicillin, cephalosporin, and monobactam to both microorganisms. This resistance can also be transferred to other microorganisms and can develop during antimicrobial therapy.

Consequently, it is fundamental to rationalize the use of antimicrobials during the neonatal period. In the choice of antimicrobials, priority should be given to drugs that are safer and present more success in therapeutics or prophylaxis; are well-tolerated and that cause less adverse effects; are less toxic and cause less selective induction on the endogenous microbes of the patient; and are more cost effective.

In addition, the understanding of the prevalence of bacteria sensitive to antimicrobials with epidemiological surveillance at each hospital unit, as well as that of the modifications in this sensitivity that occur with time are fundamental for the designing of empirical recommendations of antibacterial therapy and for a more rational use of antimicrobials.

Nursing Routine

It has been clearly demonstrated by many investigators that the most important factor for preventing the spread of hospital-associated infections in maternity ward is good hand hygiene in all members of the staff. Bar soap is likely to be contaminated after some days use, so a liquid soap should be preferred.

Bathing the newborn daily with hexachlorophene has been suggested to reduce the incidence of staphylococcal disease, but it does not reduce the incidence of infection with gram-negative organisms and severe brain damage has been reported with its use. Babies should be bathed after delivery if soiled with feces or urine. Bathtub must be cleaned and disinfected after each use. Gowns should be worn in nursery and changed daily or changed immediately if soiled. Baby powder, baby soap, soap for staff hand washing should be bacteriologically sterile.

Neonatal Wards

Same rules should be applied to babies in the neonatal wards as to the healthy babies in the maternity wards. The hands are the most important source of spread of infections and frequent hand washing is therefore the most important preventive measure.

Disposable diapers should preferably be used (may not be possible in developing countries). These should be placed in a plastic bag or some other container and not transported uncovered to the refuse bag. Mattresses should be covered with plastic, so that they can be easily wiped with a disinfectant or if possible disposable mattresses should be used.

In neonatal wards prevention of diarrhoea and care of incubators need special attention. Children with diarrhea should be isolated. Baby incubators and their nebulizers and humidifiers may readily serve as reservoirs for gram-negative microorganisms especially *Pseudomonas* species, so they must be carefully cleaned and wiped dry after each use. Baby incubators must be bacteriologically monitored after each cleaning and disinfection.

Bacteriological cultures should be taken from all suspected or proven cases of infection, and sensitivity tests performed on isolated pathogens. This will facilitate the choice of right antibiotic.

Staff Carriers and Staff Infections

Members of staff carrying Group A streptococci should be treated with penicillin for 10 days and stay off work for first 3 days. Staff carriers of *Staphylococcus aureus* must stay off work if they have a purulent skin infection. If healthy, they rarely disseminate their staphylococci to a hazardous extent.

Staff members in maternity and neonatal wards and in milk kitchens are an infection hazard if they harbor potential enteropathogens especially *Salmonella* species and *Shigella* species in their gastrointestinal tract. They should report any attack of diarrhea.

Prevention of Spread[8]

Isolation facilities are necessary for both mothers and babies. Maternal diseases that require isolation include puerperal sepsis, which may be due to *Streptococcus pyogenes* (Group A beta hemolytic), gastrointestinal infections, breast abscess and staphylococcal skin sepsis. Infected neonates should also be isolated as soon as infection is suspected. It may be necessary to separate infants from their mothers, if the later are infected, particularly in cases of maternal typhoid or *Shigella* infections.

Babies born with gastroenteritis should be isolated immediately. If an infection is severe or more than two cases occur, the ward should be closed to further admissions. The other infants should be screened and all carriers kept in one nursery. If possible separate nurses should attend babies in the infected and noninfected nurseries. Nurses preparing feeds should not handle infected babies or their contacts.

Surveillance of infection is particularly important in neonatal unit (Staphylococcal infections, those due to enterobacteriacecae, and other gram-negative bacteria), so that immediate action may be taken to prevent extension of an outbreak.

PREPARATION OF INFANT FEEDS AND USE OF MILK KITCHENS

Introduction

Milk is a good growth medium for most pathogenic bacteria, and contamination of feeds is a particular hazard in neonatal nurseries. Actually outbreaks of infection due to contaminated feeds occur very commonly, but they are not reported, hence, there is hardly any published evidence regarding it. Many organisms have been isolated in large numbers from feeds (e.g. *Salmonella* species, *Enteropathogenic* and other strains of E. *coli,* group A and other groups *of* β-hemolytic streptococci, *Candida albicans, Proteus* species, *Klebsiella* species and *Pseudomonas species, Staphylococcus aureus* and many other organisms).

All feeds must be free from intestinal pathogens. The greatest risk is from these organisms, but other bacteria (e.g. *Proteus and Klebsiella* species) may cause infection if they are abundant.

Contamination of feeds can occur due to variety of reasons: Faulty or improper disinfections of bottles, teats and other mixing and dispensing equipment. Milk, water or other additives may be contaminated prior to use. Additional contamination can occur during the preparation process or when feeding the baby. This may be from the air, from the hands of the staff or from the mother.

Usually, the initial level of contamination is low, but storage at room temperature for longer periods, allows organisms to grow and multiply. Normally, child accepts feed at room temperature, and there is no necessity of warming the feed, but if it is done, a special container should be used which should be kept for this purpose only. The container should be filled with boiled water, and then the bottle with the intact teat should be placed in the container at body temperature and the water level should be well below the neck of the bottle. After use, the container should be immediately emptied, cleaned and dried.

Preferred Methods

Two methods are available for the use of infant feeds: (1) Commercially supplied, presterilized feeds and (2) Locally produced and terminally sterilized or heat disinfected feeds.

Choice is made depending on effectiveness, economy, availability of staff and space.

Locally produced and sterilized or heat disinfected feeds—for this controls to ensure the exposure of the feed for the required time at the correct temperature is necessary. The head of the department should regularly inspect charts showing this information. Bacteriological tests should also be performed at intervals (e.g. monthly) and commercially prepared presterilized feeds, should be bacteriologically sterile provided that their control and testing process is satisfactory. Bottles and caps should be inspected before use for obvious damage, and if any doubt exists, the bottle should be discarded. Commercially supplied presterilized feeds with the teat already attached to the bottle and adequately protected from contamination are preferable or single use teats packed separately may be used.

Disinfection of Bottles and Teats

Chemical disinfectants can be used, for bottles and teats (e.g. by hypochlorite), but this method is reliable only if properly performed, and is difficult to control and is susceptible to individual staff error. The disinfectant if used, should be made up to the correct strength (hypochlorite—125 ppm available chlorine). All equipment should be completely immersed, with removal of air bubbles, and should be left for at least the recommended time. Autoclaving is more preferable to chemicals, as it is more reliable. Boiling can also be used, and is more reliable than chemical method if correctly performed, but the boiling of bottle in an open container is difficult to control and is not recommended.

Milk, Kitchen and Staff[9]

In hospitals where commercially prepared presterilized feeds are used, all that is required is a clean storeroom. But in hospitals where feeds are prepared on site, a kitchen for preparation of feeds is required. Washing of used bottles, teats and other equipment should be done in a room separate from the kitchen. A handwashing basin should be available immediately adjacent to the kitchen. Staff should be trained in the technique of feed preparation and personal hygiene. The training should include methods of preventing contamination (e.g. through cleaning of equipment, reduction of airborne transfer and contact transfer by hand to a minimum). If possible the preparation of feeds should be done by the staff that are not handling babies, and should be supervised by a senior member of the nursing staff. After preparation the feeds (unless sterilized) must be placed in the refrigerator (at 4°C) preferably within 30 minutes, and not more than 60 minutes.

Non-sterile feeds should be discarded after 24 hours. Supplements should be added to the feeds immediately before use.

Human Expressed Milk

Human milk may be required to be stored, so as to give it to the mother's own child (premature baby), or it may be a donor mother whose milk is used for other children. Human milk contains antimicrobial factors and is believed to give the infants protection against infection. This is especially valuable in case of premature infants.

Some of the factors in the milk may be heat labile, but in pasteurization relatively low temperatures (63–65°C, {145–149°F}) are used, and so the antimicrobial factors are less inactivated. Improperly collected or stored milk may be heavily contaminated with pathogens such as *Klebsiella* species, *Pseudomonas aeruginosa* and *Staphylococcus aureus*. Milk from the mother fed to her own baby may be used unpasteurized, but must be stored refrigerated The Human Milk Banking Association of North America[10,11] guidelines state that routine microbiological testing for administration to a mother's own infant is unnecessary, but they recommend freezing if it is not used within 48 hours.

When a sick newborn is not able to be breastfed, the breast milk should be carefully stored in order to prevent bacterial contamination. The mother's hands should be washed with antiseptic agents, and the milk should be collected and stored in sterilized feeding-bottles. When a breast pump is used to collect the milk, all components that get in contact with the breast milk should be washed with water and soap after each collection; they should also be sterilized every day. Breast milk should be stored in the refrigerator for 24–48 hours or frozen at –20°C for a maximum period of 6 months. When milk-based formulas are used, the utensils involved in its preparation should be sterilized, and the water should be boiled for 5 minutes. The formula should be stored in individual feeding-bottles and refrigerated for a maximum period of 24 hours; after being taken out of the refrigerator, the formula should be consumed within 4 hours. In cases of milk administration through probes, these should be changed every 24 hours, and the syringe, every 4 hours. Routine microbiological monitoring is not recommended neither for breast milk nor for milk-based formulas, except for cases in which the newborns present gastrointestinal intolerance and sepsis, among other pathologies.[6]

To have milk of an acceptable microbiological standard, careful attention may be paid to the hygienic method of collection. These high standards are more easily achieved in hospital than in home. Potential donors should have blood tests to exclude syphilis; HBV, HCV and HIV infection and should not be excreting drugs in the milk. They should be trained in aseptic practices, and supplied with suitable equipment for disinfection. Home conditions should also be hygienically acceptable. In addition, several samples of milk should be microbiologically tested before it is acceptable. Instructions on collection and storage should be clear and precise, and should include handwashing, care of the breast, and methods of cleaning, disinfection and storage of the pump. Whenever possible, sterilized equipment should be supplied. The first 5 mL of milk should be discarded and the remainder transferred to a sterile bottle, which is labeled with the time of collection, the storage time and temperature. It must be placed in a refrigerator as soon as possible at 4°C and the temperature during transport should not be allowed to rise above 10°C. The time out of the refrigerator should not exceed 2 hours, and refrigerated transport or insulated containers may be required for transport.

Although samples are collected from infection-screened mothers, pasteurization is still advisable, but excessive heat should be avoided. Exposure at 63°C and not less than 57°C for 30 minutes is recommended.[12] Any bacterial growth is unacceptable. A standard volume of milk should be treated, and should be cooled rapidly so also temperature checks and microbiological tests should be made on setting up the process and at regular intervals afterwards. Milk should be deep frozen (–9 to –18°C), as quickly as possible after collection and repeated thawing and freezing should be avoided.

Microbiological Standards

Some centers state feed raw "donor" milk to the infants. In these cases, microbiological testing of each milk sample is essential.

As the number of organisms required to infect the infant, as well as the role of relatively non-pathogenic organisms remain uncertain, suggested standards differ.

The resistance of the recipient infant to infection is also variable, and the possible deleterious effect of pasteurization is uncertain. It is generally agreed that gram-negative bacilli should be absent.

Microbiological screening of donor milk is done before (if there is no cost constraint), and as soon as possible after pasteurization. Pre-pasteurization microbiology can result in wastage of milk to the tune of about 30% in some cases. Even after pasteurization, the endotoxins of organisms are still present in the milk in some cases but they have not been found to have any clinical effect on the baby. A bacterial count of 10^5 CFU/mL or more in raw breast milk can be considered as an indicator of the poor quality of milk. Based on this and on the theoretical concern that heavily contaminated milk with specific bacteria (e.g. *S. aureus, E. coli*) may contain enterotoxins and thermostable enzymes even after pasteurization, expert panel selected 10^5 CFU/mL for total bacterial count, 10^4 CFU/mL for *Enterobacteriaceae* and *S. aureus* as threshold values, which are in consonance with milk banks operating in other parts of the world. No growth is acceptable in post-pasteurization microbiology cultures. Whole batch of culture positive container of pasteurized milk should be discarded.[12]

Storage[12,13]

Pasteurized milk awaiting culture report should be kept in dedicated freezer/freezer area taking precaution not to disburse it till the culture is negative. Storage should be done in the same container that is used for pasteurization. It is advisable not to transfer processed milk in other containers as it has risk of contamination. Culture negative processed milk should be kept at –20°C in tightly sealed container with clear mention of expiry date and other relevant data on the label. It can be preserved for 3 to 6 months. Random cultures of preserved milk before disbursal can aid quality assurance.

Although, there is no evidence of infection occurring from milk, which complies with these standards, it is believed to be safer to pasteurize all donor breast milk before use.

PRACTICAL PROCEDURES FOR PREVENTION OF HAI IN GYNECOLOGY AND OBSTETRICS[14]

Labor Room

Most of the infections occurring during delivery are usually endogenous infec-tions. These are usually due to organisms in the genitourinary tracts (vagina and endocervix) of pregnant women. Any manipulations, e.g. rectal or vaginal examination, instrumentation, or putting the physicians' hand during delivery can displace the organisms from lower genital tract to the uterus. Rectal examination has been banned presently and vaginal examinations are severely restricted during labor.

Precautions to be Observed

- All standard aseptic procedures to be meticulously observed. Instruments and materials used must be properly sterilized.
- Universal precautions must be observed by HCW's. Hands are to be thoroughly washed before putting on gloves and after removal of gloves. Use waterproof (plastic) gowns (ankle length), facemask, eye shield and protective shoe covers, since splashing of blood is likely.
- Splashing to be avoided during cutting of umbilical cord. Delayed clamping avoids splashing of blood.
- Contamination of any body part with blood and amniotic fluid should be dealt with by thorough washing of the part with soap and water.
- Placenta should be inspected with gloved hands in the tray.
- All swabs, disposables (other than sharps) and placenta should be discarded in plastic bags and sent for incineration. Sharps are discarded in puncture resistant container with tight fitting lids.

In a patient with HIV infection placenta should be handled with gloved hands only. It should be buried deep with bleaching powder around placenta. The bleaching powder should be first spread in the pit made for burial, and then on the placenta. Lime can be used in place of bleach.

- Correct obstetric procedures to be observed to reduce the need for blood transfusion.
- Safe house keeping practices to be followed:
  - Routine daily cleaning of floors with soap and water followed by cleaning with a hypochlorite.
  - Table should be cleaned thoroughly with a hypochlorite solution after each case.
  - Immediate cleaning and disinfection of any blood and body fluid spills.
  - Robust plastic jars containing hypochlorite be available to put, the blood and amniotic fluid.

Care of Newborn at Birth

- *Establishment of airway:* Throat suction done by using sterile mucus suction.
- *Emptying of stomach:* Baby stomach should be aspirated using a sterile catheter/mucus sucker.
- *Care of eyes:* Usually, eyes should be cleaned with cotton swabs soaked in sterile water or saline and nothing else advocated. Cleaning to be done from inner canthus to outer canthus and not vice versa. Putting 1% silver nitrate (for preventing ophthalmia neonatorum) may lead to chemical conjunctivitis and does not prevent chlamydial conjunctivitis. Tetracycline (1%) or erythromycin (0.5%) eye ointment prevents chemical conjunctivitis[5] and has been advocated by some to prevent both gonococcal and chlamydial conjunctivitis. Some advocate a single intramuscular injection of 125 mg ceftriaxone for preventing *Penicillin resistant gonococci.*
- *Care of umbilical stump:* Immediately after birth, the umbilical cord is clamped with a sterile clamp (or tied with a sterile tape) and cut with sterile instruments. Some investigators have advocated application of silver sulfadiazine cream or bacitracin ointment to prevent infection, but most prefer keeping the cord dry with periodic swabbing with alcohol. Recently some authors[6] have carried out a study comparing four different antiseptic solutions used in the umbilical stump care of term newborns: ethyl alcohol at

70%; iodinated alcohol at 2%; Povidone iodine; and alcoholic chlorhexidine. These authors observed a decrease in bacterial colonization (mainly by *S. aureus*) with the use of chlorhexidine. However, the use of antiseptic agents both in the umbilical stump care and in the newborn's daily bath has been restricted to situations in which high rates of colonization are associated with a high frequency of staphylococcal infection at the unit. In this case, the application of chlorhexidine is preferred, since iodophors may impair the thyroidal function when absorbed by the newborn's skin and hexachlorophene may lead to neurotoxicity in the neonatal period.

- *Care of skin:* Current view is that the so-called dry technique decreases trauma, avoids toxicity from chemical and interferes least with acquisition of normal flora. So shortly after birth, the skin is cleansed using sterile cotton sponges, and sterile water either alone or with mild soap. The diaper area is then similarly cleaned.
- *Temperature control:* Baby must be wrapped in sterile warm cloth after cleaning.

Precautions in Neonatal Nursery

Isolation facilities may be required for both mothers and babies. Maternal conditions requiring isolation are puerperal sepsis, gastrointestinal infections, and breast abscess and staphylococcal sepsis. Infected neonates should be placed in isolation as soon as an infection is suspected; infants are separated from mothers if the later are infected. If there is insufficient number of isolation rooms, cohort nursing is helpful. Separate nurses should attend babies in the infected and non-infected nurseries. Nurses preparing feeds should not handle infected babies.

Hospital Environment[5]

In relation to hospital environment, some factors associated with the acquisition of infections are physical area, nurse: patients ratio, and equipment. It is recommended that the nursery be located close to the obstetric unit and count on internal divisions, with beds for intermediary and intensive care. According to the Society of Pediatrics from São Paulo[6] recommendations, the intermediary care unit should have an area of 3.5 m^2 for each bed and a 60 cm distance between the cradles; for the intensive care unit, these measures should be of 5 m^2 and 80 cm, respectively. Concerning sinks, one sink is necessary to every five patients in medium and high-risk nurseries.

- **Strict adherence to handwashing before and after handling babies is most important for infection control in nurseries:** Washing with soap and water is usually adequate, but an antiseptic detergent should be used for handwashing in premature baby units and in outbreaks of infection, chlorhexidine detergent, povidone-iodine solution or hexachlorophene are equally suitable.

Caps and masks are not necessary routinely but gowns should be worn. Separate gowns are needed for attending each baby in the premature baby unit. But recently the *wearing of aprons* in neonatal units has given rise to controversy. The routine use of aprons by the hospital staff has not shown to be an important measure in the control of nosocomial infections, since the transmission of microorganisms usually occurs through the hands. Several studies showed that the use of aprons does not alter the bacterial colonization of the newborn or the rate of infection in neonatal units. The use of aprons is indicated in the performance of invasive procedures and in some situations of contact isolation. Wearing gloves is indicated as part of universal prevention measures whenever there is the possibility of the professional getting in contact with the patient's blood and secretions.[5]

Traditionally, linens have been sterilized by autoclaving. But routine laundering is sufficient provided there is good laundry in the hospital. Soiled linens should be placed into plastic bags, sealed and removed every 8 hours.

- Napkins should be disposed off into a bucket lined with a plastic bag, which is sealed when full and removed.
- CSSD should centrally sterilize equipment for preparing special feeds in the wards, so also the containers, teats, tube feeding equipment. Feeds should be terminally sterilized or heat disinfected. Bottles, teats and catheters for feeds should be sterilized after each use. Feeds (unless sterilized should be placed in refrigerator (4°C) within 30 minutes. Nonsterile feeds should be discarded after 24 hours.

Equipments

- Stethoscopes and thermometers should be cleaned between uses with alcohol or an iodophor solution.
- Nebulization equipment is easily contaminated. It should be autoclaved every 8 hours (if autoclavable) or sterilized by low temperature steam. Water may also be a source of bacterial proliferation (examples are *Pseudomonas* species and *Serratia* species); thus it is recommended that sterile liquids be used in nebulizers and humidifiers, and that the liquid that condenses in the ventilator circuit be thrown away, in order to prevent it from returning to the nebulizer.
- Ventilators should be cleaned externally with liquid soap and water, and the circuits should be changed every 48 hours and disinfected with glutaraldehyde at 2% (the nasal cannula should also be disinfected using this solution).
- Equipment used in neonatal resuscitation, such as balloons, masks, and laryngoscopes should be cleaned every time they are used, according to the hospital protocol.
- Cradles and incubators should be washed with water and liquid soap every day, and terminal cleaning should be performed every 7 days or after the bed is disoccupied.
- The floor, walls, windows, and other surfaces should be cleaned every day using methods that minimize the spread of dust, using chlorinated and quaternary ammonium compounds.
- The use of phenolic compounds is not indicated in neonatal units due to their absorption by the skin and to the risk for hyperbilirubinemia in newborns.
- Cleaning and disinfection of suction equipment should be done.
- Baby's incubator should be cleaned and disinfected after discharge of the patient. The inner surface of the incubator is first cleaned with paper wipe, followed by cleaning with soap and water and dried and kept dry. If necessary, it is cleaned with a disinfectant.
- The part of the X-ray equipment that comes into contact with an infant should be cleaned with an alcohol or an iodophor solution.
- Aseptic care of intravascular catheters should be taken.[5]

Collection of Breast Milk

Many mothers like to provide breast milk for their babies who are unable to nurse. Mother first scrubs her hand with an iodophor or other antiseptic. The nipple area does not need special cleaning. The milk is expressed manually or collected by a mechanical device, stored in a sterile bottle and refrigerated.

Blood

In addition to testing for HbsAg and HIV antibodies, it is also tested for CMV antibodies. The blood given to neonates must be free from all the above three diseases.

Fluids for Total Parenteral Nutrition

If fluids are mixed for fluids for total parenteral nutrition (TPN), this should be done under a positive -pressure filtered hood.

Serum Hepatitis in Mother During Pregnancy

A dose of hepatitis immunoglobulin should be given to the infant within ten days of birth.

Other Precautions

Visitors

- Parents should do the scrubbing as for HCWs before entering. A long sleeved gown must be worn over street clothing. They must not touch other babies. Parents with respiratory infections or infected lesions on hands or face should not be permitted to enter nurseries.
- Female HCWS (child-bearing age) in the nursery are tested for rubella antibodies and if found negative are given Rubella vaccine. Immunity for hepatitis B should also be investigated, and vaccination is recommended whenever necessary. Annual immunization against prevalent strains of the influenza virus is highly recommended, because the neonates, especially preterms or those with chronic pulmonary disease, are particularly vulnerable to complications when they acquire infections.[5]
- Pregnant HCWs should not handle infants infected with CMV. HCWs with active tuberculosis, pertusis, influenza, and other communicable diseases should not handle infants. HCW's with bacterial or viral lesions on exposed part of skin must be excluded from nursery. Personnel with acute diarrhea are excluded. Individuals with acute sore throat and fever are excluded until group A streptococcal infection has either been ruled out or treated.
- The use of central venous catheters in critically ill newborns is a potential source of nosocomial infection. One of the factors associated with the increase in catheter-related infections in the blood flow is its insertion method. The risk for sepsis with central venous catheters inserted surgically is three times higher in the neonatal period when compared to peripherally inserted catheters. Based on these data, percutaneous catheters have been more often used than surgical catheters. The main prevention measures for infections-related central venous catheters are the use of maximum barrier precautions, such as the use of surgical caps, masks, aprons, gloves, sterilized areas and materials, skin disinfection with alcoholic chlorhexidine, and a team specialized in the insertion and maintenance of the catheter.[5]
- Although the administration of antibiotics may be necessary as soon as infection in neonate is suspected, the widespread use of chemoprophylaxis is not recommended. Beta lactam and aminoglycoside combinations are the mainstay of therapy in newborn nurseries. Because of their widespread use in neonatal ICU and in low birth weight babies, there is emergence of resistance to aminoglycosides. Then temporarily a broad-spectrum cephalosporin (cefotaxime or ceftrioxone) is the drug of choice. It is best to monitor the prevalence of resistant bacteria in nurseries from time to time as a guide to therapy for treating undiagnosed infections in the unit.

REFERENCES

1. Gibbs RS. Obstetric and gynaecologic infections. In: Groschel D (Ed). Hospital associated infections in the general hospital population and specific measures of control. Handbook on Hospital-associated Infections, 3rd edition. Mancel Dekkar INC, New York, US; 1979.p.50-2.
2. Ohm MJ, Galask RP. Effects of antibiotic prophylaxis, alteration of microbial flora. Am J Obstet Gynaecol. 1976;125:448 Pg 53. Quoted in Ref. No. 1.
3. Gibbs RS, O'Dell TN, Mac Greger RR, Shwarz RH, Mortom H. Peurperal endometritis—a prospective microbiologic study. Am J Obstet Gynaecol. 1975;121:919 Pg 53. Quoted in Ref No. 1.

4. Centre for Disease Control, National Nosocomial Infections Study. Quarterly report, Annual Summary 1976, Issued February, 1978.
5. Baltimore RS. Neonatal Nosocomial Infections. Semin Perinatol. 1998:22:25-32. Quoted in Marisa Marcia Mussi-Pinhata, Suely Dornellas do Nascimento: Neonatal nosocomial infections (Review article). Jornal de Pediatria 0021-7557/01/77-Supl.1/S81. Accessed on 15/7/2015 from www.ped.com.br/conteudo/01-77-s81/ing.pdf.
6. Mussi-Pinhata MM, do Nascimento SD. Neonatal nosocomial infections (Review article). Jornal de Pediatria 0021-7557/01/77-Supl.1/S81. Accessed on 15/7/2015 from www.ped.com.br/conteudo/01-77-s81/ing.pdf.
7. Gibbs RS. Obstetric and gynaecologic infections. In: Groschel D (Ed). Hospital associated infections in the general hospital population and specific measures of control. Handbook on Hospital-associated Infections, 3rd edition. Mancel Dekkar INC, New York, US; 1979.p.63.
8. George R. Maternity Departments Chapter 16. In: Ayliffee GA, Fraise AP, Geddes AM, Mitchell K (Eds). Control of hospital infection-A Practical Handbook, 4th edition, Oxford University Press; 2000.p.319.
9. Burnett IA, Wardley BL, Magee JT. The Milk kitchen at Sheffield Children's Hospital—before and after a review. J Hosp Infect. 1989;13:179.
10. Human Milk Banking Association of North America (1993a). Guidelines for the establishment and operation of a Human Milk Bank. Hartford CT: HMBA North America. Quoted in Ref No. 7.
11. Human Milk Banking Association of North America (1993b). Recommendations for Collection, Storage and Handling of a mother's milk for her own infant in the hospital setting. Hartford CT: HMBA North America. Quoted in Ref No. 7.
12. Royal College of Paediatricians and Child Health Working Party (1999). Guidelines for the establishment of human Milk Banks in the UK, London: Royal College of Paediatrics and Child Health. Quoted in Ref No. 6.
13. Bharadva, et al. Human milk banking guidelines. For the infant and young child feeding chapter, Indian Academy of Pediatrics. Indian Paediatrics. 2014;51:472. Accessed on 14th July 2015. From www.indianpaediatrics.net/june2014/469.pdf.
14. Aggarwal DS. Microbiology Department, University of Medical Sciences and GTB Hospital, Delhi. Guidelines for Nosocomial Infections. Surveillance and Control World Health Organization. South-East Asia Regional Office. New Delhi.

Chapter 14

Intensive Care Unit—Problems and Management

Chapter Outline

- General Problems and Management in ICU
- Control of Infection
- Transmission-based (Isolation) Precautions
- Antibiotic Utilization Policies
- Surveillance
- Prevention of Specific Infection Sites
- *Clostridium difficile* Infections
- Nosocomial Sinusitis
- Decolonization
- Design of the Unit
- Furniture and Fitting
- Cleaning of Environment
- Handling of Patients
- Procedures in ICU
- Equipment in ICU
- Antibiotic Prophylaxis
- Administrative Aspects
- Visitor Policy and Use of Protective Shoe Covers
- Practical Aspects for Infection Control in Intensive Care Areas

GENERAL PROBLEMS AND MANAGEMENT IN ICU

Infection is one of the principal hazards to which patients in intensive care units (ICUs) are exposed. Patients admitted to ICU are those who require intensive care in the form of support of a vital function until the disease process is arrested.

These patients are likely to have poor resistance to infection. This may be due to immunosuppressive or steroid therapy, or due to depression of immunological response (often seen in patients with multiple organ failure). In addition to being more susceptible, they are exposed in the intensive care unit to greater hazards of contamination and cross infection than most patients in the ordinary wards. This is due to the fact that they receive much more nursing attention and handling and various forms of instrumentation particularly tracheostomy, mechanical ventilation, aspiration of bronchial secretions, catheterization of the urinary tract, treatment of open wounds, and central venous catheterization. The host defenses are by passed by the invasive devices and there are greater chances of infection with endogenous flora.

Special difficulties arise in emergencies (e.g. respiratory obstruction requiring immediate clearing of the patients' airway) and the sudden excessive pressure of work, which occurs when several patients are admitted at the same time. In such circumstances, it may be difficult or impossible to observe all the recommendations of asepsis. Intensive therapy requires an excessive number of trained nursing staff, and if this is not available, nurses inevitably have to move rapidly between patients without having time even to wash hands. The amount of technical assistance and the number of domestic staff in intensive units is much greater than it is in normal wards, but these are essential if nursing skills are to be used effectively and if meticulous cleanliness of equipment is to be maintained.[1]

Microorganisms involved in HAI, in almost all cases previously colonized the host, coming from an exogenous or an endogenous source. In the first case transmission from an exogenous source usually takes place via direct contact or airborne droplets transmission, while in the second case, it is commonly associated with a normal barrier derangement.[2]

The microorganisms which cause infection in intensive care units include any of those which are associated with hospital infection, but as the patients are often deficient in resistance to infection, many organisms which have little or no pathogenicity to healthy individuals and tissues are potentially important as causes of infection in intensive care patients. The commonest infecting organisms in ICU are *S. aureus* (including MRSA),

S. epidermidis, E. coli, P. aeruginosa, Klebsiella species, *Proteus* species, *Acinetobacter* species, *Enterobacter* species and *Candida* species. Endogenous infection with coliform bacilli and sometimes *Bacteroides* species and other anaerobic non-sporing bacteria is a hazard in patients with abdominal wounds.

The reduction of gastric acid by the use of H_2 blockers may be followed by colonization of the stomach with gram-negative bacilli. Aspiration of stomach contents may lead to colonization of the oropharynx and the respiratory tract and possibly to bronchopneumonia.

Staphylococcal infection may be transmitted by contact or by air, and epidemic strains of MRSA are a particular hazard. Gram-negative bacteria, when not acquired from the patients' own flora of skin, gut or upper respiratory tract, are most likely to be acquired by contact and from solutions and medicament, food, humidifiers of mechanical ventilators, etc. Airborne infection with gram-negative bacilli is a remote risk, except from aerosols produced by a contaminated nebulizer, or less commonly from removal of dressings (e.g. of burns) on which heavily contaminated exudate has dried.

Expectoration by patients with tracheostomies or endotracheal tubes may cause heavy local contamination with bronchial mucus, but the air of an Intensive care unit has been found to be usually free from *P. aeruginosa*, even when several patients with respiratory and urinary tract *Pseudomonas* infection are in the ward. The suggestion that the expired air of all the patients undergoing artificial ventilation in the unit should be filtered or exhausted seems unnecessary.

The infection rate in ICU is generally 5–10 times greater than general wards. The main sites of infection are urinary tract, lower respiratory tract (Pneumonia), intravascular cannula entry site infection, primary bacteremia and gastrointestinal tract.[3]

Because of the increased rate of emerging multidrug-resistant pathogens multidisciplinary infection control programs have become a necessity in order to suppress antibiotic resistance and to improve the outcome of critically ill patients. Infection control in ICU is based on general control measures, transmission-based (isolation) precautions, antibiotic utilization policies, surveillance and decolonization of patients. Hand disinfection remains the cornerstone of the bundle of actions apart from general infection control measures and transmission-based precautions, must have antibiotic utilization restriction policy as a priority. So also specific infections' prevention strategies should be implemented, emphasizing on ventilation-associated pneumonia and bloodstream infections. Systematic surveillance reflects a tool with which the infection rates and the effectiveness of different measures could be evaluated.[2]

CONTROL OF INFECTION[2]

The general principles of aseptic care and hospital hygiene must be meticulously applied with certain additional procedures of intensive care unit. The infection control programs in the ICU are based on general infection control measures for the prevention of microbial transmission among patients and healthcare workers (HCW), transmission-based precautions and antimicrobial policy-surveillance methods for the restriction of the emergence of MDR pathogens and their source control.

General Control Measures for Infections Prevention[2]

The purpose of general control measures is to prevent the transmission of infectious agents among patients and HCW. They are applied uniformly to all patients, regardless of the microorganisms by which they are colonized or infected, including mainly hand hygiene and barrier precautions (gloves, masks and gowns).

Hand Hygiene

Hand hygiene is the most important measure for the avoidance of microbial transmission in the hospital setting among patients, HCW and different surfaces. Hand disinfection should take place before and after every contact with a patient or his surrounding, whether there is a body fluid exposure or not. The alcohol- based products are the cornerstone for handwashing as they are more effective than antimicrobial liquids or plain soap and water and are less time consuming, involve less hand drying and show higher rates of compliance with the guidelines (only in *Clostridium difficile* infections is handwashing with soap the only effective measure against the produced spores). Although, there are no strict guidelines, many experts recommend also the avoidance of artificial fingernails and hand jewelry.

Gloves, Gowns, Face and Respiratory Protection

Gloves, gowns and face protection accessories, such as masks, goggles and face shields, are characterized as personal protective equipment. They are used as barriers for the skin, mucous membranes, airway and clothing protection from contamination.

Gloves: These should always be used when a direct contact with blood, body fluids, mucous membranes, non-intact skin or possibly contaminated patient equipment or surfaces is anticipated and in every direct contact with patients who are colonized with pathogens transmitted by the contact route [Vancomycin-resistant enterococci (VRE), methicillin-resistant *Staphylococcus aureus* (MRSA), etc]. They are used in order to protect from infectious agents transmission from patient to HCWs and vice versa, as well as to reduce the chance of colonization of the hands of HCW.

Masks: These are recommended for the protection of HCWs' from the patients' respiratory secretions and body fluid aerosols and for the protection of patients from HCW-produced respiratory aerosols during sterile procedures (e.g. lumbar puncture).

Goggles and face shields: These are used for eye or face protection in the context of specific procedures where a splash or spray or other biological fluid is likely.

For respiratory protection: The Centers of Disease Control and Prevention (CDC) currently recommends N95 or higher-level respirators when exposure to patients with a suspected or confirmed tuberculosis is anticipated as well as in cases of other diseases possibly transmitted through the airborne route such as influenza, severe acute respiratory syndrome (SARS) and smallpox.

Personal protective equipment accessories should always be disposed in designated containers after removal and hand hygiene should necessarily follow as last precaution.

TRANSMISSION-BASED (ISOLATION) PRECAUTIONS[2]

These precautions are applied when specific epidemiologically important pathogens are suspected or proved to be present in order to prevent transmission to other patients (source control). They are performed when general infection control measures are not adequate for transmission control and are always used in addition to them, singly or in combination, depending on the pathogen and their route of transmission.

- *Contact precautions:* Contact precautions are required in cases of epidemiologically important pathogens, such as MDR bacteria. Patients who require contact isolation should be placed in a private room or cohorted with other patients sharing the same colonization or infection and they should never share medical equipment with other patients. HCW must apply general infection measures before and after contact with the patient or the patient's environment.
- *Droplet precautions:* Droplets are particles of respiratory secretions larger than five micron that remain suspended in the air for limited periods. Human-to-human transmission of droplet-borne pathogens (such as *Neisseria meningitis*, *Bordetella pertussis*, human influenza virus, *Mycoplasma pneumoniae*, rubella, mumps, *Haemophilus influenzae* type b, SARS, *Streptococcus* group A) usually requires exposure within less than one meter (sometimes up to two meters) When droplet precautions are needed, single patient room is preferred and the use of face masks by HCW within two or three meters of the patient is advised. Patient themselves should wear facemasks when they are moved outside their rooms. Special air-handling systems and higher level respirator masks are not required.
- *Air-borne transmission:* Air-borne droplets are particles of respiratory secretions smaller than five microns that can be suspended in the air for longer periods, constituting an infectious source. *Mycobacterium tuberculosis* is the most characteristic pathogen of this type, as well as measles, varicella and perhaps small-pox. In those cases special air-handling and ventilation systems should be applied. Patients with air-borne droplet infections must be isolated in rooms with negative air pressure and a minimum of six to twelve air changes per hour with closed doors must be performed. All persons entering the room must wear respirators offering filtering capacity of 95% with a tight seal over the nose and mouth.

ANTIBIOTIC UTILIZATION POLICIES[2]

Multidrug antibiotic resistance has increased dramatically among gram-positive and gram-negative bacteria worldwide, while antimicrobial agents with new mechanisms of actions are lacking. As a result infections by MDR pathogens are rising and they are associated with significant morbidity, mortality and financial costs. This phenomenon particularly affects Intensive care-units where patients have multiple risk factors (long hospital stay, prior use of antibiotics, severity of illness, absence of normal anatomical barriers, high frequency of medical and nursing interventions). Extended spectrum beta-lactamases (ESBL) enterobacteriaceae, carbapenems resistant *Pseudomonas aeruginosa*, VRE and MRSA represent the most commonly reported MDR pathogens in the ICU. Apart from general infection control measures that are considered valuable and irreplaceable, strict antibiotic hospital policies are of urgent need. Several methods have been proposed for the restriction of broad-spectrum antibiotics use, including antibiotic cycling, broad empiric antibiotic treatments, prompt de-escalation according to cultures' results and shorter courses of antibiotic treatment. Clinicians do not always comply with guidelines, mainly due to the lack of convincing evidence. This however gives a good excuse to the antibiotic evaluation committees for a strict surveillance of staff compliance.

SURVEILLANCE[2]

The surveillance techniques are considered as prerequisite for effective HAI prevention predominantly in high-risk hospital settings such as the ICUs. Surveillance is defined as the systematic and continuous investigation for the early detection of single cases or cluster of HAI by epidemiologically important infectious agents. The analysis and presentation of the collected information aims towards the adequate and appropriate treatment of HAI in order to improve the related morbidity and mortality. Surveillance allows the early recognition and management of epidemics and outbreaks, the recognition of systemic faults in daily clinical practice and the evaluation of infection control programs.

Colonization surveillance has been proposed as an important tool of surveillance systems in the ICU, where the high incidence of MDR pathogens make the empirical antimicrobial treatment of septic patients a difficult decision. The hypothesis is that nosocomial pathogens predominate early on patient's flora before they induce infection and if the intensivist is informed about the type of pathogens by which the septic patient is colonized, he could add early and appropriate empirical therapy while waiting for the results from the taken cultures. The collection of cultures for surveillance purposes is not extensively studied and no specific guidelines have been reported regarding the best sites and the frequency of screen. A cost-effective policy has not yet been proved and even if there are several studies reporting the significance of colonization surveillance programs, it is still not clear if there is a positive impact on mortality rates. However, surveillance provides an accurate screening method for the detection of patients who are colonized with MDR pathogens at the time of their admission, allowing for early contact and isolation measures to be applied.

PREVENTION OF SPECIFIC INFECTION SITES[2]

Ventilator-associated Pneumonia

Ventilator-associated pneumonia (VAP) is the most common infection in the ICU leading to increased morbidity and mortality, prolonged hospitalization in ICU, increased number of days on mechanical ventilation and prolonged duration of antimicrobial use.

The prevention of VAP is based on specific and general measures.

The general control measures include hand hygiene, surveillance methods performance and staff education.

The specific measures include:

- Short duration of ventilation (avoidance of mechanical ventilation if possible)

- Preference of noninvasive ventilation whenever possible
- Daily efforts to wean
- The prevention of aspiration (maintenance of semi-recumbent position
- Avoidance of gastric over- distension
- Avoidance of unplanned extubation
- Maintenance of endotracheal cuff pressure of at least 20 cm H_2O
- Strategies for reduction of aerodigestive colonization (orotracheal intubation performance)
- Avoidance of H_2-blocking agents and proton-pump inhibitors
- Usage of oral antiseptics and silver-coated endotracheal tubes with subglotic aspiration ports)
- Appropriate cleansing and disinfection of ventilator equipment.

Catheter-related Bloodstream Infections[2]

Catheter-related bloodstream infections also reflect a significant cause of infection in ICU. A significant percentage of those infections can be prevented by using the general proposed measures which includes:

- Education of healthcare personnel on indications, insertion procedures and infection control measures.
- Nursing staff adequacy is considered crucial in the catheter-related bloodstream infections (CRBSI) control as high patient-to-nurse ratios are associated with more CRBSI.
- The continuous assessment of knowledge and adherence to guidelines.
- Surveillance for CRBSI rates, clusters and epidemics.
- The routine monitoring for the detection of wrong practices.
- Feedback and communication of the collected data.

The prevention of CRBSI are focused mainly on:

- The selection of the catheter type and site of insertion
- Hand hygiene procedures
- Aseptic techniques and barrier precautions
- Skin preparation and site dressing regimens
- Cleansing and surveillance
- Upper extremities are preferred for central venous catheter (CVC)
- Maximal sterile barrier precautions should be undertaken for the insertion of CVCs (cap, mask, sterile gloves, sterile full-body drape).
- Skin preparation should be done with chlorhexedine (>0.5%) with alcohol before CVC insertion and during dressing changes (tincture of iodine, iodophor, 70% alcohol are alternatives.
- Catheter insertion site should be evaluated daily by palpation and visually when changing the dressing, depending on the clinical situation of the individual patient, if patients have tenderness at the insertion site, fever without obvious source, or other manifestations suggesting local or bloodstream infection, the dressing should be removed to allow thorough examination of the site.
- Chlorhexidine-impregnated sponge dressing for temporary short-term catheters should be used in patients more than two months old if CRBSI rate is not decreasing despite adherence to basic prevention measures.
- CVCs should not be routinely replaced or removed on the basis of fever alone, but only after clinical judgment.
- Guidewire exchanges should not be used to prevent infection or when infection is suspected, but only to replace a malfunctioning non-tunneled catheter if no evidence of infection is present and always with sterile gloves.
- Administration sets should be replaced no frequently than at 96 hours intervals but at least every seven days.
- Ultrasound guidance to place CVCs (if this technology is available) is associated with a reduction in the number of cannulation attempts and mechanical complications and therefore this technique must be only used by fully-trained physicians.

- The use of a sutureless securement device to reduce the risk of infection for intravascular catheters is allowed, while the use of chlorhexidine/silver sulfadiazine or minocycline, rifampin-impregnated CVC is recommended in patients whose catheter is expected to remain in place more than five days after successful implementation of a comprehensive strategy to reduce rates of CRBSI if their rate is not decreasing.

Urinary Tract Infections[2]

Urinary tract infections are relatively common in critically ill patients, almost exclusively related to the use of an indwelling urinary catheter or to invasive urinary tract procedures. UTIs include symptomatic UTI, asymptomatic bacteriuria and other infections of the urinary tract. The recognized risk factors for the development of UTI include female gender, duration of catheterization, immunodeficiency and length of ICU stay. UTIs are often associated with increased morbidity, but not mortality, while the preventive measures are:

- General measures (education of staff concerning the correct techniques of catheter insertion and manipulation, hand hygiene and aseptic methods for inserting the catheter and obtaining urine samples.
- Catheterization only when necessary
- Maintenance of a closed drainage system
- Maintenance of unobstructed urine flow and
- The use of silver-coated catheters.
- A practice that must be avoided is the use of prophylactic antibiotics.
- Finally, it is very important to remember that asymptomatic bacteriuria is a distinct condition which does not need antibiotic treatment compared to symptomatic UTI.

CLOSTRIDIUM DIFFICILE INFECTIONS[2]

C. difficile-related diarrhea is the most common cause of nosocomial diarrhea, associated with the prior use of antibiotics (mainly clindamycin, beta-lactamase inhibitors, third generation cephalosporins). The severity of diarrhea varies from mild diarrhea to fatal pseudomembranous enterocolitis, while treatment includes the use of metronidazole or vancomycin orally, as well as the discontinuation of the causative agent.

Precautionary measures include:

- Prevention of ingestion of *C. difficile* (hand hygiene, isolation of patients).
- Reduction of the incidence of infection after ingestion through antimicrobial stewardship.
- Environmental control, room disinfection and
- Barrier precautions.
- Prophylaxis with antimicrobial agents and treatment of asymptomatic carriers are not recommended, while the use of probiotics remains controversial.

NOSOCOMIAL SINUSITIS[2]

Nosocomial sinusitis appears to occur due to impaired drainage of the sinus cavity, slowed venous drainage due to positive pressure ventilation and the presence of nasogastric and nasotracheal tubes. Sinusitis is a risk factor for the development of pneumonia. The prevention of sinusitis in the ICU setting is the systematic use of orotracheal intubation

DECOLONIZATION[2]

Many of the serious HAIs often originate from endogenous sources such as patients' own flora. Thus, eradication of the colonizing bacteria that potentially could cause infections in the critically ill patients reflects a strategy often performed in ICUs. Decolonization policies commonly focus on:

- Eradication/reduction of MRSA carriage on the skin and mucus membrane using different regimens. The local use of mupirocin alone as a 2% ointment must be avoided because of significant relapse episodes or high reinfection rates. Better results have been reported with the combined use of mupirocin, chlorhexidine baths and systemic therapy such as rifampin, doxycycline and trimethoprim-sulfamethoxazole, although recolonization may occur. The intact skin and underlying good health status are very important determinants of success.

- Screening and decolonization of healthcare workers remains controversial.
- Another method of decontamination is the selective digestive decontamination (SSD) aiming to prevent colonization by gram-negative bacteria, *S. aureus* and yeasts in intensive care patients through the application of non-absorbable antimicrobial agents in the gastro-intestinal tract. The most commonly used antibacterials include a parenteral third-generation cephalosporin (e.g. cefotaxime), an enteral polymixin, an aminoglycoside and an antifungal agent. The aim of this intervention is to maintain patients' anaerobic bacteria, although concerns about the development of highly resistant bacteria have limited its adoption.

To conclude, ICU-acquired infections are a major cause of increased morbidity and mortality, prolonged hospitalization and high cost especially when MDR pathogens are involved. The cornerstone for their treatment is the early recognition of causative pathogens and sites of infection. Infection control in ICU is based on hand hygiene, surveillance programs and adequate and appropriate antibiotics use. These methods present an effective manner to reduce the incidence of ICU infections.[2]

DESIGN OF THE UNIT[1]

- Because of the need for quick and unimpaired access of staff to the patients, it is usually inappropriate for the patients to be in single bed isolation room, but one or two isolation rooms are required (e.g. in a 8 bed unit, there could be 2–3 bed wards or divisions of a ward and two isolation rooms).
- There should be adequate space (e.g. 10–12 feet between bed centers) to allow easy access of staff and equipment.
- In the "Open" section retractable water-proof curtains between beds may have some value in preventing contamination of adjacent beds with expectorated mucus. Curtains should be changed weekly and between patients.
- The isolation rooms should be suitable for use by either the infected patient (source isolation) or hypersusceptible patients who must be given maximum protection against infection (protective isolation) or for combined source and protective isolation, e.g. by plenum ventilation into the room and extraction of air, when required from the room to the outside of the hospital. It is probably desired that the open section of the unit should have mechanical ventilation with a turnover of air (e.g. 10 air changes (Ayliffee) to 15–20 airchanges/hour (Agarwal DS), sufficient to prevent a build up of bacteria released by individuals in the unit and to keep the airborne bacteria at low level. It is desirable to have a positive pressure mechanical ventilation with 15–20 air changes per hour. The incoming air passes through HEPA filters. However, an ICU may be reasonably safe without plenum ventilation, or with a degree of mechanical ventilation to provide maximum comfort.
- Washbasins should be located in convenient places to facilitate hand washing.
- Housekeeping should be as in wards.

FURNITURE AND FITTING[1]

- Floors and walls should be washable.
- Furniture should be reduced to a minimum.
- Monitoring equipment should be clear of the floor and easily moved and cleaned.

- Suction apparatus and sphygmomanometers should be well mounted but detachable.

CLEANING OF ENVIRONMENT

It should be done as in wards.

HANDLING OF PATIENTS[1]

- A high standard of aseptic care must be used by nurses, doctors, pathology technicians, microbiologist, radiologist, etc. in handling patients in the ICU.
- Hands should be washed with an antimicrobial detergent or preferably disinfected with 70% alcohol rubbed to dryness, which is rapid and effective.
- Plastic disposable (non-sterile) gloves should be worn for bronchial and oral toilet, and as many as possible of the procedures (e.g. oral toilet), should always be performed before dirty procedures (e.g. taking rectal temperature).
- Protective clothing (gowns or plastic aprons) should be worn when attending to a patient. All members of staff or visitors should wear a gown or apron used for the patient only. Overshoes are unnecessary, but masks (deflector type) should be worn when attending to patients with tracheostomies or extensive wounds.
- Non-essential visiting should be discouraged, but relatives or close friends should be allowed to visit the patient. They must have almost unrestricted access to prevent disorientation of the patient, which can prevent severe psychological disturbance one of the major problems for those who survive.

Furthermore, there is good evidence that infection is more likely to be acquired from a member of the hospital staff who attends to other patients, than from a (healthy) visitor, who visits only one patient in the ward.

PROCEDURES IN ICU[1]

Tracheostomy and Endotracheal Intubation

Though tracheostomy is a procedure, which benefits the patient as the exudates can be aspirated and mechanical ventilation can be established, it has a disadvantage, i.e. the risk of infection.

Colonization of the oral cavity and trachea may sometimes lead to the development of bronchopneumonia caused by various organisms, but predominantly by gram-negative bacilli introduced into the respiratory tract at the time of aspiration of exudate or during mechanical ventilation or humidification, or *Staphylococcus aureus* from inspired air.

Tracheostomy is used for patients who require long-term ventilation, however most patients can be ventilated using endotracheal tubes. These may also be a channel of contamination, but they have the advantage of avoiding the need for an operation, with possible infection of the operation wound. There is usually no difficulty in reintubating patients and aspirations can be easily aspirated from an endotracheal tube as from a tracheostomy.

Control of infection in patients with tracheostomy or endotracheal tube is difficult. When any patient in the unit has multiresistant gram-negative infection (of the respiratory tract or of a wound) infection may spread to other patients in the unit. Care is needed during removal of endotracheal tubes, and nonsterile plastic gloves should be worn.

The most important procedure for reducing the spread of infection is handwashing between patients.

Intravenous Catheters

(See intravenous catheter-associated infections).

Ventilatory Equipment

Prevention of infection from this source is very important. Various methods of decontamination are available (see chapters on Sterilization and Disinfection). The designs of all modern lung ventilators have the ability either to isolate the ventilator completely from the patient by bacterial filters, or for the patient's circuit and humidifier to be easily removed for autoclaving or both. It has been suggested that placing a filter between the patient and the circuit may reduce colonization of ventilatory equipment and thus reduce the incidence of pneumonia, although conclusive evidence to support this hypothesis is lacking.

Urine Drainage

A fluid balance is required as a part of management of patients in the intensive care unit. Drainage bags must be changed or emptied twice daily under aseptic conditions, and the urine collected for 24 hours analysis must not be stored at bed side.

EQUIPMENT IN ICU[1]

All equipment used in intensive care units should be kept meticulously clean and dry. In a study on sources of infection, washing bowls used by patients in an ICU were often found to be contaminated with *Pseudomonas aeruginosa* in residues of moisture. Individual bowls that have been heat disinfected or at least thoroughly washed and dried after use are desirable. Shaving brushes should be avoided and electric razors used on one patient and then on another are also potential vectors of infection. An individual shaving kit is desirable. Proper disinfection of ventilators, nebulizers, humidifiers and suction equipment should be done. Food mixers are also a potential source of infection. Water in flower vases is frequently contaminated with *Pseudomonas* species, although this is an unlikely source of infection. Storage of equipment in fluids should be avoided.

ANTIBIOTIC PROPHYLAXIS[1]

Antibiotic prophylaxis should generally be avoided to reduce the risk of selecting multi-resistant opportunistic organisms. However, selective decontamination of the oropharynx and gastrointestinal tract with antibiotics has been used successfully in several studies, to prevent colonization with aerobic gram-negative bacilli. One such regime includes applications of a paste containing polymixin B, tobramycin and amphoterecin B to the oral pharynx, the introduction of these agents into the stomach with a nasogastric tube, and the systemic administration of cefotaxime.[2] Respiratory infection has been shown to be significantly reduced by this regime. Other studies have shown similar results, although there is less evidence that mortality is reduced. Further studies over a longer time period are still required to determine the specific applications for this routine, and to determine whether selective decontamination will also select highly resistant strains.

ADMINISTRATIVE ASPECTS[4]

- Sufficient numbers of frequently used instruments should be available to allow time for cleaning and sterilization or disinfection.
- Since ICU demands a high level of nursing care and strict application of rigid barrier nursing, adequate number of nurses should be provided. A nurse-to-patient staffing ratio of 1:1 has been recommended.
- HCWs in ICU must be well trained in intensive care. They also need periodic updates.
- A mechanism of monitoring the quality of care should be developed to keep a check on compliance with recommended guidelines.
- Only patients who benefit from high intensity, high-risk care should be admitted to ICU.

Patients should be discharged from ICU as soon as possible to decrease the risk of infection.

VISITOR POLICY AND USE OF PROTECTIVE SHOE COVERS[5-10]

ICUs experience higher infection rates due to the severity of illness of the patient and frequent use of invasive devices. Hand hygiene and use of Personal protective barrier (Gloves, Personal protective eye wear, Apron, Gown, Shoe covers and a Cap/Hair cover) are important for prevention of transmission of infection. PPE should be chosen in accordance to the risk of exposure. Healthcare workers should assess whether they are at risk of exposure to blood, body fluids, excretions or secretions and choose their items of personal protective equipment according to the assessed risk. Disposable caps and protective foot wear should be used when there is a likelihood that patient's blood, body fluids, secretions or excretions might splash, spill or leak onto the hair or shoes.

Many of the hospitals in India do not comply with the hand hygiene measures, small number implement the use of personal protective equipment for infection prevention. Most hospitals do not have a policy regarding restricted access of visitors in intensive care units and a shoe change policy. Hand hygiene and barrier precautions have been proved to be important measures for infection control in hospitals, but there is still a controversy regarding restricted access of visitors and a shoe change policy. It has been concluded by some of these studies that the use of shoe covers in critical care area is not helpful in preventing infections of common ICU pathogens; nor has it decreased the mortality and length of stay in ICU patients.[5,7]

As regards visitor's policy, it is stated that critical care areas manage patients who are critically ill and hence associated with a situation of panic, anxiety, loss of control and crisis functioning. In such situation, not only patients, but also families need support to cope positively and stay informed. This advocates a more liberalized policy for ICU.[8] A study on beliefs and attitudes on ICU nurses has shown interesting findings. Nurses believed that open visiting hampers nursing care, interferes with direct nursing care and causes nurses to spend more time in providing information to the patient's families. Another study on nurses beliefs concluded that liberal visiting policy reduces the tension and anxiety of patients and helps nurses to carry out quality care.[9] However, unrestricted entry to ICU can result in noise and thereby cause distraction of nursing staff. Besides variable communication skills of the nursing staff can lead to confusion and misinterpretation of facts by relatives which can subsequently result in conflict and may even lead to legal repercussions.

Visiting times can be influenced by local decisions regarding structural requirements of planning and design aspects[10] the most important being provision of day and overnight facilities for relatives, more important being that the position of the relatives' room must prevent relatives from having continuous access to staff and should be outside the area of medical and nursing staff areas. In this case, an open visitors' policy may be feasible.

Most of the studies have however concluded that in spite of all controversies, there should be a visitor policy for the ICUs and other critical areas in order to ensure adequate rest to the patient, to undertake the required care and treatment by the nursing staff, keep the ward environment clean, control the spread of infection and to have some degree of consistency of rules across the hospital. The policy thus adopted should consider the hours of visiting, the number of visitors allowed per patient, and who can visit.

However, it requires more scientific studies to be carried out regarding aspects such as shoe change practices, restricted access, etc., so that definite policies can be laid down. A universal policy can be implemented for visitors in ICUs at a national level for critical care areas. However, if not feasible some standard policies may be developed with due consideration to the sociocultural-educational-religious factors of the local population and the overall hygiene and sanitary environment of the hospital. While developing such policies, an integrated approach should be made by both the administrators and clinicians to achieve optimum result on implementation of the same.

PRACTICAL ASPECTS FOR INFECTION CONTROL IN INTENSIVE CARE AREAS[11]

Design and Layout

- Doors and windows should be well sealed.
- Single room should be divided into separate units with toilet facilities.
- Protective clothing should be available for staff and visitors.
- Handwashing facility should be available at the entrance and also a alcohol/chlorhexidine scrub.
- Airflow should be monitored.
- Coarse filters (7 microns) and Hepa filters (0.3 microns) should be provided in the air conditioning system. These should be cleaned every 3 to 4 months.
- Ideally 20 to 30 air changes are recommended.
- Microbiological environmental monitoring should be carried out after changing/cleaning of filters.
- Patient should be provided sterile water.

Surveillance in ICUs[12]

- Monitoring of device associated infections should be done regularly. The basic indicators require ventilator-associated pneumonia (VAP), catheter-related blood stream infections (CRBSI) and catheter-associated urinary tract infection (CAUTI). VAP, CRBSI and CAUTI episodes are monitored.
- Regular active surveillance is recommended through the emergence/clustering of positive culture cases or similar clinical case clustering.
- In case of surveillance following surveillance specimens must be collected:
  Surveillance samples:
  - Clinical material
    - Central line tips with blood culture
    - ET tube secretions for microscopy and culture
    - Urine samples from catheterized patients
    - Others
  - Environmental sampling
    - Water samples from humidifiers
    - Samples from nebulizers
    - Samples from ventilators
    - Samples from suction tubing
    - Disinfectants on dressing trolleys.

    Samples (random samples) are sent to microbiology department. Records are maintained and results of these presented during the monthly HICC meeting.
  - Swabs from various sites in the ICU like bed, trolley, equipment are sent after cleaning and disinfection of the ICU on a regular basis and whenever there is an outbreak.
  - Environmental monitoring
    If ICU has filters; monitoring of filters as per manufacturer's instructions (checking the air flow/air changes, etc.).
  - Staff with cough, cold, fever, skin infection or any communicable disease should not be allowed to enter the ICU.
  - In case of an outbreak, patients should be screened weekly for bacterial pathogens. Sites to be screened are nose and perineal swabs
  - Records are to be maintained by the ICU nursing in charge.

Screening for MRSA

Screening for methicillin-resistant *Staphylococcus aureus* (MRSA)(nasal swab/perineal swab/axillary swab-usually only nasal swab is preferred as it is convenient) on admission to ICU may be indicated in the following:

- Patients who have been admitted for more than five days in the ICU
- Patients with previous positive cultures for MRSA either in the blood, tracheal aspirate or urine
- Patients admitted from other hospital
- Patients admitted from long-term care institutions, e.g. nursing homes
- Patients on chronic renal dialysis.

Policies for the Burns Unit[11]

- Waterproof cover is recommended for mattresses.
- Cover should be cleaned with hypochlorite/any disinfectant when necessary.
- Sterilize dressing material separately for each patient.

Cleaning

All areas should be cleaned daily with clean damp cloth and separate cloth for each patient. Mop should be cleaned thoroughly and dried.

Pharmaceutical Products

- All drugs and IV therapy must be prepared in the laminar flow cabinet by a person using sterile protective clothing.
- Left over product should be discarded.

Microbiological

- Patient should be screened weekly for bacterial pathogens.
- Sites to be screened are nose, throat, perineal swab, hair, urine and feces.
- Environmental monitoring is necessary when filters are cleaned or changed.
- Microbiological investigations are done when infection is clinically noted.
- Staff with cough, cold, fever, skin infection or any communicable disease should not be allowed to enter the room.

REFERENCES

1. Ayliffe GAJ, Fraise AP, Geddes AM, Mitchell K. Control of Hospital Infection—A Practical Handbook. 4th edition, Oxoford University Press; 2000.p.297.
2. Kaziani K, Poulakou G, Lerikou M, Peros E, Dimopoulos G. Infection control in the intensive care unit. European Infectious Disease. 2011;5(2):121-4.
3. Van Saene HKF, Stoutenbeek LP, Hart CA. Selective decontamination of the digestive tract (SDD) in intensive care patients—A critical evaluation of clinical, bacteriological and epidemiological benefits. J Hosp Infect. 1991;18:261.
4. Aggarwal DS. Guidelines for nosocomial infection—Surveillance and control. 32:109.
5. Misra UB, Kant S, Rao SKM, Murli JS. A study of visitor policies in ICUs of various hospitals at Mumbai, New Delhi and Chandigarh. Journal of Academy of Hospital Administration. 2010;22:1-2.
6. Ali Z, Quadeer A, Akhtar A. To determine the effect of wearing shoe covers by medical staff and visitors on infection rates, mortality and length of stay in intensive care units. Pak J Med Sci. 2014;30:2 www.pjms.com.pk).
7. Gupta A, Anand AC (VSM), Chumber SK, Sashindran VK, Patrikar SR. Impact of Protective Footwear on Floor and Air Contamination of Intensive Care Units. Med J Armed Forces India. 2007;63(4):334-6. doi:10.1016/S0377-1237(07)80009-8.
8. Berti D, Ferdinande P, Moons P. Beliefs and attitudes of intensive care nurses towards visits and open visiting policy. Intensive Care Medicine. 2007;33(6):1060-5.
9. Ghyasvandian S, et al. The effect of open visiting care nurses' belief. Research Journal of Biological Sciences. 2009;4(1):4-70.
10. Scothis Health Planning Note 27. Intensive care unit. NHS in Scotland, P and EFEx. September 2000;25-35.
11. Protocol for Intensive Care Areas/Burns Unit. In Manual for Hospital Infection Control compiled by Hospital Infection Control Committee LTMGH and LTMMC. Pg 17.
12. Gaind R, Deb M. Infection Control Policy, Vardhaman Mahavir Medical College and Safdarjung Hospital. New Delhi. August 2010. Accessed from www.vmmc.sjh.nic.in/.../Infection_Control_Policy.5967286291pdf on 8th Dec 15.

Chapter 15

Intravenous Catheter/Cannulation-associated Infection

Chapter Outline

- Terminology and Estimates of Risk
- Pathogenesis
- Etiological Agents—Epidemiology and Microbiology in Adult and Pediatric Patients
- Strategies for Prevention of Catheter-related Infections in Adult and Pediatric Patients
- Practical Approach for Prevention of Catheter-associated Infection
- CRBSI Summary (Including CRBSI Bundle)

INTRODUCTION[1,2]

Infections due to intravenous catheterization have increased due to an increase in the proportion of patients receiving therapy and supportive care intravenously. The trend is particularly evident in centers specializing in intensive care, burn injuries and cancer, where 80% of in-hospital treatment is delivered by the intravenous route. Both venous and arterial devices are used. They are used to deliver sterile fluids, medications and nutritional products, as well as for central monitoring of blood pressure and other hemodynamic functions.

Because catheters inserted into the venous or arterial bloodstream bypass the normal skin defense mechanism, these devices provide a way for microorganisms to enter the blood stream from:

- The device at the time of insertion
- Subsequent contamination of the device or attachments (e.g. tubing connected to the blood monitoring apparatus or the fluids being administered), or
- Pathogens on the skin surrounding the insertion site.

Unfortunately, IV therapy is associated with regular and unavoidable complications, the most prevalent of which is the introduction of microorganisms into the vascular system. Sepsis—sometimes associated with suppurative thrombophlebitis or septic thrombosis, is a life-threatening condition. Furthermore, length of hospitalization and hospital costs are significantly increased. It is therefore important that infectious complications of modern IV therapy are minimized by strict guidelines and infection control measures.

Intravenous cannulas are either rigid steel needle or flexible catheters made of plastic or silicone elastomer. They are usually inserted in the veins of the upper extremities or into the subclavian or jugular veins. Lower extremity cannulation has been viewed with disfavor because of the distressing incidence of septic and embolic complications.

TERMINOLOGY AND ESTIMATES OF RISK[1]

The terminology used to identify different types of catheters is confusing, because many clinicians and researchers use different aspects of the catheter for informal reference. A catheter can be designated by the type of vessel it occupies (e.g. peripheral venous, central venous, or arterial); its intended life span (e.g. temporary or short-term versus permanent or long-term); its site of insertion [e.g. subclavian, femoral, internal jugular, peripheral, and peripherally inserted central catheter (PICC)]; its pathway from skin to vessel (e.g. tunneled versus nontunneled); its physical length (e.g. long versus short); or some special characteristic of the catheter (e.g. presence or absence of a cuff, impregnation with heparin, antibiotics or antiseptics, and the number of lumens). To accurately define a specific type of catheter, all of these aspects should be described (Table 15.1).

Catheter-related bloodstream infection (CRBSI) is a clinical definition, used when diagnosing and treating patients, that

Table 15.1: Catheters used for venous and arterial access

Catheter type	Entry site	Length	Comments
Peripheral venous catheters	Usually inserted in veins of forearm or hand	<3 inches	Phlebitis with prolonged use; rarely associated with bloodstream infection
Peripheral arterial catheters	Usually inserted in radial artery; can be placed in femoral, axillary, brachial, posterior tibial arteries	<3 inches	Low infection risk; rarely associated with bloodstream infection
Midline catheters	Inserted via the antecubital fossa into the proximal basilic or cephalic veins; does not enter central veins, peripheral catheters	3–8 inches	Anaphylactoid reactions have been reported with catheters made of elastomeric hydrogel; lower rates of phlebitis than short peripheral catheters
Nontunneled central venous catheters	Percutaneously inserted into central veins (subclavian, internal jugular, or femoral)	≥8 cm depending on patient size	Account for majority of CRBSI
Pulmonary artery catheters	Inserted through a Teflon® introducer in a central vein (subclavian, internal jugular, or femoral)	≥30 cm depending on patient size	Usually heparin bonded; similar rates of bloodstream infection as CVCs; subclavian site preferred to reduce infection risk
Peripherally, inserted central venous catheters (PICC)	Inserted into basilic, cephalic, or brachial veins and enter the superior vena cava	≥20 cm depending on patient size	Lower rate of infection than nontunneled CVCs
Tunneled central venous catheters	Implanted into subclavian, internal jugular, or femoral veins	≥8 cm depending on patient size	Cuff inhibits migration of organisms into catheter tract; lower rate of infection than nontunneled CVC
Totally implantable	Tunneled beneath skin and have subcutaneous port accessed with a needle; implanted in subclavian or internal jugular vein	≥8 cm depending on patient size	Lowest risk for CRBSI; improved patient self-image; no need for local catheter-site care; surgery required for catheter removal
Umbilical catheters	Inserted into either umbilical vein or umbilical artery	≤6 cm depending on patient size	Risk for CRBSI similar with catheters placed in umbilical vein versus artery

requires specific laboratory testing that more thoroughly identifies the catheter as the source of the bloodstream infection (BSI). CLABSI (Central Line-associated Bloodstream Infection) is a term used by CDC's National Healthcare Safety Network (NHSN).[3] A CLABSI is a primary BSI in a patient that had a central line within the 48-hour period before the development of the BSI and is not bloodstream related to an infection at another site. However, since some BSIs are secondary to other sources other than the central line (e.g. pancreatitis, mucositis) that may not be easily recognized, the CLABSI surveillance definition may overestimate the true incidence of CRBSI.

PATHOGENESIS[1]

There are four recognized routes for contamination of catheters (Fig. 15.1):

1. Migration of skin organisms at the insertion site into the cutaneous catheter tract and along the surface of the catheter with colonization of the catheter tip; this is the most common route of infection for short-term catheters—more common in early period following insertion in less than 7 days.
2. Direct contamination of the catheter or catheter hub by contact with hands or contaminated fluids or devices—more common after 7 days, intraluminal contamination.
3. Less commonly, catheters might become hematogenously seeded from another focus of infection.
4. Rarely, infusate contamination might lead to CRBSI.

Important pathogenic determinants of CRBSI are:

1. The material of which the device is made.
2. The host factors consisting of protein adhesions, such as fibrin and fibronectin, that form a sheath around the catheter.
3. The intrinsic virulence factors of the infecting organism, including the extracellular polymeric substance (EPS) produced by the adherent organisms.

Some catheter materials also have surface irregularities that enhance the microbial adherence of certain species (e.g. *S. epidermidis* and *C. albicans*). Catheters made of these materials are especially vulnerable to microbial colonization and subsequent infection. Due to the formation of the fibrin sheath, silastic catheters are associated with higher risk of catheter infections than polyurethane catheters. On the other hand, biofilm formation by *C. albicans* occurs more readily on silicone elastomer catheter surfaces than polyurethane catheters. Modification of the biomaterial surface properties has been shown to influence the ability of *C. albicans* to form biofilm. Additionally, certain catheter materials are more thrombogenic than others, a characteristic that also might predispose to catheter colonization and infection. This association has led to emphasis on preventing

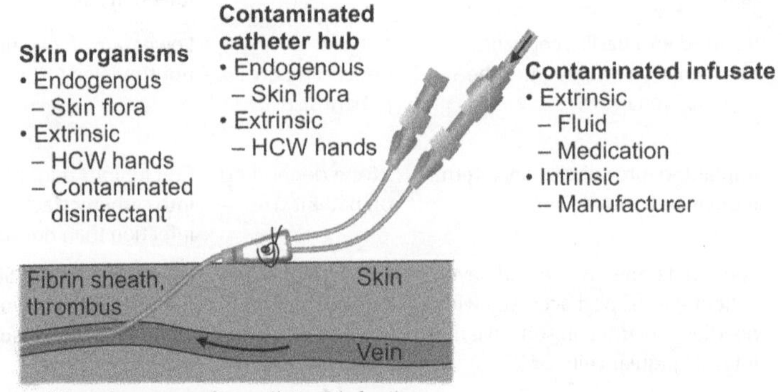

Fig. 15.1: Sources and sites of catheter-associated bloodstream infections[17]

catheter-related thrombus as an additional mechanism for reducing CRBSI.

The adherence properties of a given microorganism in relationship to host factors are also important in the pathogenesis of CRBSI. For example, *S. aureus* can adhere to host proteins (e.g. fibrinogen, fibronectin) commonly present on catheters by expressing clumping factors (ClfA and Clf B) that bind to the protein adhesins. Furthermore, adherence is enhanced through the production by microbial organisms, such as coagulase negative staphylococci, *S. aureus*, *Pseudomonas aeruginosa*, and *Candida* species of an extracellular polymeric substance (EPS) consisting mostly of an exopolysaccharide that forms a microbial biofilm layer. This biofilm matrix is enriched by divalent metallic cations, such as calcium, magnesium and iron, which make it a solid enclave in which microbial organisms can embed themselves. Such a biofilm potentiates the pathogenicity of various microbes by allowing them to withstand host defense mechanisms (e.g. acting as a barrier to engulfment and killing by polymorphonuclear leukocytes) or by making them less susceptible to antimicrobial agents (e.g. forming a matrix that binds antimicrobials before their contact with the organism cell wall or providing for a population of metabolically quiescent, antimicrobial tolerant "persister" cells). Some *Candida* species, in the presence of dextrose-containing fluids, produce slime similar to that of their bacterial counterparts, potentially explaining the increased proportion of BSIs caused by fungal pathogens among patients receiving parenteral nutrition fluids.

EPIDEMIOLOGY AND MICROBIOLOGY IN ADULT AND PEDIATRIC PATIENTS[1]

Both gram-negative bacteria and staphylococci are primary causes of catheter-related infections. Approximately, 50% of all cases of cannula-related septicemia is caused by *S. aureus*. Virtually, all common bacteria and fungi have been reported in association with cannula infections. The incidence of fungemia especially with *Candida,* is particularly striking with catheters used for parenteral nutrition, and is increasingly reported with the advent of HIV infections. The most commonly reported causative pathogens by CDC are coagulase-negative staphylococci, *Staphylococcus aureus*, enterococci and *Candida* species.

Suppurative phlebitis is one of the most serious complications of intravenous therapy. *S. aureus* and gram-negative bacilli (particularly *E. Coli*, *Klebsiella* species and *Enterobacter* species) are the most frequent isolates in this complication.

Some microorganisms especially *coagulase-negative Staphylococcus aureus* and *Pseudomonas* and *Acinetobacter* species adhere to the fibrin film that forms on the inside wall of catheters within days of insertion. As a consequence, infection with these organisms is quite common, especially if the infection occurs within 10 days of insertion.

For all common pathogens causing CLABSIs, antimicrobial resistance is a problem, particularly in ICUs. Although methicillin-resistant *Staphylococcus aureus* (MRSA) now account for more than 50% of all *Staphylococcus aureus* isolates obtained in ICUs, the incidence of MRSA CLABSIs has decreased in recent years, perhaps as a result of prevention efforts. For gram-negative rods, antimicrobial resistance to third-generation cephalosporins among *Klebsiella pneumoniae* and *E. coli* has increased significantly as has imipenem and ceftazidime resistance among *Pseudomonas aeruginosa*. *Candida* species are increasingly noted to be fluconazole resistant. The incidence of fungemia especially with *Candida,* is particularly striking with catheters used for parenteral nutrition, and is increasingly reported with the advent of HIV infections.

STRATEGIES FOR PREVENTION OF CATHETER-RELATED INFECTIONS IN ADULT AND PEDIATRIC PATIENTS[1]

Education, Training and Staffing

Recommendations

1. Educate healthcare personnel regarding the indications for intravascular catheter use, proper procedures for the insertion and maintenance of intravascular catheters, and appropriate infection control measures to prevent intravascular catheter-related infections (*Category 1A*).
2. Periodically assess knowledge of and adherence to guidelines for all personnel involved in the insertion and maintenance of intravascular catheters (*Category 1A*).
3. Designate only trained personnel who demonstrate competence for the insertion and maintenance of peripheral and central intravascular catheters (*Category 1A*).
4. Ensure appropriate nursing staff levels in ICUs (*Category 1B*).

Selection of Catheters and Sites

Peripheral and Midline Catheter Recommendations

1. In adults, use an upper-extremity site for catheter insertion. Replace a catheter inserted in a lower extremity site to an upper extremity site as soon as possible (*Category 2*).
2. In pediatric patients, the upper or lower extremities or the scalp (in neonates or young infants) can be used as the catheter insertion site (*Category 2*).
3. Select catheters on the basis of the intended purpose and duration of use, known infectious and non-infectious complications (e.g. phlebitis and infiltration), and experience of individual catheter operators (*Category 1B*).
4. Avoid the use of steel needles for the administration of fluids and medication that might cause tissue necrosis if extravasation occurs (*Category 1A*).
5. Use a midline catheter or peripherally inserted central catheter (PICC), instead of a short peripheral catheter, when the duration of IV therapy will likely exceed six days (*Category 2*).
6. Evaluate the catheter insertion site daily by palpation through the dressing to discern tenderness and by inspection if a transparent dressing is in use. Gauze and opaque dressings should not be removed if the patient has no clinical signs of infection. If the patient has local tenderness or other signs of possible CRBSI, an opaque dressing should be removed and the site inspected visually (*Category 2*).
7. Remove peripheral venous catheters if the patients develop signs of phlebitis (warmth, tenderness, erythema or palpable venous cord), infection, or a malfunctioning catheter (*Category 1B*).

Central Venous Catheters Recommendations

1. Weigh the risks and benefits of placing a central venous device at a recommended site to reduce infectious complications against the risk for mechanical complications (e.g. pneumothorax, subclavian artery puncture, subclavian vein laceration, subclavian vein stenosis, hemothorax, thrombosis, air embolism, and catheter misplacement) (*Category 1A*).
2. Avoid using the femoral vein for central venous access in adult patients (*Category 1A*).
3. Use a subclavian site, rather than a jugular or a femoral site, in adult patients to minimize infection risk for nontunneled CVC placement (*Category 1B*).

4. No recommendation can be made for a preferred site of insertion to minimize infection risk for a tunneled CVC (*Unresolved Issue*).
5. Avoid the subclavian site in hemodialysis patients and patients with advanced kidney disease, to avoid subclavian vein stenosis (*Category 1A*).
6. Use a fistula or graft in patients with chronic renal failure instead of a CVC for permanent access for dialysis (*Category 1A*).
7. Use ultrasound guidance to place central venous catheters (if this technology is available) to reduce the number of cannulation attempts and mechanical complications. Ultrasound guidance should only be used by those fully-trained in its technique (*Category 1B*).
8. Use a CVC with the minimum number of ports or lumens essential for the management of the patient (*Category 1B*).
9. No recommendation can be made regarding the use of a designated lumen for parenteral nutrition (*Unresolved Issue*).
10. Promptly remove any intravascular catheter, i.e. is no longer essential (*Category 1A*).
11. When adherence to aseptic technique cannot be ensured (i.e. catheters inserted during a medical emergency), replace the catheter as soon as possible, i.e. within 48 hours (*Category 1B*).

Type of Catheter Material[1]

Polytetrafluoroethylene (Teflon®) or polyurethane catheters have been associated with fewer infectious complications than catheters made of polyvinyl chloride or polyethylene. Steel needles used as an alternative to catheters for peripheral venous access have the same rate of infectious complications as do Teflon® catheters. However, the use of steel needles frequently is complicated by infiltration of intravenous fluids into the subcutaneous tissues, a potentially serious complication if the infused fluid is a vesicant.

Hand Hygiene and Aseptic Technique[1]

Recommendations

1. Perform hand hygiene procedures, either by washing hands with conventional soap and water or with alcohol-based hand rubs (ABHR). Hand hygiene should be performed before and after palpating catheter insertion sites as well as before and after inserting, replacing, accessing, repairing, or dressing an intravascular catheter. Palpation of the insertion site should not be performed after the application of antiseptic, unless aseptic technique is maintained (*Category 1B*).
2. Maintain aseptic technique for the insertion and care of intravascular catheters (*Category 1B*).
3. Wear clean gloves, rather than sterile gloves, for the insertion of peripheral intravascular catheters, if the access site is not touched after the application of skin antiseptics (*Category 1C*).
4. Sterile gloves should be worn for the insertion of arterial, central, and midline catheters (*Category 1A*).
5. Use new sterile gloves before handling the new catheter when guidewire exchanges are performed (*Category 2*).
6. Wear either clean or sterile gloves when changing the dressing on intravascular catheters (*Category 1C*).

Maximal Sterile Barrier Precautions

Recommendations

1. Use maximal sterile barrier precautions, including the use of a cap, mask, sterile gown, sterile gloves, and a sterile full body

drape, for the insertion of CVCs, PICCs, or guidewire exchange (*Category 1B*).
2. Use a sterile sleeve to protect pulmonary artery catheters during insertion (*Category 1B*).

Skin Preparation

Recommendations

1. Prepare clean skin with an antiseptic (70% alcohol, tincture of iodine, an iodophor or chlorhexidine gluconate) before peripheral venous catheter insertion (*Category 1B*).
2. Prepare clean skin with a >0.5% chlorhexidine preparation with alcohol before central venous catheter and peripheral arterial catheter insertion and during dressing changes. If there is a contraindication to chlorhexidine, tincture of iodine, an iodophor, or 70% alcohol can be used as alternatives (*Category 1A*).
3. No comparison has been made between using chlorhexidine preparations with alcohol and povidone-iodine in alcohol to prepare clean skin (*Unresolved Issue*).
4. No recommendation can be made for the safety or efficacy of chlorhexidine in infants aged <2 months (*Unresolved Issue*).
5. Antiseptics should be allowed to dry according to the manufacturer's recommendation prior to placing the catheter (*Category 1B*).

Background

Two well-designed studies evaluating the chlorhexidine (2%) containing cutaneous antiseptic regimen in comparison with either povidone iodine (10%) or alcohol (70%) for the care of an intravascular catheter insertion site have shown lower rates of catheter colonization or CRBSI associated with the chlorhexidine preparation. (The comparison of chlorhexidine gluconate alcohol to povidone iodine alcohol has not been done). While chlorhexidine has become a standard antiseptic for skin preparation for the insertion of both central and peripheral venous catheters, 5% povidone iodine solution in 70% ethanol was associated with a substantial reduction of CVC-related colonization and infection compared with 10% aqueous povidone iodine.

Catheter Site Dressing Regimens[1]

Recommendations

1. Use either sterile gauze or sterile, transparent, semipermeable dressing to cover the catheter site.
2. If the patient is diaphoretic or if the site is bleeding or oozing, use gauze dressing until this is resolved.
3. Replace catheter site dressing if the dressing becomes damp, loosened, or visibly soiled.
4. Do not use topical antibiotic ointment or creams on insertion sites, except for dialysis catheters, because of their potential to promote fungal infections and antimicrobial resistance.
5. Do not submerge the catheter or catheter site in water. Showering should be permitted if precautions can be taken to reduce the likelihood of introducing organisms into the catheter (e.g. if the catheter and connecting device are protected with an impermeable cover during the shower).
6. Replace dressings used on short-term CVC sites every 2 days for gauze dressings.
7. Replace dressings used on short-term CVC sites at least every 7 days for transparent dressings, except in those pediatric patients in which the risk for dislodging the catheter may outweigh the benefit of changing the dressing.
8. Replace transparent dressings used on tunneled or implanted CVC sites no more than once per week (unless the dressing is soiled or loose), until the insertion site has healed.

9. No recommendation can be made regarding the necessity for any dressing on well-healed exit sites of long-term cuffed and tunneled CVCs (*Unresolved Issue*).
10. Ensure that catheter site care is compatible with the catheter material.
11. Use a sterile sleeve for all pulmonary artery catheters.
12. Use a chlorhexidine-impregnated sponge dressing for temporary short-term catheters in patients older than 2 months of age if the CLABSI rate is not decreasing despite adherence to basic prevention measures, including education and training, appropriate use of chlorhexidine for skin antisepsis, and MSB (Maximum Sterile Barrier Precautions).
13. No recommendation is made for other types of chlorhexidine dressings. (*Unresolved Issue*).
14. Monitor the catheter sites visually when changing the dressing or by palpation through an intact dressing on a regular basis, depending on the clinical situation of the individual patient. If patients have tenderness at the insertion site, fever without obvious source, or other manifestations suggesting local or bloodstream infection, the dressing should be removed to allow thorough examination of the site.
15. Encourage patients to report any changes in their catheter site or any new discomfort to their provider.

Patient Cleansing

Recommendation

Use a 2% chlorhexidine wash for daily skin cleansing to reduce CRBSI.

Catheter Securement Devices

Recommendation

Use a sutureless securement device to reduce the risk of infection for intravascular catheters.

Background

Catheter stabilization is recognized as an intervention to decrease the risk for phlebitis, catheter migration and dislodgement, and may be advantageous in preventing CRBSIs. Pathogenesis of CRBSI occurs via migration of skin flora through the percutaneous entry site. Sutureless securement devices avoid disruption around the catheter entry site and may decrease the degree of bacterial colonization. Using a sutureless securement device also mitigates the risk of sharps injury to the healthcare provider from inadvertent needlestick injury.

Antimicrobial/Antiseptic Impregnated Catheters and Cuffs[1]

Recommendation

Use a chlorhexidine/silver sulfadiazine or minocycline/rifampin-impregnated CVC in patients whose catheter is expected to remain in place >5 days if, after successful implementation of a comprehensive strategy to reduce rates of CLABSI, the CLABSI rate is not decreasing. The comprehensive strategy should include at least the following three components: (1) educating persons who insert and maintain catheters, (2) use of maximal sterile barrier precautions, and (3) a >0.5% chlorhexidine preparation with alcohol for skin antisepsis during CVC insertion.

Background

These catheters have been approved by FDA for use in patients weighing >3 kg. Two non-randomized studies in pediatric ICU patients suggest that these catheters might reduce risk of catheter-associated infection. No antiseptic or antimicrobial impregnated catheters currently are available for use in infants weighing <3 kg.

Chlorhexidine/silver sulfadiazine: Catheters coated with chlorhexidine/silver sulfadiazine only on the external luminal surface have been studied as a means to reduce CRBSI. Two meta-analyses of first-generation catheters demonstrated that such catheters reduced the risk for CRBSI compared with standard non-coated catheters. A second-generation catheter is now available with chlorhexidine coating the internal surface extending into the extension set and hubs while the external luminal surface is coated with chlorhexidine and silver sulfadiazine. The external surface has three times the amount of chlorhexidine and extended release of the surface bound antiseptics than that in the first, generation catheters. All three prospective, randomized studies of second-generation catheters demonstrated a significant reduction in catheter colonization, but they were underpowered to show a difference in CRBSI. Prolonged anti-infective activity provides improved efficacy in preventing infections. Although rare, anaphylaxis with the use of these chlorhexidine/silver sulfadiazine catheters has been observed.

Chlorhexidine/silver sulfadiazine catheters are more expensive than standard catheters. Use of these catheters might be cost effective in ICU patients, burn patients, neutropenic patients, and other patient populations in which the rate of infection exceeds 3.3 per 1,000 catheter days.

Minocycline/rifampin: In a multicenter randomized trial, CVCs impregnated on both the external and internal surfaces with minocycline/rifampin were associated with lower rates of CRBSI when compared with the first-generation chlorhexidine/silver sulfadiazine impregnated catheters. The beneficial effect began after day 6 of catheterization. Silicone minocycline/rifampin impregnated CVCs with an average dwell time of over 60 days have been shown to be effective in reducing CRBSI. No minocycline/rifampin-resistant organisms were reported in these studies. Two trials demonstrated that use of these catheters significantly reduced CRBSI compared with uncoated catheters. No comparative studies have been published using the second-generation chlorhexidine/silver sulfadiazine catheter. Although, there have been concerns related to the potential for development of resistance, several prospective clinical studies have shown that the risk is low. Further, no resistance to minocycline or rifampin related to the use of the catheter has been documented in the clinical setting. Two studies using decision model analysis revealed these catheters were associated with superior cost savings compared with first-generation chlorhexidine/silver sulfadiazine catheters. Such analysis needs to be done compared with the second-generation catheters. However, as baseline rates of infection decrease and the cost of catheters decrease, the cost-benefit ratio will likely change.

The decision to use chlorhexidine/silver sulfadiazine or minocycline/rifampin impregnated catheters should be based on the need to enhance prevention of CRBSI after bundled standard procedures have been implemented (e.g. educating personnel, using maximal sterile barrier precautions, and using >0.5% chlorhexidine preparation with alcohol for skin antisepsis) and then balanced against the concern for emergence of resistant pathogens and the cost of implementing this strategy.

Systemic Antibiotic Prophylaxis[1]

Recommendation

Do not administer systemic antimicrobial prophylaxis routinely before insertion or during use of an intravascular catheter to prevent catheter colonization or CRBSI.

Antibiotic/Antiseptic Ointments

Recommendation

Use povidone iodine antiseptic ointment or bacitracin/gramicidin/polymyxin B ointment at the hemodialysis catheter exit site after catheter insertion and at the end of each dialysis session only if this ointment does not interact with the material of the hemodialysis catheter as per manufacturer's recommendation.

Replacement of Peripheral and Midline Catheters

Recommendations

1. There is no need to replace peripheral catheters more frequently than every 72–96 hours to reduce risk of infection and phlebitis in adults.
2. No recommendation is made regarding replacement of peripheral catheters in adults only when clinically indicated (*Unresolved Issue*).
3. Replace peripheral catheters in children only when clinically indicated.
4. Replace midline catheters only when there is a specific indication.

Replacement of CVCs, Including PICCs and Hemodialysis Catheters

Recommendations

1. Do not routinely replace CVCs, PICCs, hemodialysis catheters, or pulmonary artery catheters to prevent catheter-related infections.
2. Do not remove CVCs or PICCs on the basis of fever alone. Use clinical judgment regarding the appropriateness of removing the catheter if infection is evidenced elsewhere or if a noninfectious cause of fever is suspected.
3. Do not use guidewire exchanges routinely for non-tunneled catheters to prevent infection.
4. Do not use guidewire exchanges to replace a non-tunneled catheter suspected of infection.
5. Use a guidewire exchange to replace a malfunctioning non-tunneled catheter if no evidence of infection is present.
6. Use new sterile gloves before handling the new catheter when guidewire exchanges are performed.

Umbilical Catheters

Recommendations

1. Remove and do not replace umbilical artery catheters if any signs of CRBSI, vascular insufficiency in the lower extremities, or thrombosis are present.
2. Remove and do not replace umbilical venous catheters if any signs of CRBSI or thrombosis are present.
3. No recommendation can be made regarding attempts to salvage an umbilical catheter by administering antibiotic treatment through the catheter (*Unresolved Issue*).
4. Cleanse the umbilical insertion site with an antiseptic before catheter insertion. Avoid tincture of iodine because of the potential effect on the neonatal thyroid. Other iodine-containing products (e.g. povidone iodine) can be used.
5. Do not use topical antibiotic ointment or creams on umbilical catheter insertion sites because of the potential to promote fungal infections and antimicrobial resistance.
6. Add low-doses of heparin (0.25–1.0 U/mL) to the fluid infused through umbilical arterial catheters.
7. Remove umbilical catheters as soon as possible when no longer needed or when any sign of vascular insufficiency to the lower extremities is observed. Optimally, umbilical artery catheters should not be left in place >5 days.
8. Umbilical venous catheters should be removed as soon as possible when no longer needed, but can be used up to 14 days if managed aseptically.
9. An umbilical catheter may be replaced if it is malfunctioning, and there is no other indication for catheter removal, and the

total duration of catheterization has not exceeded 5 days for an umbilical artery catheter or 14 days for an umbilical vein catheter.

Peripheral Arterial Catheters and Pressure Monitoring Devices for Adult and Pediatric Patients

Recommendations

1. In adults, use of the radial, brachial or dorsalis pedis sites is preferred over the femoral or axillary sites of insertion to reduce the risk of infection.
2. In children, the brachial site should not be used. The radial, dorsalis pedis, and posterior tibial sites are preferred over the femoral or axillary sites of insertion.
3. A minimum of a cap, mask, sterile gloves and a small sterile fenestrated drape should be used during peripheral arterial catheter insertion.
4. During axillary or femoral artery catheter insertion, maximal sterile barriers precautions should be used.
5. Replace arterial catheters only when there is a clinical indication.
6. Remove the arterial catheter as soon as it is no longer needed.
7. Use disposable, rather than reusable, transducer assemblies when possible.
8. Do not routinely replace arterial catheters to prevent catheter-related infections.
9. Replace disposable or reusable transducers at 96-hour intervals. Replace other components of the system (including the tubing, continuous-flush device, and flush solution) at the time the transducer is replaced.
10. Keep all components of the pressure monitoring system (including calibration devices and flush solution) sterile.
11. Minimize the number of manipulations of and entries into the pressure monitoring system. Use a closed flush system (i.e. continuous flush), rather than an open system (i.e. one that requires a syringe and stopcock), to maintain the patency of the pressure monitoring catheters.
12. When the pressure monitoring system is accessed through a diaphragm, rather than a stopcock, scrub the diaphragm with an appropriate antiseptic before accessing the system.
13. Do not administer dextrose-containing solutions or parenteral nutrition fluids through the pressure monitoring circuit.
14. Sterilize reusable transducers according to the manufacturers' instructions if the use of disposable transducers is not feasible.

Replacement of Administration Sets

Recommendations

1. In patients not receiving blood, blood products or fat emulsions, replace administration sets that are continuously used, including secondary sets and add-on devices, no more frequently than at 96-hour intervals, but at least every 7 days.
2. No recommendation can be made regarding the frequency for replacing intermittently used administration sets (*Unresolved Issue*).
3. No recommendation can be made regarding the frequency for replacing needles to access implantable ports (*Unresolved Issue*).
4. Replace tubing used to administer blood, blood products, or fat emulsions (those combined with amino acids and glucose in a 3-in-1 admixture or infused separately) within 24 hours of initiating the infusion.
5. Replace tubing used to administer propofol infusions every 6 or 12 hours, when the vial is changed, per the manufacturer's recommendation.[4]
6. No recommendation can be made regarding the length of time a needle used to access implanted ports can remain in place (*Unresolved Issue*).

Needleless Intravascular Catheter Systems

Recommendations

1. Change the needleless components at least as frequently as the administration set. There is no benefit to changing these more frequently than every 72 hours.
2. Change needleless connectors no more frequently than every 72 hours or according to manufacturers' recommendations for the purpose of reducing infection rates.
3. Ensure that all components of the system are compatible to minimize leaks and breaks in the system.
4. Minimize contamination risk by scrubbing the access port with an appropriate antiseptic (chlorhexidine, povidone iodine, an iodophor, or 70% alcohol) and accessing the port only with sterile devices
5. Use a needleless system to access IV tubing.
6. When needleless systems are used, a split septum valve may be preferred over some mechanical valves due to increased risk of infection with the mechanical valves.

Performance Improvement

Recommendation

Use hospital-specific or collaborative-based performance improvement initiatives in which multifaceted strategies are "bundled" together to improve compliance with evidence-based recommended practices.

PRACTICAL APPROACH FOR PREVENTION OF CATHETER-ASSOCIATED INFECTION

These are commonly performed invasive procedures administered either by the peripheral or central routes.

Definitions (Fig. 15.2)[5]

- *Exit site infection (microbiologic diagnosis)*: Clinical infection in which culture of the discharge (pus or fluid) at the exit site yields a microorganism, with or without microbiologic evidence of blood stream infection.

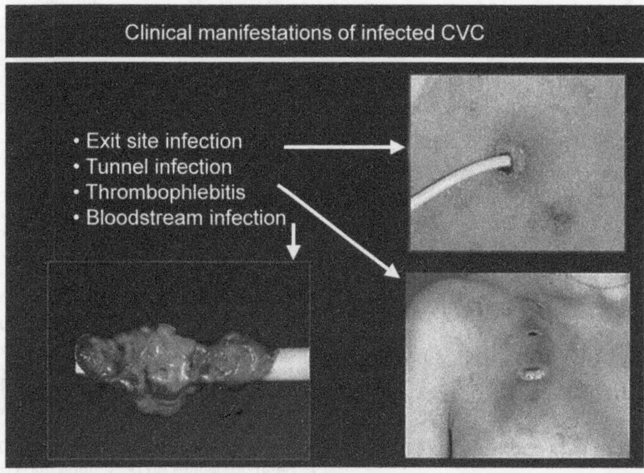

Fig. 15.2: Clinical manifestations of central venous catheter-associated infections *(For color version, see Plate 1)*

- *Phlebitis:* Area of swelling, redness, warmth and tenderness of the skin around the site where the intravascular catheter comes out of the skin (the exit site). If phlebitis is associated with other signs of infection such as fever and pus coming from the exit site, it is classified as **clinical exit site infection.**
- *Pocket infection:* Infected fluid isolated from the area around a totally implanted intravascular device, with or without microbiologic evidence of bloodstream infections.
- *Tunnel infection:* Tenderness, redness and swelling for more than 2 cm along the tract of an intravascular catheter, with or without microbiologic evidence of local or bloodstream infection.

Risk Factors[6]

Factors Related to Equipment and Fluids

- Cannula material itself may be thrombogenic, e.g. polyethylene and polypropylene which is more reactive than Teflon, which in turn is more reactive than steel or silicone coated Teflon.
- Intravenous infusion fluids prepared without proper sterile precautions.
- Contaminated administration sets or fluids.
- Hypodermic needles used as air inlets.
- Disconnected IV cannulas—source of aerial influx.
- Three way stop cocks.
- Contaminated splints used for sprained/operated joints.
- Large bandages over the insertion site (contaminated by patients' blood and fluids).

Factors Related to Insertion and Duration

- Skin flora and inadequate disinfection.
- Skin flora/transient flora of staff/other patients/visitors.
- Contaminated disinfectants.
- Unstable cannulae—movement increases the risk of bacterial contamination.
- Cannula left in for over 72 hours.
- Alternate arms should be used for IV therapy that lasts longer than 72 hours.
- Pre-existing infection/venous thrombus/septic focus.

Key Factors for All Vascular Catheters (Tables 15.2 and 15.3)[5,7]

These include:

- Avoiding catheterization unless there is a medical indication.
- Maintaining a high level of asepsis for catheter insertion and care.
- Limiting the use of catheters to as short a duration as possible.
- In adults, use an upper-extremity site for catheter insertion.
- Use a midline catheter or peripherally inserted central catheter (PICC), instead of a short peripheral catheter, when the duration of IV therapy will likely exceed six days.

Table 15.2: Prevention of IV catheter-associated infections

Infection risks with IV catheters	Prevention
Catheter system	To be avoided unless indicated
Duration	Prolonged catheterization to be avoided
Skin preparation	Strict aseptic technique to be used
Infection or colonization of catheter	Catheter should be removed
Technique	Surgical asepsis
Dressing change	Frequency of dressing change to be limited
Type of catheter	Antibiotic coated catheter for CVC when it is expected to remain for >5 days, and the CLABSI rate is not decreasing despite the usual measures

Source: Adapted from intravascular catheter related infections page 34 in guidelines on prevention and control of hospital associated infections WHO regional office for South-east Asia, New Delhi[5] modified acc to CDC manual.

Table 15.3: Effective methods in prevention of catheter-associated infections

Proven effective	Proven not effective
All catheters	
Closed system	Antimicrobial creams for skin preparation except at the hemodialysis catheter exit site after catheter insertion and at the end of each dialysis session
Limit duration	Systemic antimicrobial prophylaxis routinely before insertion or during use of an intravascular catheter to prevent catheter colonization or CRBSI
Local skin preparation	
Aseptic technique at insertion	
Removal if infection suspected	
Central lines	
Surgical asepsis for insertion	
Limitation of frequency of dressing change	
Antibiotic-coated catheter for CVC when it remains for >5 days, and the CLABSI rate is not decreasing despite the usual measures	

Vascular device infections[7]

Source: Adapted from prevention of common nosocomial infections, page 38 from prevention of hospital-acquired infections 2nd edition WHO.

- Remove peripheral venous catheters if the patients develop signs of phlebitis, infection, or a malfunctioning catheter.
- Preparing fluids aseptically and immediately before use.
- Training of personnel in catheter insertion and care.

General Guidelines[8]

- A high level of aseptic technique should be used for insertion and handling of catheters.
- Hands must be washed before all catheter care, using hygienic hand wash or rub.
- Skin at the insertion site must be washed and disinfected with an antiseptic solution.
- Hand hygiene is a must even if you wear gloves.
- Hand hygiene to be observed before and after palpating the catheter insertion sites; before and after inserting, replacing, accessing, repairing or dressing IV catheter. Do not palpate after application of antiseptic unless aseptic technique is maintained.
- Maximal sterile barrier precautions including cap, mask, sterile gown, sterile gloves and a sterile full body drape are required for insertion of CVCs, PICCs or guidewire exchange.
- Periodic assessment of knowledge of adherence to guidelines for all those who insert and manage IV catheters is essential.
- Surveillance in ICU and other patient populations should be conducted to determine CRBSIs and monitor trends. Express ICU data as number of catheter-associated BSIs per 1000 catheter days.

Dressings[8]

- Use either sterile gauze or a sterile transparent, semi-permeable dressing.
- Wear clean or sterile gloves when changing the dressing.
- Change the dressing weekly for adults and adolescents based on individual patient circumstances.
- Replace dressings when damp, loose or visibly soiled.
- Replace dressing on short PIV catheters when the catheter is removed or replaced.
- Remove a bulky peripheral IV dressing daily to evaluate site if dressing prevents ability to palpate or directly visualize site, and apply new dressing.
- Replace dressings on short-term CVC sites every 2 days for a gauze dressing and at least every 7 days for transparent dressings,

except in pediatrics in which the risk for dislodging the catheter may outweigh the benefit of changing the dressing.
- Replace dressings on tunneled or implanted CVC sites no more than once a week until insertion site has healed.
- A gauze dressing is preferred when site is bleeding or oozing or when patient is diaphoretic.

Site/Line Care[8,9]

- Palpate insertion site through the dressing daily.
- Inspect through a transparent dressing daily.
- Remove an opaque/gauze dressing and inspect visually, if patient develops local tenderness or signs of infection.
- Remove any intravascular device, i.e. is no longer essential.
- Replace a catheter as soon as possible or within 48 hours, when aseptic technique during insertion cannot be ensured (as in emergency).
- Replace IV tubing including add- on devices and secondary sets, no more frequently than 72 hours unless a catheter related infection is suspected.
- Replace tubing used for blood products or lipid emulsions within 24 hours of initiating the infusion.
- Clean access port with appropriate anti-septic and access port only with a sterile device.
- Clean injection ports with 70% alcohol, Povidone-iodine or an Iodophor before accessing.
- Cap all stopcocks when not in use.
- Disinfect clean skin with appropriate antiseptic before insertion and at the time of dressing change—2% chlorhexidine is preferred.
- Allow antiseptics to remain on insertion site and air dry—povidone iodine should be allowed to air dry for 2 minutes or longer.
- Do not apply organic solvent (acetone or ether) to skin before insertion and at dressing change.

Peripheral Vascular Catheter/ Midline Catheters[8]

- Avoid use of steel needles.
- Use upper extremity insertion sites for adults and hand, scalp, or foot for pediatrics.
- Replace adult short peripheral IV catheters at least every 72–96 hours. For pediatrics, leave catheter in place until treatment completed, unless complication occurs.
- Use a midline or PICC when duration of therapy is expected to exceed 6 days.
- Remove peripheral venous catheters if the patients develop signs of phlebitis, infection, or a malfunctioning catheter.

Peripheral Arterial Catheters/ Pressure Monitoring Devices.[8]

- In adults radial, brachial or dorsalis pedis sites is preferred over the femoral or axillary sites of insertion to reduce the risk of infection.
- In children, the brachial site should not be used. The radial, dorsalis pedis and posterior tibial sites are preferred over the femoral or axillary sites of insertion.
- Replace arterial catheters only when there is a clinical indication.
- Use disposable rather than reusable, transducers.
- Replace disposable or reusable transducers, tubing, flush devices and flush solutions at 96 hours interval.
- Keep all components of the pressure monitoring system (including calibration devices and flush solution) sterile.

Central Venous Catheters and Pulmonary Artery Catheters[8]

- Clean the insertion site with an antiseptic solution.
- Do not apply antimicrobial ointment to the insertion site.
- Masks, cap and sterile gloves and gown must be worn for insertion by HCWs.

- The introduction of the catheter and the subsequent catheter dressings require a surgical hand wash or rub.
- Follow appropriate aseptic care in accessing the system, including disinfecting external surfaces of hubs and ports.
- An increased number of catheter lumens may increase the risk of infection. A single lumen catheter is preferred wherever possible.
- Use subclavian site in preference to jugular or femoral sites.
- Use ultrasound guidance to place central venous catheters (if this technology is available) to reduce the number of cannulation attempts and mechanical complications. Ultrasound guidance should only be used by those who are fully trained in the technique.
- Use antimicrobial or antiseptic-impregnated CVCs in adults whose catheter will remain in place for >5 days if after implementing a comprehensive strategy to reduce rates of CRBSI, the CRBSI rate remains above the goal set by the institution.
- Use totally implantable devices for long-term, intermittent access and PICCs or tunneled CVCs for frequent or continuous access.
- Replace any short-term CVC, if there is any purulence at the insertion site.
- Use sterile sleeve for pulmonary artery catheters.

Hemodialysis Catheters[8,9]

- Avoid using subclavian site in hemodialysis patients and in patients with advanced kidney disease to avoid subclavian stenosis.
- Place catheters for hemodialysis and pheresis in jugular or femoral veins vs subclavian veins.
- Use a fistula or graft in patients with chronic renal failure instead of a CVC for permanent access for dialysis.
- Use cuffed CVCs if access is needed for greater than three weeks.
- Use povidone-iodine ointment or bacitracin/gramicidin/polymyxin B ointment at the hemodialysis exit site after catheter insertion and at the end of each dialysis session and at each dressing change.
- Do not use for blood drawing or applications other than hemodialysis, except in emergencies or during dialysis.

Not Recommended[8,9]

- Do not use chlorhexidine sponge dressings in neonates less than 7 days or gestational age less than 26 weeks.
- Do not routinely use in-line filters or antibiotic lock solutions.
- Do not routinely replace central venous, pulmonary artery, PICC, hemodialysis, midline or arterial catheters.
- Do not change catheters over guidewire when catheter-related infection (CRI) is clinically suspected.
- Do not routinely culture catheter tips.
- Do not routinely administer intranasal or systemic prophylactic antimicrobials.
- Do not routinely use topical antimicrobial ointments or creams on insertion sites, except when using hemodialysis catheter.
- Do not submerge catheter under water. Showering is permitted if catheter and connecting device are protected with impermeable cover.

IDSA Practice Guidelines for the Diagnosis and Management of Intravascular Catheter-related Infection (2009)[10]

If catheter is removed:

1. Catheter cultures only if catheter removed for suspected CRBSI; catheter cultures should not be obtained routinely.
2. Qualitative broth culture of catheter tips not recommended.
3. For central venous catheters (CVCs), catheter tip cultured, not subcutaneous segment.

4. For cultures of an anti-infective catheter tip, use specific inhibitors in culture media.
5. Less than 15 colony-forming units (CFU) from 5 cm segment of catheter tip by semiquantitative (roll-plate) culture OR $<10^2$ CFU from a catheter by quantitative (sonication) broth culture reflects catheter colonization.
6. If catheter infection suspected and there is catheter exit site exudate, collect specimen for culture and Gram staining.
7. For short-term catheter tip cultures, roll plate technique recommended.
8. For suspected pulmonary artery catheter infection, culture introducer tip.

CRBSI SUMMARY (INCLUDING CRBSI BUNDLE)[11,12]

Definition

- *Catheter-related bloodstream infection (CRBSI):* That requires specific laboratory testing that more thoroughly identifies the catheter as the source of the bloodstream infection (BSI).
- *Central line-associated bloodstream infection (CLABSI):* A CLABSI is a primary BSI in a patient that had a central line within the 48 hour period before the development of the BSI and is not bloodstream related to an infection at another site.

How to Identify an Infection Clinically

- *Exit site infection:* Clinical infection in which culture of the discharge (pus or fluid) yields a microorganism with or without evidence of bloodstream infection.
- *Phlebitis:* Area of swelling, redness, warmth and tenderness of the skin around the site where the intravascular catheter comes out of the skin (the exit site). If phlebitis is associated with other signs of infection such as fever and pus—it is said to be a clinical exit site infection.
- *Pocket infection:* Infected fluid isolated from the area around a totally implanted intravascular device with or without microbiologic evidence of bloodstream infections.
- *Tunnel infection:* Tenderness, redness and swelling for more than 2 cm along the tract of an intravascular catheter, with or without microbiologic evidence of local or bloodstream infection.
- Patient has fever not related to infection at any other site.
- Positive blood culture report (one or more blood cultures).

Signs to be Looked for

- Local redness, tenderness, warmth.
- Swelling at the site from where the catheter comes out.
- Discharge/pus from exit site.
- Fever.

Laboratory-confirmed Bloodstream Infection Criteria

LCBI 1

Must meet one of the following criteria:

- Patient has a recognized pathogen cultured from one or more blood cultures
  and
- Organism cultured from blood is not related to an infection at another site.

LCBI 2

- Patient has at least one of the following signs or symptoms: fever (>38°C), chills, or hypotension
  and
- Positive laboratory results are not related to an infection at another site.
  and
- The same common commensal [i.e. diphtheroids (*Corynebacterium* species not *C. diphtheriae*), *Bacillus* species (not *B. anthracis*), *Propionibacterium* species, coagulase-negative staphylococci

(including *S. epidermidis*), viridans group streptococci, *Aerococcus* species, and *Micrococcus* species] is cultured from two or more blood cultures drawn on separate occasions.

LCBI 3

- Patient ≤1 year of age has at least one of the following signs or symptoms: fever (>38°C core), hypothermia (<36°C core), apnea, or bradycardia
  and
- Positive laboratory results are not related to an infection at another site.
  and
- The same common commensal [i.e. diphtheroids (*Corynebacterium* species not *C. diphtheriae*), *Bacillus* species (not *B. anthracis*), *Propionibacterium* species, coagulase-negative staphylococci (including *S. epidermidis*), viridans group streptococci, *Aerococcus* species, *Micrococcus* species] is cultured from two or more blood cultures drawn on the same or consecutive days and separate occasions.

Prevention

- Hand hygiene.
- Remove unnecessary lines.
- Use of maximal barrier precautions.
- Chlorhexidine for skin antisepsis.
- Avoid femoral lines.

Review of Bundle Components (Fig. 15.3)

Hand Hygiene

- Before and after palpating* catheter insertion sites.
- Before and after inserting, replacing, accessing, repairing, or dressing a catheter.
- When hands obviously soiled or contamination suspected.
- Before and after invasive procedures.
- Between patients.
- Before donning and after removing gloves.

****Note:*** palpation of insertion site should not be performed after application of antiseptic unless aseptic technique maintained.

Maximal Barrier Precautions

- Wear cap, mask, sterile gown and sterile gloves.
  (Both the line inserter and immediate assistant)
- Cover patient from head to toe with sterile drape with small opening for site of insertion.

Chlorhexidine Skin Antisepsis

Allow time to dry completely before puncturing site.

Optimal Catheter Site Selection

Subclavian vein the preferred site for non-tunneled catheters in adults.

Daily Review of Central Line Necessity with Prompt

- Removal of unnecessary lines.
- Risk of infection increases with duration of line.
- Examples of appropriate uses: receipt of TPN, chemotherapy, extended use of antibiotics, or hemodialysis.

CDC Prevention Strategies

Core Strategies

- High levels of scientific evidence.
- Demonstrated feasibility.
- Should become standard practice.

Supplemental Strategies

- Some scientific evidence.

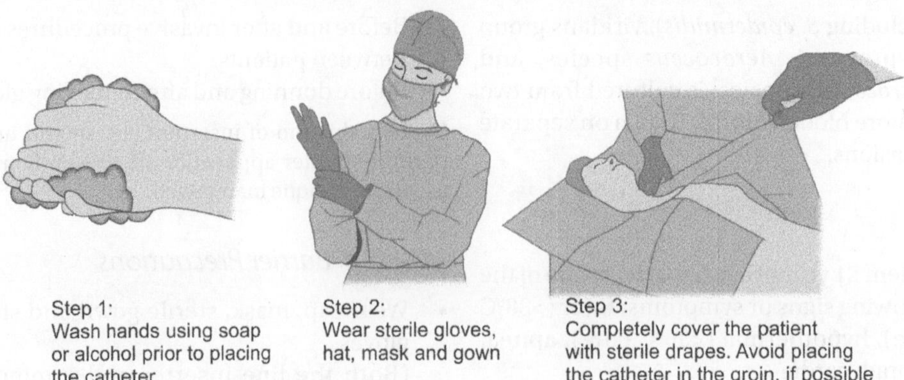

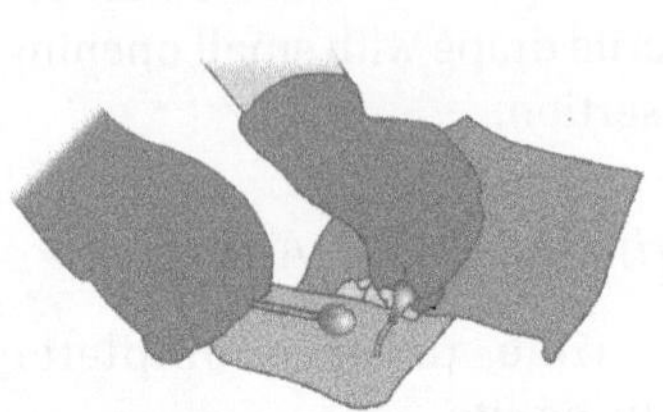

Step 4:
Clean the insertion site on the patient's skin with chlorhexidine antiseptic solution

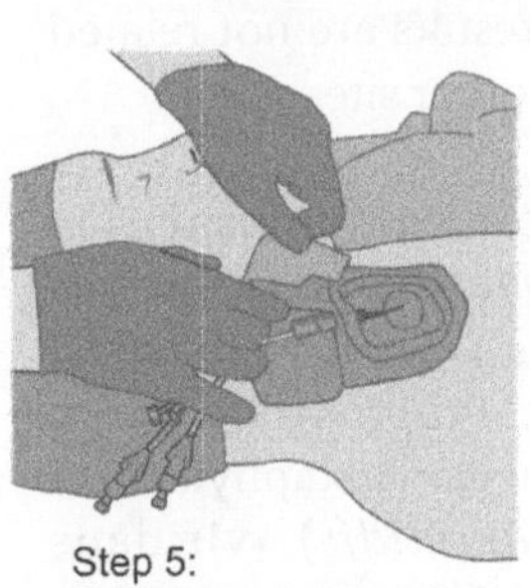

Step 5:
Remove catheters when they are no longer needed

Fig. 15.3: Five steps to prevent central line infections[19]

- Variable levels of feasibility.
- Consider implementing in addition to Core when infections persist or rates are high.

CLABSI Prevention Strategies

Core (Always, Every Time)

- Remove unnecessary central lines.
- Proper insertion practices.
- Hand hygiene.
- Skin antisepsis.
- Lower risk insertion sites.
- Hub and access port disinfection.
- Educate on central line insertion and maintenance.

Supplemental

- Chlorhexidine bathing.
- Antimicrobial-impregnated catheters.
- Chlorhexidine-impregnated dressings.

Considerations for Supplemental Prevention Strategies

Chlorhexidine Bathing

- Daily bathing with 2% chlorhexidine decreased BSI rate in ICU compared to soap and water (single study).
- No data outside the ICU.

Chlorhexidine Dressings

- Chlorhexidine dressings have been shown to decrease CLABSI rates in some studies, not in others.
- May be an option when core interventions have not decreased CLABSI rates to established goals.

Antimicrobial Catheters

- May be appropriate for patient's catheter expected to be used for >5 days

- When core strategies have not decreased CLABSI rates to established goals.
- Studies show some supporting evidence for catheters with minocycline-rifampin and chlorhexidine-silver sulfadiazine
- Platinum-silver catheters available but less evidence to support use.

Central Line Site Selection

- Whenever possible, and not contra-indicated, the subclavian line site should be preferred over the jugular and femoral sites for non-tunneled catheters in adult patients
- For tunneled catheters-no recommendation
- For hemodialysis—subclavian not to be used.

How to Look for Infection Locally Peripheral Venous Catheter

- If dressing is transparent—site is inspected visually.
- If gauze or opaque dressing applied—look for tenderness on palpation, remove dressing if tenderness present and look for redness, erythema, infection or malfunctioning catheter (signs of phlebitis).

Replacement of Catheters

- Replace peripheral catheters every 72 to 96 hours.
- Replace peripheral catheters in children only when indicated.
- Remove peripheral venous catheters if patients develop signs of phlebitis, infection or a malfunctioning catheter.
- Replace midline catheters only when there is specific indication.
- Do not routinely replace CVCs, PICCs and hemodialysis or pulmonary artery catheters.
- Remove and do not replace umbilical artery or venous catheters if any signs of CRBSI or vascular insufficiency to lower extremities,or thrombosis are present.
- Umbilical catheters should not be left in place for >5 days and venous catheters >14 days.
- Replace transducers disposable or reusable at 96 hours interval (including its components).
- Sterilize transducers (reusable) according to manufacturer's instructions.

Replacement of Administration Sets, Tubings

- Replace administration sets (in patients not receiving blood, blood products, fat emulsions) every 96 hours or at least every 7 days.
- Replace tubings used for the above (blood, blood products, fat emulsions) within 24 hours.
- Replace tubing used to administer propofol infusion every 6 to 12 hours.
- Replace needleless intravascular catheter sets every 72 hours.

Type of Dressings and Change of Dressings

- Use sterile gauze or a sterile transparent, semi-permeable dressing.
- Replace dressing on short PIV catheter when the catheter is removed or replaced.
- Replace dressings on short-term CVC sites every 2 days for a gauze dressing and at least every 7 days for transparent dressings, except in pediatrics in which the risk for dislodging the catheter may outweigh the benefit of changing the dressing.
- A gauze dressing is preferred when there is bleeding or oozing.
- Replace dressings when damp, loose or visibly soiled.

Samples for Culture and Sensitivity

Peripheral Venous Catheter

Send catheter tip for culture and peripheral blood culture from other side.

Central Venous Catheter

- Catheter tip culture and peripheral blood culture from other side.
- Send blood culture from the central line as well as blood culture from peripheral site.

Laboratory Diagnosis of Catheter-related Bloodstream Infections[13]

- When the blood culture obtained from the catheter is positive, but the percutaneous blood sample is negative, it indicates colonization of the catheter rather than CRBSI.
- The diagnosis of CRBSI requires a positive culture of blood from a peripheral vein and clear evidence that the catheter is the source. CRBSI means a patient with an intravascular catheter has at least one positive blood culture obtained from a peripheral vein, clinical manifestations of infections (i.e. fever, chills, and/or hypotension), and no apparent source for the BSI, except the catheter.
- In addition, one of the following is also present: A positive semi-quantitative (>15 CFU/catheter segment)[14] or quantitative (>10^3CFU/catheter segment)[15] catheter tip culture, also, the same organism (species and anti-biogram) is isolated from the catheter segment and peripheral blood culture.
- Simultaneous quantitative paired blood cultures with a >5:1 ratio CVC versus peripheral, or differential time to positivity, whereby a non-quantitative blood culture drawn from the CVC that becomes positive at least 2 hours earlier than the peripheral blood culture, is a new method for the diagnosis of CRBSI without removing the catheter.[16]

CRBSI and CLABSI Infection Rates

Catheter-related Blood stream Infection Rate

$$\text{CRBSI rate} = \frac{\text{Number of catheter-related BSI}}{\text{Number of patients on IV line-days}} \times 100$$

Central Line-associated Infection Rate (per 1,000 Central Line Days)

$$\text{CLABSI rate} = \frac{\text{CLABSI}}{\text{CL Days}} \times 1000$$

REFERENCES

1. CDC Guidelines for the Prevention of Intravascular Catheter-related Infections, 2011. Available at http://www.cdc.gov/hai/prevent/prevent-pubs.html accessed on 5/2/2014.
2. Ayliffe GAJ, Fraise AP, Geddes AM, Mitchell K. Control of Hospital Infection. A Practical Handbook. 4th edition. Oxford University Press, New York; 2000.p.140.
3. Horan TC, Andrus M, Dudeck MA. CDC/NHSN surveillance definition of healthcare-associated infection and criteria for specific types of infections in the acute care setting. Am J Infect Control. 2008;36:309-32.
4. Bennett SN, McNeil MM, Bland LA, et al. Postoperative infections traced to contamination of an intravenous anesthetic, propofol. N Engl J Med. 1995;333:147-54 (CR 186 in Ref 1).
5. Intravenous catheter-related infections. In Guidelines on Prevention and Control of Hospital-associated Infections. WHO, Regional Office for Southeast Asia, New Delhi; Pg 33-4.
6. Prevention of IV Catheter-associated Infection. In Manual for Hospital Infection Control Compiled by Hospital Infection Control Committee LTMGH and LTMMC; Pg. 23.
7. Ducel G, Fabry J, Nicolle L. Prevention of hospital-acquired infections. A practical guide, 2nd edition; 2000.pp.38-41.
8. CDC Guidelines for the Prevention of Intravascular Catheter-related Infections, 2011. Available at http://www.cdc.gov/hai/prevent/prevent-pubs.html accessed on 5/2/2014.
9. Newsletter of Hospital Infection Society, Mumbai Forum. 5th Issue. Guidelines for the prevention of intravascular catheter-associated infection, Quick summary: 2002 CDC-HICPAC IV Infection Control Guidelines; 2004.p.16.
10. Mermel LA, et al. IDSA Practice Guidelines for the Diagnosis and Management of Intravascular Catheter-related Infection: 2009 Clinical Infectious Diseases. 2009;49:1-45. Acessed from www.uphs.upenn.edu/bugdrug/

antibiotic_manual/idsacathinfect2009.pdf. on 4th Oct 2016.

11. Kallen A. Division of Healthcare Quality Promotion. Centers for Disease Control and Prevention. Central Line-associated Bloodstream Infections (CLABSI) in Non-Intensive Care Unit (Non-ICU) settings Toolkit. Activity C: ELC Prevention Collaboratives. Accessed on 23/1/2015. Available at www.cdc.gov/hai/ppt/CLABSItoolkit3242010ppt.
12. Vicki Brinsko RN, CIC. Central Line-associated Bloodstream Infections. Tennessee Center for Patient Safety. Accessed on 23/1/2015. Available at www.tnpatientsafety.com/central%20Line%20Associated%20 Bloodstr.
13. Gahlot R, Nigam C, Kumar V, Yadav G, Anupurba S. Catheter-related bloodstream infections. Int J Crit Illn Inj Sci. 2014;4(2):162-7. Accessed from www.ncbi.nlm.nih.gov › NCBI › Literature › PubMed Central (PMC).
14. Maki DG, Weise CE, Sarafin HW. A semi-quantitative culture method for identifying intravenous-caheter-related infection. N Engl J Med. 1977;296:1305-9.
15. Brun-Buisson C, Abrouk F, Legrand P, Huet Y, Larabi S, Rapin M. Diagnosis of central venous catheter-related sepsis—critical level of quantitative tip cultures. Arch Intern Med.1987;147:873-7.
16. Seifert H, Cornely O, Seggewiss K, Decker M, Stefanik D, Wisplinghoff H. Bloodstream infection in neutropenic cancer patients related to short-term non-tunnelled catheters determined by quantitative blood cultures, differential time to positivity, and molecular epidemiological typing with pulsed-field gel electrophoresis. J Clin Microbiol. 2003;41:118.23. [PMC free article]
17. Accessed from http://www.doh.wa.gov/portals/1/images/5000/CLABSIPathogenesis2.png on 2nd October 2016.
18. Accessed from http://images.slideplayer.com/23/6814133/slides/slide_6.jpg on 2nd October 2016.
19. Accessed from https://cdn2.vox-cdn.com/uploads/chorus_asset/file/3852280/medical-errors-steps2_1024.0.png on 2nd October 2016.

Chapter 16

Respiratory Infections

Chapter Outline

- Pathogenesis
- Etiological Agents
- Treatment
- Risk Factors
- Prevention and Control Measures
- Summary of Ventilator-associated Pneumonia (VAP) Including VAP Bundle

INTRODUCTION

Hospital-acquired pneumonias (HAPs) are defined as pneumonias occurring ≥48 hours after admission. Any infection that is incubating at the time of admission is not considered as hospital-acquired pneumonia.

Pneumonia has accounted for approximately 15% of all hospital-associated infections.[1] This incidence will vary according to the type of hospital. It has been the second most common hospital-associated infection after that of the urinary tract. The primary risk factor for the development of hospital-associated bacterial pneumonia is mechanical ventilation (with its requisite endotracheal intubation). In high-risk areas such as surgical or medical intensive care units; the incidence of nosocomial pulmonary infection may be much higher. The mortality rate of hospital-acquired gram-negative pneumonia is more than 50% and in spite of treatment may approach 90–100%.[2]

Ventilator-associated pneumonia (VAP) is defined as pneumonia occurring more than 48 hours after endotracheal intubation and initiation of mechanical ventilation (MV) including pneumonia after extubation.[3] VAP is the most frequent ICU-acquired infection, occurring in 9 to 27% of patients intubated for longer than 48 hours.[3] VAP occurs in an average of 10 to 41.7 per 1000 ventilator days.[3] Mechanically-ventilated patients are 6–21 times more likely to develop nosocomial pneumonia than non-ventilated patients, because the endotracheal tube bypasses upper respiratory tract defenses, allowing pooling of oropharyngeal secretions and prevents effective cough.[4] The intensive care unit (ICU) length of stay in patients with VAP is increased by an average of 6.1 days and increases the cost of hospitalization per patient.[5] The mortality rates for HAP vary between 14% and 20% and for VAP between 33% and 50%[6] and may be as high as 70% when infections are caused by multi-resistant invasive pathogens.[7]

VAP has been classified into either early-onset pneumonia (EOP), if pneumonia develops within 96 hours (4 days) of the patient's admission to an ICU or intubation for mechanical ventilation, and late-onset pneumonia (LOP), if pneumonia develops after 96 hours (4 days) of the patient's admission to an ICU or intubation for mechanical ventilation. Early onset VAP, which occurs during first four days of mechanical ventilation, is usually less severe, associated with a better prognosis, and is more likely to be caused by antibiotic sensitive bacteria such as *Escherichia coli, Klebsiella* species, *Proteus* species, *S. pneumoniae, H. influenzae,* and oxacillin-sensitive *S. aureus.* Late onset VAP which develops five or more days after mechanical ventilation, is caused by multidrug-resistant (MDR) pathogens and has been associated with *Pseudomonas aeruginosa,* oxacillin-resistant *S. aureus*[1] and *Acinetobacter* species strains that are usually multi-antibiotic-resistant and is associated with increased morbidity and mortality.[7]

PATHOGENESIS

It is well-known fact that the hospital environment has a profound effect on the bacterial flora of the oropharynx, gastrointestinal tract, and skin of patients, and to a lesser degree, of hospital personnel. In these individuals the usual nonpathogenic bacteria such as *Streptococcus viridans, Branhamella catarrhalis* and a variety of microaerophilic and anaerobic organisms are replaced by *Staphylococcus aureus* and more commonly gram-negative bacilli. Colonization is not always accompanied by clinical or laboratory evidence of disease. The affected patients may simply be asymptomatic carriers. It has been found however, that bacterial pneumonia is usually preceded by colonization.

Bacterial infections of the lower respiratory tract like purulent tracheobronchitis and pneumonia are usually preceded by bacterial colonization. The high incidence of gram-negative bacillary pneumonia in hospitalized patients appears to be the result of factors that promote colonization of the pharynx by gram-negative bacilli and the subsequent entry of these microorganisms into the lower respiratory tract. Although aerobic gram-negative bacilli are recovered infrequently or are found in small numbers in pharyngeal cultures of healthy persons, colonization dramatically increases in patients with acidosis, alcoholism, azotemia, coma, diabetes mellitus, hypotension, leukocytosis, leukopenia, pulmonary disease, or endotracheal or nasogastric tubes in place, and in patients given antimicrobial agents.

In addition to the oropharynx, the stomach has been postulated to be an important reservoir of organisms that cause healthcare-associated pneumonia, although the exact role of the stomach in the causation of healthcare-associated pneumonia, specifically VAP, has been critically investigated and debated. It appears, however, that the stomach's role may vary depending on the patient's underlying condition(s) and on the prophylactic or therapeutic interventions that the patient receives. In healthy persons, few bacteria entering the stomach survive in the presence of hydrochloric acid at pH <2. However, when gastric pH increases from the normal levels to >4, microorganisms are able to multiply to high concentrations in the stomach. This can occur in patients with advanced age), achlorhydria, ileus, or upper gastrointestinal disease, and in patients receiving enteral feeding, antacids, or histamine-2 (H-2) antagonists. The contribution of other factors (e.g. duodenogastric reflux and the presence of bile) to gastric colonization in patients with impaired intestinal motility also has been suggested.[1]

The relative importance of oropharyngeal colonization over that of gastric colonization in the development of VAP has been strongly suggested.[1] In one of the studies, mechanically ventilated patients who received selective oropharyngeal decontamination without concurrent decontamination of the stomach had a 60% lower risk of VAP compared to those who did not have such a treatment.[1]

The greatest incidence of purulent tracheobronchitis and pneumonia as nosocomial infections is in patients who have received ventilatory assistance. Outbreaks of nosocomial pneumonia have been traced to contaminated nebulizers of respiratory assist devices. If the nebulizer reservoir contains bacteria, the organisms may be contained in the aerosol and infectious particles of appropriate size may reach the terminal airway. Simple humidifiers, on the other hand, are unlikely to aerosolize bacteria, in spite of being contaminated. With intubation or tracheostomy, a valuable primary defense mechanism, the upper respiratory tract with its ciliary epithelium is bypassed. The presence of a semirigid tube in the trachea is associated with a diminished cough reflex and reduced clearing of secretions, which accumulate, serving as a medium for bacterial growth. The initial inoculums of bacteria into the lungs are often the result of direct implantation by faulty, unsterile technique during suctioning, although aspiration may also occur around endotracheal tubes. Sedated or unconscious patients with impaired cough reflex are likely to develop aspiration pneumonia whether or not they are intubated.

Most of the patients who have nosocomial infections are infants, young children, persons more than 65 years of age, persons who have underlying disease, immunosuppression, depressed sensorium or cardiopulmonary disease and persons who have had thoracoabdominal surgery.

Although patients receiving mechanically-assisted ventilation do not represent a major proportion of patients who have nosocomial pneumonias, they are highest risk of acquiring that infection.

Most bacterial pneumonias occur by aspiration if bacterial colonization occurs in the oropharynx or upper gastrointestinal tract of the patient. It has been seen that oropharyngeal colonization is rare in healthy individuals (<10%), but it increases to 35% in moderately ill patients and up to 75% in critically ill patients.[8] It is obvious therefore that colonization and pneumonia coexist.[9] Because intubation and mechanical ventilation alter first line defenses, they greatly increase the risk for nosocomial bacterial pneumonia.

Pneumonia by *Legionella* species, *Aspergillus* species and influenza virus are often caused by inhalation of contaminated aerosols. RSV infection occurs after viral inoculation of conjunctiva or nasal mucosa by contaminated hands.[10]

Rarely, bacterial pneumonia can result from hematogenous spread of infection to the lung from another infection site, e.g. pneumonia resulting from purulent phlebitis or right-sided endocarditis.

ETIOLOGICAL AGENTS

Gram-negative Aerobic Bacilli

The common gram-negative bacilli that cause hospital-acquired pneumonia *are Pseudomonas* species, *Acinetobacter baumannii* and *Klebsiella pneumoniae* followed by *E. coli* and *Staphylococcus aureus,* however, the principal infecting organisms vary from one hospital to another depending on resident flora and almost any gram-negative bacillus may be implicated. Highly resistant organisms amongst gram-negative bacilli are *Psuedomonas* species and *Acinetobacter and Klebsiella* species.[11-14] In Asia hospital-associated pneumonia (HAP) and ventilator-associated pneumonia (VAP) are commonly due to gram-negative organisms.

A number of studies from India have investigated the causative organisms of VAP. *Pseudomonas* species, *Acinetobacter* species, *Escherichia coli, Klebsiella pneumoniae* and *Staphylococcus aureus* were identified as the common pathogens with varying prevalence. Upto 40% of these infections were polymicrobial. *Pseudomonas* species, *Acinetobacter* species, and even *Enterobacteriaceae* are quite often multidrug-resistant due to production of β-lactamases (ESBL), Amp C β-lactamases (Amp C) or metallo-β-lactamases (MBL). The etiological agents of VAP will vary with different patient populations and types of ICUs. Therefore, the local microbial flora needs to be studied in each setting to guide more effective rational utilization of antimicrobial agents.[12]

Anaerobic Bacteria

Respiratory infection due to anaerobic bacteria is usually related to aspiration of oropharyngeal contents, although several cases of secondary hematogenous pneumonia have been reported following pelvic infections.

When aspiration occurs outside the hospital, anaerobic bacteria are almost uniformly present and are the only organisms isolated in more than half of the cases. By contrast, aspiration in the hospital is more likely to contain aerobic bacteria, particularly gram-negative bacilli. However, a mixed infection including aerobes and anaerobes or purely anaerobic aspiration pneumonia is relatively common.

Staphylococcus aureus

In United states and other Western countries gram-positive organisms especially methicillin-resistant *S. aureus* plays a major role in HAP and VAP. *Staphylococcus aureus,* still causes nosocomial pneumonia. The carrier rate for these organisms is high among both patients and hospital personnel. Infections can therefore be due to patients' own strains, or those transmitted to patients by person-to-person contact. Air-borne transmission of *S. aureus* is thought to occur only infrequently. Mild to moderate pneumonia is usually caused by *Methicillin-sensitive S. aureus,* whereas severe HAPs are due to MRSAs.

Other Bacteria

Virtually every other pathogenic bacterium can be expected to cause pneumonia. However, *Streptococcus pneumoniae* (*Pneumococcus*) and *Meningococcus Streptococcus pyogenes* and *Haemophilus influenzae* are other organisms, which should be considered.

Mycobacterium tuberculosis

Because of the recent trend towards treating tuberculosis in general hospitals rather than sanatoria, the possibility of spread of this infection in the hospital must be re-evaluated. Usually, hospitalized patients who are known to have tuberculosis and who are being treated are unlikely to be contagious. By contrast, unsuspected cases of tuberculosis are a potential danger to other patients and hospital personnel alike. Transmission of tuberculosis is by droplet aerosol.

Fungi

True fungi rarely cause nosocomial infection, because the infective (yeast) form is acquired in nature, whereas the mycelial form, which invades, mammalian tissue is not contagious. Yeasts on the other hand, commonly colonize hospitalized patients. Factors predisposing to colonization by *Candida* species include diabetes mellitus, broad-spectrum antibiotics, or immunosuppressive therapy of any type. Infection of pharynx, trachea and esophagus are relatively common, in contrast, true pulmonary infection due to *Candida* species is rare.

Necrotizing pneumonia due to *Aspergillus* species is a serious problem usually in immunosuppressed patients and those with widespread malignancy. Infections are usually thought to be endogenous. Other organisms such as *Pneumocystis carinii* and

Nocardia have on occasion been thought to be hospital acquired.

Viruses

The problem of hospital-acquired viral infections is probably most severe during influenza epidemics. Influenza virus is transmitted by droplets and hospitalized individuals may acquire infection from visitors, other patients, or the medical and nursing staff. Since morbidity and mortality due to influenza is greatest in elderly patients and those who have underlying cardio-pulmonary disease, the consequences of this infection are particularly severe in hospitalized patients.

Other hospital-acquired viral diseases such as rubella; chickenpox and measles may be seen in pediatric wards. Recently, attention has been given to nosocomial infection due to parainfluenza and respiratory syncytial virus. These diseases are rarely severe, but pneumonia has been reported, and in any case, they contribute to the duration of hospitalization and therefore to the morbidity.

Cytomegalovirus infection occurs in a high percentage of patients undergoing organ or bone marrow transplantation.

TREATMENT

The treatment of HAP and VAP in Asian countries differs from that in United states.[6,15] The predominant pathogens in Asian countries are *A. baumanii, P. aeruginosa* and *K. pneumoniae,* but in United States and other Western countries, it is MRSA. The causative organisms of VAP tend to be more resistant than HAP. Therefore, higher potential antimicrobials to cover drug-resistance organisms were recommended.[15] Fourth-generation cephalosporin, e.g. cefepime or cefpirome, was preferred over ceftazidime as initial empiric treatment of agent for early onset VAP. Other alternative antibiotics were imipenem, meropenem or piperacillin-tazobactam and should be used in combination with aminoglycosides or fluoroquinolones. For late-onset VAP, carbapenems or piperacillin-tazobactam are preferred over third- or fourth-generation cephalosporins because these have greater activity against ESBL producing gram-negative bacilli, *Pseudomonas* and *Acinetobacter.*[15] Piperacillin-tazobactam does not induce ESBL production in gram-negative bacteria unlike cefepime.[15] Antibiotic regimens containing sulbactam compound (cefoperazone-sulbactam and ampicillin-sulbactam) are especially recommended for MDR *Acinetobacter* in some Asian countries.[15] They were also recommended for use in combination with aminoglycosides or fluoroquinolones.[15] For aminoglycosides, amikacin is preferred over gentamycin, and netilmicin had broad antimicrobial activity against aerobic gram-negative bacilli including *Acinetobacter* strains.

The recommended treatment for MDR pathogens in Asia are as follows:[15] For MDR *P. aeruginosa* the drug of choice are piperacillin-tazobactam or carbapenems with or without aminoglycosides or fluoroquinolones (ciprofloxacin), and the second choice is polymixin B or Colistin with or without ciprofloxacin. For MDR *Acinetobacter,* the drugs of choice are cefoperazone-sulbactam and/or tigecycline and the second choice is polymixin B or Colistin; for ESBL producing *Klebsiella pneumoniae,* the drugs of choice are carbapenems or tigecycline and second choice is piperacillin-tazobactam. For MRSA, the drugs of choice are vancomycin or teicoplanin, and second choice is linezolid or tigecycline.

RISK FACTORS[1]

Potential risk factors for healthcare-associated bacterial pneumonia have been examined in several large studies. Although specific risk factors may differ slightly between study populations, they can be grouped into the following general categories:

1. Factors that enhance colonization of the oropharynx and/or stomach by

microorganisms, e.g. administration of antimicrobial agents, admission to the ICU, or presence of underlying chronic lung disease.
2. Conditions favoring aspiration into the respiratory tract or reflux from the gastrointestinal tract (e.g. initial or repeat endotracheal intubation; insertion of nasogastric tube; supine position; coma; surgical procedures involving the head, neck, thorax, or upper abdomen; and immobilization due to trauma or illness).
3. Conditions requiring prolonged use of mechanical ventilatory support with potential exposure to contaminated respiratory devices and/or contact with contaminated or colonized hands, mainly of healthcare personnel.
4. Host factors such as extremes of age, malnutrition, and severe underlying conditions, including immunosuppression.

Oropharyngeal, Tracheal, and Gastric Colonization

The association between a patient's predisposition to gram-negative bacillary pneumonia and bacterial colonization of the patient's oropharynx, trachea, or stomach prompted attempts by researchers to prevent the infection by various means, mainly by local and/or systemic antimicrobial prophylaxis.

Oropharyngeal and/or Tracheal Colonization

Local bacterial interference and aerosolized antimicrobial agents

Bacterial interference (with alpha-hemolytic streptococci) was successfully used by some investigators to prevent oropharyngeal colonization by aerobic gram-negative bacilli. However, the efficacy of this method for general use has not been evaluated. In small studies, aerosolization of antimicrobial agents has been shown to eradicate common gram-negative bacillary pathogens from the upper respiratory tract and/or decrease the incidence of gram-negative-bacillary pneumonia or VAP; however, no effect on patient mortality rate has been shown and superinfection occurred in some patients receiving the therapy. The use of intratracheal colistin was shown to significantly decrease the incidence of gram-negative bacillary and polymicrobial pneumonia in critically ill patients who were compared to historic controls. There was, however, no effect on mortality, and although no increase was detected in the number of cases infected with colistin-resistant microorganisms, the follow-up period was relatively short.

Selective oropharyngeal decontamination with antimicrobial agents

It has been observed that by selectively modulating the bacterial colonization of the oropharynx only [without modulating the gastric and intestinal colonization and without the concomitant use of systemic antimicrobial agent(s)] ,with the use of a topical prophylactic preparation containing gentamicin, colistin, and vancomycin resulted in the eradication of oropharyngeal and tracheal colonizers and also prevented acquisition of new oropharyngeal colonizers and lowered the incidence of VAP. However, the use of the topical preparation was not associated with shorter duration of ventilation or ICU stay or longer survival in study patients.

Oropharyngeal cleaning and decontamination with an antiseptic agent

It has been found that there have been a decrease in rates of pneumonia, including VAP, upon implementation of a comprehensive oral-hygiene program for patients or residents, respectively. The oral hygiene programs consisting of frequent toothbrushing and mouth-swabbing with an antiseptic agent; and in the ICU, frequent suctioning of the mouth and subglottic areas of patients receiving mechanically assisted ventilation. More randomized, controlled studies are needed to determine the role of a comprehensive oral-hygiene program in the prevention of VAP or NHAP. However, in the interim, it is prudent for healthcare facilities to implement such a program.

Oral chlorhexidine rinse in adult patients undergoing cardiac surgery

The antiseptic chlorhexidine gluconate (0.12%) is used successfully as a perioperative oral rinse to decrease the overall incidence of nosocomial respiratory tract infections in patients of cardiac surgery. However, its use for preventing healthcare-associated pneumonia in other groups of patients at high-risk for this infection has not been evaluated.

Oropharyngeal and Gastric Colonization

"Selective" decontamination of the digestive tract

Selective decontamination of the digestive tract (SDD) is one of the most studied strategies designed to prevent lower respiratory tract infection in critically ill and/or mechanically ventilated patients by preventing bacterial colonization of the digestive tract. SDD is aimed at preventing oropharyngeal and gastric colonization with aerobic gram-negative bacilli and *Candida* species, without altering the digestive tract's anaerobic flora. Various SDD regimens include a combination of locally administered nonabsorbable antimicrobial agents, such as polymyxin or colistin, and an aminoglycoside (tobramycin, gentamicin, or, rarely, neomycin) or a quinolone (norfloxacin or ciprofloxacin), coupled with either amphotericin B or nystatin several times a day. The local antimicrobial preparation is applied as a paste to the oropharynx and, and rarely given orally or via the nasogastric tube for gastric decontamination.

SDD has not been shown to decrease significantly the duration of mechanical ventilation or ICU stay; however, a decrease in overall antimicrobial use and mortality has been observed. SDD will probably be found cost-effective for use on subsets of ICU patients, such as trauma and/or critically ill surgical patients. However, there are concerns about the potential for increased bacterial antimicrobial resistance and superinfection with multi-drug resistant pathogens in patients.

Sucralfate, H-2 Receptor Antagonists, Antacids, and Stress-Bleeding Prophylaxis

The administration of antacids and/or H-2 receptor antagonists for prevention of stress bleeding in critically ill, postoperative, or mechanically ventilated patients has been associated with gastric bacterial overgrowth and increased risk for pneumonia. Sucralfate, a cytoprotective agent that has little effect on gastric pH and may have bactericidal properties of its own, has been suggested as a substitute for antacids and H-2 receptor antagonists. The results of clinical trials comparing the risk of pneumonia in patients receiving sucralfate with that in patients given H-2 receptor antagonists and/or antacids have been variable.

Acidified Enteral Feeding

Because enteral feeding can increase gastric pH and result in gastric colonization, acidification of enteral solutions has been advocated to prevent gastric and tracheal colonization in patients receiving such treatment. The absence of "pathogenic" bacteria from the stomachs of patients given acidified enteral feeding has been shown; however, the effect on the incidence of pneumonia has not been evaluated.

Continuous versus Intermittent Enteral Feeding

Continuous enteral feeding of mechanically ventilated patients, a common practice in ICUs, has been associated with increased gastric pH, subsequent gastric colonization with gram-negative bacilli, and a high incidence of pneumonia; whereas intermittent enteral feeding has been associated with lower gastric pH and lower rates of pneumonia.

However, in a cross-over study of intermittent enteral feeding of patients who had just had continuous enteral feeding, intermittent feeding had no lowering effect on gastric pH or gastric microbial colonization. In another study that compared intermittent and continuous enteral feeding, intermittent feeding resulted in decreased gastric pH during the "off-feeding" interval; however, the oropharyngeal and tracheal colonization rates and the incidence of VAP were similar in patients who received either treatment. More studies are needed to determine the effect of intermittent enteral feeding on the incidence of pneumonia.

Aspiration of Oropharyngeal and Gastric Flora and Nasal Sinus Secretions

Clinically important aspiration usually occurs in patients who have one or more of the following conditions: a depressed level of consciousness; dysphagia due to neurologic or esophageal disorders; an endotracheal (naso- or orotracheal), tracheostomy, or enteral (naso- or orogastric) tube in place; and receipt of enteral feeding. Placement of an enteral tube may increase nasopharyngeal colonization, cause reflux of gastric contents, or allow bacterial migration via the tube from the stomach to the upper airway. Gross contamination of the enteral solution during its preparation may lead to gastric colonization with gram-negative bacilli. Prevention of pneumonia in such patients may be difficult; however, placing the patient in a semi-upright position (by elevating the head of the bed at an angle of 30–45°) has been beneficial, probably by preventing aspiration.

On the other hand, other measures that theoretically might be beneficial have yielded either negative or equivocal results in studies involving small numbers of patients: the use of flexible, small-bore nasogastric tubes did not reduce the incidence of gastroesophageal reflux or microaspiration; and placement of the enteral tube below the stomach (e.g. in the jejunum) had variable effects on the rate of aspiration and the incidence of pneumonia.

Direct correlations have been reported between nasotracheal (rather than orotracheal intubation) and the occurrence of nosocomial maxillary sinusitis and high incidence of pneumonia. These findings suggest that the entry site for endotracheal intubation may affect the incidence of VAP.

Mechanically-assisted Ventilation and Endotracheal Intubation

The increased risk for pneumonia in intubated, mechanically ventilated patients is partly due to the carriage of oropharyngeal microorganisms via passage of the endotracheal tube into the trachea during intubation, as well as to depressed host defenses secondary to the patient's severe underlying illness. In addition, bacteria can aggregate on the surface of the endotracheal tube over time and form a glycocalyx (i.e. biofilm) that protects the bacteria from antimicrobial agents or host defenses. Some investigators believe that these bacterial aggregates may become dislodged by ventilation flow, tube manipulation, or suctioning and subsequently embolize into the lower respiratory tract and cause focal pneumonia.

Drainage of Subglottic Secretions

In the intubated patient, leakage around the cuff of the endotracheal tube allows bacteria laden secretions (which pool below the glottis and above the endotracheal-tube cuff) direct access to the lower respiratory tract. The effect of using an endotracheal tube that has a separate dorsal lumen which allows drainage (i.e. removal by suctioning) of the subglottic secretions has shown a lower incidence as well as delayed onset of VAP as compared to that of a conventional endotracheal tube.

Noninvasive Ventilation: Noninvasive Positive-pressure Ventilation

Noninvasive ventilation (NIV) of patients in acute respiratory failure due to various causes is emerging as a potentially more advantageous method of delivering positive-pressure ventilation than endotracheal tube placement. Noninvasive positive-pressure ventilation (NPPV) has been shown to reduce the need for, and duration of, intubation, and has resulted in improved survival, particularly in patients with hypercapnic acute respiratory failure due to exacerbation of chronic obstructive pulmonary disease (COPD). The use of NPPV results in a decreased risk for pneumonia.

Repeat Endotracheal Intubation

Repeat insertion of the endotracheal tube soon after it is removed from a patient who is taken off ventilatory support has been shown to be a risk factor for pneumonia. Using NIV instead may help reduce the risk.

Cross-colonization Via Hands of Personnel

Pathogens causing healthcare-related pneumonia, such as gram-negative bacilli and *S. aureus*, are ubiquitous in health-care settings, especially in intensive- or critical-care areas. Transmission of these microorganisms to patients frequently occurs via healthcare personnel's hands that become contaminated or transiently colonized with the microorganisms. Procedures such as tracheal suctioning and manipulation of ventilator circuit or endotracheal tubes increase the opportunity for cross-contamination. The risk of cross-contamination can be reduced by using aseptic technique and sterile or disinfected equipment when appropriate and eliminating pathogens from the hands of personnel.

In theory, handwashing is an effective way of removing transient bacteria from the hands; however, in general, personnel compliance with handwashing has been poor. New guidelines for hand hygiene that promote the use of alcohol-based antiseptic preparations may result in increased personnel compliance and decreased incidence of hand-transmitted infections.

Gloving also helps prevent cross-contamination. Routine gloving (in addition to gowning) was associated with a decrease in the incidence of healthcare-related RSV infection and infections occurring in the ICU. Gloves, however, can be colonized by pathogens prevalent in the healthcare setting, and outbreaks have been traced to healthcare personnel who did not change gloves after contact with one patient and before providing care to another. In addition, gloved hands may get contaminated via leaks in the gloves. Thus, personnel should use gloves properly and decontaminate their hands after gloves are removed.

Contamination of Devices Used on the Respiratory Tract

Devices used on the respiratory tract for respiratory therapy (e.g. nebulizers, endotracheal tubes), diagnostic examination (e.g. bronchoscopes or spirometers), or administration of anesthesia are potential reservoirs or vehicles for infectious microorganisms. Routes of transmission may be from device to patient, from one patient to another, or from one body site to the lower respiratory tract of the same patient via hand or device.

Contaminated reservoirs of aerosol-producing devices, e.g. nebulizers, can allow the growth of hydrophilic bacteria that may be subsequently aerosolized during device use. Gram-negative bacilli (e.g. *Pseudomonas* species or *Flavobacterium* species; *Legionella* species) and nontuberculous mycobacteria can multiply to high concentrations in nebulizer fluid and increase the device user's risk of acquiring pneumonia. Proper cleaning and sterilization or disinfection of reusable equipment are important components of a program to reduce infections associated with devices used for respiratory therapy, pulmonary diagnostic tests, or delivery of anesthesia.

Most devices or parts of devices used on the respiratory tract have been categorized as semicritical in the Spaulding classification system for appropriate sterilization or disinfection of medical devices because they come into direct or indirect contact with mucous membranes but do not ordinarily penetrate body surfaces, and the associated infection risk following the use of these devices in patients is less than that associated with devices that penetrate normally sterile tissues.

Thus, after they are thoroughly cleaned, they can be subjected to high-level disinfection by either using liquid chemical disinfectants that are cleared by the Food and Drug Administration (FDA) for use on medical instruments or by pasteurization at >70°C for 30 minutes. Sterile water is preferred to tap or unsterilized distilled water for rinsing off residual liquid chemical disinfectant from a respiratory device that has been chemically disinfected for reuse, because tap or distilled water may harbor microorganisms that can cause pneumonia.

However, when rinsing with sterile water is not feasible, rinsing with tap water or filtered water (water passed through 0.2 μ filter), followed by an alcohol rinse and forced-air drying, may be done. Forced-air drying has been shown to markedly lower the level of microbial contamination of stored endoscopes, most likely by removing the wet environment favorable for bacterial growth.

Mechanical Ventilators, Breathing Circuits, Humidifiers, Heat-moisture Exchangers, and In-line Nebulizers

a. Mechanical ventilators

The internal machinery of mechanical ventilators used for respiratory therapy has not been reported as an important source of bacterial contamination of inhaled gas. Thus, routine sterilization or high-level disinfection of the internal machinery is considered unnecessary.

b. Breathing circuits, humidifiers, and heat-moisture exchangers

Most US hospitals use ventilators that provide inspired-gas humidification with either bubble-through or wick humidifiers. Because bubble-through humidifiers produce insignificant amounts of aerosol and wick humidifiers produce no aerosol, they do not pose an important risk for pneumonia in patients. In addition, bubble-through humidifiers are usually heated to temperatures that reduce or eliminate bacterial pathogens. In general, however, sterile water is still used to fill these humidifiers because of the potential presence in tap or distilled water, of microorganisms (e.g. *Legionella* species) that are more heat-resistant than other bacteria.

The potential risk for pneumonia in patients using mechanical ventilators with heated bubble-through humidifiers primarily results from the formation of condensate in the inspiratory phase tubing of unheated ventilator circuits due to the difference in the temperatures of the inspiratory-phase gas and ambient air. The condensate and tubing can rapidly become contaminated, usually with bacteria that originate from the patient's oropharynx. In a study, 33% of inspiratory circuits were colonized with bacteria from patients' oropharynx within 2 hours, and 80% within 24 hours, of use. Spillage of the contaminated condensate into the patient's tracheobronchial tree can occur with procedures during which the tubing may be moved (e.g. suctioning, adjusting the ventilator setting, or feeding or giving hygienic care to the patient) and may increase the patient's risk for pneumonia. Thus, in many healthcare facilities, personnel are trained to prevent such spillage and drain and discard the fluid periodically.

Microorganisms contaminating ventilator-circuit condensate can be transmitted to other patients via hands of the healthcare personnel handling the fluid, especially if the personnel fail to decontaminate their hands after handling the condensate.

The role of ventilator-tubing changes in preventing pneumonia in patients using mechanical ventilators is variable and therefore the previous CDC recommendation to change ventilator circuits routinely on the basis of duration of use should be changed to one that is based on visual and/or known contamination of the circuit.

Condensate formation in the inspiratory-phase tubing of a ventilator breathing circuit can be decreased by elevating the temperature of the inspiratory-phase gas with a heated wire in the inspiratory-phase tubing. However, it can result in tube blockage by dried patient secretions, attributed to the decrease in the relative humidity of inspired gas that results from the elevation of the gas temperature. Therefore, users of heated ventilator tubing should be aware of the advantages and potential complications of using heated tubing.

Condensate accumulation can also be eliminated by using a heat-moisture exchanger (HME). An HME recycles heat and moisture exhaled by the patient and eliminates the need for a humidifier. In the absence of a humidifier, no condensate forms in the inspiratory phase tubing of the ventilator circuit. Thus, bacterial colonization of the tubing is prevented; and periodic, routine changing of the tubing is not necessary. An HME, however, increases the dead space and resistance to breathing, may leak around the endotracheal tube, and may result in drying of sputum and blockage of the tracheobronchial tree. Its effect on the work of breathing and the ventilatory drive may cause increased inspiratory neuromuscular activity from the patients, which, if sustained during acute respiratory failure, may lead to inspiratory muscle fatigue. Thus, consideration of the economic advantages of the use of an HME should be balanced with its possible negative respiratory effects.

Recently, an HME with an active humidifier (i.e. external heat and moisture added at the patient side of the HME) was designed to offset the device's negative effects (i.e. drying of patient's secretions and increased resistance to airflow).

Small-volume (in-line) and hand-held medication nebulizers

Small-volume (in-line) medication nebulizers that are inserted in the inspiratory circuit of mechanical ventilators and hand-held liquid-medication nebulizers can produce bacterial aerosols. If in-line nebulizers become contaminated by condensate in the inspiratory tubing of the breathing circuit, they can increase the patient's risk of pneumonia because the nebulizer aerosol is directed through the endotracheal tube and bypasses many of the normal host defenses against infection. Handheld small-volume medication nebulizers have been associated with healthcare-associated pneumonia, including Legionnaires disease, as a result of their contamination with medications from multidose vials or with *Legionella*-contaminated tap water used for rinsing and filling the reservoir. Thus, when nebulized liquid medications are used, unit-dose vials are preferable to multidose vials. If multidose medication vials are used, the persons who handle, dispense, and store such medications should closely follow the medications' manufacturers' directions to prevent equipment and medication contamination.

Suction Catheters

Endotracheal suction catheters can introduce microorganisms into a patient's lower respiratory tract. Currently, two types of suction-catheter systems are used in US hospitals: the open single-use catheter system and the closed multiuse catheter system. The closed-suction system has the potential advantages of decreased environmental contamination as well as lower costs, especially if it can be corroborated that, notwithstanding the manufacturer-recommended daily catheter changes, the catheter can remain unchanged for an indefinite period without increasing the patient's risk of VAP. However, studies that compared the effect of the open single-use catheter system and that of the closed multiuse catheter system on the incidence of VAP have yielded equivocal results. More studies are needed to determine the effect of the type of suction system on the incidence of VAP.

Resuscitation Bags, Ventilator Spirometers and Temperature Probes

Reusable resuscitation bags are particularly difficult to clean and dry between uses; microorganisms in secretions or fluid left in the bag may be aerosolized or sprayed into the lower respiratory tract of the patient on whom the bag is used; in addition, contaminating microorganisms may be transmitted from one patient to another via hands of staff members. Ventilator spirometers and temperature probes have been associated with outbreaks of gram-negative bacillary respiratory tract colonization and pneumonia resulting from patient-to-patient transmission of microorganisms. Devices such as these require sterilization or high-level disinfection between uses on different patients. Education of physicians, respiratory therapists, and nursing staff about the appropriate care and handling of these devices (in addition to appropriate hand decontamination between patients) is essential.

Anesthesia Equipment

The contributory role of anesthesia equipment in outbreaks of healthcare-associated pneumonia was reported before hospitals implemented routine after-use cleaning and disinfection/sterilization of reusable components of anesthesia-equipment that may become contaminated with pathogens during use.

a. *Anesthesia machine*: The internal components of anesthesia machines (e.g. the gas sources and outlets, gas valves, pressure regulators, flow meters, and vaporizers) are not considered important sources of bacterial contamination of inhaled gases. Thus, routine sterilization or high-level disinfection of the internal machinery is considered unnecessary.
b. *Breathing system or patient circuit:* The breathing system or patient circuit through which inhaled and/or exhaled gases flow to and from a patient can become contaminated with microorganisms that may originate from the patient's oropharynx or trachea. The breathing system includes the tracheal tube or face mask, inspiratory and expiratory tubing, y-piece, CO_2 absorber and its chamber, the anesthesia ventilator bellows and tubing, humidifier, adjustable pressure limiting valve, and other devices and accessories. Recommendations for in-use care, maintenance, and reprocessing (i.e. cleaning and disinfection or sterilization) of the components of the breathing system have been published. In general, reusable components of the breathing system that directly touch the patient's mucous membranes (e.g. face mask or tracheal tube) or become readily contaminated with the patient's respiratory secretions (e.g. y-piece, inspiratory and expiratory tubing and attached sensors) are cleaned and subjected to high-level disinfection or sterilization between patients. The other parts of the breathing system (e.g. carbon dioxide absorber and its chamber) for which an appropriate and cost-effective schedule of reprocessing has not been firmly determined are changed, cleaned, and sterilized or subjected to high-level disinfection periodically, according to published guidelines and manufacturers' instructions.

Using high-efficiency bacterial filters at various positions in the patient circuit (e.g. at the y-piece or on the inspiratory and expiratory sides of the patient circuit) has been advocated and shown to decrease contamination of the circuit.). However, the efficacy of bacterial filters in preventing healthcare-associated pneumonia has not been shown.

Pulmonary Function Testing Equipment

In general, pulmonary function testing devices (e.g. spirometers, peak flow meters) have not been considered an important source of bacterial contamination of inhaled gas. However, because of concern about possible carry-over of bacteria from an infectious user of the device to the next patient-user(s), placement of bacterial filters that remove exhaled bacteria between the patient and the testing equipment has been advocated. Randomized controlled studies have not been done to evaluate the efficacy of these filters in preventing healthcare associated pneumonia.

Whereas high-level disinfection of spirometer tubing and mouthpieces was recommended in the past because these spirometer parts could become contaminated with secretions during patient use, recent routine use of filters has obviated the need for such disinfection. Instead, the mouthpiece and the filter are changed between uses by different patients.

Postoperative State

A preoperative risk index for predicting postoperative pneumonia was recently developed. The following significant risk factors were identified: type of surgery (abdominal aortic aneurysm repair, thoracic surgery, and emergency surgery); use of general anesthesia; age >60 years; totally dependent functional status; weight loss greater than 10%; steroid use for chronic conditions; recent history of alcohol use; history of chronic obstructive pulmonary disease; smoking within one year of surgery; impaired sensorium; history of cerebrovascular accident with residual neurologic deficit; low (<8 mg/dL) or high (>22 mg/dL) blood urea nitrogen level; and receipt of more than 4 units of blood before surgery.

Interventions aimed at reducing the postoperative patient's risk for pneumonia and other pulmonary complications have been developed; most measures have been geared towards clearing secretions and increasing lung expansion. These include deep breathing exercises, chest physiotherapy, use of incentive spirometry and continuous positive airway pressure by face mask.

Other Prophylactic Measures

Immunomodulation

a. Pneumococcal vaccination

Although pneumococci are not a major cause of healthcare-associated pneumonia, they have been identified as etiologic agents of serious healthcare-associated pulmonary infection and bacteremia. The following factors render patients at high risk for complications from pneumococcal infections: >65 years of age, chronic cardiovascular or pulmonary disease, diabetes mellitus, alcoholism, cirrhosis, cerebrospinal fluid (CSF) leaks, immunosuppression, functional or anatomic asplenia, or HIV infection.

Strains of drug-resistant *S. pneumoniae* have become increasingly common in the United States and in other parts of the world. In certain areas of the US, approximately 35% of invasive isolates have intermediate (MIC = 0.1–1.0 μg/mL) susceptibility or high-level (MIC >2 μg/mL) resistance to penicillin. Because many of the penicillin-resistant strains of pneumococci are also resistant to other antimicrobial agents [e.g. erythromycin, trimethoprim-sulfamethoxazole (TMPSMZ), and extended-spectrum cephalosporins], therapeutic management of invasive pneumococcal infections (e.g. pneumonia) becomes difficult and expensive.

The 23-valent vaccine is cost-effective and protective against invasive pneumococcal disease when administered to immunocompetent persons aged >5 years, and although not as effective for immunocompromised patients as for immunocompetent persons, its potential benefits and safety justify its use on this group of patients. The Advisory Committee on Immunization Practices (ACIP) recommends the administration of the vaccine to the following: (a) immunocompetent persons >65 years of age, persons aged >2–64 years who have chronic cardiovascular disease (e.g. congestive heart failure or cardiomyopathy), chronic pulmonary disease (e.g. COPD or emphysema, but not asthma), diabetes mellitus, alcoholism, chronic liver disease (cirrhosis), or CSF leaks; persons aged >2–64 years who have functional or anatomic asplenia; and persons aged >2–64 who are living in special environments or social settings; and (b) immunocompromised persons aged >2 years with HIV infection, leukemia, lymphoma, Hodgkin's disease, multiple myeloma, generalized malignancy, chronic renal failure, nephrotic syndrome, or other conditions associated with immunosuppression, such as solid-organ or human-stem-cell transplantation, and persons receiving immunosuppressive chemotherapy, including long-term systemic corticosteroids.

Because the 23-valent vaccine does not protect children aged <2 years, the age group with the highest rate of invasive (e.g. bacteremia, meningitis) and noninvasive pneumococcal disease (i.e. community-acquired pneumonia, acute otitis media, and sinusitis), a 7-valent pneumococcal polysaccharide protein-conjugate vaccine has been recommended for use in all children aged <2 years and for children aged 24–59 months who are at increased risk for pneumococcal disease (e.g. children with sickle cell disease, HIV infection, and other immunocompromising or chronic medical conditions).

b. Use of immune globulin or granulocyte colony-stimulating factor

Intravenous immune globulin (given at 400 mg/kg body weight, once a week) was shown to be efficacious in reducing the overall incidence of nosocomial infections, including gram-negative bacillary pneumonia, in postoperative patients.

The use of hyperimmune globulin (100 mg/kg) against exotoxin A, *Klebsiella* species, and *Pseudomonas aeruginosa* has not been shown to prevent infections due to these microorganisms.

Granulocyte colony-stimulating factor (GCSF) increases the immune response of granulocytopenic patients to infections. It has been administered to patients with chemotherapy induced febrile neutropenia and to those with acute traumatic brain injury or cerebral hemorrhage to decrease the incidence of healthcare-associated infections in general.

c. Use of glutamine-enriched enteral feeding

Deficiency of glutamine, an essential amino acid that is needed for adequate lymphocyte and enterocyte function, may develop in times of severe illness, and contribute greatly to depression of the immune response and increased gut permeability. The intravenous administration of glutamine has been shown to help maintain integrity of the intestines and glutamine-enriched enteral feeding was associated with lower incidences of VAP and bacteremia in multiple-trauma patients.

Administration of Antimicrobial Agents

a. Prophylactic systemic antimicrobial administration

Studies that evaluated the effect of systemic administration of an antimicrobial agent on the prevention of healthcare-associated pneumonia have had conflicting results. In addition, prophylaxis with systemic antibiotics can potentially cause the emergence of and superinfection with antimicrobial-resistant microorganisms.

b. Periodic scheduled change in the class of antimicrobial agents used for empiric therapy of infections

The incidence of VAP in the ICU caused by antibiotic-resistant gram-negative bacilli decreased significantly when (1) a scheduled change was made in the class of antimicrobial agents; (2) restriction of the use of ceftazidime and ciprofloxacin for empiric or definitive therapy; (3) rotation of antimicrobial agents for use in the unit; and (4) supervision and control of antibiotic use by designated personnel.[16,17]

Turning or Rotational Therapy

Turning or rotational therapy is used to prevent pulmonary and other complications of prolonged immobilization or bed rest as occur in patients with acute stroke, critical illness, head injury or traction, blunt chest trauma, and/or mechanically-assisted ventilation. In the last two decades, automated beds or cushions have been used to provide turning therapy to immobilized patients. These equipment fall into 2 general classes based on the turning angle: the "kinetic" bed (i.e. one that achieves a 62°-angle turn), and the continuous lateral rotational therapy (CLRT) bed (i.e. one that turns <40° along its longitudinal axis). Among the hypothesized benefits of using these beds are improved drainage of secretions within the lungs and lower airways, increased tidal volume, and reduction of venous thrombosis and its sequela, pulmonary embolization.

PREVENTION AND CONTROL MEASURES[1,18]

Staff Education and Involvement in Infection Prevention

Educate healthcare workers regarding the epidemiology of, and infection control procedures for, preventing healthcare-associated bacterial pneumonia.

Infection and Microbiologic Surveillance

Conduct surveillance for bacterial pneumonia in ICU patients who are at high risk for healthcare-associated bacterial pneumonia (e.g. patients with mechanically-assisted ventilation or selected postoperative patients) to determine trends and help identify outbreaks and other potential infection-control problems. Include data on the causative microorganisms and their antimicrobial susceptibility patterns. Express data as rates (e.g. number of infected patients or infections per 100 ICU days or per 1,000 ventilator days) to facilitate intra-hospital comparisons and trend determination.

Prevention of Transmission of Microorganisms

Sterilization or Disinfection and Maintenance of Equipment and Devices

1. General measures

a. Thoroughly clean all equipment and devices to be sterilized or disinfected.
b. Whenever possible, use steam sterilization (by autoclaving) or high level disinfection by wet heat pasteurization at >158°F (>70°C) for 30 minutes for reprocessing semicritical equipment or devices (i.e. items that come into direct or indirect contact with mucous membranes of the lower respiratory tract) that are not sensitive to heat and moisture. Use low-temperature sterilization methods for equipment or devices that are heat- or moisture-sensitive. After disinfection, proceed with appropriate rinsing, drying, and packaging, taking care not to contaminate the disinfected items in the process.
c. Preferentially use sterile water for rinsing reusable semicritical respiratory equipment and devices when rinsing is needed after they have been chemically disinfected. If this is not feasible, rinse the device with filtered water (i.e. water that has been through a 0.2 μ filter) or tap water, and then rinse with isopropyl alcohol and dry with forced air or in a drying cabinet.

2. Mechanical ventilators

Do not routinely sterilize or disinfect the internal machinery of mechanical ventilators.

3. Breathing circuits, humidifiers, and HMEs

A. Breathing circuits with humidifiers

1. Do not change routinely on the basis of duration of use the breathing circuit (i.e. ventilator tubing and exhalation valve and the attached humidifier) that is in use on an individual patient. Change the circuit when it is visibly soiled or mechanically malfunctioning.
2. Breathing-circuit-tubing condensate
   a. Periodically drain and discard any condensate that collects in the tubing of a mechanical ventilator, taking precautions not to allow condensate to drain toward the patient.
   b. Wear gloves to perform the above procedure or handle the fluid.
   c. Decontaminate hands with soap and water (if hands are visibly soiled) or with an alcohol-based hand rub, after performing the procedure or handling the fluid.
3. *No recommendation* can be made for placing a filter or trap at the distal end of the expiratory-phase tubing of the breathing circuit to collect condensate. This is still an (*Unresolved Issue*).
4. Humidifier fluids
   a. Use sterile (not distilled, non-sterile) water to fill bubbling humidifiers.
   b. *No recommendation* can be made for the preferential use of a closed, continuous-feed humidification system (*Unresolved Issue*).

B. Ventilator breathing circuits with HMEs

1. *No recommendation* can be made for the preferential use of either HMEs or heated humidifiers to prevent pneumonia in patients receiving mechanically assisted ventilation (*Unresolved Issue*).
2. Changing HMEs
   a. Change an HME that is used on a patient when it malfunctions mechanically or becomes visibly soiled.
   b. Do not routinely change more frequently than every 48 hours an HME that is in use on a patient.
3. Do not change routinely (in the absence of gross contamination or malfunction) the breathing circuit attached to an HME while it is in use on a patient.
4. Oxygen humidifiers
   a. Follow manufacturers' instructions for use of oxygen humidifiers.
   b. Change the humidifier-tubing (including any nasal prongs or mask) that is in use on one patient when it malfunctions or becomes visibly contaminated.
5. Small-volume medication nebulizers: in-line and hand-held nebulizers
   a. Between treatments on the same patient: clean, disinfect; rinse with sterile water (if rinsing is needed), and dry small-volume in-line or hand-held medication nebulizers.
   b. Use only sterile fluid for nebulization, and dispense the fluid into the nebulizer aseptically.
   c. Whenever possible, use aerosolized medications in single-dose vials. If multidose medication vials are used, follow manufacturers' instructions for handling, storing, and dispensing the medications.
6. Mist-tents
   a. Between uses on different patients, replace mist-tents and their nebulizers, reservoirs, and tubings with those that have been subjected to sterilization or high-level disinfection.
   b. *No recommendation* can be made about the frequency of routinely changing mist-tent nebulizers, reservoirs, and tubings while in use on one patient (*Unresolved Issue*).
   c. Subject mist-tent nebulizers, reservoirs and tubings that are

used on the same patient to daily low-level disinfection (e.g. with 2% acetic acid) or pasteurization followed by air-drying.

7. Other devices used in association with respiratory therapy
   a. Respirometers and ventilator thermometers between their uses on different patients, sterilize or subject to high-level disinfection portable respirometers, and ventilator thermometers.
   b. Resuscitation bags
      i. Between their uses on different patients, sterilize or subject to high-level disinfection reusable hand-powered resuscitation bags.
      ii. *No Recommendation* can be made about the frequency of changing hydrophobic filters placed on the connection port of resuscitation bags (*Unresolved Issue*).
8. Anesthesia machines and breathing systems or patient circuits
   a. Do not routinely sterilize or disinfect the internal machinery of anesthesia equipment.
   b. Between uses on different patients, clean reusable components of the breathing system or patient circuit (e.g. tracheal tube or face mask; inspiratory and expiratory breathing tubing; y-piece; reservoir bag; humidifier; and tubing) and then sterilize or subject them to high-level liquid chemical disinfection or pasteurization in accordance with the device manufacturers' instructions for their reprocessing.
   c. *No recommendation* can be made about the frequency of routinely cleaning and disinfecting unidirectional valves and carbon dioxide absorber chambers. (*Unresolved Issue*).
   d. Follow published guidelines and manufacturers' instructions about in use maintenance, cleaning, and disinfection or sterilization of other components or attachments of the breathing system or patient circuit of anesthesia equipment.
   e. *No recommendation* can be made for placing a bacterial filter in the breathing system or patient circuit of anesthesia equipment (*Unresolved Issue*).
9. Pulmonary-function testing equipment
   a. Do not routinely sterilize or disinfect the internal machinery of pulmonary-function testing machines between uses on different patients.
   b. Change the mouthpiece of a peak flow meter or the mouthpiece and filter of a spirometer between uses on different patients.
10. Room-air "humidifiers" and faucet aerators
   a. Do not use large-volume room-air humidifiers that create aerosols (e.g. by Venturi Principle, ultrasound, or spinning disk, and thus actually are nebulizers) unless they can be sterilized or subjected to high-level disinfection at least daily and filled only with sterile water.
   b. Faucet aerators
      i. *No recommendation* can be made about the removal of faucet aerators from areas for immunocompetent patients (*Unresolved Issue*).
      ii. If *Legionella* species are detected in the water of a transplant unit and until *Legionella* species are no longer detected by culture, remove faucet aerators in the unit.

Prevention of Person-to-Person Transmission of Bacteria

Standard precautions

a. Hand hygiene
Decontaminate hands by washing them with either antimicrobial soap and water or with nonantimicrobial soap and water (if hands are visibly dirty or contaminated with proteinaceous material or are soiled with blood or body fluids) or by using an alcohol-based antiseptic agent (e.g. hand rub) if hands are not visibly soiled after contact with mucous membranes, respiratory secretions, or objects contaminated with respiratory secretions, whether or not gloves are worn.
Decontaminate hands as described previously before and after contact with a patient who has an endotracheal or tracheostomy tube in place, and before and after contact with any respiratory device that is used on the patient, whether or not gloves are worn.

2. Gloving
   a. Wear gloves for handling respiratory secretions or objects contaminated with respiratory secretions of any patient.
   b. Change gloves and decontaminate hands as described previously between contacts with different patients; after handling respiratory secretions or objects contaminated with secretions from one patient and before contact with another patient, object, or environmental surface; and between contacts with a contaminated body site and the respiratory tract of, or respiratory device on, the same patient.
3. Gowning
When soiling with respiratory secretions from a patient is anticipated, wear a gown and change it after soiling occurs and before providing care to another patient.

Care of patients with tracheostomy

1. Perform tracheostomy under aseptic conditions.
2. When changing a tracheostomy tube, wear a gown, use aseptic technique, and replace the tube with one that has undergone sterilization or high-level disinfection.
3. *No recommendation* can be made for the daily application of topical antimicrobial agent(s) at the tracheostomy site (*Unresolved Issue*).

Suctioning of respiratory tract secretions

1. *No recommendation* can be made for the preferential use of either the multiuse closed-system suction catheter or the single-use open system suction catheter for prevention of pneumonia (*Unresolved Issue*).
2. *No recommendation* can be made about wearing sterile rather than clean gloves when performing endotracheal suctioning (*Unresolved Issue*).
3. *No recommendation* can be made about the frequency of routinely changing the in-line suction catheter of a closed-suction system in use on one patient (*Unresolved Issue*).
4. If the open-system suction is employed, use a sterile single-use catheter.
5. Use only sterile fluid to remove secretions from the suction catheter if the catheter is to be used for re-entry into the patient's lower respiratory tract.

Modifying Host Risk for Infection

Increasing Host Defense Against Infection: Administration of Immune Modulators

1. Pneumococcal vaccination. Vaccinate patients at high risk for severe pneumococcal infections:
   a. Administer the 23-valent pneumococcal polysaccharide vaccine to persons aged >65 years; persons aged 5-64 years who have chronic cardiovascular disease (e.g. congestive heart failure or cardiomyopathy), chronic pulmonary disease (e.g. COPD

or emphysema, but not asthma), diabetes mellitus, alcoholism, chronic liver disease (cirrhosis), or cerebrospinal fluid (CSF) leaks; persons aged 5-64 years who have functional or anatomic asplenia; persons aged 5-64 years who are living in special environments or social settings; immunocompromised persons aged >5 years with HIV infection, leukemia, lymphoma, Hodgkin's disease, multiple myeloma, generalized malignancy, chronic renal failure, nephritic syndrome, or other conditions associated with immunosuppression (e.g. receipt of HSCT, solid-organ transplant, or immunosuppressive chemotherapy, including long-term systemic corticosteroids); and persons in long-term care facilities.

b. Administer the 7-valent pneumococcal polysaccharide protein conjugate vaccine to all children aged <2 years and to children aged 2 to 5 years who are at increased risk for pneumococcal disease [e.g. children with sickle-cell disease and other hemoglobinopathies or children who are functionally or anatomically asplenic; children with HIV infection; children who have chronic disease, including chronic cardiac or pulmonary disease (except asthma), diabetes mellitus, or CSF leak; and children with immunocompromising conditions including malignancies, chronic renal failure or nephritic syndrome, immunosuppressive chemotherapy, including long-term corticosteroids, and receipt of solid-organ transplant].

c. In nursing homes and other long-term care facilities, establish an SOP for the administration of 23-valent vaccine to persons at high risk of acquiring severe pneumococcal infections, including pneumococcal pneumonia.

2. *No recommendation* can be made for the routine administration of preparations of GCSF or intravenous gamma globulin for prophylaxis against health-care-associated pneumonia (*Unresolved Issue*).
3. *No recommendation* can be made for the routine enteral administration of glutamine for prevention of healthcare-associated pneumonia (*Unresolved Issue*).

Precautions for Prevention of Aspiration

1. As soon as the clinical indications for their use are resolved, remove devices such as endotracheal, tracheostomy, or enteral (i.e. oro- or nasogastric, or jejunal) tubes from patients for prevention of aspiration associated with endotracheal intubation.
   a. Use of noninvasive ventilation (NIV) to reduce the need for and duration of endotracheal intubation
      i. When feasible and not medically contraindicated, use noninvasive positive-pressure ventilation delivered continuously by face or nose mask, instead of performing endotracheal intubation in patients who are in respiratory failure and are not needing immediate intubation (e.g. those who are in hypercapnic respiratory failure secondary to acute exacerbation of COPD or cardiogenic pulmonary edema).
      ii. When feasible and not medically contraindicated, use NIV(non-invasive ventilation as part of the weaning process (from mechanically-assisted ventilation) in order to shorten the period of endotracheal intubation.
   b. As much as possible, avoid repeat endotracheal intubation in patients who have received mechanically-assisted ventilation.
   c. Unless contraindicated by the patient's condition, perform orotracheal rather

than nasotracheal intubation on patients.

d. If feasible, use an endotracheal tube with a dorsal lumen above the endotracheal cuff to allow drainage (by continuous or frequent intermittent suctioning) of tracheal secretions that accumulate in the patient's subglottic area.

e. Before deflating the cuff of an endotracheal tube in preparation for tube removal, or before moving the tube, ensure that secretions are cleared from above the tube cuff.

2. Prevention of aspiration associated with enteral feeding
   i. In the absence of medical contra-indication(s), elevate at an angle of 30–45 degrees, the head of the bed of a patient at high risk for aspiration pneumonia (e.g. a person receiving mechanically-assisted ventilation or who has an enteral tube in place).
   ii. Routinely verify appropriate placement of the feeding tube.
   iii. *No recommendation* can be made for the preferential use of small bore tubes for enteral feeding (*Unresolved Issue*).
   iv. *No recommendation* can be made for preferentially administering enteral feedings continuously or intermittently (*Unresolved Issue*).
   v. *No recommendation* can be made for preferentially placing the feeding tubes (e.g., jejunal tubes) distal to the pylorus (*Unresolved Issue*).
3. Prevention or modulation of oropharyngeal colonization
   a. Oropharyngeal cleaning and decontamination with an antiseptic agent: Develop and implement a comprehensive oral-hygiene program (that might include the use of an antiseptic agent) for patients in acute-care settings or residents in long-term care facilities who are at high risk of developing healthcare-associated pneumonia
   b. Chlorhexidine oral rinse
      i. *No recommendation* can be made for the routine use of an oral chlorhexidine rinse for the prevention of healthcare-associated pneumonia in all postoperative or critically ill patients or other patients at high risk for pneumonia (*Unresolved Issue*).
      ii. Use a oral chlorhexidine gluconate (0.12%) rinse during the perioperative period on adult patients who undergo cardiac surgery.
   c. Oral decontamination with topical antimicrobial agents
      No recommendation can be made for the routine use of topical antimicrobial agents for oral decontamination to prevent VAP (*Unresolved Issue*).
4. Prevention of gastric colonization
   a. *No recommendation* can be made for the preferential use of sucralfate, H2-antagonists, or antacids for stress-bleeding prophylaxis in patients receiving mechanically-assisted ventilation (*Unresolved Issue*).
   b. *No recommendation* can be made for the routine administration of SDD (selective decontamination of digestive tract) to all critically ill, mechanically ventilated, or ICU patients (*Unresolved Issue*).
   c. *No recommendation* can be made for routine acidification of gastric feeding (*Unresolved Issue*).

Prevention of Postoperative Pneumonia

1. Instruct preoperative patients, especially those at high risk for contracting pneumonia, about taking deep breaths and ambulating as soon as medically indicated in the postoperative period. Patients at high-risk include those who will have abdominal aortic aneurysm repair, thoracic surgery, or emergency surgery; who are receiving general anesthesia; age >60 years; with totally dependent

functional status; a weight loss >10%; using steroids for chronic conditions; with recent history of alcohol use, history of COPD, or smoking during the preceding year; with impaired sensorium, a history of cerebrovascular accident with residual neurologic deficit, or low(<8 mg/dL) or high (>22 mg/dL) blood urea nitrogen level; and those who will have received more than 4 units of blood before surgery.

2. Use incentive spirometry on postoperative patients at high risk for developing pneumonia.
3. *No recommendation* can be made about the routine use of chest physiotherapy on all postoperative patients at high risk for pneumonia (*Unresolved Issue*).

Other Prophylactic Procedures for Pneumonia

1. Administration of antimicrobial agents other than in SDD
   a. Systemic antimicrobial prophylaxis
      No recommendation can be made about the routine administration of systemic antimicrobial agent(s) to prevent pneumonia in critically ill patients and/or in those receiving mechanically-assisted ventilation (*Unresolved Issue*).
   b. Scheduled changes in the class of antimicrobial agents used for empiric therapy.
      No recommendation can be made for scheduled changes in the class of antimicrobial agents used routinely for empiric treatment of suspected infections in a particular group of patients (*Unresolved Issue*).
2. Turning or rotational therapy
   No recommendation can be made for the routine use of turning or rotational therapy, either by "kinetic" therapy or by continuous "lateral rotational therapy (i.e. placing patients on beds that turn on their longitudinal axes intermittently or continuously) for prevention of healthcare-associated pneumonia in critically ill or immobilized patients (*Unresolved Issue*).

Practical Approach for Prevention of Lower Respiratory Tract Infection (Tables 16.1 and 16.2)[19,20]

Nosocomial pneumonia is mainly associated with intubation and mechanical ventilation in patients in intensive care units. Equipments and hands contaminated with secretions, aerosols or droplets are the main routes of transmission of microorganisms.

Mode of Acquisition of Nosocomial Pneumonia[17]

- Respiratory: Droplets—inhalation of aerosols.
- Oropharyngeal: Hands of staff-colonization—aspiration.
- Gastric: Reduced pH—colonization—aspiration.

Risk Factor for Nosocomial Pneumonia

- Condition of patient
- Severely ill (e.g. septic shock)
- Age (elderly or neonate)
- Surgical operation (chest/abdomen)
- Major injuries
- Coronary bypass surgery
- Existing cardiopulmonary disease
- Cerebrovascular accidents
- Coma
- Heavy smoker
- Immunosuppressed patients with malignancy.

Therapy

- General anesthesia
- Tracheal intubation
- Tracheostomy, artificial ventilation, external feeding
- Length of time of ventilation
- Antibiotic therapy, antacids and histamine type 2 blockers.

Table 16.1: Prevention of ventilator-associated respiratory infections

Ventilator-associated respiratory infections	Prevention
Risk factors	
Duration of intubation	Limit duration
Invasive ventilation	Noninvasive ventilation is preferred
Ventilation procedures	
Intubation and suction	Aseptic technique should be used
Water for oxygen and aerosol therapy	Water should be sterile and changed regularly
Tracheal toilet	Aseptic technique should be followed
Tubing, respirators and humidifiers	Appropriate cleaning and disinfection to limit contamination and subsequent infection Change breathing circuits, humidifiers, HME only when visibly soiled
Suction tubes	Sterile, aseptic technique should be used
Humidifier bottles	Should be sterilized between use and should not be topped up
Portable respirometers and ventilator thermometers	Between their uses on different patients, sterilize or subject to high-level disinfection
Reusable resuscitation bags	Between their uses on different patients, sterilize or subject to high-level disinfection
Reusable components of the breathing system or patient circuit (e.g. tracheal tube or face mask; inspiratory and expiratory breathing tubing; y-piece; reservoir bag; humidifier; and tubing)	Clean and then sterilize or high-level disinfect between patients
Mouthpiece of a peak flow meter or the mouthpiece and filter of a spirometer	Change between use on different patients
Small-volume medication nebulizers	Between treatments on the same patient: clean, disinfect; rinse with sterile water (if rinsing is needed)

Source: Adapted from guidelines for prevention and control of Hospital- associated infections WHO January 2002 and modified according to CDC guidelines for preventing health care associated pneumonia,2003.[1]

Table 16.2: Effective methods for prevention of ventilator-associated pneumonia

Proven effective	Proven not effective
Aseptic intubation and suctioning	Digestive decontamination for all patients
Limit duration	Changes of ventilator circuit every 48–72 hours
Noninvasive ventilation	
Orotracheal rather than nasotracheal intubation on patients use an endotracheal tube with a dorsal lumen above the endotracheal cuff to allow drainage of tracheal secretions that accumulate in the patient's subglottic area	
A comprehensive oral-hygiene program	
Others	
Influenza vaccination for staff	
Isolation policy	
Sterile water for oxygen and aerosol therapy	
Prevention of *Legionella* and *Aspergillus* during renovations	

- Immunosuppressive and cytotoxic drugs
- Insertion of nasogastric tube/orogastric tube
- Contaminated respiratory devices (nebulizers, endotracheal tubes, bronchoscopes, spirometer, humidifiers, suction catheters)
- And/or contact with contaminated or colonized hands, mainly of healthcare personnel.
- Enteral feeding
- Steroid use for chronic conditions
- History of chronic obstructive pulmonary disease.

Methods of Prevention

- To prevent cardiopulmonary illness—clear airways, oral cavity care at least 6 times a day.

Other Important Measures

- Hand washing before and after contact with patients, whether or not gloves are worn.
- Disposable or reprocessed gloves and sterile or disinfected catheters for tracheal aspiration and tracheostomy care.
- Education of staff in patient's care and cleaning and disinfection of respiratory equipment.

Prevention of aspiration pneumonia in hospital:

- Comatose patients must be positioned on their side to limit the potential for aspiration.
- Oral feeds should be avoided in patients with neurological or swallowing abnormalities.
- Medications which impair consciousness (sedatives, narcotics) must be limited.

Prevention of pneumonia after surgical procedures:

- All invasive devices used during anesthesia must be sterile.
- Anesthetists must use gloves and masks when undertaking invasive tracheal care.
- Disposable filters (for individual use) for endotracheal intubation effectively prevent the transmission of micro-organisms among patients by ventilators.
- Preoperative physiotherapy helps to prevent nosocomial pneumonia in patients with chronic respiratory disease.

SUMMARY OF VENTILATOR-ASSOCIATED PNEUMONIA INCLUDING VAP BUNDLE [21]

Definition

Ventilator-associated pneumonia (VAP) is defined as pneumonia occuring more than 48 hours after endotracheal intubation and initiation of mechanical ventilation (MV) including pneumonia after extubation.

Types of VAP

- Early-onset pneumonia [<96 hours (4 days) of intubation or ICU admission]
  - Usually community acquired
  - Pathogens:
    - *Streptococcus pneumoniae*
    - *Haemophilus influenzae*
    - *Staphylococcus aureus*
    - *E. coli, Klebsiella* species, *Proteus* species
    - Are antibiotic—sensitive
- Late-onset pneumonia [> 96 hours (i.e. >4 days) of intubation or ICU admission]
  - Hospital acquired
  - Pathogens:
    - *Pseudomonas aeruginosa*
    - Methicillin-resistant *Staphylococcus aureus* (MRSA)
    - *Acinetobacter*
    - *Enterobacter*
  - Are antibiotic-resistant.

Diagnosis of VAP

Diagnosis is imprecise and usually based on a combination of:

- Clinical factors-fever or hypothermia; change in secretions; cough; apnea/bradycardia; tachypnea.
- Microbiological factors-positive cultures of blood/sputum/tracheal aspirate/pleural fluids.
- Radiological factors—new or changing infiltrates.

CDC National Healthcare Safety Network Definition for Ventilator-associated Pneumonia[22]

Radiological Signs

Two or more serial chest radiographs with at least one of the following:

- New or progressive and persistent infiltrate
- Consolidation
- Cavitation.

Clinical Signs

At least one of the following:

- Fever (temperature >38°C with no other recognized cause).
- Leucopenia (<4000 WBCs/μL)
- Adults 70 years or older—altered mental status with no other recognized cause.

Plus at least two of the following:

- New onset of purulent sputum, or change in character of sputum, or increased respiratory secretions, or increased suctioning requirements.
- New onset or worsening cough, or dyspnea, or tachypnea.
- Rales or bronchial breath sounds.
- Worsening gas exchange [e.g. O_2 desaturations (e.g. decreased PF ratio—PaO_2/FiO_2 ≤240), increased O_2 requirements, or increased ventilatory demand].

Microbiological Criteria (Optional)

At least one of the following:

- Positive growth in blood culture not related to another source of infection.
- Positive growth in culture of pleural fluid.
- Positive quantitative culture from bronchoalveolar lavage ≥10^4 colony-forming units/mL) or protected brush specimen (≥10^3 colony-forming units/mL)
- Five percent or more of cells with intracellular bacteria on direct microscopic examination of gram-stained bronchoalveolar lavage fluid.
- Histopathological evidence of pneumonia.

Risk Factors for Nosocomial Pneumonia

- Major risk factor = mechanical ventilation
- Factors that enhance colonization of the oropharynx and/or stomach:
  - Administration of antibiotics
  - Admission to ICU
  - Underlying chronic lung disease.
- Conditions favoring aspiration into the respiratory tract or reflux from GI tract:
  - Supine position
  - Nasogastric tube placement
  - Intubation and self-extubation
  - Immobilization
  - Surgery of head/neck/thorax/upper abdomen.
- Conditions requiring prolonged use of mechanical ventilatory support with potential exposure to contaminated respiratory devices and/or contact with contaminated hands.
- Host Factors:
  - Extremes of age
  - Malnutrition
  - Immunocompromised
  - Underlying conditions/disease process
  - Neurological/neuromuscular disease
  - Burns, trauma.

VAP Antibiotic Selection

- Considerations in making selection
  - Setting (Community, hospital)
  - Suspected organisms (GNBs, GPCs)
  - Host factors (immunosuppression)
  - Local susceptibility patterns.

- Initial empiric and broad; subsequent narrow spectrum
  - Concept is to 'Not Miss' the organism with initial coverage and then de-escalate when able.

Ventilator Care Bundle

- Key components of the bundle are:
  - Elevation of the head of the bed (30–45°).
  - Daily 'sedation vacations' and assessment of readiness to extubate
  - Peptic ulcer prophylaxis (for high-risk patients only).
  - Deep vein thrombosis prophylaxis.
- Additional protocols could include:
  - A structured oral care protocol
  - A patient mobility component
  - Weaning protocols.

Strategies to Prevent VAP

Physical Strategies

1. Strict infection control including hand hygiene with alcohol based hand disinfectants, gowning and gloving minimizes person-to-person transmission of pathogens.
2. Adequate ICU staffing.
3. Minimize endotracheal intubation where possible.
   - Orotracheal route preferred to nasotracheal route.
   - Maintenance of orotracheal cuff pressure >20 cm H_2O (but <30).
   - Subglottic secretion drainage via ETT with a dorsal lumen (in patients ventilated for >72 hours).
   - Use of a closed endotracheal suctioning system for safety considerations only (decrease transmission of infection-resistant organisms) does not prevent VAP.
   - Closed endotracheal suctioning system changed between patients, or as clinically indicated.
4. Minimize the duration of mechanical ventilation
   - Daily interruption of sedation.
   - Standardized weaning protocols.
   - Circuit changes only if the circuit becomes soiled or damaged, and between patients.
   - Changing of heat-moisture exchangers (HMEs) every 5–7 days or as clinically indicated (clogged with secretions) if in use.
   - Use of water bath humidification or a heated humidifier is acceptable.
   - Bacterial filters are only indicated for use in patients with infectious diseases such as TB.
5. Consider non-invasive ventilation, if possible.
6. Consider rotating beds, if available (kinetic bed therapy).
7. Semi-recumbent positioning (30–45° head up) is protective, especially during enteral feeding (prevents gastroesophageal reflux and aspiration).
8. Begin enteral feeding slowly, especially during the 48 hours after initiating mechanical ventilation, to minimize gastric reflux and potential aspiration risk.
9. The gastric route for feeding is recommended (post-pyloric route not superior).
10. Oral care.

Pharmacological Strategies

- Oropharyngeal decontamination with a topical antiseptic such as chlorhexidine has been proven to be beneficial.
- Oral decontamination with povidone-iodine oral antiseptic only in patients with severe head injuries.
- Limit stress ulcer prophylaxis to high-risk patients (avoid antacids and histamine type 2 antagonists, sucralfate and proton pump inhibitors (PPIs) preferable).
- Limit red blood cell transfusions in trauma and the critically ill.

- Targeted antibiotic administration strategies such as de-escalation and antibiotic rotation or 'cycling'.

Note: Selective decontamination of the digestive tract (SDD) with topical or systemic antibiotics or antiseptics has not been shown to provide benefit and may increase the incidence of MDR infections, and is therefore not recommended for general use.

Strategies that have not proved beneficial include:

- A systematic search for prevention of sinusitis (unless patient is intubated via the nasotracheal route)
- Prone positioning
- Prophylactic antibiotics (aerosolized, nasal or intravenous)
- Aerosolized antibiotics
- Intranasal mupirocin
- Topical antibiotics
- Postpyloric feeding.

Educational Strategies

- Staff education program.
- Prevention.

Diagnosis and Treatment of VAP: Recommendations

Diagnosis

- Noninvasive techniques, e.g. endotracheal aspirates with non-quantitative cultures, are recommended for the diagnosis of VAP in immunocompetent patients as the initial diagnostic strategy.

Treatment

Initial treatment

- Empiric antimicrobial therapy where there is a clinical suspicion of VAP.
- Choice of antibiotics based on patient factors and local resistance patterns.

Duration of treatment

- Maximum of 8 days' antibiotic therapy in patients who received adequate initial antibiotic therapy.
- Longer duration of antibiotic therapy for cases of VAP caused by a non-fermenting gram-negative bacillus such as *Pseudomonas or Acinetobacter,* e.g. 14–15 days.
- De-escalation of antibiotic therapy to culture-directed sensitive therapy.

How to Calculate VAP Rate and Ventilator Utilization Rate

- **VAP rate**

$$= \frac{\text{Number of ventilator-associated pneumonia}}{\text{Number of patients on ventilator-days}} \times 1000$$

- **Ventilator utilization rate**

$$\frac{\text{Number of ventilator days}}{\text{Number of patient days}} \times 100$$

REFERENCES

1. Guidelines for preventing healthcare-associated pneumonia, 2003. Recommendations of CDC and the healthcare infection control practices Advisory Committee. Taken from website:www.cdc.gov/hai/prevent/prevent-pubs.html. Accessed on 5/2/2014.
2. Thorsteinsson SB, Musher DM. Respiratory infections. In: Groschel D (Ed). Hospital-associated infections in the general hospital population and specific measures of control. Handbook on Hospital-associated Infection, 3rd edition. Marcel Dekker Inc, New York, US; 1979.p.73.
3. Chastre J, Fagon JY. Ventilator-associated pneumonia. Am J Respir Crit Care Med. 2002;165:867-903. Quoted by Joseph NM, Sistla S, Dutta TK, Badhe AS, Rasitha D, Parija SC. Ventilator-associated pneumonia in a tertiary care hospital in India: role of multidrug resistant pathogens. J Infect Dev Ctries. 2010;4(4):218-25.
4. Torres A, Aznar R, Gatell JM, et al. Incidence, risk and prognosis factors of nosocomial pneumonia in mechanically ventilated patients. Am Rev Respir Dis. 1990;142:523-8. Quoted by Reechaipichitkul W, Phondongnok

S, Bourpoem J, Chaimanee P. Causative agents and resistance among hospital-acquired and ventilator-associated pneumonia patients at Srinagarind Hospital, Northeastern Thailand. Southeast Asian J Trop Med Punlic Health. 2013;44:3. Accessed from net site: www.tm.mahidol.ac.th/seamea/2013-44-3-full/17-5333-12.pdf.

5. Safdar N, Dezfulian C, Collard HR, Saint S. Clinical and economic consequences of ventilator-associated pneumonia: a systematic review. Crit Care Med. 2009;33:2184-93.
6. American Thoracic Society (ATS) and the Infectious Disease Society of America (IDSA). Guidelines for the management of adults with hospital-acquired, ventilator-associated, and healthcare-associated pneumonia. Am J Respir Crit Care Med. 2005;171:388-416.
7. Niederman MS, Craven DE. Guidelines for the management of adults with hospital acquired, ventilator-associated and healthcare-associated pneumonia. Am J Respir Crit Care Med. 2005;171:388-416.
8. Johanson WG, Pierce AK, Sanford JP. Changing pharyngeal bacterial flora of hospitalized patients: emergence of gram-negative bacilli. N Eng J Med. 1969;281:1137-40.
9. Johanson WG, Pierce AK, Sanford JP, Thomas GD. Nosocomial respiratory infections with gram-negative bacilli: the significance of colonization of the respiratory tract. Ann Intern Med. 1972;77:701-6.
10. Guidelines for prevention of nosocomial pneumonia—center for disease control and prevention. MMWR Recomm Rep. 1997;46(RR-1):1-79.
11. Rakshit P, Nagar VS, Deshpande AK. Incidence, clinical outcome and risk stratification of ventilator-associated pneumonia—a prospective cohort study. Indian J Crit Care Med. 2005;9:211-6.
12. Joseph NM, Sistla S, Dutta TK, Badhe AS, Rasitha D, Parija SC. Ventilator-associated pneumonia in a tertiary care hospital in India: role of multidrug-resistant pathogens. J Infect Dev Ctries. 2010;4(4):218-25.
13. Singh S, Pandya Y, Patel R, Paliwal M, Wilson A, Trivedi S. Surveillance of device-associated infections at a teaching hospital in rural Gujrat-India. Indian J Med Microbiol. 2010;28:342-7. Available from http://www.ijmm.org/text.asp?2010/28/4/342/71830.
14. Reechaipichitkul W, Phondongnok S, Bourpoern J, Chaimanee P. Causative agents and resistance among hospital-acquired and ventilator-associated pneumonia patients at Srinagaring Hospital, Northeastern Thailand. Available at http/:www.tm.matialol.ac.th/seamea/2013-44-3-full/17-5333-12.pdf. Accessed on 14/2/2014.
15. Song JH, the Asian HAP working group. Treatment recommendations of hospital-acquired pneumonia in Asian countries: first consensus report by the Asian HAP working group. Am J Infect Control. 2008;36:S83-92.
16. Kollef MH, Vlasnik J, Sharpless L, Pasque C, Murphy D, Fraser V. Scheduled change of antibiotic classes: a strategy to decrease the incidence of ventilator-associated pneumonia. Am J Respir Crit Care Med. 1997;156:1040-8. (Cross reference in Ref No.1).
17. Gruson D, Hilbert G, Vargas F, et al. Rotation and restricted use of antibiotics in a medical intensive care unit. Impact on the incidence of ventilator-associated pneumonia caused by antibiotic-resistant gram-negative bacteria. Am J Respir Crit Care Med. 2000;162:837-43. (Cross reference in Ref No .1).
18. Guidelines for Preventing Healthcare-associated Pneumonia, 2003. Recommendations of CDC and Healthcare Infection Control Practices Advisory Committee. MMWR Recommendations and Reports. 2004;53(RR03):1-36.
19. Manual for Hospital Infection Control: Compiled by Hospital Infection Control Committee LTMGH and LTMMC. Courtesy Johnson and Johnson professional products.
20. Guidelines on Prevention and Control of Hospital-associated Infections. WHO; 2002.
21. Gillespie R. Prevention and management of ventilator-associated pneumonia—the care bundle approach, Department of Anaesthesia and Critical Care, Groote Schuur Hospital and University of Cape Town. SAJCC. 2009;25:2.
22. Klompas M. Does this patient have ventilator-associated pneumonia? JAMA. 2007;297(14):1583-93. Quoted in Ref No. 21.

Chapter 17

Burns and Open Traumatic Wounds

Chapter Outline

- Etiological Agents
- Transmission of Infection
- Outbreaks in Burn Units
- Other Infections in Burns Patients
- Open Wounds
- Culture and Surveillance
- Design of Units
- Prevention of Infection
- Category-specific Precautions
- Environmental Issues
- Special Problems of Sterilization and Immunization
- Methicillin-resistant *Staphylococcus aureus*
- Homografts as Vectors of Infection
- Silver-based Applications

INTRODUCTION

Burns are at first virtually free from bacteria, which have been killed by the heat. But soon the layer of dead tissue and exudates becomes heavily colonized by bacteria, unless effective measures are taken to exclude them. In small superficial burns and in many deeper and more extensive burns, the bacteria do not cause any apparent ill effects, although this depends on the types of bacteria present and on the patient's resistance.[1] In more extensive burns, bacterial infection is the most important cause of illness and death.

ETIOLOGICAL AGENTS

The most common isolate in burns is *Staphylococcus aureus,* followed by *Pseudomonas aeruginosa*. However, *Acinetobacter* species are now said to be isolated more frequently than *Pseudomonas aeruginosa.*[2] *Streptococcus pyogenes,* when present, will usually cause complete failure of skin grafts and delay healing. Today, it rarely causes invasive infection, although it may cause fever. Of the other bacteria, *Pseudomonas aeruginosa* has proved to be the most important cause of septicemia and toxemia. It can also cause failure of skin grafts, but to a smaller extent than *Streptococcus pyogenes*. Other gram-negative bacilli (*Proteus* species, *Klebsiella* species, *Serratia* species and *Acinetobacter* species), etc. are also isolated and they can occasionally cause septicemia in severely burned patients. Methicillin-resistant *Staphylococcus aureus* (MRSA) is a common cause of colonization of burns. These strains may be rare causes of clinical infection at some places, but at other places may be responsible for major infection problems. Nowadays, coagulase-negative staphylococi have also been implicated in these patients. Rarer pathogens include *Enterobacter cloacae* and *Aeromonas hydrophila*, and fungi like *Candida albicans*, *Aspergillus* species and, gas gangrene, tetanus bacilli and herpes virus.

The worldwide emergence of antimicrobial resistance among a wide variety of human bacterial and fungal burn wound pathogens, particularly nosocomial isolates, limits the available therapeutic options for effective treatment of burn wound infections. MRSA, methicillin-resistant coagulase-negative staphylococci, vancomycin-resistant enterococci, and multiply resistant gram-negative bacteria that possess several types of beta-lactamases, including extended spectrum beta-lactamases (ESBL), amp C beta-lactamases, and metallobeta-lactamases (MBL), have been emerging as serious pathogens in hospitalized patients.[3]

TRASMISSION OF INFECTION

In burn patients, the primary mode is direct or indirect contact, either via the hands of the personnel caring for the patient or from contact with inappropriately decontaminated equipment.[3] *Pseudomonas aeruginosa* and other bacteria are usually acquired from the burns of other patients in the ward, transmitted on the hands of nurses by various fomites and by air. Air is a less significant route, especially for gram-negative bacilli, but it may be important if large dressings are changed in open wound.

The two areas most likely to become contaminated when caring for the burn patient are the hands and apron area of the person, as the surfaces (e.g. beds, side rails, tables, equipment) are often heavily contaminated with organisms from the patient. Likewise all equipment used on the patient (e.g. blood pressure cuffs, thermometers, wheelchairs, IV pumps) are also heavily contaminated and may be transmitted to other patients if strict barriers are not maintained and appropriate decontamination carried out. In fact, a single cause is uncommon in a burn unit outbreak; in almost all instances, multiple factors contribute to its occurrence and perpetuation.[4]

OUTBREAKS IN BURN UNITS[4]

Outbreaks of cross colonization and infection are a major challenge in burn units. In almost all cases the colonized patient is thought to be a major reservoir for the epidemic strain. Other important sources include contaminated hydrotherapy equipment, common treatment areas, and contaminated equipment such as mattresses, which appear to pose unique risks of cross contamination in the burn environment.

Risks associated with care of the burn wound, such as hydrotherapy and common treatment rooms, are related to the use of water sources that are frequently contaminated by gram-negative organisms intrinsically, and may also be contaminated by organisms from other patients. This aquatic environment is difficult to decontaminate because of continuous reinoculation of organisms from the patients' wound flora and because of the organisms' ability to form a protective glycocalyx in water pipes, drains, and other areas, making them resistant to the actions of disinfectants. Adequate decontamination of this equipment (e.g. tanks, plinths, shower tables, straps) is difficult to achieve between patients using this equipment on a daily basis and monitoring techniques are insufficient to provide timely detection of contamination. In addition, the patient's own flora may be spread through the water and by caregivers to colonize other sites on the patient that are at increased risk of infection. For example, organisms from the wound may migrate to a central venous catheter site or bowel flora may be transferred to the burn wound.

OTHER INFECTIONS IN BURNS PATIENT

In addition to the burn, the urinary tract, respiratory tract and intravenous infusion sites are important portals of entry and sites of infection. Invasive devices, such as endotracheal tubes, intravascular catheters and urinary catheters, bypass the body's normal defense mechanisms. In general, pediatric patients have fewer problems with pneumonia than do adults because they are less likely to have pre-existing lung damage. Infection from intravascular catheters is of particular concern in burn patients, as often these lines must be placed directly through or near burn injured tissue. Catheter-associated bloodstream infection (BSI) is caused by organisms which migrate along the catheter from the insertion site and colonize the catheter tip. Catheter tips are also susceptible to colonization from hematogenous seeding of organisms from the colonized burn wound.[4]

OPEN WOUNDS

Open wounds resemble burns, but there is usually less necrotic tissue in which small number of bacteria can multiply. Contaminants acquired at the time of injury, including tetanus and gas gangrene, are more likely to play a role in the infection of open wounds than of burns, but hospital-acquired infection (both exogenous and endogenous) is potentially more important than contamination at time of injury.

CULTURING AND SURVEILLANCE

Culturing and surveillance guidelines are more stringent for the burn patient, particularly the patient with larger injuries, because of the increased propensity for transmission and infection in this population. Burn wound flora and antibiotic susceptibility patterns change during the course of the patient's hospitalization, so that the purposes of obtaining routine surveillance cultures are:

- To provide early identification of organisms colonizing the wound
- To monitor the effectiveness of current wound treatment
- To guide perioperative or empiric antibiotic therapy
- To detect any cross-colonizations which occur quickly so that further transmission can be prevented.

Routine surveillance wound cultures should be obtained when the patient is admitted and at least weekly until the wound is closed. Many burn centers recommend obtaining wound cultures two or three time a week for patients with large burn injuries. Admission cultures are particularly important for patients transferred from other facilities, as they may be colonized with multiply resistant organisms and serve as an unsuspected reservoir for cross-transmission to other patients in the unit. For pediatric patients, admission throat cultures are also recommended as about 5% of the population will be colonized with group A beta-hemolytic *Streptococcus* (*S. pyogenes*) which can have serious consequences if it is transmitted to the burn wound.[4]

Methods of burn wound culturing include obtaining a semi-quantitative swab culture or a quantitative biopsy specimen. Semi-quantitative swab cultures provide information on the type of organisms present on the burn wound, as well as the approximate amount and antimicrobial susceptibility. A general rule is to obtain a swab culture for each 10% of open burn to identify organisms of significance on the wound. Quantitative cultures are used to define invasive infection based on bacterial count of 100,000 colonies or more per gram of tissue. However, further study has revealed that this technique is not precise, as 50% of patients with quantitative counts of greater than 100,000 organisms do not have histologic evidence of invasive infection. Furthermore, quantitative culturing is more costly and labor-intensive than swab cultures, and their routine use to identify colonizing organisms on *appropriately* debrided wounds is rarely indicated. Accurate diagnosis of invasive burn wound infection is best determined by clinical criteria, supported when possible by histopathologic examination if the patient's condition is suspicious for this infection.[4]

Surveillance of infection has been shown to diminish the rate of nosocomial infection as well as reduce cost. Surveillance of infection in burn patients should be done to monitor incidence and rates which have been appropriately risk adjusted by size of burn injury and invasive device use. At a minimum, surveillance should include collection of data on burn wound infection, urinary tract infection, pneumonia, and bloodstream infection. Systematic collection of data allows the burn unit to monitor changes in infection rates over time, identify trends, and evaluate current treatment methods.[4]

DESIGN OF UNITS[5]

A burns unit should if possible be self-contained with its own operating theater and intensive care facilities. It should preferably be a part of a teaching or District General Hospital with ready access to other specialist activities (e.g. renal dialysis).

The number of rooms and beds depend on the work load. Single room should be available for isolation and at least two of them should be equipped to intensive care standards. Washbasins for washing hands should be adjacent to all beds in the unit. Filtered air should be provided to isolation rooms and the dressing room and extracted to the exterior. Several options for ventilating rooms are available.[5]

PREVENTION OF INFECTION

Mortality from sepsis and other causes has decreased in recent years, but infection is still a major problem.

Main Requirements for Reducing Infection and Mortality

These are as follows:

- Barrier techniques
- Isolation: The open burn wound increases the environmental contamination present around the patient, which is the major difference in burn versus non-burn patients. The degree or amount of contamination is roughly proportional to the size of the open wound and amount of colonization present and is inversely proportional to the distance from the patient.
- Standard precautions include appropriate handwashing, removal of garbage immediately upon leaving the room.
- Changing gloves that become contaminated with patient secretions or excretions before contact with another site, and addition of sterile gloves, caps and masks when caring for an open burn wound or other sterile procedures.
- Equipment and surfaces are considered contaminated following use and should be appropriately decontaminated before storage or use on other patients. Appropriate protective wear should also be worn when decontaminating this equipment.
- Adequate resuscitation.[6]
- Early excision and grafting of burn.[2]
- Use of topical antibacterial agents.
- Routine microbiological surveillance.
- Rapid and effective treatment of clinical infection.
- Good aseptic techniques.

The bacterial flora of all burns should be examined on admission and at all changes of dressing for *Streptococcus pyogenes, Pseudomonas aeruginosa* and often-common bacteria. If *Streptococcus pyogenes* is present the patient must be treated with penicillin, flucloxacillin, or erythromycin (if allergic to penicillin), and grafting operations must be postponed until the burn is free of this organism. Benzyl or phenoxymethyl penicillin is not suitable if *Staphylococcus aureus* is present, because they are likely to be inactivated by penicillinase from other bacteria colonizing the same burn. Prophylaxis against infection of burns can be divided into two lines of defense.[7]

First Line of Defense

The first line of defense (i.e. methods of protecting the patient against microbial contaminants) includes the following:

1. Primary excision (within 5 days, and preferably earlier) and skin grafting (only suitable for relatively small burns of full thickness) or on application of a dermal template (e.g. Integra).
2. Antisepsis (i.e. application of antibacterial substance to the burn).
3. Asepsis.[8]

Antisepsis

Local treatment with appropriate antimicrobial agents have been shown in controlled trials to protect burns against colonization of *Pseudomonas aeruginosa, Streptococcus pyogenes, Staphylococcus aureus* and other bacteria, and to reduce the septic consequences of infection, including skin graft failure and mortality. The qualities looked for in such prophylactic agents are effectiveness against all strains of significant burn pathogens, minimal local or systemic toxicity, and failure to select resistant variants in patients under treatment. There is no ideal preparation that fulfils all requirements. Silver sulfadiazine cream has been widely adopted as a standard prophylactic application, but a preponderant flora of sulfonamide resistant gram-negative bacilli has been found to emerge where silver sulfadiazine was in regular use for several years. However silver sulfadiazine may delay wound healing and therefore other topical applications like (Bacitracin and polysporin), chlorhexidine or mafenide could be used. Mafenide can however result in acidosis.[9] In patients with extensive burns, silver nitrate compresses (0.5%) have proved highly effective, especially against *Pseudomonas aeruginosa* and *Proteus* species, but patients who receive this treatment need supplements of electrolytes by mouth and laboratory control of serum electrolytes to avoid imbalance. This method is not suitable for infants. A further disadvantage is the black staining of all items that come into contact with the silver solution (including the walls). Silver sulfadiazine when acceptable is more suitable for smaller burns and for children, and although less active against *Pseudomonas aeruginosa* and *Proteus* species, it is more active against some gram-negative bacilli. Chlorhexidine 0.2% or cerium nitrate may be added to silver sulfadiazine or silver nitrate cream. For minor burns (especially these treated in outpatient units, a tulle gras containing 0.5% chlorhexidine (Bactigras) has been found to be appropriate. Burns treated by the exposure method have a physical protective barrier against infection once a dry eschar has formed. This can be anticipated and supplemented by topical chemoprophylaxis with povidone-iodine (7.5% with 0.75% available iodine), or with aqueous silver nitrate (0.5%) dabbed on three or four times a day for 6–8 days. Mafenide acetate (11%) cream can be used as an alternative, but it is painful on burns in which the nerve endings are not destroyed, and may cause acidosis, and patients require daily baths to remove the dried cream.

Antibiotics should preferably not be used for topical prophylaxis because of risk of emergence of resistant organisms and of toxic or allergic effects in the patients.[10]

Monitoring of the sensitivity of burns flora is an important routine procedure in a burns unit. This is performed at every dressing change. Also, if antibacterial treatment is necessary, awareness should be heightened for the possibility of superinfection with resistant organisms, yeasts, or fungi.

Systemic antimicrobials are indicated to treat documented infections, such as pneumonia, bacteremia, wound infection, and urinary tract infection (UTI). Empiric antimicrobial therapy to treat fever should be strongly discouraged because burn patients often have fever secondary to the systemic inflammatory response to burn injury.

Prophylactic antimicrobial therapy is recommended only for coverage of the immediate perioperative period surrounding excision or grafting of the burn wound when it is used to cover the documented increase in risk of transient bacteremia. Treatment should be started immediately prior to the procedure and generally discontinued within 24 hours, assuming restoration of normal cardiovascular hemodynamics. Prophylactic penicillin therapy in the early post-burn period may be recommended if there is a delay in quick identification and treatment of pediatric patients colonized with group A beta-hemolytic streptococci.[4]

Sites of Infection and Prevention Techniques[3]

Specific sites of infection that are particularly important for burn patients include bloodstream infection, pneumonia, burn wound infection and urinary tract infection. Fever, a highly specific indicator of infection for many patient populations, often does not correlate well with the presence of infection in patients with burn injuries, particularly large injuries. In burn injuries, the skin and core temperatures increase, and there is an increase in heat production, which is associated with the onset of a hypermetabolic response. The core temperature is commonly "reset" to a higher level [38° to 39°C (100.4° to 102.2°F)]. Because of this response, fever alone, without other signs and symptoms, is not indicative of infection.[3]

Asepsis

Dressing of burns in a ventilated dressing room, barrier nursing, source and protective isolation of patients and good ward hygiene contribute to the control of infection. The dressing may be carried out in a single isolation room provided that the ventilation system and facilities are adequate. For patients with burns in hospital, a dressing technique with two nurses should be used if possible in a room with combined source and protective isolation (e.g. plenum ventilation with an exhaust ventilated airlock). Exposure treatment, which is clinically desirable for many burns of the trunk and the face, provides some protection by the development of a dry eschar on which bacteria cannot grow (but which may cover a zone of heavy growth and suppuration). Exposure treatment is better than moist application with no antibacterial activity.

Second Line of Defense

This consists of preventing invasion of the tissues and bloodstream by bacteria growing on the burns. This includes antibiotic therapy, active and passive immunization and general supportive measures (treatment of diabetes, anemia, etc.). Systemic treatment of all *Streptococcus pyogenes* infections with an appropriate antibiotic protects all patients in the ward by eliminating reservoirs of infection during a major outbreak. In rare circumstances, all patients in the ward whether infected or not, may be treated prophylactically. Severely burned patients who have acquired heavy growths of *Pseudomonas aeruginosa* may be given protection with a systemic antipseudomonal agent (e.g. ceftazidine or a quinolone). A more promising procedure would be the use of a polyvalent *Pseudomonas* vaccine which has been found to give early protection and reduced mortality in patients with severe burns. Hyperimmunoglobulin prepared from immunized human volunteers has also provided valuable protection, but commercial preparations are not available. Prophylaxis against tetanus by use of a "boosting" dose of toxoid when the patient is known to be actively immune, or by means of antiserum (human antitetanus globulin), if there is no evidence of active immunity, should be given to all patients with burns who are admitted to the hospital.

CATEGORY-SPECIFIC PRECAUTIONS[4]

Two groups of burn patients are unique and require additional precautions, patients with larger burn injuries [>25–30% of total burn surface area (TBSA)] and those colonized with multiply resistant organisms

- Patients with greater than 30% TBSA burn injuries are more immunocompromised, due to the larger size of their injury. This, in combination with their loss of physical defenses and need for invasive devices, significantly increases their risk of infection. These patients also represent a significant risk for contamination of their surrounding environment with organisms, which may then be spread to other patients on the unit. These may include multiply resistant organisms, if broad spectrum antibiotic treatment has been required to treat infectious complications. For these reasons, it is recommended that patients with larger burn injuries be isolated in private rooms or other enclosed bed spaces to ensure physical separation from other patients on the unit. Such isolation has been associated with a decrease in cross transmission of organisms. Laminar airflow units, in place of private rooms, can be used for infection control purposes, either method can provide effective isolation if their use is strictly adhered to.
- Special attention is also required for patients with smaller burn injuries who are colonized or infected with multiply resistant organisms (e.g. MRSA, VRE, multiply resistant gram-negative organisms). This is especially true for patients with wound drainage that cannot be adequately contained in dry, occlusively wrapped outer dressings or pediatric patients who cannot comply with hand washing or other precautions. Patients transferred to the burn unit after treatment in another hospital should also be included in this group until the results of their admission cultures are known. These patients are frequently colonized with resistant organisms and may serve as an unsuspected reservoir for transmission to other patients unless they are isolated. Isolation for this group of patients generally includes placement in a private room on contact precautions, with the addition of droplet precautions in some circumstances.
- Patients colonized with multiply resistant organisms must frequently have their need for isolation balanced against their need for rehabilitation. In general, if the patient's wound cannot be occlusively wrapped in a dry outer dressing, the patient should not be taken to the rehabilitation department for therapy when other patients will be present in the same area. If rehabilitation needs cannot be met in the patient's room, then sufficient time should be scheduled in the rehabilitation department to allow for the patient's treatment followed by thorough cleaning of all equipment and surfaces afterwards before the area is used by other patients. The rehabilitation therapy staff should wear appropriate attire during therapy.

ENVIRONMENTAL ISSUES[4]

- Disinfection and sterilization guidelines for patient care equipment must take into account the presence of sometimes extensive, open wounds which is the major difference separating this population from other patient populations. Many items such as blood pressure cuffs, stethoscopes, bedpans, if used on areas without dry, occlusive dressings, may need high-level disinfection as a semicritical item or may need to be restricted to an individual patient.

- Plants and flowers should not be allowed in units with burn patients because they harbor gram-negative organisms, such as *Pseudomonas* species, other enteric gram-negative organisms, and fungi. Many of these organisms are intrinsically resistant to multiple antibiotics, which may serve as reservoirs to colonize the burn wound.
- Pediatric burn patients should also have policies restricting the presence of non-washable toys such as stuffed animals and cloth objects. These can harbor large numbers of bacteria and are difficult to disinfect. Toys should be nonporous and washable, designated for individual patient use, and thoroughly disinfected after use and before being given to another child to use. Paper items, such as storybooks and coloring books, should always be designated for single patient use and should be disposed of if they become grossly contaminated or when the child is discharged.
- Routine environmental surveillance culturing is not generally recommended on units with burn patients. The exception may be the hydrotherapy room and common treatment room used in burn wound care. Environmental culturing is important as part of any outbreak investigation which is done on the burn unit.

SPECIAL PROBLEMS OF STERILIZATION AND IMMUNIZATION

The outside of electric equipment, cardiac monitoring equipment, portable lights, diathermy, X-ray machines, suction apparatus and respiratory ventilators may be cleaned after use because of heavy contamination (e.g. with 70% alcohol).

The disinfection of respiratory ventilators and anesthetic apparatus is discussed in chapter on ICU. Water circulating mattresses may be disinfected with a chlorine-releasing agent, and the body temperature recorders may be disinfected with 70% alcohol. Mattress covers may be damaged by repeated application of phenolic disinfectants or by silver nitrate treatment of patients. Gram-negative bacilli are likely to grow in the mattresses. Mattresses therefore should be inspected regularly for damage.

Beds that provide air support systems are sometimes used for the management of extensive injuries, including burns, or in the care of the patients who are at special risk of ulcer formation. One type of bed (the fluidized-bead-bed has a trough filled with silica beads and covered with a special sheet, through which air is pumped. Another type (the low air loss bed) is constructed from a series of inflatable cushions, air being continuously pumped through these, with pneumatic controls to vary the elevation.

The risk of dispersing bacteria into the environment from these beds, even when heavily infected patients occupy them, has been shown to be no greater than of a standard hospital bed. If these beds are colonized with *Enterococci* it has been suggested that the heat tolerance of this organisms allows it to survive decontamination procedures. This has been identified as a risk factor for transmission of vancomycin-resistant enterococci. Otherwise normal cleaning procedures (e.g. with cloth moistened with a detergent solution) are generally adequate.[11,12] If the external surfaces are contaminated, they should be cleansed with a chlorine-releasing agent, rinsed and allowed to dry. The air sacs of low air-loss bed should be machine washed at a temperature of 60°C (but this may be inadequate for *enterococci*). The advice of the manufacturer should be sought when internal ducting has become contaminated, and also with regard to appropriate agents for disinfection.

Baths are a potential source of gram-negative infection, particularly *Pseudomonas aeruginosa*. Adequate cleaning and disinfection of baths should be carried out.

METHICILLIN-RESISTANT *STAPHYLOCOCCUS AUREUS*

Attempts at eradication of epidemic MRSA from a burns unit usually fail, and are rarely cost effective. However, the introduction of full control measures may be necessary if clinical infections are causing a problem.

Large burns should be protected from colonization whenever possible and particular care is required in the management of intravenous lines. Staff should preferably not work in other wards, and routine screening of staff should only be carried out if an eradication program is indicated.

Screening and isolation of patients from other countries or hospitals with a known MRSA problem should be carried out if possible, but MRSA carriers should not be refused admission to a specialized burns unit if admission is clinically indicated.

HOMOGRAFTS AS VECTORS OF INFECTION

Homografts are potentially sources of infection with pathogenic bacteria. HIV can be transmitted in this way from a donor who is a carrier and it is probable that other viruses (e.g. HBV, HCV and cytomegalovirus) can be also be transmitted on skin homografts.

Homografts are now mainly processed in skin banks in UK Cadaver donors are screened for infections and grafts are stored as non-viable glycerolized skin or cryopreserved viable skin.

SILVER-BASED APPLICATIONS[13]

Usually, silver-based applications are used for application on burns' patients. Silver-based applications are either liquid (silver nitrate) or incorporated in a cream (silver sulfadiazine) or mafenide acetate is used. Presently silver coated dressings (ACTICOAT antimicrobial barrier dressing) has been introduced. Though mafenide acetate showed largest zones of inhibition in conducted studies, it had highest MIC and MBC, and a significant number of bacteria survived after 6 hours. Zones of inhibition were similar with silver sulfadiazine, silver nitrate and silver-coated dressing, but viable bacteria were undetectable 30 minutes after inoculation with the dressing in case of the silver-coated dressing, whereas bacteria remained viable for upto 2 hours with silver nitrate and silver sulfadiazine. Also silver-coated dressing (ACTICOAT) showed the lowest MIC and MBC.

ACTICOAT is non-crystalline silver-based dressing and is active against *P. aeruginosa* as well as have a broad-spectrum antifungal activity.[14]

REFERENCES

1. Ayliffee and Lawrence. Burns and open traumatic wounds. In: Ayliffe GAJ, Fraise AP, Geddes AM, Mitchell K (Eds). Control of Hospital Infection—A Practical Handbook. 4th edition. Oxford University Press, Inc. New York; 2000.p.301.
2. Papini RPG, Wilson APR, Steer JA, et al. Wound management in burns centre in UK. Br J Surg. 1995;82:505.
3. Sharma M, Taneja N. Burns, antimicrobial resistance and infection control (Commentary). Indian J Med Res. 2007;126:505-7. Accessed from www.medind.nic.in/iby/107/i12/ibyt07i12p505.pdf.on 6th August 2015.
4. Weber J. Infection control in burns patients. International Society for Burn Injuries. Accessed from www.worldburn.org/documents/infection.control.pdf.on 6th August 2015.
5. Working party of the British Burn Association and Hospital Infection Research Society. Principles of design of burns unit, report of a working party of the British Burn Association

and Hospital Infection Research Society. J Hosp Infec. 1991;19:63.
6. Nguyen TT, Gilpin DA, Meyer NA, et al. Current treatment of severely burned patients. Annals of Surgery. 1996;223:14.
7. Lowbury EJL. Special problems in hospital antisepsis. In: Russel AD, Huge WB, Ayliffe GAJ (Eds). Principles and practice of disinfection, preservation and sterilization. 2nd edition. Oxford: Blackwell Scientific Publications; 1992.p.310 (Quoted by Ref. No. 1).
8. Newson SWB. Special problems in hospital antisepsis. In: Russel AD, Huge WB, Ayliffe GAJ (Eds). Principles and practice of disinfection, preservation and sterilization. 3nd edition. Oxford: Blackwell Science Publications; 1998.p.416 (Quoted by Ref. No. 1).
9. Long B. Minor burn management and controversies of silver sulfadiazine. Available at www.emdocs.net/minor-burn-management-and controversies -of –silver-s. Accessed on 2nd July 2015.
10. Lowbury EJL. Prophylaxis and treatment for infection of burns. Br J Hosp Med. 1976;16:566.
11. Gould FH, Freeman R. Nosocomial infection with microsphere beads. Lancet. 1993;342:241.
12. Bradley CR, Fraise AP. Heat and chemical resistance of enterococci. J Hosp Infec. 1996;34:191.
13. Yin HQ, Langford R, Burrel RE. Comparative evaluation of the antimicrobial activity of Acticoat. Antimicrobial Barrier Dressing: in beneficial effects of silver on burn infection. Available at http://www.burnsurgery.org/betaweb/modules/silver/section5_b.htm.
14. Wright JB, Lam K. From Net www.burnsurgery.org/Betaweb/modules/silver/section 5b).

Chapter 18

Human Immunodeficiency Virus

Chapter Outline

- Transmission and Prevalence
- Diagnosis
- HIV-2 Infections
- Prevention of Spread of Blood-borne Viral Infections in Hospitals
- Contaminated Sharps
- Determination of PEP Recommendation
- Drug Regimen
- Testing and Counseling
- Duration of PEP
- Pregnancy and PEP
- Side Effects of these Drugs
- Steps to be Taken by Infection Control Officer on Receiving Information About Exposure
- Primary Side Effects Associated with Antiretroviral Agents
- Occupational Transmission of HIV
- Monitoring and Management of PEP Toxicity
- Counseling and Education

INTRODUCTION

This virus as is already known infects the CD4+ *T. lymphocytes* and leads to immunodeficiency primarily due to deficiency of the T cells. The initial or primary infection is associated with a glandular fever type seroconversion illness, which includes flu like symptoms, widespread rash, diarrhea as well as generalized lymphadenopathy. This is followed by a long and variable asymptomatic period, during which the total CD4 count declines. During this period quantitative plasma human immunodeficiency virus (HIV) RNA assays demonstrate a very large viral burden, representing a rapid turnover of infected cells. This 'steady state' viral load established during primary infection is predictive of the rapidity of the progression of HIV disease. The data generated by these new assays also shows that the HIV infected patients are infectious to others throughout their infection.

Although, it is said that HIV inevitably leads to acquired immune deficiency syndrome (AIDS), the natural history of the infection is changing due to effective prophylactic therapies that reduce the risk of opportunistic infections such as pneumocystis and tuberculosis and the use of range of antiretroviral drugs. These reverse transcriptase and protease inhibitors lead to dramatic reductions of circulating viral load when used in combination. This correlates with long-term clinical benefit. Therefore, the HIV-infected individuals are now living longer with an improved quality of life.[1]

TRANSMISSION AND PREVALENCE

The major routes of transmission of HIV infection include, sexual intercourse, vertical spread and blood-borne spread. Widespread screening of donors has reduced the rate of transfusion-acquired infection. The prevalence of HIV infection is variable not only between countries but also within one country. The prevalence in blood donors in some central African countries have been reported to be upto 10%, and similar figures have been cited for prostitutes in Bombay. In UK homosexual men form the largest HIV positive group, although now the incidence of heterosexually-acquired infection is growing rapidly. In India, HIV infection is more common in the heterosexual group.

A number of studies on occupational exposure show that the risk to (HCW) from percutaneous route from HIV-infected patients are approximately 0.32%[2] and after a mucous membrane exposure, approximately 0.09%. Factors, which predicted the transmission of infection, were: deep injuries, visible blood on the device before injury, devices that were used on an artery or vein before injury and exposure to a person with AIDS.[3] If we also consider that the risk of viral transmission from mother to infant is increased with a higher maternal load, it becomes evident that transmission is a function of the inoculum of the virus as well as the route of entry.

DIAGNOSIS[1]

Generally, the presence of HIV specific antibodies indicates infection. It may take 3-6 months for these antibodies to become detectable. This is called as 'window period'. During this window period, this infection can be detected by detection of HIV antigen and RNA in the blood. As stated previously HIV RNA quantitation is routinely used to monitor infected individuals and this determines when the antiretroviral drugs would be initiated, and when drug therapy is failing.

Tests Used

Food and Drug Administration (FDA) approved rapid tests can produce HIV test results within 30 minutes, with sensitivities and specificities similar to those of first and second generation enzyme immunoassays (EIAs). Third-generation chemiluminescent immunoassays, run on automated platforms and can detect HIV specific antibodies two weeks sooner than conventional EIAs and generate test results in an hour or less. Fourth-generation combination P24 antigen-antibody (Ag/Ab) tests produce both rapid and accurate results and their P24 antigen detection allows identification of most infections during the window period. All above tests are acceptable for determination of source patient HIV status.[4]

HIV-2 INFECTIONS

HIV-2 was originally prevalent in West Africa and now is reported from number of cases in India, a few cases have been diagnosed in UK. HIV-2 infection also progresses to AIDS, but the speed of progress is slower. Rate of infection control implications of HIV-2 are similar to those for HIV-1, although the viruses show rare differences in antiretroviral drug susceptibilities, which will have a bearing on post-exposure prophylaxis regimens.

PREVENTION OF SPREAD OF BLOOD-BORNE VIRAL INFECTIONS IN HOSPITALS[1]

There are two views:

1. Whether to view all patients as potential sources of infection.
2. Whether to use a two-tier level of protection based on the knowledge of which patients are infected with these agents.

In the former approach, known as 'universal precautions' we take it for granted that risk is associated with a particular procedure (e.g. venepuncture, lumbar puncture, laboratory testing, etc.). In the two-tier approach, the risk is associated with a particular patient.

The approach of universal precautions involves the routine use of gloves, double-gloving for invasive operations and if need be wearing of masks, gown and eye protection. The major problem is the availability of all these, even then arguments are strongly in favor of this approach because (1) all patients infected with HBV, HCV or HIV may not be aware of their infection (as these patients are asymptomatic for long periods), so the two tier system of approach of infection control means that such individuals will be treated as safe; (2) Newly acquired blood-borne infections, which have yet to be identified, may spread to HCW, and this can be reduced by implementation of universal precautions.

CONTAMINATED SHARPS

Steps to be Taken Immediately Following an Exposure

- Needle-sticks and cuts should be washed with soap and water.
- Splashes to the nose, mouth or skin should be flushed with water.
- Eyes should be irrigated with clean water, saline or sterile irrigants.
- Pricked finger should not be put into mouth reflexly.

Note: Although no scientific evidence exists to the fact that the use of antiseptics for wound care or squeezing the wound will reduce the risk of transmission of HIV, however, this practice is always recommended. The use of a caustic agent such as bleach is not recommended.

Reporting of the Exposure

Report the exposure to the appropriate authority and condition must be treated as an emergency, prompt reporting is essential because in some cases, HIV postexposure prophylaxis (PEP) may be recommended and it should be started as soon as possible, preferably within a few hours. Initiating treatment after 72 hours of exposure is not recommended.

Postexposure Prophylaxis

The decision to start PEP is made on the basis of degree of exposure to HIV and the HIV status of the source from whom the exposure/infection has occurred. Although concerns have been expressed about HIV-negative sources that might be in the "window period" it is unnecessary for determining whether HIV PEP is indicated unless acute retroviral syndrome is clinically suspected. Rapid HIV testing of source patients facilitates timely decision making regarding the need for administration of HIV PEP after occupational exposures to sources whose HIV status is unknown.[5]

- Exposure code can be defined as per the Figure 18.1. It may be classified into three categories, EC1, EC2 and EC3, depending upon the nature of exposure.

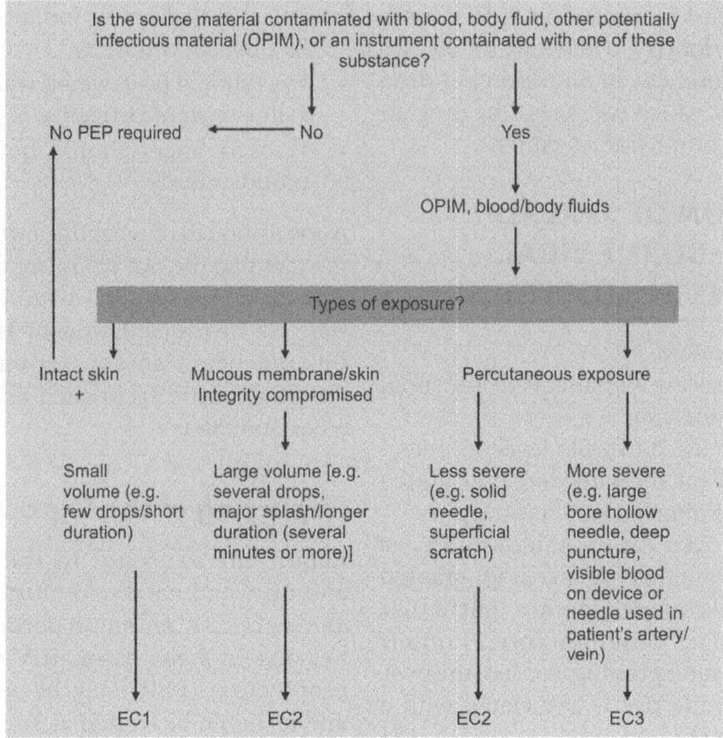

Fig. 18.1: Exposure code (EC)[6]

Determination of HIV Status Code (HIV SC)

The main purpose of determining HIV status code is to know the HIV status of source of exposure. It may be classified into three categories—HIV SC1, HIV SC2 and HIVSC unknown (Fig. 18.2).

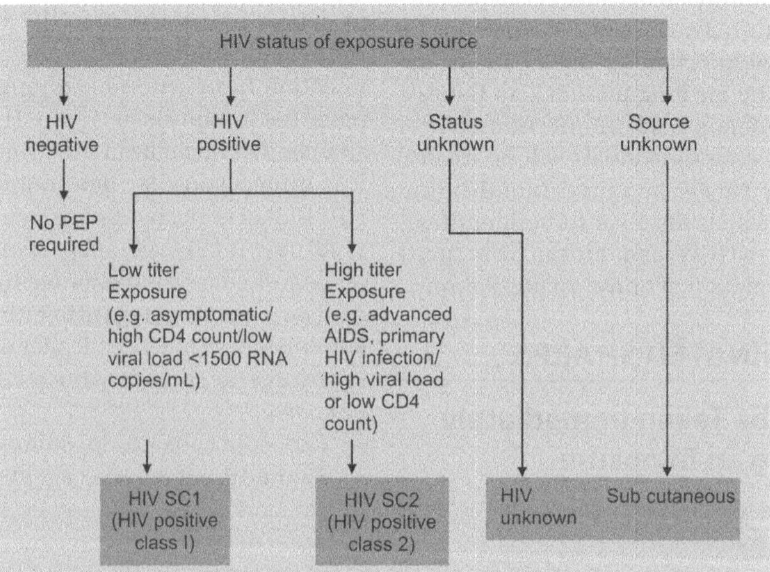

Fig. 18.2: HIV status code[6,7]

- Status unknown (e.g. deceased person with no samples available for HIV testing).
- Unknown source (e.g. a needle from a sharps disposal container).
- 'Consider' PEP indicates that PEP is optional and should be based on an individualized decision between the exposed person and the treating clinician.

DETERMINATION OF PEP RECOMMENDATION[6,7]

EC	HIV SC	PEP recommendation
1	1	(PEP may not be warranted) "Consider" basic 2 drug PEP
1	2	Consider basic regimen (Negligible risk)
2	1	Recommend basic regimen (Most exposures are in this category)
2	2	Recommend expanded regimen
3	1 or 2	Recommend expanded regimen
2/3	Unknown	If setting suggests a possible risk (epidemiological risk factors) and EC is 2 or 3, consider basic regimen
1/2	Unknown (status or source)	Generally no PEP warranted; however, consider basic 2 drug PEP for source with HIV risk factors. Generally, no PEP warranted, however, consider 2 drug PEP in settings where exposure to HIV-infected persons is likely

If source is HIV-negative, whatever be the EC—no PEP warranted.

If PEP is offered and taken and the source is later determined to be HIV-negative, PEP should be discontinued.

DRUG REGIMEN[6]

Basic regimen: Zidovudine (AZT)—600 mg in divided doses (300 mg/twice a day or 200 mg/thrice a day for 4 weeks)

\+

Lamivudine (3 TC)—150 mg twice a day for 4 weeks

Expanded regimen: Basic regimen (4 weeks therapy) +

Indinavir—800 mg/thrice a day.

Or any other protease inhibitor

TESTING AND COUNSELING[6,7]

The healthcare provider should be tested for HIV as per the following schedule:

i. Baseline HIV test—at time of exposure.
ii. Repeat HIV test—at six weeks following exposure.
iii. 2nd repeat HIV test—at twelve weeks following exposure.
iv. 3rd repeat HIV test—at 6 months following exposure.
v. 4th repeat test—12 months (if coinfected with HCV).

On all occasions, HCW must be provided with a pretest and post-test counseling. HIV testing should be carried out on three ERS (Elisa/Rapid/Simple) test kits or antigen preparations. The HCW should be advised to refrain from donating blood, semen or organs/tissues and abstain from sexual intercourse, in case sexual intercourse is undertaken a latex condom be used consistently. In addition, women HCW should not breastfeed their infants during the follow-up period.

DURATION OF PEP[6]

PEP should be started, as early as possible, after an exposure. It has been seen that PEP started after 72 hours of exposure is of no use and hence is not recommended. The optimal course of PEP is not known, but 4 weeks of drug therapy appears to provide protection against HIV.

If the HIV test is found to be positive at anytime within 12 weeks, the HCW should be referred to a physician for treatment.

PREGNANCIES AND PEP[6,7]

Based on limited information, antiretroviral therapy taken during 2nd and 3rd trimester of pregnancy has not caused serious side effects in mothers or infants. There is very little information on the safety in the 1st trimester. If the HCW is pregnant at the time of exposure to HIV, the designated authority/physician must be consulted about the use of the drugs for PEP.

Recent data suggested that limited data is available on the potential effects of antiretroviral drugs on the developing fetus or neonate. But in vitro studies have shown many of these drugs to be carcinogenic or mutagenic. Various drugs are toxic; effects like progressive neurologic disease have also been reported but most of these were seen in HIV infected women taking the drugs for more than 4 weeks.

Therefore, if the HCW is pregnant at the time of exposure to HIV, the designated authority/physician must be consulted about the use of drugs.

Certain drugs should be avoided in pregnant women. Because teratogenic effects were observed in primary studies, EFV (Efavirenz) is not recommended during pregnancy. Reports of fatal lactic acidosis in pregnant women treated with a combination of d4t (Stavudine) and ddl (Didanosine) have prompted warnings about these drugs during pregnancy. Because of the risk of hyperbilirubinemia in newborns, IDV (Idinavir) should not be administered to pregnant women shortly before delivery.

Administration of antiretroviral triple drug regimens to breastfeeding HIV-infected women has been shown to reduce the risk of transmission to their infants and infant toxicity has been minimal. Prolonged maternal antiretroviral drug use during breastfeeding has been associated with increase risk of infant hematologic toxicity, but limited exposure during 4 weeks of PEP may also limit the risk of drug toxicity to the breastfeeding infant. To completely eliminate any risk of HIV transmission to her infant, the healthcare provider may want to stop breastfeeding. Ultimately, the lactating women with occupational exposure to HIV who will take antiretroviral medications as PEP must be counseled to weigh the risks and benefits of continued breastfeeding both while taking PEP, and while being monitored for seroconversion.[4]

SIDE-EFFECTS OF THESE DRUGS[6,7]

Most of the drugs used for PEP have usually been tolerated well except for nausea, vomiting, tiredness, or headache. Side effects are more common when a 3-drug combination is used.

STEPS TO BE UNDERTAKEN BY THE INFECTION CONTROL OFFICER ON RECEIVING INFORMATION ABOUT EXPOSURE[6]

- All needle-stick/sharp injuries should be reported to the State AIDS Control societies giving the Exposure Code and the HIV Status code.
- The State AIDS Societies should in-turn inform National AIDS Control Organization (NACO) about the cases periodically.
- A register should be maintained in all hospitals and at the level of the State AIDS Control societies.
- NACO has decided to supply PEP drugs to all cases in government hospitals through the State AIDS Control societies.
- Infection control officers in all hospitals have been directed to ensure that PEP drugs are available at all times.

PRIMARY SIDE EFFECTS ASSOCIATED WITH ANTIRETROVIRAL AGENTS (TABLE 18.1)[7]

Table 18.1: Primary side effects associated with antiretroviral agents

Antiretroviral class/agent	Primary side effects and toxicities
Nucleoside reverse transcriptase inhibitors (NRTIs)	
Zidovudine (Retrovir™; ZDV; AZT)	Anemia, neutropenia, nausea, headache, insomnia, muscle pain and weakness
Lamivudine (Epivir™; 3TC)	Abdominal pain, nausea, diarrhea, rash and pancreatitis
Stavudine (Zerit™; d4T)	Peripheral neuropathy, headache, diarrhea, nausea, insomnia, anorexia, pancreatitis, increased liver function tests (LFTs), anemia and neutropenia
Didanosine (Videx™; ddl)	Pancreatitis, lactic acidosis, neuropathy, diarrhea, abdominal pain and nausea
Abacavir (Ziagen™; ABC)	Nausea, diarrhea, anorexia, abdominal pain, fatigue, headache, insomnia and hypersensitivity reactions
Nonnucleoside reverse transcriptase inhibitors (NNRTIs)	
Nevirapine (Viramune™; NVP)	Rash (including cases of Stevens-Johnson syndrome), fever, nausea, headache, hepatitis, and increased LFTs
Delavirdine (Rescriptor™; DLV)	Rash (including cases of Stevens-Johnson syndrome), nausea, diarrhea, headache, fatigue, and increased LFTs
Efavirenz (Sustiva™; EFV)	Rash (including cases of Stevens-Johnson syndrome), insomnia, somnolence, dizziness, trouble concentrating and abnormal dreaming
Protease inhibitors (PIs)	
Indinavir (Crixivan™; IDV)	Nausea, abdominal pain, nephrolithiasis and indirect hyperbilirubinemia
Nelfinavir (Viracept™; NFV)	Diarrhea, nausea, abdominal pain, weakness, and rash
Ritonavir (Norvir™; RTV)	Weakness, diarrhea, nausea, circumoral paresthesia, taste alteration and increased cholesterol and triglycerides
Saquinavir (Fortovase™; SQV)	Diarrhea, abdominal pain, nausea, hyperglycemia, and increased LFTs
Amprenavir (Agenerase™; AMP)	Nausea, diarrhea, rash, circumoral paresthesia, taste alteration and depression
Lopinavir/Ritonavir (Kaletra™)	Diarrhea, fatigue, headache, nausea and increased cholesterol and triglycerides

OCCUPATIONAL TRANSMISSION OF HIV[7]

Risks of Occupational Transmission

The average risk of HIV transmission after percutaneous exposure has been estimated to be 0.3% and after mucous membrane exposure, it is approximately 0.09%.[6] The risk of transmission after non-intact skin exposure has been documented but not been quantified. So also the risk of transmission after exposure to fluid or tissues other than HIV-infected blood has not been quantified but is much lower than for blood exposures.

MONITORING AND MANAGEMENT OF PEP TOXICITY[7]

If PEP is used, HCW should be monitored for drug toxicity by testing at baseline and again 2 weeks after starting PEP.

Minimal laboratory monitoring for toxicity should include:

1. Complete blood count
2. Renal and hepatic function tests.
3. Blood sugar levels for hyperglycemia if the drug regimen include protease inhibitors.
4. Monitoring for crystalluria, hematuria, hemolytic anemia and hepatitis if IDV (Idinavir is used).

Clinical Monitoring for Toxicity

Symptoms to be reported without delay are:

- Rash, fever, back or abdominal pain
- Pain on urination or blood in urine or symptoms of hyperglycemia (increased thirst and/or frequent urination).

Most of the times HCW may fail to complete the recommended regimen due to side effects like nausea and diarrhea. These symptoms can be managed by giving anti-motility and anti-emetic agents or other indications that target the specific symptoms.

If toxicity is noted modification of the regimen should be considered after expert consultation and further diagnostic studies may be indicated.

COUNSELING AND EDUCATION[7]

HIV-exposed HCW should be advised to use the following measures to prevent secondary transmission during the follow-up period especially the first 6–12 weeks after the exposure when most HIV-infected persons are expected to seroconvert.

1. Exercise sexual abstinence or use condoms to prevent sexual transmission.
2. To avoid pregnancy.
3. To refrain from donating blood, plasma, organ, tissue or semen.
4. If women are breastfeeding, she should be counseled about the risk of transmission through breast milk and discontinuation of breast milk should be considered especially for high-risk procedures. Also drugs like nucleoside reverse transcriptase (NRTTs) are known to pass into break milk whether this is true for other antiretroviral drugs are not known.
5. Any illness should be reported to the physician (especially if characterized by fever, myalgia; fatigue, malaise or lymphadenopathy.
6. They should be told that although short-term toxicity is limited, serious adverse reactions have occurred in persons taking PEP.
7. All drugs for PEP may be stopped by the exposed person (HCW) who experience HIV occupational exposures for which PEP is not recommended and he/she should be informed that the potential side effects and toxicity of taking PEP outweigh the negligible risk of transmission posed by the type of exposure.

Recent Update

"Updated US Public Health Service Guidelines for the Management of Occupational Exposure to HIV and Recommendations for Postexposure Prophylaxis "prepared by US Public Health Service Working Group.[4]

A summary of their recommendations is given below:

1. PEP is recommended when occupational exposure to HIV occurs.
2. Determine the HIV status of the exposure source patient to guide need for HIV PEP, if possible.
3. Start PEP medication regimens as soon as possible after occupational exposure to HIV and continue them for 4-week duration.
4. New Recommendations PEP medication regimens should contain 3 (or more) antiretroviral drugs (listed in Appendix) for all occupational exposures to HIV
5. Expert consultation is recommended for any occupational exposures to HIV and at a minimum for situations described in Box 18.1.
6. Provide close follow-up for exposed personnel (Box 18.2) that includes counseling, baseline and follow-up HIV testing and monitoring for drug toxicity. Follow-up appointments should begin within 24 hours of an HIV exposure.
7. New Recommendation: If a newer 4th generation combination HIV p24 antigen-antibody test is utilized for follow-up HIV testing of exposed HCP, HIV testing may be concluded at 4 months after exposure (Box 18.2). If a newer testing platform is not available, follow-up HIV testing is typically concluded at 6 months after an HIV exposure.

Box 18.1: Situations for which expert consultation for human immunodeficiency virus (HIV) postexposure prophylaxis (PEP) is recommended[4]

Delayed (that is later than 72 hours) exposure report
- Interval after which benefits from PEP are undefined

Unknown source (e.g. needle in sharps disposal container or laundry)
- Use of PEP to be decided on a case-by-case basis
- Consider severity of exposure and epidemiologic likelihood of HIV exposure
- Do not test needles or other sharp instruments for HIV

Known or suspected pregnancy in the exposed person
- Provision of PEP should not be delayed while awaiting expert consultation

Breastfeeding in the exposed person
- Provision of PEP should not be delayed while awaiting expert consultation

Known or suspected resistance of the source virus to antiretroviral agents
- If source person's virus is known or suspected to be resistant to one or more of the drugs considered for PEP, selection of drugs to which the source person's virus is unlikely to be resistant recommended
- Do not delay initiation of PEP while awaiting any results of resistance testing of the source person's virus

Toxicity of the initial PEP regimen
- Symptoms (e.g. GI symptoms and others) often manageable without changing PEP regimen by prescribing antimotility or antiemetic agents
- Counseling and support for management of side effects is very important as symptoms are often exacerbated by anxiety

Serious medical illness in the exposed person
- Significant underlying illness (e.g. renal disease) or an exposed provider already taking multiple medications may increase the risk of drug toxicity and drug-drug interactions

Box 18.2: Follow-up of healthcare personnel (HCP) exposed to known or suspected human virus (HIV)—positive sources[4]

Counseling (at the time of exposure and at follow-up appointments): Exposed HCP should be advised to use precautions (e.g. use of barrier contraception, avoid blood or tissue donations, pregnancy and if possible, breastfeeding) to prevent secondary transmission, especially during the first 6–12 weeks postexposure

For exposures for which PEP is prescribed, HCP should be informed regarding:
- Possible drug toxicities (e.g. rash and hypersensitivity reactions which could initiate acute HIV seroconversion and the need for monitoring
- Possible drug interactions, and
- The need for adherence to PEP regimens

Early evaluation after exposure: Regardless of whether a healthcare provider is taking PEP, reevaluation of exposed HCP within 72 hours after exposure is strongly recommended, as additional information about the exposure or source person may be available

Follow-up testing and appointments: Follow-up testing at a minimum should include:
- HIV testing at baseline, 6 weeks, 12 weeks, and 6 months postexposure, alternatively if the clinician is certain that a 4th generation combination HIV p24 antigen-HIV antibody test is being utilized, then HIV testing could be performed at baseline, 6 weeks and concluded at 4 months postexposure
- Complete blood counts. Renal and hepatic function tests (at baseline and 2 weeks postexposure; further testing may be indicated if abnormalities were detected)

HIV testing results should preferably be given to the exposed healthcare provider at face-to-face appointments

APPENDIX:

HIV Postexposure Prophylaxis Regimens[4]

<table>
<tr><td colspan="2">Preferred HIV PEP Regimen
Raltegravir (Isentress®, RAL) 400 mg PO twice daily
Plus
Truvada™, 1 PO once daily
[Tenofovir DF (Viread®; TDF) 300 mg + emtricitabine (Emtriva™ FTC) 200 mg]</td></tr>
<tr><td colspan="2">Alternative Antiretroviral Agents for Use as PEP Only with Expert Consultation
Abacavir (Ziagen® ;ABC)
Efavirenz (Sustiva®; EFV)
Enfuvirtide (Fuzeon™; T20)
Fosamprenavir (Lexiva®; FOSAPV)
Maraviroc (Selzentry®; MVC)
Saquinavir (Invirase®; SQV)
Stavudine (Zerit®; d4T</td></tr>
<tr><td colspan="2">Alternative Regimens
(May combine one drug or drug pair from the left column with one pair of nucleoside/nucleotide reverse transcriptase inhibitors from the right column. Prescribers unfamiliar with these agents/regimens should consult physicians familiar with the agents and their toxicities.)</td></tr>
<tr><td>Raltegravir (Isentress®, RAL)</td><td>Tenofovir DF (Viread®; TDF) + emtricitabine (Emtriva™ FTC)]; available as Truvada™</td></tr>
<tr><td>Darunavir (Prezista®; DRV + Ritonavir (Norvir®; RTV)</td><td>Tenofovir DF (Viread®; TDF) + lamivudine (Epivir®; 3TC)</td></tr>
<tr><td>Etravirine (Intelence®; ETR</td><td>Zidovudine (Retrovir™; ZDV; AZT) + lamivudine (Epivir®; 3TC); available as Combivir®</td></tr>
<tr><td>Rilipivirine (Endurant™; RPV)</td><td>Zidovudine (Retrovir™; ZDV; AZT) + emtricitabine (Emtriva™; FTC)</td></tr>
<tr><td>Atazanavir (Reyataz®; ATV) + Ritonavir (Norvir®; RTV)</td><td></td></tr>
<tr><td>Lopinavir/ritonavir (Kaletra®; LPV/RTV</td><td></td></tr>
<tr><td colspan="2">The following alternative is a complete fixed-dose combination regimen and no additional antiretrovirals are needed: Stribild™ (elvitegravir, cobicistat, tenofovir DF, emtricitabine)</td></tr>
<tr><td colspan="2">Antiretroviral Agents Generally Not Recommended for use as PEP
Didanosine (Videx EC®; ddl)
Nelfinavir (Viracept®; NFV)
Tipranavir Aptivus®; TPV)</td></tr>
<tr><td colspan="2">Antiretroviral Agents Contraindicated as PEP
Nevirapine (Viramune®; NVP)</td></tr>
</table>

REFERENCES

1. Pillay D. Control of viral hepatitis and human immunodeficiency virus (HIV) infection. In: Ayliffee GAJ, Fraise AP, Geddes AM, Mitchell K (Eds). Control of hospital infection. A Practical Handbook. 4th edition. Oxford University Press, New York; 2000.pp.211-4.
2. Centers for Disease Control. Case control study of HIV seroconversion in healthcare workers after percutaneous exposure to HIV infected blood—France, United Kingdom and United States, January 1988 to August 1994. Morbidity and Mortality Weekly Report. 1995;44:929.
3. Beckmann SE, Vlahore D, Koziol DE, et al. Temporal association between implementation of universal precautions and a sustained progressive decrease in percutaneous exposures to blood. Clin Infec Disc. 1994;18:562.
4. Kulhar DT, Henderson DK, Struble KA, et al. Updated US Public Health Service Guidelines for the Management of Occupational Exposures to HIV and Recommendations for Postexposure Prophylaxis. US PHS Guidelines for the Management of Occupational Exposures to HIV. Prepared by US Public Health Service Working Group. CDC National Center for Emerging and Zoonotic Infections. Division of Healthcare Quality Promotion. Accessed on 9th Nov 2013. Available at www.//stacks.cdc.gov/view/cdc/20711.
5. Updated US Public Health Service Guidelines for the Management of Occupational Exposures to HIV and Recommendations for Postexposure Prophylaxis. In MMWR Morbidity and Mortality Weekly Report. Recommendations and Reports. 2005;54:RR-9. US Dept of Health and Human Services CDC, Atlanta. GA 30333. From Net www.cdc.gov/mmwr//mmwr/pdf/rr/rr5409.pdf. Accessed on October 25th 2013.
6. Management of occupational exposure and post-exposure prophylaxis. In Manual for Control of Hospital-associated Infections. Standard Operative Procedures. National AIDS Control Organisation. Ministry of Health and Family Welfare. Govt of India; Pg. 67-73.
7. Updated US Public Health Service, Guidelines for the management of occupational exposures to HBV, HCV and HIV and Recommendations for Post-exposure Prophylaxis. In MMWR Morbidity and Mortality Weekly Report. Recommendations and Reports. 2001; 50:RR-11. US Dept of Health and Human Services CDC, Atlanta. GA 30333. From Net www.cdc.gov/mmwr/preview/mmwrhtml/rr5011a1.htm-101k. Accessed on 16th August 2013.

Chapter 19

Control of Hepatitis Virus Infections in Healthcare Settings

Chapter Outline

Control of Hepatitis A Virus Infection
- Diagnosis and Transmission of Hepatitis A Virus Infection
- Prophylaxis for HAV Infection
- Postexposure Prophylaxis

Control of Hepatitis B Virus Infection
- Hepatitis B Markers and their Implication
- Incidence of Hepatitis B
- Needlestick Injury from HbeAg Positive Blood and Transmission of Infection
- Treatment
- Prevention Strategies
- HBV Vaccination in Healthcare Workers
- Candidates for Hepatitis B Vaccination
- Side Effects (Adverse Reaction) of Vaccine

Control of Hepatitis C Virus Infection
- Diagnosis of Hepatitis C Virus Infection
- Treatment and Vaccine
- Risk of Occupational Transmission of HCV
- Management of Exposures to HCV

Control of Hepatitis D Virus Infection
- Diagnosis
- Treatment and Prevention

Control of Hepatitis E Virus Infection
- Diagnosis
- Vaccines

CONTROL OF HEPATITIS A VIRUS INFECTION

INTRODUCTION

Infection with hepatitis A virus (HAV) may be asymptomatic or symptomatic. The former is more common in children. The incubation period is 15-50 days. The illness may be short lived with symptoms including fever, malaise nausea, vomiting, and pain in abdomen in the preicteric stage followed by, dark urine and jaundice of acute onset. Very rarely HAV can lead to fulminant hepatitis. Virus is excreted in the stool with peak levels shed in 2 weeks preceding onset of the disease. The levels of virus decline after this time, although children can shed virus for longer periods of time.

DIAGNOSIS AND TRANSMISSION OF HEPATITIS A VIRUS INFECTION

Definitive diagnosis of HAV infection is made by the detection of HAV-specific IgM in serum. Long-lasting immunity is conferred by specific IgG. The virus is spread by the fecal-oral route, and is thus highly prevalent in areas of poor sanitation, where the water quality is low. Most individuals in such areas have acquired asymptomatic infection during childhood.

Usually, patients admitted to the hospital with acute HAV show minimal viral shedding, and therefore, there is little risk to the staff. Even then strict hygienic precautions are recommended, as spread is possible, especially in association with fecal incontinence. Although outbreaks of HAV are common in the community, they are usually rare in health care settings.[1]

PROPHYLAXIS FOR HAV INFECTION (TABLES 19.1 AND 19.2)

Protection against HAV is by passive immunization with intramuscular normal immunoglobulin or with hepatitis A vaccine. This is an inactivated vaccine and is highly immunogenic. The efficacy of both methods of protection is good when used as timely prophylaxis or postexposure prophylaxis in outbreaks.[2]

Candidates for Hepatitis A Vaccination[3]

Routine Vaccination

Children living in areas with high incidence rates of hepatitis A, check with your health department to see if this applies to your area.

High-risk Populations

- Travelers to developing countries with high rates of hepatitis A.
- Homosexuals.
- Users of illegal drugs.
- People who work with hepatitis A virus in research settings.
- People who work with infected nonhuman primates.
- Recipients of clotting factor concentrates.

People with chronic liver disease (because of risk of fulminant hepatitis.

Table 19.1: HAVRIX*

Age	No. of doses	Schedule	Dose
Children age 2 to 18 years	2	0 and 6–12 months	720 ELISA units (0.5 mL)
Adults 18 years and older	2	0 and 6–12 months	1440 ELISA units (1.0 mL)

*Inactivated vaccine. Manufactured by Smith Kline Beecham Biologicals.

Table 19.2: VAQTA**

Age	No. of doses	Schedule	Dose
Children age 2 to 17 years	2	0 and 6–18 months	25 units (0.5 mL)
Adults 17 years and older	2	0 and 6 months	50 units (1.0 mL)

** Inactivated vaccine. Manufactured by Merck & Company, Inc.

POSTEXPOSURE PROPHYLAXIS

Immune globulin is more than 85% effective in preventing hepatitis A virus infection when given within 2 weeks of exposure to the hepatitis A virus. The dose is 0.02 mL/kg injected into the gluteal muscle in adults or the anterolateral thigh muscle in children less than 2 years. Concurrent hepatitis A vaccination may also be appropriate in individuals above 2 years.

CONTROL OF HEPATITIS B VIRUS INFECTION

INTRODUCTION[1]

General Introduction (Table 19.3)

Hepatitis B infection and HIV infection are the two major infections, which may create problems in healthcare settings. They are blood-borne viral infections, and therefore transmission of these viral infections from one person to the other is very likely to occur unless proper precautions are taken. Together with these two viruses hepatitis C virus is also becoming a major concern. The hepatitis infections also include hepatitis A and E viruses which spread by feco-oral route, and hepatitis D, which requires the presence of hepatitis B in order to replicate. Thus, all the infection control implications of hepatitis B virus are relevant to hepatitis D virus.

Introduction Specific to Hepatitis B Infection[1,4]

Hepatitis B

This disease has an incubation period about 40-160 days (1 month to 6 months), often about 90 days. The serum concentration of the virus may reach 10^8–10^9 viral genome copies/mL, and virus can be detected in saliva, semen and vaginal secretions. The commonest mode of infection all throughout the world is transmission from mother to the neonate.

Table 19.3: Risks from occupational exposure to HBV, HCV and HIV

Virus	Risk of infection from percutaneous contact (%)
HBV	2–40
HCV	3–10
HIV	0.2–0.5

Adopted from Centers for Disease Control (1995).[2,5]

These infants have a high risk of becoming lifelong carriers of the virus (defined as the presence of hepatitis B surface antigen (HbsAg) in serum for more than 6 months). Such individuals are also at higher risk of developing the severe hepatic sequelae of HBV infection. Adults who acquire infection may be asymptomatic or suffer from acute hepatitis. However, they are likely to clear the virus (95% of cases) and become naturally immune.

HEPATITIS B MARKERS AND THEIR IMPLICATION (TABLE 19.4)[1]

Three different components of the virus may be detected in the serum of infected individuals. The presence of HbsAg defines an infection. HbsAg positive individual may also have "e" antigen, which is associated with a highly infectious state. In contrast, the absence of "e" and the presence of antibody to "e" suggests low infectivity. Finally, serum HBV DNA can be detected and quantitated. All these sensitive assays have been used to predict and assess the response to drug therapy. However, the HbeAg/Ab status can sometimes be misleading criteria of infectivity (because there are certain viral variants which do not code for the e protein). Hence, it is likely that these markers will be replaced by HBV DNA quantitation (viral load in future). Antibodies to core antigen (HbcAb) develop soon after infection and persist whether the infection is cleared or a carrier state develops. The presence of core-antigen specific IgM (i.e. anti-HBV antibodies (IgM type) indicates a recent acquisition of infection. By contrast

Table 19.4: Serological markers of hepatitis B infection[3,6]

Clinical condition	Hbs Ag	Hbe Ag	Anti HBs	Anti HBe	Anti-HBC		HBV DNA
					IgM	IgG	
Incubation period	+	+	-	-	-	-	+
Acute hepatitis	+	+	-	-	+	+	+
Chronic active hepatitis	+	+	-	-	+	+	+
Asymptomatic carrier stage	+	-	-	+	-	+	-
Past infection (Natural immunity)	-	-	+	-	-	+	-
Immunization without infection (Post-vaccine immunity)	-	-	+	-	-	-	-

antibodies to HbsAg develop with clearance of surface antigen, and therefore signifying immunity. Since HBV vaccine is composed of hepatitis B surface antigen (HbsAg) alone, response to the vaccine is also assessed by presence of these antibodies.

INCIDENCE OF HEPATITIS B[1,4]

The incidence of hepatities B virus (HBV) infection ranges from 0.1 to 1% in UK, USA and Nothern Europe (low) to 4–5% in Southern Europe (Medium), and more than 10% in the Far East and some areas of Africa (High). In India, the incidence due to screening of donated blood for HbsAg has minimized the risk of transfusion-associated HBV infection. Groups which are at high risk of acquiring this infection are intravenous drug users, homosexual men, renal dialysis and where healthcare precautions are suboptimal. The incidence in India ranges from 2 to 10% (Intermediate/medium).[4,7] The number of HbsAg carrier rate in India has been estimated to be over 40 million (4 crores).

NEEDLESTICK INJURY FROM HbeAg POSITIVE BLOOD AND TRANSMISSION OF INFECTION[1,4]

Following a needlestick injury with blood from an "e" Ag-positive HBV-infected patient, the risk of infection for a susceptible individual is estimated to be up to 22–40%,whereas in an HBeAg negative individual the risk is only 1 to 6%. HCW who are most at risk of infection are those involved in invasive procedures, such as gynecologists, who often perform, blind deep pelvic surgery in which they may have small innocuous cuts on their hands with suture needle which occur commonly although non-apparent infections through mucous membranes may also occur.

HBV infections may be due to risk activity outside work. As stated above virus can be detected in saliva, but at 1000–10,000 fold lower concentrations than in serum. Transmission of HBV via bites has been documented, but mucosal contact with saliva has been said to pose very little risk. In UK, it has been recommended that HbeAg postive HBV carrier must not perform procedures, where there is risk of injury to themselves, which would result in their blood contaminating a patient's open tissues. This follows previous evidence that transmission of HBV from HCW to patient was limited to such HbeAg positive staff. However, transmission from HbeAg negative surgeons have recently been documented, and a review of current guidance is being undertaken within UK (Anon, 1997).

According to a recent update of CDC Recommendations (July 2012)[8] for Management of hepatitis B infected healthcare-providers (HCP) and students state the following:

They reaffirm the 1991 CDC recommendations that HBV infection alone should not disqualify infected persons from practice or study of surgery, dentistry, medicine or allied health fields.

Following changes have also been made in these recommendations:

1. No prenotification of patients of a health-care provider or students' HBV status is necessary. Previously according to 1991 recommendations on HBV-infected HCP who performed exposure prone procedures an infected HCP or student was supposed to notify patients in advance regarding their seropositivity. This is because scientific data and clinical experience since 1991 demonstrates that the risk for HBV and other blood-borne virus transmission from HCP to patients is extremely low.
2. Serum DNA levels rather than HBeAg status to be used to monitor infectivity. HBV DNA levels provide better information to serve as a predictive indicator of infectivity than is provided by monitoring HBeAg status.
3. According to SHEA guidelines (US) 2010, HCP should have levels of HBV DNA $\leq 10^4$ genome equivalents GE/mL (approximately 2,000 IU/mL) without a requirement for HBeAg negativity to perform exposure prone procedures,whereas according to UK guidelines HBV infected HCP who are HBe Ag negative require those health care providers to achieve or maintain HBV DNA levels of $\leq 10^3$ GE/mL (approximately 200 IU/mL) should be achieved by HCP to perform exposure prone procedures.
4. Exposure prone procedures are those procedures likely to pose an increased risk of percutaneous injury to HCP that have resulted in provider to patient transmission of HBV (e.g. digital palpation of needle tip in a body cavity and/or simultaneous presence of healthcare provider's fingers and a needle or other sharp instrument or object (e.g. a bone spicule) in a poorly visualized or highly confined anatomic sites. Therefore, these procedures are limited to major abdominal, cardiothoracic, orthopedic surgery, repair of major traumatic injuries, abdominal and vaginal hysterectomy, ceserian section,vaginal deliveries, major oral and/or oral maxillofacial surgery (e.g. fracture reductions).
5. Guidance is usually given by Expert Review Panels set up at each institute. Usually, HCP, residents, medical and dental students with active HBV infection (i.e. those who are HBsAg positive) who do not perform exposure prone procedures, no restriction should be imposed on their activities or study. It is not necessary that they achieve low or undetectable levels of serum HBV DNA, HBeAg negativity or have review or oversight by an expert panel, as recommended for those HCP or students who perform exposure prone procedures. However, they should receive medical care for condition by clinicians in their health care setting.
6. Expert panel oversight and restrictions however are recommended for surgeons including oral surgeons, obstetricians and gynecologists, surgical residents and others who perform exposure prone procedures depending on their HBV DNA levels.

Improvements in infection control practices into effect since 1991 in the US and other developed countries have enhanced protection from exposure to blood and blood-borne viruses. Universal Precautions practices and double gloving during surgical procedures have eliminated completely the low risk of transmission of HBV as well as hepatitis C virus (HCV) and human immunodeficiency virus (HIV).

Symptomatic acute HBV infections in US have declined by 85% from early 1990s to 2009 following the adoption of Universal infant vaccination and catch-up vaccination for children and adolescent. Patient to HCP transmission of HBV has also declined markedly.

TREATMENT[1,4]

Medications for hepatitis B have been improving continually and are usually effective in reducing viral load markedly or nearly to undetectable levels. Currently, seven therapeutic agents are approved by the Food and Drug Administration for the treatment of chronic hepatitis B, including two formulations of interferon (interferon alpha and pegylated interferon) and five nucleotide analogs (lamivudine, telbivudine, abacavir, entecavir and tenofovir). Among the approved analogs, both entecavir and tenofovir have potent antiviral activity as well as very low rates of drug resistance. Treatment with these agents reduces HBV DNA levels to undetectable or nearly undetectable levels in most treated persons. Virtually all treated patients, even those still receiving the older agents (e.g. lamivudine), can expect to achieve a reduction of HBV DNA viral load to very low levels within weeks or months of initiating therapy.

However, vaccination against HBV is the most important tool for eradication of this virus. The vaccine does not contain any genetic material and is safe and effective. Passive immunization with hyperimmuneglobulin may be useful as an adjunct to active vaccination in the postexposure prophylaxis.

PREVENTION STRATEGIES[8]

Strategies to promote patient safety and to prevent transmission of blood-borne viruses in health care settings include hepatitis B vaccination of susceptible healthcare personnel and the use of primary prevention (i.e. preventing exposures and therefore infection) by strict adherence to the tenets of standard (universal) infection control precautions, the use of safer devices (engineering controls) and the implementation of work practice controls (e.g. not recapping needles) to prevent injuries that confer risks for HBV transmission to patients and their providers.

- Standard (Universal Precautions): Public health officials in United States-based standard precautions on the premise that all blood and blood containing body fluids are potentially infectious. Since 1996, CDC has specified the routine use of Standard Precautions that include the use of protective equipment in appropriate circumstances, implementation of both work practice controls and engineering controls, and adherence to meticulous standards for cleaning and reusing patient care equipment. For example, double-gloving now is practiced widely.
- Use of safer devices (Engineering Controls) include:
  1. Practice of not resheathing needles.
  2. Use of puncture-resistant needle and sharp object disposal container.
  3. Avoidance of unnecessary phlebotomies.
  4. Avoidance of unnecessary needle and sharp object use.
  5. Use of ports and other needleless vascular access when possible.
  6. Avoidance of unnecessary IV catheters by using needleless or protected needle infusion systems.
- Work practice controls
- Adherence to meticulous standards for cleaning and reusing patient care equipment, e.g. double gloving is now practiced widely.

HBV VACCINATION OF HEALTHCARE WORKERS[1,4]

All staff (HCW like Medical, Dental, Nursing and Ancillary), who have potential contact with blood, or blood-stained body fluids, or with patient's tissues should receive immunization. According to the current UK Department of Health Guidelines, healthcare worker (HCW) should not start work, until it is made sure that they are not infected with HBV, or before getting involved in exposure prone procedures. It must be made sure that they show adequate HBV response.

According to the Updated CDC Recommendations 2012, it is stated that the employer should make available the hepatitis B vaccine and vaccine series to all employees who have occupational exposure and that

Table 19.5: Follow-up of HBV vaccines

Post-vaccine anti- Hbs level (mIU/mL)	Action
<10	Nonresponse
10–100	Booster 1 year
>100	Booster 5 years

postexposure evaluation and follow-up be provided to all employees who have an exposure incident.

A full course of a recombinant HBV vaccine consists of 3 injections into the deltoid at 0,1, and 6 months. Two months after the last dose, a blood sample should be tested for antibodies to HbsAg, to know the level of response to the vaccine. A level of 10-50 mIU/mL is thought to be protective against infection, and 100 m IU/mL is therefore used as a safe cut-off value for determining good vaccine response (Table 19.5).

It is usually expected that 90% of HCW will respond to the vaccine. One reason for non-response is existing chronic HBV infection, and this should be checked for in non-responders. In such cases, it is necessary to check the postvaccine blood sample for HB core antibodies (Fig. 19.1). If a positive result is obtained, consent should be obtained before proceeding to HbsAg testing. However, most non-responders will be HB antibody negative, and therefore not infected. A number of new HBV vaccine, incorporating additional immunogenic epitopes, are currently being evaluated, and should be available for those who do not respond to current vaccines.

Management of exposure prone health care workers with non-response to HBV vaccine.

Hepatitis B causes death in 1 to 2% of patients. Most people with hepatitis B recover completely, but approximately 6 to 10% become chronic carriers of the virus. Most of these people have no symptoms but can continue to transmit the disease to others. Some patients may develop chronic active hepatitis and cirrhosis. HBV also is a causative factor in the development of liver cancer.

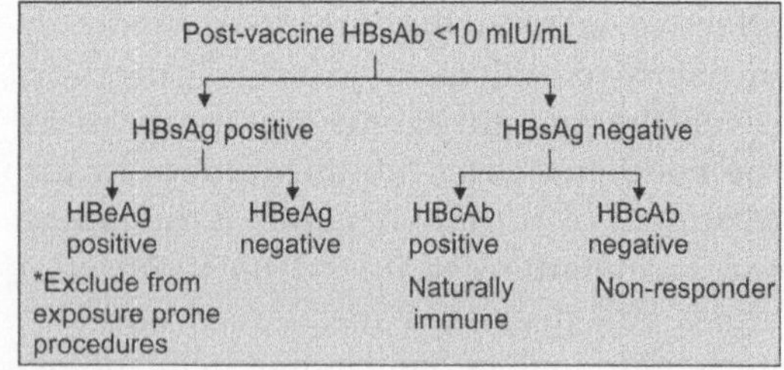

Fig. 19.1: Management of exposure prone health care workers with non-response to HBV vaccine

* Currently under review

Immunization against hepatitis B can prevent hepatitis B and its sequelae including cirrhosis and liver cancer.

CANDIDATES FOR HEPATITIS B VACCINATION—DOSES AND SCHEDULES OF HEPATITIS B (TABLE 19.6)[6]

Routine Vaccination

All infants, children, and adolescents.

High-risk Populations

- People with multiple sex partners and those who have been recently diagnosed with a sexually transmitted disease.
- Sex partners and household contacts of HBV carriers.
- Homosexuals.
- Injection drug users.
- Travelers to countries with high rates of hepatitis B (staying longer than 6 months).
- People with occupational exposure to blood.
- Clients and staff in institutions for the developmentally disabled.
- Patients with chronic kidney failure (including those on chronic hemodialysis).
- Patients receiving clotting factor concentrates.
- Inmates of long-term correctional facilities.

Table 19.6: Doses and schedules of hepatitis B[6,11]

Age	Nos of doses	Schedule	Dose recombivax HB*	Dose engerix B**
Infants with HbsAg-negative mother	3	0 to 2, 1 to 4, and 6–18 months	5.0 mg (0.5 mL)	10 mg (0.5 mL)
Infants with HbsAg-positive mother	3	Hepatitis B immune globulin and vaccination within 12 hours of birth, then vaccine at 1–2 and 6 months	5.0 mg (0.5 mL)	10 mg (0.5 mL)
Children and adolescents age 1–19 years	3	0, 1 to 2 and 4–6 months	5.0 mg (0.5 mL)	10 mg (0.5 mL)
Adolescents 11–15 years	2	0 and 4–6 months	10 mg (1.0 mL)	N/A
Adults 20 years and older	3	0, 1 to 2, and 4–6 months	10 mg (1.0 mL)	20 mg (1.0 mL)
Immunocompromised adults	3 4	0, 1 and 6 months 0, 1, 2 and 6 months	40 mg (1.0 mL) N/A	N/A 40 mg (2.0 mL)

Note: There should be at least 1 month between the first and second doses, at least 2 months between the second and third doses, and at least 4 months between the first and third doses. For infants, the third dose should not be given before 6 months of age.

* Recombinant vaccine. Manufactured by Merck and Company, Inc.

** Inactivated vaccine. Manufactured by SmithKline Beecham Biologicals.

SIDE EFFECTS (OR ADVERSE REACTIONS) OF VACCINE[5,9]

1. Usually, side effects are mild that is mild fever with local pain and tenderness at the injection site, urticaria and angioedema may occur. Anaphylactic reactions although rare have been reported.
   Studies have claimed an association of the vaccine and demyelinating diseases including multiple sclerosis, but available data does not demonstrate a cause association.
2. HBIG prepared from human plasma is screened for HbsAg and antibodies to HIV and HCV. Since 1996, the final product has been tested for HCV RNA by PCR to see that it is free of HCV. The process used to prepare HBIG inactivates and eliminates HIV from the final product.
   PEP for HBV during pregnancy—HBIG is not a contraindication for pregnant or lactating women. The vaccine contains non-infectious HbsAg particles and should pose no risk to fetus. In fact HBV infection during pregnancy might result in severe disease.

Management of Needlestick Injury or Exposure in Other Way (Tables 19.7 and 19.8)[6,11]

1. Wash the site as soon as possible under running water and soap, and allow free flow of blood.
2. Mucous membranes should be flushed with water.
3. Immediately report the incident to the concerned infection control officer incharge of PEP.
4. Blood samples should be taken from the HCW and the patient with relevant counseling. It is mandatory that blood should be obtained in all cases.

Important Points Regarding Hepatitis B Viral Transmission[5,9]

1. Transmission rate is more if source is both HBsAg and HBeAg positive . This increases the risk of developing clinical hepatitis in exposed person and is up to 22-31% and of developing serological evidence of HBV infection is 37-62%. If source is only HbsAg positive risk of developing

Table 19.7: Recommended postexposure prophylaxis for exposure to hepatitis B virus[5,9]

Vaccination and antibody response status of exposed workers*	Treatment		
	Source HbsAg ^ positive	Source HbsAg ^ negative	Source unknown or not available for testing
Unvaccinated	HBIG@X1 and initiate HB vaccine series#	Initiate HB vaccine series	Initiate HB vaccine series If known high-risk source, may treat as if source were HBsAg positive
Previously vaccinated			
Known responder**	No treatment	No treatment	No treatment
Known Non-responder$$	HBIGx1 and initiate revaccination Or HBIG x 2^^ with second dose separated from first dose by 4 weeks***	No treatment	If known high-risk source, treat as If source were HbsAg positive
Antibody response unknown	Test exposed person For anti-HBs## 1. If adequate,** no treatment is necessary 2. If inadequate,$$ administer HBIG x 1 and vaccine booster Recheck HBsAb in 3–4 months. If titer is still inadequate for immunity, complete full second series of vaccinations	No treatment	Test exposed person for anti-HBs 1. If adequate,# no treatment is necessary 2. If inadequate,# administer vaccine booster and recheck titer of HBsAb in 1–2 months. If titer is still inadequate for immunity, complete full second series of vaccinations

*Persons who have previously been infected with HBV are immune to reinfection and do not require postexposure prophylaxis.
^Hepatitis B surface antigen.
@Hepatitis B immune globulin; dose is 0.06 mL/kg intramuscularly.
#Hepatitis B vaccine.
**A responder is a person with adequate levels of serum antibody to HbsAg (i.e. anti-HBs $\geq$10 mIU/mL).
$$A nonresponder is a person with inadequate response to vaccination (i.e. anti-HBs <10 mIU/mL).
^^The option of giving one dose of HBIG and reinitiating the vaccine series is preferred for nonresponders who have not completed a second 3 dose vaccine series. For persons, who previously completed a second vaccine series but failed to respond, two doses of HBIG are preferred.
##Antibody to HbsAg.

Note: Both HBIG and the first dose of hepatitis B vaccine should be ideally administered within 24 hours of exposure. HBIG should not be given later than 14 days post-exposure (can be given up to 7 days for occupational exposures and 14 days for sexual exposures). The three dose vaccine series is given at 0, 1 to 2 months, and 6 months. It is best to give hepatitis B vaccine within 3 days; giving hepatitis B vaccine after that timeframe is better than not giving it. Hepatitis B antibodies should be obtained 1–2 months after completion of the third dose of the vaccine.

Initiation of HBV vaccine series within 12–24 hours of an exposure has been demonstrated to be 70–90% effective in preventing HBV infection. The combination of vaccine and HBIG achieves a similar level of efficacy. Among known non-responders to vaccination, one dose of HBIG is 70–90% effective in preventing HBV when administered within 7 days of percutaneous HBV exposure, and multiple doses have shown to be 75–95% effective.[10]

Table 19.8: Exposure and treatment of needlestick injury

Exposure	Treatment
1. Perinatal	One dose of HBIG given with the first hepatitis B vaccine dose
2. Percutaneous or permucosal	HBIG and vaccination depending on vaccination and exposure status
3. Sexual	Exposure to acute hepatitis—HBIG with or without vaccination Chronic exposure—vaccination alone
4. Household contact	HBIG with vaccination—Acute hepatitis in infants under age 12 months Chronic—only vaccination

clinical hepatitis in the exposed persons is 1-6% and risk of developing serological evidence 23–37%.

2. HBV has been demonstrated to survive in dried blood at room temperature on environmental surfaces for at least one week. Therefore, sometimes the HCW may not give any history of exposure, but contact with such environmental surfaces may have inoculated HBV into cutaneous scratches, abrasions, burns or other lesions.
3. a. Potentially infectious fluids are—blood (most infectious), cerebrospinal fluids, synovial fluid, pleural fluids, peritoneal fluid and amniotic fluid.
   b. Feces, nasal secretions, saliva, sputum, sweat, tears, urine and vomitus are not considered potentially infectious unless they contain blood.
4. Most body fluids are not efficient vehicles of transmission, because they contain low quantities of infectious HBV, despite the presence of HBsAg (the concentration of HbsAg may be 100–1000 fold higher than the concentration of infectious HBV particles.

CONTROL OF HEPATITIS C VIRUS INFECTION

INTRODUCTION (SOURCE AND TRANSMISSION)

This is also one of the major causes of post-transfusion hepatitis. It was previously labeled as non-A, non-B hepatitis virus. Hepatitis C infection is also followed by a long-term carriage, with up to 60–70% of infected individuals developing chronic liver disease after 20–30 years. Acute infection is often asymptomatic and infection is therefore likely to remain unidentified at this stage. It is estimated that there are 100 million HCV carriers world wide, with a prevalence of 0.5–2% among the general population in Europe.[12] Very high rates are observed in intravenous drug users, hemophiliacs and to a lesser extent in hemodialysis patients. Transmission is therefore parenteral although sexual and perinatal transmission has also been documented, with far less frequency than hepatitis B.

Around 40–50% diagnosed HCV infections are of unknown source. Unlike HBV, the prevalence of HCV infection in HCW is not much greater than in general population, although needlestick transmission from patients to HCW has been described and is a potential risk.

DIAGNOSIS OF HEPATITIS C VIRUS INFECTION

Hepatitis C infection is diagnosed by the detection of antibodies to HCV. Infection diagnosed in this way should always be confirmed by further tests, as some antibody assays have less than optimal specificity. So confirmation is done by detection of HCV viral genome in serum by polymerase chain reaction (PCR) and the presence of virus in blood infers a potential risk to others.

TREATMENT AND VACCINE

Combinations of interferon and ribavirin have good efficacy in clearing HCV from the circulation, although there is a significant rate of recurrence following cessation of treatment.[13] This proven benefit of treatment may be seen by some as a rationale for actively following HCW who have been infected with HCV.

No vaccine is currently available and there is no efficacy data for postexposure prophylaxis.

RISK OF OCCUPATIONAL TRANSMISSION OF HCV[14]

The average incidence of anti-HCV seroconversion after accidental percutaneous exposure from an HCV-positive source is 1.8% (range: 0–7%). HCV however is not transmitted efficiently through occupational exposures to blood.

One study indicates that transmission occurred only through hollow-bored needles compared with sharps. Transmission rarely occurs from mucous membrane exposures to blood, and no transmission in HCV has been documented from intact or non-intact skin exposures to blood. The risk of transmission through environmental contamination with HCV-infected blood is not significant as compared to HBV except in hemodialysis unit. The risk of transmission from exposure to fluids or tissues has not been quantified, but is expected to be low.

MANAGEMENT OF EXPOSURES TO HCV[14]

Recommendations

- Clinicians should consider concurrent exposure to HCV when exposed workers present with an HIV exposure.
- Neither immunoglobulin nor antiviral agents are recommended for HCV post-exposure prophylaxis.
- When HCV infection is identified, the exposed worker should be referred for medical management to a clinician with experience in treating HCV.

Healthcare professionals who are looking after persons exposed to HCV in the occupational setting should be knowledgeable regarding the risk for HCV infection and appropriate counseling, testing and medical follow-ups.

Ig and antiviral agents are not recommended for PEP after exposure to HCV-positive blood. In addition no guidelines exist for administration of therapy during the acute phase of HCV infection. However, if an individual becomes acutely infected with hepatitis C and is diagnosed at that time, immediate referral to a specialist experienced in the treatment of hepatitis C is strongly recommended. Recent data suggests that early treatment of acute hepatitis C with interferon is highly effective, perhaps as high as 98%.[12] The best regimen or duration of therapy is unknown. However, observation for a period of 8 to 12 weeks post-infection is reasonable to assess for possible spontaneous resolution of acute hepatitis C.[12]

Baseline Management

Recommendations

- Following exposure to blood or body fluid, the clinician should assess the risk for exposure to HCV. Wounds should be washed with soap and water, and should not be squeezed. Mucous membranes should be flushed with water.
- Once the clinician has determined that exposure to blood or body fluid has occurred, the following baseline tests should be obtained (Table 19.8)
- Source patient:
  - HCV antibody test (e.g: EIA/ELISA), and if positive, HCV RNA test or recombinant immunoblot assay (RIBA).
- Exposed worker:
  - Liver panel including liver enzymes
  - HCV antibody, and if positive HCV RNA test.

If the source patient is tested with EIA/ELISA and found to be positive, then follow-up testing is necessary to confirm the source patient's status. According to the most recent updated US Public Health Service Guidelines for the Management of Occupational Exposures to HBV, HCV, and HIV and Recommendations of Postexposure Prophylaxis (2001), either HCV RNA or RIBA may be used as a confirmatory test. However, most clinicians currently obtain HCV RNA testing, instead of RIBA to confirm a positive antibody screening result. When the source patient tests positive by either RIBA or HCV RNA test, the exposed worker should be managed as though the source has chronic HCV.[15]

If at any time the serum ALT level is elevated in the exposed worker, the clinician

Table 19.9: Hepatitis C postexposure management according to baseline test results[15]

Sl. No.	Clinical scenario	Follow-up
1.	Source patient is HCV antibody negative	No further testing or follow-up is necessary for the source patient or the exposed worker
2.	Source patient is unavailable or refuses testing	Exposed worker: Follow-up HCV antibody at 3 and 6 months
3.	Source patient is HCV-antibody positive and HCV RNA negative	Manage the exposed worker as if the source patient has chronic hepatitis C
4.	Source patient is positive for both HCV antibody and HCV RNA And Exposed worker is HCV antibody negative	Source patient: Counsel and manage as chronic hepatitis C regardless of status of exposed worker Exposed worker: Follow-up as outlined in post-exposure follow-up for HCV, below
5.	Exposed worker tests positive for both HCV antibody and HCV RNA	Counsel and manage as chronic hepatitis C

should test for HCV RNA to assess for acute HCV infection. A single negative HCV RNA result does not exclude active infection.

Postexposure Follow-up for HCV (Table 19.9)[15]

Recommendations

- If the source patient is known to be positive for HCV RNA, the follow-up schedule for the exposed worker should be as follows:
  - Week 4: HCV RNA and liver panel (LFT)
  - Week 12: HCV RNA and liver panel (LFT)
  - Week 24: Liver panel and HCV antibody.
- If at any time the serum ALT is elevated, the clinician should repeat HCV RNA testing to confirm acute HCV infection.
- At any time that exposed workers test positive for HCV RNA, the clinician should refer the exposed worker for medical management and possible treatment by a clinician with experience in treating HCV.

For individuals exposed to hepatitis C-infected source patients, regular follow-up with HCV RNA testing is recommended in addition to HCV antibody testing, because HCV RNA testing can identify acute infection within 2 weeks of exposure, whereas accuracy of the antibody test can be delayed up to several months after acute infection (i.e. window period).[15]

Seroconversion with the ELISA antibody test occurs in 50% of the patients within 9 weeks of exposure, in 80% of patients within 15 weeks of exposure, and in at least 97% of patients within 6 months of exposure. The ELISA test is highly sensitive but relatively nonspecific, resulting in low positive predictive value in low-prevalence populations. Positive HCV ELISA antibody test results require confirmation by a quantitative viral load assay, such as HCV PCR.[15]

CONTROL OF HEPATITIS D VIRUS INFECTION

INTRODUCTION

This virus can infect individuals in association with HBV. Hepatitis D virus (HDV) (HDV) infection is distributed worldwide although not uniformly.[16] It is estimated that 5% of HBsAg carriers are also infected with HDV, which signifies that there might be between 15 and 20 million HDV-infected individuals. This is however a very rough number because it lacks data from areas where HBV is highly prevalent and HDV is poorly studied.[17]

HDV is highly endemic in Mediterranean countries, the Middle East, northern parts of South America and central Africa. HDV also has a high prevalence in Turkey, Central Asia, the Amazon region of western Brazil and southern Europe.

Based on nucleotide sequence analysis eight genotypes have been defined. HDV genotype 1 is the commonest, prevalent worldwide, present mainly in Europe, Middle East, North America, North Africa. It is associated with both severe and mild forms of disease. Genotype 2 is more common in Far East, present in Japan, Taiwan and parts of Russia. Genotype 2 is associated with a milder course. HDV genotype 3 is found exclusively in Amazon Basin and has been associated with more aggressive forms of HDV infection. The combined infection with HDV Genotype 3 and HBV Genotype F was associated with fulminant hepatitis in South America. Genotype 4 present in Japan and Taiwan has variable pathogenicity. Genotype 4 isolated from Okinawa, Japan, has been associated with greater progression to cirrhosis than the Genotype 4 predominant in Taiwan. Genotypes 5 to 8 were found in African patients who had migrated to Northern Europe.[17]

In India, prevalence of HDV varies between 20 and 38% in high-risk population (multiple transfusions, CRF and asymptomatic HBsAg carriers and medical professionals), and it varies between 16 and 19% in hepatitis B related liver diseases. Blood transfusion is probably the most common mode of transmission suggesting a need for blood screening for HDV.[18,19]

Delta hepatitis is the least common form of chronic viral hepatitis and is the form most likely to lead to cirrhosis. Despite the higher rates of progression to cirrhosis, not all published studies refer to an increase in rate of hepatocellular carcinoma. This may be due to the suppression of HBV replication by HDV, since other studies assert that higher HBV DNA serum levels correlate with greater risk of carcinoma.[17]

For an HBV and HDV acute coinfection, the most common outcome is viral clearance, however it can be more severe than acute HBV monoinfection, resulting in some cases in acute liver failure. HDV superinfection of chronic HBV patients also cause severe acute hepatitis, but in this case in 80% of cases, it progresses to chronicity, if this HDV is not ultimately cleared, then chronic infection is established and the preexisting liver disease is usually aggravated. Patients with HDV superinfection suffer a more rapid progression to cirrhosis, increased liver decompensation and death.[17]

DIAGNOSIS

Diagnosis of this infection is very important because knowing the presence of HDV infection in a HBV-infected individual allows a more accurate prognosis. HDV infection effects the response of patients to antiviral therapy and a higher dosage of antiviral is needed than of cases with chronic hepatitis B alone. HDV infection occurs only in HBV infection and is diagnosed by IgM anti-HDV for acute and IgG anti-HDV for chronic infection. In some patients, markers of HBV infection may not be detected because of rapid HBsAg clearance in fulminant or acute hepatitis cases or due to inhibitory effect of HDV on HBV replication.[20]

HDV RNA is another important marker of HDV infection in patients with chronic infection as well as acute infection in which it is a early marker. It is detected by RT-PCR which is very sensitive and can detect as few as 10 genomic copies. HDV RNA is also useful for antiviral therapy monitoring. A rise in serum alfa-feto protein (AFP) in a HDV-infected patient indicates the probability of HCC.[20]

Although detection of HDAg in the liver by immunostaining is the gold marker of diagnosis of HDV infection, this test is not used for routine practice. Serum HDAg is usually detected by enzyme-linked (EIA) or radioimmunoassay (RIA).

TREATMENT AND PREVENTION

The aim of treatment of hepatitis D is to eradicate or to achieve long-term suppression of both HDV and HBV. The only drug approved at present for treatment of chronic hepatitis D is interferon alfa (IFNa/IFNα). Currently, PEG-IFN-α is recommended for one year, if the patients can tolerate the adverse effects of this therapy. However, most importantly alternative treatments need to be explored, as the efficacy of the current therapies is clearly unsatisfactory.[17,20]

Prevention of HDV infection is the same as for control of hepatitis B.

CONTROL OF HEPATITIS E VIRUS INFECTION

INTRODUCTION

Hepatitis E virus (HEV) is also spread through enteric route as with HAV, and also has a similar clinical presentation, apart from the manifestation in the last trimester of pregnancy, when it is associated with 15% mortality. Fecal shedding of the virus is maximum prior to the onset of symptoms. This infection is endemic in India and Pakistan, Africa and South America. Diagnosis is by detection of HEV- specific IgM in serum. The risk of nosocomial infection is rare, although hospital cases should be dealt with as for hepatitis A.

In the recent past, a significant number of studies have been published regarding the threat HEV poses to blood safety. There are studies which provide evidence of transmissibility of this virus through transfusions. However, the extent of transmission and its clinical relevance are issues under debate at present. Initially known to spread only by feco-oral route, now it has been shown to have a zoonotic transmission too. So also parenteral and perinatal routes have been implicated.

HEV hepatitis has varied manifestations ranging from acute self-limiting illness to fulminant hepatic failure.[21] There is increasing evidence from endemic regions that asymptomatic infections comprise a major chunk of the disease burden. Although HEV hepatitis has been clinically described as an acute illness, recently there have been reports of chronicity in immunocompromised patients. Fulminant hepatic failure due to massive liver necrosis is seen in a small subset of patients where mortality is very high. Pregnant women especially in the third trimester are at a disproportionately high risk of developing fulminant hepatic failure with adverse outcome for mother and fetus. Mortality rate up to 20% is seen in these patients.

Another patient group having high morbidity and mortality associated with HEV are patients with preexisting liver disease (such as chronic hepatitis B and C, Wilson's disease, autoimmune and cryptogenic liver disease).[21] Chronic HEV infection leading to cirrhosis and liver failure has been described in liver transplant recipient. Hepatitis E-related cirrhosis has been seen in other solid organ transplant recipients.

Natural history of HEV infection differs in developed and developing countries. With an almost equivalent seroprevalence among population, no outbreaks have been reported from developed countries suggesting predominantly subclinical infection.

In order to be transmissible through blood there should be a period of asymptomatic viremia or the infection should be subclinical in a proportion of the infected population. Viremia in HEV infected individuals is usually of short duration with a brief incubation period followed by symptomatic phase. The viremia disappears before complete resolution of symptoms and there is no chronic carrier state. However, prolonged viremia has been seen to extend beyond three years in renal transplant patients and in those on immunosuppressive therapy although they do not pose a threat to blood safety as they would not be eligible as donors. However, in recent years, viremia has been shown in blood donors who are suggestive of ongoing subclinical infection. These blood donors had elevated ALT and some had detectable

HEV RNA. In non-endemic area no clear association of HEV with previous transfusion was seen, however, in endemic areas, the studies have suggested the possibility of transmission through blood transfusion.[21]

The effects of transmission of HEV through blood have not been described in patients at high risk of fulminant hepatitis such as pregnant females and patients with preexisting liver disease and solid organ transplants. These patients may not have an uneventful recovery and may need more comprehensive preventive measures against HEV.[21]

So the most important question remains that is, "Is transfusion transmitted HEV preventable through donor screening?" Are there quick reliable and affordable tests available to screen the virus in blood?

DIAGNOSIS

HEV can easily be diagnosed through simple laboratory serological tests.

Detection of IgM Antibodies

By screening for IgM antibodies of donated blood, transmission may be prevented. IgM antibodies to HEV are present during the acute phase of infection and disappear within several weeks after symptoms have resolved. Serological based assays especially IgM detection have good sensitivity and specificity.[21]

Detection of IgG Antibodies

These are also very strongly detected during the acute phase of infection and known to persist for several months.

Two HEV antibody assays commercially available are Abbott Immunoglobulin G assay (Abbott laboratories, Germany) and Gene labs IgG assay (Gene labs Diagnostics, Singapore) have been evaluated and found to have adequate sensitivity and specificity.[21]

Molecular assays based on HEV RNA detection are not warranted for screening or even diagnosis of infection. They are usually used for epidemiological studies and genotyping of virus. It has many limitations in being less sensitive, labor intensive, cumbersome and expensive. Moreover HEV viremia is short lived approximately 20 days and always coincidental with acute phase of illness. Another test is immune electron microscopy which again requires a specialized laboratory facilities and is used in research studies only.[22]

Hence by careful screening by reliable serological tests, HEV infection clinical or subclinical can be detected. At present, IgM ELISA would cost around ₹100–150 per assay and can be carried out within 2–3 hours in routine blood bank setting.

VACCINES

A vaccine based on recombinant viral proteins was developed in the 1990's and tested in high-risk population (military personnel of Nepal) in 2001. The vaccine appeared effective and safe, but development stopped for economical reasons, since hepatitis E is rare in developed countries. There is no licensed hepatitis E vaccine in the US. There is only one hepatitis E vaccine developed by Chinese scientists which was available at the end of 2012, called as HEV 239 and sold as Hecolin by its developer Xiamen Innovax Biotech. This was approved by the Chinese Ministry of science and Technology. It proved effective following a phase 3 trial. The first vaccine came out of Innovax in late October 2012.[23]

In the light of present knowledge there is no clear cut association of transfusion with HEV infection as exists for HBV or HCV, but nevertheless transmission of HEV does occur and may be more common in endemic areas. There is no evidence of significant morbidity in most recipients and as of now the screening of all blood for HEV is not warranted.

However, knowledge regarding the serious consequences of HEV in certain class of patients and taking into consideration that there are no definitive treatment modalities for HEV hepatitis and no licensed vaccine available at present, serious consideration should be given to selective screening for patients at high risk for fulminant hepatic failure or chronicity.

REFERENCES

1. Pillay D. Control of Viral Hepatitis and Human Immunodeficiency Virus (HIV) infection. Chapter 10. In: Ayliffee GAJ, Fraise AP, Geedes AM, Mitchell K (Eds). Control of Hospital Infection. A Practical Handbook, 4th edition, Oxford University Press, New York; 2000.p.217.
2. Centres for disease control. Prevention of Hepatitis A through active or passive immunization. Morbidity and Mortality Weekly Report. 1996;45:15.
3. Vaccination for Hepatitis A&B NIDDK National Digestive diseases clearinghouse. Pages 1&2. http//www.niddk.nih.gov/health/digest/pubs/.vacc4hep/vacc4hep.htm.
4. Pillay D. Control of Viral Hepatitis and Human Immunodeficiency virus (HIV) infection. In: Ayliffe GAJ, Fraise AP, Geddes AM, Mitchell K (Eds). Control of hospital infection. A practical handbook. 4th edition. Oxford University Press, Inc. New York; 2000.pp.207-16.
5. Centers for Disease Control (1995). Case Control Study of HIV seroconversion in healthcare workers after percutaneous exposure to HIV infected blood—France, United Kingdom and United States. January 1988 - August 1994. MMWR 44(50);929-933. Publication date: 12/22/1995. CDC Web Search: http://www.cdc.gov/search htm or http://wonder.cdc.gov/wonder/prevguid/moo39830/moo39830.asp
6. Arora DR. Textbook of Microbiology. 2nd edition. CBS Publishers and Distributors, New Delhi; 2003.p.577.
7. World Health Organization, Representative to India. Introducing Hepatitis B under Universal immunization program. Frequently asked questions about Hepatitis B Disease and Vaccine. www.whoindia.org/CHS/HepB/FAQ.asp.
8. Updated US. Public Health Service Guidelines for the management of occupational exposures to HBV, HCV and HIV and Recommendations for Post-exposure prophylaxis. Pg.22. from CDC MMWR Morbidity and Mortality Weekly Report June 29, 2001;50:RR-11. US Dept of Health and Human Services CDC. Atlanta. From Net. www.cdc.gov/mmwr/preview/mmwrhtml/rr5011a1.htm-101k.
9. Vaccination for hepatitis A and B NIDDK (National digestive diseases information clearing house.) Pg 2-4 from net http//www.niddk.nih.gov/health/digest/pubs/vacc4hep.htm.
10. Updated CDC Recommendations for management of Hepatitis B virus-infected Healthcare Providers and Students. CDC MMWR Recommendations and Reports. 2012;61:3. Accessed from www.cdc.gov/mmwr/pdf/rr/rr6103.pdf on 5th August 2013.
11. Zingman BS. HIV Prophylaxis following Occupational Exposure: Guideline and Commentary. Accessed from www.medscape.com/view article/778035-11 on 13th August 2013.p.3.
12. Pillay D. Control of Viral Hepatitis and Human Immunodeficiency Virus (HIV) infection. Chapter 10. In: Ayliffee GAJ, Fraise AP, Geedes AM, Mitchell K (Eds). Control of Hospital Infection. A practical Handbook, 4th edition, Oxford University Press, New York; 2000. pp.211-6.
13. Liang JT. Combination therapy for Hepatitis C infection. New Eng J Med. 1998;339:1549.
14. Occupation transmission of HCV pages 6, 7 and 21 in MMWR Morbidity and Mortality Weekly Report (Updated Public Health Service Guidelines) for the Management of Occupational Exposures to HBV, HCV and HIV and Recommendations for Post-exposure Prophylaxis. June 29, 2001;50(No.RR-11)from net www.cdc.gov/mmwr/preview/mmwrhtml/rr5011a1.htm-101K.
15. Zingman BS. HIV Prophylaxis following Occupational Exposure: Guideline and Commentary. Accessed from www.medscape.com/view article/778035-11 on 13th August 2013.p.5.
16. Pillay D. Control of Viral Hepatitis and Human Immunodeficiency Virus (HIV) infection. Chapter 10. In: Ayliffee GAJ, Fraise AP, Geedes AM, Mitchell K (Eds). Control of Hospital

Infection. A practical Handbook, 4th edition, Oxford University Press, New York; 2000.p.210.
17. Alves C, Branco C, Cunha C. Hepatitis Delta Virus: A Peculiar Virus. Advances in virology. 2013.pp.1-11. Accessed on 15/10/2013.Website:www.hindawi.com/journals/av/2013/560105,http://dx.doi.org/10.1155/2013/560105.
18. Amarapurkar DN, Vishwanath N, Kumar A, Shankaran S, Murti P, Kalro RH, et al. Prevalence of delta virus infection in high risk population and hepatitis B virus related liver diseases. Indian J Gastroenterol. 1992;11(1):11-2. Accessed on 19/10/2013 .Website:http://www.ncbi.nlm.nih.gov/pubmed/1551704.
19. Shah LJ, Mulla SA. Prevalence of hepatitis D virus (HDV) in South Gujarat. National Journal of Medical Research. 2012;2(2)117-20. Accessed on 19/10/2013.Web site: njmr.in/home/download/60.
20. Hajiani E, Alavi SM. A review on epidemiology,diagnosis and treatment of hepatitis D virus infection. Jundishapur J Microbiol. 2011;4(Supplement 1):S1-S8. Accessed on 15/10/2013. Website: microbial.con/4133pdf.
21. Bajpai M, Gupta E. Transfusion transmitted Hepatitis E virus—Is screening warranted? Indian Journal of Medical Microbiology, 2011;29(4):353-8.
22. Hepatitis E Fact sheet. Updated July 2013. World Health Organization. Accessed on !5/10 2013 from website: http://www.who.int/mediacentre/factsheets/fs280/en.
23. Hepatitis E. Symptoms Virology Prevention Epidemiology From Wikipedia, the free encyclopedia. Accessed on 17/10/2013 from http//www.en.wikipedia.org/wiki/Hepatitis_E.

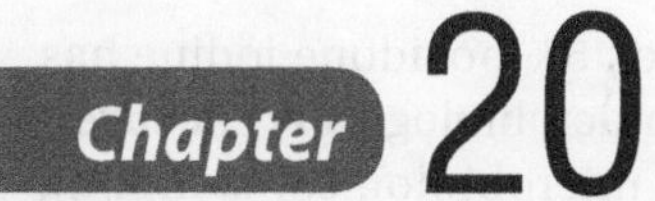

Infection Control in Specialty Clinics

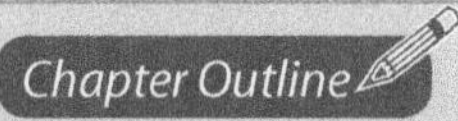

OPHTHALMIC DEPARTMENT

INTRODUCTION

Nosocomial infection of the eye is an uncommon complication acquired during the course of hospital management.

Infections of eye can occur as a result of trauma leading to corneal injuries or corneal ulcers, and also following surgeries, which may be intraocular, orbital surgery or intraocular surgery. The greatest risk from contamination occurs in intraocular operations, and also in patients who have corneal injuries or ulcers. The transparent, ocular media have no direct blood circulation and are deficient in antibodies. However, they are well-oxygenated and provide good culture media for exogenous microorganisms (In particular *Pseudomonas aeruginosa*).[1]

Eyes are in general susceptible to infection with gram-negative bacilli, fungi, adenoviruses and herpes simplex virus and organisms which are often or always resistant to antibiotics, sometimes used for prophylaxis. In some studies, it has been noted that *Staphylococcus aureus, Staphylococcus epidermidis* and *Pseudomonas aeruginosa* are the most frequently isolated bacteria.[2]

Traumatic wounds and surgical operations increase or determine the risk of severe infection with these organisms. Endophthalmitis is still a significant worldwide problem and remains a potentially devastating complication after ocular surgery.

CONTROL OF INFECTION

Preoperative Disinfection of the Conjunctiva

Usually antibiotic drops are used (Gatifloxacin or moxifloxacin, Cefazolin or cefuroxime and topical neomycin-polymixin B-gramicidin); they are instilled into the eye preoperatively and postoperatively. Use of disinfectants is uncertain, as disinfectants are not well tolerated, however, 5% povidone iodine has been used and is microbiologically effective.

Preoperative microbiological sampling may be performed, but its value is limited, and it may delay the operation unnecessarily. With solutions, eye drops, ointments the greatest risk of intraocular infection are associated with the use of contaminated fluids, either due to inadequate sterilization or to recontamination due to improper handling or multiple use containers.

In corneal grafts, cornea is the only tissue from the eye, which is transplanted. Donors should be tested for HIV, HCV and HBV.

Sterilization of Instruments and Appliances

Although autoclaving is satisfactory for sterilization of instruments, some instruments, e.g. cataract knives have delicate cutting edge and may therefore be damaged by this method. Therefore, sterilization by dry heat at 160°C for 1 hour or lower temperatures for longer periods are preferred by most authorities. Gamma sterilized disposable knives and autoclaved diamond knives are now solving some of these problems. Ethylene oxide has been used for sterilization of cryothermy leads and other heat labile items. As the gas must be allowed to escape from the sterilized pack for at least 24 hours before use of the equipment on patients, this method requires reserve supplies of essential apparatus to cover the 'turnover' of sterilization (especially where transport to another center adds further delay).

Newer alternatives to ethylene oxide (e.g. gas plasma sterilization) are still being evaluated. Vitrectomy and other infusion/aspirations apparatus also requires sterilization, as the vitreous provides an ideal nidus for colonization by microorganisms.

The adjustment of the operating microscope and other equipment by the surgeon requires special precautions. The provision of dry sterile guards is usually considered satisfactory, and most microscopes, can now be adjusted by the foot or other methods, that do not require direct handling by the surgeon. The equipment must be kept meticulously clean, as cleaning during the operation is not possible.

Surgical Technique

Ideally operative procedures should be carried out with a gloved hand, if gloves are not used (as some surgeons believe they can have a finer control with an ungloved hand) then the hands should be absolutely dry and never touch the operating area or the operating ends of the instruments. Regular and repeated use of an effective detergent antiseptic (e.g. 4% chlorhexidine detergent (Hibiscrub) or 0.5% alcoholic chlorhexidine) is a particularly important precaution if gloves are not worn. Most surgeons now prefer to wear gloves, because by using an ungloved hand, there is a risk of infection either due to accidental contact or from dry epidermal scales which are likely to fall from the hands during the course of a long operation. By using gloves, the disastrous consequences of a postoperative infection can be avoided if the edges of the wound are properly opposed, then the wound is secure, and there is little risk of intraocular contamination from the exterior from about 48 hours after the operation.

During operation, instruments also should be held in such a way that the part which comes into contact with the eye should not be touched. Instruments are more effectively, controlled, when they are regularly used with an operating microscope, which is also an effective mechanism for excluding foreign material from the operating area.

WARDS

Sterile dressing packs (supplied from SSD) should be used. Also individual droppers, which are provided as single use sterile containers, should be preferably used. Multidose eye drops bottles should not be used for more than 7 days.

CARE OF CONTACT LENSES

Hard lenses are difficult to contaminate and simple hygiene is usually sufficient. However, they may be disinfected with benzalkonium chloride (0.01% w/v). This method is not suitable for soft lenses. Low-water content soft lenses can be satisfactorily disinfected by heating to 80°C for 20 minutes daily. High water content lenses may be damaged by heating and require chemical disinfection. Stabilized hydrogen peroxide (3%) is commonly used. This should be thoroughly washed off or preferably neutralized. Saline solutions used for storage should be changed daily.

POSTOPERATIVE ENDOPHTHALMITIS

Postoperative endophthalmitis is a rare complication of ECCE (Extracapsular cataract extraction) and IOL (Intraocular lens implantation). It was found that infection resulted from the introduction of organisms from patient's skin or ocular surface tissues. But sometimes infection with the same microorganisms in multiple patients can result from a common source, such as contaminated saline, lens, or lens solution. Therefore, there is need for (1) strict quality control for the procedures of such solutions; (2) strict adherence by the users of commercial products to product-storage procedures, specified by manufacturers instructions; and (3) increased surveillance by ophthalmologist and other infection control personnel for cases of postoperative endophthalmitis associated with invasive ocular operations.[3]

USE OF VANCOMYCIN FOR PROPHYLAXIS

Recently, ophthalmologists have been using vancomycin for prophylaxis in routine uncomplicated intraocular surgeries. Vancomycin is added routinely to irrigating solutions. At the same time, there has been a growing problem of vancomycin resistance, which calls for restriction of the use of vancomycin. There has been a sudden increase in the infections and colonization with vancomycin resistant enterococci. The Van A gene which is frequently plasmid borne confers a high-level resistance to vancomycin (most strains of VRE are resistant to all standard enterococcal drugs, including gentamicin and ampicillin), which can be transferred from enterococci to a variety of gram-positive cocci (especially to *S. aureus* and *S. epidermidis*, and this may carry serious implications in future).

Therefore, CDC in 1995 has called for prudent use of vancomycin to prevent and control the spread of vancomycin resistance. They discourage the use of vancomycin for routine surgical prophylaxis except for use in patients with a documented life-threatening allergy to beta-lactam antibiotics.[4]

CONTROL OF INFECTION IN OPHTHALMIC PRACTICE[5]

- Consider ALL patients **and** staff a potential infection risk.
- Staff **and** patients should wash hands with soap before commencing any examination.
- Wash hands with soap before and after every clinical procedure, even if gloves are worn.
- Staff **and** patients with any broken skin, however, small, must wear an occlusive dressing.
- Staff with any known or suspected infection should not have direct patient contact.

Equipment

- Applanation tonometer prisms (**tips only**), diagnostic contact lenses, A-scan probes, occluders and pin-holes should be wiped with disposable paper tissue after each use. Store in sodium hypochlorite 1%, in a non-metallic pot, for 10 minutes, rinse in sterile water and dry before re-use.
- Slit lamp-chin rest, head rim, handgrips and table top should be washed with detergent and water between each patient examination.

Surgical Instruments and Decontamination Procedures

- Loaded needle holders-lie point down on trolley and table tops.
- Pass sharp instruments to colleagues with verbal warning and eye contact communication.
- Sharp instruments should not project beyond the surface edge.
- Ensure surgical instruments are thoroughly cleaned before being passed for sterilization or disinfection.
- Choose the appropriate sterilization or disinfection method for the specific instrument.
- Emphasize care of instruments and sterilization and disinfection procedures in training programs.

Clinical Practice and Safety Issues

- Critically review work practices regularly.
- Include control of infection policies in training programs.
- Implement and emphasize strict adherence to universal control of infection policies.
- Teach correct hand-washing technique and display a written procedure in all relevant areas (see below).
- Eye drops and ointments—provide individual containers for each patient.
- Eye dressings—following removal, dispose of immediately, by burning.
- Eye shields—if removed from a knowingly infected patient, **never** re-use.
- Pathological specimens—dispose of needles and blades used to obtain corneal and conjunctival material into 'sharps' container.

Eye Drops[6]

- Eye drop medications must be discarded and replaced with a new bottle when the manufacturer's expiration date is exceeded unless the product becomes contaminated.
- The bottle should be dated when opened.
- When administering eye drops, do not touch the dropper to the eye. Discard the bottle if the dropper comes in contact with the eye, including eye lashes.

Retrobulbar Injections

- After administering retrobulbar injections, immediately place the needle and syringe into the sharps container.
- All instruments used during retrobulbar injections are disposable.

Disinfection of Tonometer Prisms

- Tonometer prisms must be disinfected after each patient use.
- Saturate a cotton ball with 70% ethyl alcohol and mechanically disinfect the prism. Allow it to air dry before use.

EAR, NOSE AND THROAT (ENT) DEPARTMENT

INTRODUCTION[7]

Patients admitted to the ENT department are of two types, those admitted for a short stay like for tonsillectomy. These patients are vulnerable to endemic hospital organisms like staphylococci or B hemolytic streptococci, and other community type organisms, which are brought into the hospital by patients. Viruses such as measles, which are spread by droplet infection, are also especially hazardous in the operative period.

Other patients are the long stay patients, who are those who suffer from a serious illness like carcinoma of the larynx where the tissues are more susceptible to infections. So also in these patients, operative procedures such as tracheostomy provide an alternative route for colonization and ultimately infection by hospital strains of *Pseudomonas aeruginosa* and other gram-negative bacilli. The mode of spread in these cases is usually by contact. Medical apparatus such as suction tubing or ventilators may also be important.

Apart from these, many patients with community-acquired infections may be admitted to the wards, further increasing the risks. These include patients with tonsillitis, quinsy, or acute otitis media (caused by streptococci, pneumococci, hemophilis or staphylococci) and patients with chronic external otitis (often heavily colonized with gram-negative bacilli, staphylococci, yeasts or fungii).

PREVENTION OF INFECTION

- Isolation facilities are essential in the ENT department:
  - For isolation of infected cases.
  - To protect those that are particularly susceptible.
- Long stay patients with tracheostomy should be ideally nursed in separate rooms.
- Patients with streptococcal infections, if admitted at all, must be in a room separate from the patients who require operation.
- Children admitted for tonsillectomy and found to have pyrexia, are best isolated, or as a common practice sent home.
- Patients with chronic ear disease do not require isolation, although the organisms present are often highly resistant to antibiotics, and care should be taken to prevent contact spread, particularly by fomites. However, most of these patients are treated as outpatients.
- Children and adults should be preferably in separate wards.

CARE DURING OPERATIVE PROCEDURES

Most of the operations on the ear, nose and throat require incision through colonized mucous membranes and surface disinfection is therefore required, but these may pose considerable difficulties. Some of these agents may damage the membranes, or may lead to fistula formation if they gain access to the middle ear.

Patients who require operation in the middle ear may require intensive outpatient treatment of infection if present. At the time of operation, many surgeons use 1% aqueous cetremide as membrane disinfectant, but this agent has poor activity against *Pseudomonas aeruginosa*, and an alternative (e.g. an aqueous solution of iodine or idophor) should be considered.

Care of tracheostomy is described in the section on intensive care units. The other hospital hygiene problems are the same as in any other ward. The apparatus used for examination of patients or other minor procedures should be sterile. Nasal and aural specula should be used on one patient only and then decontaminated or sterilized. Decontamination of small items can be done in the clinic or ward itself. This can be done by boiling in water for 5–10 minutes, or less desirably by immersion for 5 minutes in 70% alcohol. However sterilization by autoclave is preferable. In each case, the specula should be allowed to dry and be stored covered in the dry state. Tracheostomy tubes, suction catheters and similar apparatus must be supplied sterile from CSSD (central sterile supply department) or commercial presterilized packs can be used. Most laryngoscopes are capable of withstanding autoclave temperatures and so can be autoclaved. Whereas fiberoptic bronchoscopes are usually disinfected with glutaraldehyde.

Wiping with 70% ethyl alcohol is the most effective method of disinfection of operating microscopes.

Risks to and from the personnel in the department are similar to those in other wards, however there are two important infections, which need mention. One is streptococcal infection, which is especially hazardous in the ENT department, so staff with sore throats should be excluded. Second is tuberculous laryngitis, which can lead to dissemination of many tubercle bacilli into the air, so that a tuberculin test, and routine health checks for nurses and doctors working in the unit is essential. Tuberculin negative staff should not be employed.

PEDIATRIC DEPARTMENT

SPECIAL PROBLEMS OF INFECTION IN PEDIATRIC DEPARTMENT[8]

Children from a special group, as they are easily susceptible to community-acquired infections, as many of them have not developed immunity to the common infections and many a times children who are suffering from one of these infections or who are in the incubating phase may be admitted to the wards. Some of these infections (like respiratory virus infections, severe gastroenteritis and infected skin lesions) are difficult to keep under control.

Most of the children's ward also has patients who are particularly susceptible (like those with malnutrition, blood disorders, or receiving steroids). So also the use of invasive techniques has been associated with more infections, including the emergence of coagulase-negative staphylococci.

Organisms involved in cross-infections are many, like bacteria which include group A streptococci, enteropathogenic *E. coli*, *Campylobacter* species, viruses like respiratory syncytial virus (RSV), varicella-zoster virus, gastroenteritis viruses such as rotavirus, fungi, such as *Candida albicans*, dermatophytes that affect scalp, and even skin or intestinal parasites (e.g. *Cryptosporidium*), *Pseudomonas aeruginosa*, *Pseudomonas cepacia* and *Staphylococcus aureus* occasionally cross-infect children suffering from cystic fibrosis. Outbreaks of tuberculosis have occasionally occurred in pediatric wards. Infections are usually contracted from staff. It is safe to isolate children with 'closed TB' as well as 'Open TB', until the source is identified.

Isolation and barrier nursing is particularly important in pediatric departments.

The types of nosocomial infections in children vary depending on the child's age, hospital unit, and instrumentation devices in use. The most common include viral upper and lower respiratory tract infections, gastroenteritis, bloodstream infections, and ventilator-associated pneumonia.[9]

There are many differences between children and adults with respect to nosocomial infections. Factors unique to pediatric patients include differences in the process of care, such as the type and amount of physical contact between patients and health care workers (e.g. feeding and diapering); differences in developmental immunity; congenital anomalies that disrupt anatomic barriers; different sources of infection, such as the maternal genitourinary tract; increased susceptibility to certain pathogens (e.g. varicella-zoster virus, parvovirus); and social interactions that may increase the transmission of microbes, such as sibling visitation, playroom exposures, and pets used for therapeutic purposes.[9]

The types of pathogens and sites of nosocomial infection also differ from those in adults. Viral infections of the upper respiratory and GI systems are the most common type of nosocomial infection among patients hospitalized on the general pediatric ward; in contrast, urinary tract infections are the most common type of nosocomial infection in adult patients. Among neonatal and pediatric ICU patients, the bloodstream is the most common site of nosocomial infection, followed by the lower respiratory tract; among adult ICU patients, the lower respiratory tract is the most common site.[9]

Nosocomial transmission of micro-organisms occurs by three main routes: contact, droplet, and airborne. Contact transmission may occur by either direct contact or indirect contact via an inanimate object. Agents spread via droplet transmission include *B. pertussis*, group A *Streptococcus*, *Neisseria meningitidis*, adenovirus, and influenza virus. Special air handling and ventilation are not required to prevent droplet transmission because droplets do not remain suspended in the air for prolonged periods. Measles virus, varicella-zoster virus, and *Mycobacterium tuberculosis* are spread via airborne transmission. Because organisms carried by airborne transmission may be spread over long distances and remain suspended in air for long periods, special ventilation and air handling are required.[9]

There are two levels of isolation precautions recommended by the Hospital Infection Control Practices Advisory Committee: standard and transmission-based. Standard precautions are recommended for the care of all hospitalized patients. Transmission-based precautions are recommended for patients with suspected or documented infections with highly transmissible agents for which measures in addition to standard precautions are necessary to prevent nosocomial transmission.[9]

RSV is the most common cause of lower respiratory tract infection in young infants, infecting 50–70% of children during their first year of life. During community outbreaks, RSV is a common cause of nosocomial infection. RSV survives readily on environmental surfaces. RSV can be cultured from hands for up to 25 minutes after contact with contaminated surfaces. RSV RNA was detected in 63% of patients' room air samples. The ubiquitous nature of RSV, along with its prolonged survival, explains its threat as a nosocomial pathogen.[9]

The spread of RSV occurs through contact with infected secretions, either from direct contact with contaminated surfaces or by large-particle aerosols. Respiratory secretions are the only body fluid that contains infectious virus. Current CDC guidelines recommend contact precautions for hospitalized patients with RSV infection. The efficacy of several additional strategies for the prevention of nosocomial RSV infection has been studied, including gown and glove barrier precautions and aggressive screening and cohorting on admission.[9]

RSV is easily inactivated by a variety of dishwashing detergents, antibacterial soaps, 1:10 bleach solutions, and 70% ethanol. Alcohol hand disinfectant is effective against enveloped viruses but has not been tested specifically against RSV. Thus, frequent cleaning of environmental surfaces, toys, and hands with commonly used disinfectants should effectively kill RSV.[9]

Rotavirus is found in 50% of stool specimens from children hospitalized with gastroenteritis and is the most common cause of nosocomial gastroenteritis, causing up to 43% of cases. Rotavirus infection presents as explosive, watery, copious diarrhea, with or without vomiting and fever. The most severe disease occurs in children younger than 2 years, with hospitalization rates reaching 5% in this age group. From 24–50% of children younger than 2 years test positive during rotavirus season. Most children have serologic evidence of infection by 2 years of age. Recurrent infection is common, and 30–50% of adult contacts acquire infection. Rotavirus is shed in the stool for several days preceding symptoms, and shedding may persist for 10–12 days; however, shedding can persist for more than a month in immunocompromised children.[9]

Rotavirus is transmitted via the fecal-oral route. During periods of viral shedding, stool may contain up to 100 billion viral particles per gram of feces. The infectious dose for the small intestine is only 10 viral particles per milliliter. Rotavirus survives for up to 7 months on surfaces, for weeks in water, and for up to 4 hours on human hands. It is resistant to many antibacterial agents. During one rotavirus outbreak in a child-care center, 19% of inanimate objects tested had detectable rotavirus RNA. Thus, there are many potential reservoirs. In addition to fecal-oral spread, rotavirus may be spread by the respiratory route. The evidence to suggest small-particle aerosol spread includes detection of rotavirus RNA in air samples from patients' rooms, detection of rotavirus in respiratory secretions from patients with pneumonia, and respiratory symptoms and otitis media in up to 50% of patients with rotavirus infection.[9]

Current CDC recommendations for hospitalized patients with rotavirus infection include contact isolation along with standard precautions. Rotavirus is effectively destroyed by routine cleaning of toys and surfaces with preparations that contain either chlorhexidine or a quaternary ammonium agent in combination with a high proportion of ethanol (70% weight per volume), ethanol 95% by volume, Lysol disinfectant spray, or bleach (1:10 solution). When investigators compared different compounds, they found virus could not be transmitted to hands from surfaces cleaned with bleach, phenolic acid, or disinfectant spray. A glutaraldehyde-containing solution and povidone iodine also reduce the viral inoculum by 99.9%. Plain soap, however, is ineffective against rotavirus. Outbreaks of rotavirus have occurred on pediatric wards where routine cleaning of toys did not occur.[9]

B. pertussis is a gram-negative bacillus that causes a prolonged, severe respiratory illness in unimmunized children and young infants, and whooping cough and prolonged coughing illness in adults. Only 30–50% of young children with pertussis have the classic paroxysmal cough and inspiratory whoop. Young infants may present with apnea, bradycardia, and poor feeding. Of children who die of pertussis, 75% are younger than 1 year, and most are 2 to 4 months old. The incubation period is typically 6–10 days (range, 5–21 days).[9]

Vaccination provides protection against disease for 2–3 years; by 10–12 years after vaccination, minimal immunity remains. Moreover, infection does not confer lifelong immunity. Attack rates among household contacts can be decreased by the administration of a macrolide. Vaccination of adults against pertussis is not currently recommended; however, vaccination of health care workers to prevent nosocomial transmission of pertussis may be recommended after further studies are performed.[9]

Hospitalized patients with documented or suspected pertussis should be placed on droplet precautions in a private room until they have received 5 days of treatment with erythromycin. Household and hospital contacts should receive 14 days of erythromycin treatment.[9]

The incidence of nosocomial infection among pediatric ICU patients has been reported to range from 2.6–25%, with a range of 15–20% in neonatal ICUs. The most common site of nosocomial infection in pediatric and neonatal ICU patients is the bloodstream, followed by the lower respiratory tract.

In children, it is often difficult to meet the criteria for catheter-related bloodstream infection (BSI) using comparative colony counts between central and peripheral cultures, because frequently only 1 set of blood cultures is obtained in order to minimize iatrogenic blood loss, particularly in neonates. Nosocomial BSIs in pediatric and neonatal ICU patients are most frequently caused by coagulase-negative staphylococci, *Staphylococcus aureus*, *Candida* species, and *Enterobacter* species.[9]

The diagnosis of VAP is particularly difficult to make. Biopsies may be indicated in the critically ill child in whom pneumonia is suspected, but negative results should be interpreted cautiously. Cultures of endotracheal aspirates may be used, recognizing that catheters may become contaminated with oropharyngeal flora and thus may not reflect lower respiratory tract microbiology but rather upper tract colonization. Organisms most commonly isolated from endotracheal aspirates of pediatric ICU patients with VAP include *Pseudomonas aeruginosa*, *Klebsiella pneumoniae*, *S. aureus*, and *Haemophilus influenzae*; in neonatal ICU patients, the most commonly isolated organisms are *S. aureus*, coagulase-negative staphylococci, *P. aeruginosa*, and *Enterococcus* species.[9]

Risk factors for nosocomial infections in pediatric ICU patients include parenteral nutrition and use of antimicrobial therapy for more than 10 days. Length of stay, device utilization ratio, postoperative status, immune dysfunction, use of H_2-receptor blockers, and Pediatric Risk of Mortality score (a weighted severity-of-illness score based on 17 physiologic variables) have all been associated with increased odds of infection developing.[9]

Nosocomial infection is common in the neonatal ICU, with an overall incidence of 15–20%. BSIs account for approximately 50% of nosocomial infections in this population, and nearly 90% are associated with central venous catheters. The lower respiratory tract and the urinary tract are the next most common sites (13% each). Nosocomial infection rates are highest in very low-birth-weight infants, with 40–60% of patients with birth weights of less than 1100 g affected. Gestational age is also correlated with nosocomial infection risk.[9]

Risk factors for infection in neonatal ICU patients include the presence of a central venous catheter, use of total parenteral nutrition, use of mechanical ventilation, prior receipt of antibiotics, and low birth weight. In another study, the overall nosocomial infection rate correlated with length of stay and device.[9]

Viral pneumonitis caused by RSV, parainfluenza virus, varicella-zoster virus, or adenovirus is associated with high mortality in neonates and other immunocompromised patients; therefore, careful screening of visitors for respiratory symptoms and varicella exposure (within 10–21 days) is prudent. Health care workers should receive annual influenza vaccinations. If they have viral respiratory symptoms, they should not care for neonates, patients with congenital heart disease, or immunocompromised patients.[9]

Within 96 hours of exposure to varicella, susceptible patients at risk for severe disease should receive varicella-zoster immune globulin (VZIG). Exposures that warrant VZIG prophylaxis include occupying the same 2- to 4-bed room, face-to-face contact, and visit by a contagious person. High-risk newborns should also receive VZIG. Patients at risk include hospitalized premature infants of less than 28 weeks of gestation or weighing 1000 g or less, irrespective of maternal varicella history; hospitalized premature infants of 28 weeks of gestation or more without maternal history or serologic evidence of prior varicella; newborns whose mother had onset of varicella within 5 days before or 48 hours after delivery; immunocompromised persons without prior history of varicella; and susceptible pregnant women.[9]

Visitation of healthy newborns and chronically-ill children by their siblings occurs frequently on pediatric wards. Guidelines for sibling visitation include assessment of the visiting child's health status by a trained health professional before the visit to evaluate for recent exposure to highly communicable diseases; supervision of the sibling's activity during the visit; and limiting the sibling to the patient's room only. Any child with fever, acute respiratory or GI symptoms, or recent varicella exposure (10–21 days prior) should be excluded. Siblings' hands should be carefully washed before and after contact with the hospitalized family member.[9]

PREVENTION OF INFECTION

General Measures

- Hand hygiene remains the single most effective measure.
- Adherence to isolation guidelines, catheter care guidelines,
- Varicella and influenza vaccination recommendations
- Screening visitors and health care workers for illness
- Enough isolation facilities should be provided in pediatric wards.
- Because of risk of gastroenteritis, there should not be more than four infants in one room.
- Ideally, there should be cubicles with only one or two cots.
- Adequate washing facilities should be provided in each cubicle.
- Each ward must have a separate examination room.
- There should be beds available for the parents to sleep in the hospital.

Outbreaks of rotavirus infection and RSV are particularly common in pediatric wards. Handwashing is important in the control of these infections. Rotavirus infection is associated with heavy environmental contamination, and the large number of organisms may be difficult to remove from hands. The use of gloves is recommended when handling excreta or contaminated material. An alcoholic handrub following hand washing is also effective. Prevention of RSV infection to the staff is also important, and in addition to hand washing, staff should be advised to avoid touching the nose and eyes. The use of goggles that cover the nose and eyes of staff has been associated with a reduction in infection in USA, although the acceptability of this device is still uncertain.

Infections at intravenous sites often caused by coagulase-negative staphylococci are mainly associated with central venous catheterization and parenteral feeding. To prevent this efficient skin disinfection and care of the site is important.

Parents may be allowed to visit their children frequently, as this does not significantly affect the infection rates. However, in case the parents are suffering from any infection, they should consult the ward sister/doctor in charge, so as to protect other children within the unit where resistance may be poor. So also their (siblings) with minor respiratory infection (however trivial) should be barred from visiting the child admitted, as these may be prodromal signs of measles.

If any of the visitors to the hospital develops a transmissible infection within 7 days of visiting, or a patient develops infection within the week of discharge, it should be notified to the staff of that ward. This enables susceptible contacts to be traced.

Parents nursing children with gastroenteritis should wear gowns or plastic aprons, and hand-washing facilities should be available to them.

Visiting of children with dangerous infections, such as diphtheria, poliomyelitis, and meningococcal meningitis should be restricted to the parents for the first 48 hours. Visitors of infectious patients should avoid contact with other patients.

Crockery and cutlery need to be clean, it can be domestically washed, but washing machine at 70–80°C is preferable, and is essential in isolation wards.

Toilet Arrangement

As intestinal infections are very common in children, the toilet areas should be maintained with a high standard cleanliness. The toilet seat should be washed daily and if required more frequently. The toilet seat and cistern handle should be sprayed with 70% alcohol or with hypochlorite solution after each patient especially during outbreaks of viral gastroenteritis. But even more important is proper hand washing. Bedpans should be washed with hot water capable of destroying vegetative forms of bacteria.

Laundry

Used napkins are put in plastic bags and sealed for transport with a label "Used Napkins", depending on the laundry policy. Disposable napkins are a standard practice in developed countries.

Personnel

Staff may acquire communicable diseases from patients, if they are not immune, and may in turn pass it on to the other patients and visitors. In developed countries an important infection, which is passed on in this way, is Rubella. Therefore, in those countries screening of staff of both sexes for immunity to Rubella is important, they have to be immunized if they are not immune, because of number of pregnant women who visit children in the hospital.

Acquisition of *Salmonella* and *Shigella* by the nursing staff, have also lead to outbreaks of infection in the hospital. Herpes simplex infection in attendants may produce a variety of lesions and may cause severe infections in children. Staff with herpetic lesions should not handle babies.

SURVEILLANCE SYSTEM

A list of patients with infection admitted to the ward or acquired in the ward is useful in the investigation if there is spread of infection. The infections most commonly recorded are those due to *Shigella,* rotavirus and other gastrointestinal pathogens, *MRSA,* group A streptococci, respiratory syncitial virus (RSV) and the common infectious diseases (particularly chickenpox).

DERMATOLOGICAL WARDS

INTRODUCTION, SOURCES AND TRANSMISSION OF INFECTION[10]

Usually patients with skin lesions are not very ill, but their skin condition may lead to some mental stress. If source isolation is considered, it may be explained to the patient that with certain exceptions, skin conditions like eczema and psoriasis is in itself not infectious and will not spread to the rest of the family or visitors. But in case of septic lesions like impetigo, there is a definite risk of transfer to healthy subjects.

In dermatological wards, patients often have general desquamating lesions which are colonized heavily with *Staphylococcus aureus.* These patients are heavy dispersers, and cross infection is frequent, though these staphylococci rarely cause clinical sepsis.

However when such a patient is admitted to the surgical ward, he may be responsible for widespread nasal colonization and wound sepsis. These strains are often resistant to two or more antibiotics, and MRSA is a particular hazard. Children admitted with clinically apparent staphylococcal lesions like impetigo, not only spread the infection to other children, but can also lead to pyogenic lesions in the staff. These strains are usually acquired outside the hospital initially, and are resistant to penicillin only. Some of the infections are caused by b haemolytic streptococci (which are often associated with *Staphylococcus aureus*) and may similarly spread to other patients. Cross infection with gram-negative bacilli (e.g. *Pseudomonas aeruginosa* and *Proteus* species) is also common in dermatological wards, and these organisms are usually found in varicose ulcers, but clinical sepsis is unusual.

Candida infections are also seen, but cross infection with Candida is less evident. Patients with dermatophyte infections are not usually admitted to the hospital, but the risk of cross-infection exists (e.g. tinea corporis and *Tinea pedis*, which may not be clinically obvious). Transmission of *Tinea corporis* can also spread in children in the wards like it spreads in schools.

The spread of virus infection is not a risk in dermatological wards.

There are quite a few dermatological diseases that can be spread and if proper measures are not applied can result in epidemic of these diseases.

Skin Diseases with Potential for Spread

- Scabies.
- Chickenpox.
- Tinea infections (scalp and skin).
- Pediculosis.
- Measles.
- Warts.

Types of Skin Infections[11]

- Primary skin infections.
- Infections secondary to irritation, allergy or hypersensitivity are common.
- Skin infections reflecting systemic disorders also occur.
- By far the most common organism involved is *Staphylococcus aureus*, followed by *Streptococcus pyogenes*.

Factors associated with the spread of skin infections include:

- Close skin-to-skin contact.
- Openings in the skin such as cuts or abrasions.
- Contaminated items and surfaces.
- Crowded living conditions.
- Poor hygiene.

Staphylococcus aureus, often are bacteria commonly carried on the skin or in the nose of healthy people. Approximately 25–30% of the population is colonized (when bacteria are present, but not causing an infection) in the nose.

Most of these skin infections are minor (such as pimples and boils) and can be treated with local antibiotics.

However, bacteria (staph and strep) can cause serious infections (such as cellulitis. erysepilas, surgical wound infections, bloodstream infections).

Epidemic of pityriasis versicolor have been seen commonly during war.

Tinea capitis, pediculosis capitis continues to be a major problem in USA schools.

In our educational institutions, scabies is a major problem. Recently loads of children are coming with pityriasis versicolor and other fungal infections from swimming pools.

CONTROL OF INFECTION[11]

Purpose

The purpose of infection control is to reduce the occurrence or spread of skin infections spread by:

- Human to human contact.
- Animal to human contact.
- Human contact with an infected surface. (Pityriasis versicolor from pools).
- Airborne transmission through tiny droplets of infectious agents suspended in the air.

Staphylococcal infection in dermatological wards spreads both by contact and air. The environment may also be so heavily contaminated that prevention of cross-infection is difficult, however, some effective measures can certainly be taken:

1. Children with clinical sepsis must be isolated in separate rooms, whether in general or dermatological wards.
2. Patients with diffuse desquamating lesions should be kept in separate room if admitted to general hospital wards.
3. General hospitals should if possible have wards kept solely for dermatological patients.
4. When isolation is required, it must be complete (i.e. patients should not leave the ward to visit other patients).

Other Measures to be Taken

- Clean your hands. You, your family, and others in close contact should wash their hands frequently with: Soap and warm water. Use an alcohol-based hand sanitizer especially after changing the bandage or touching the infected wound. Avoid contact with other people's wounds or bandages.
- Cover your wound. Keep wounds (infected eczemas and cellulitis) that are draining or have pus covered with clean, dry bandages. Pus from infected wounds can contain staph and MRSA, so keeping the infection covered will help prevent the spread to others.
- Do not share personal items.
- Avoid sharing personal items such as towels, washcloths, razors, clothing, or uniforms that may have had contact with the infected wound or bandage.
- Wash sheets, towels, and clothes that become soiled with water and laundry detergent. Drying clothes in a hot dryer, rather than air-drying also helps kill bacteria.

Hand Care

Hands should be washed:

- Before and after treating each patient.

Health care workers who have exudative lesions or weeping dermatitis, fungal (Nails), herpes infection should refrain from all direct patient care and from handling patient-care equipment until condition resolves.

Immunization/Infection Control

- Mandatory immunizations should be made available to all healthcare personnel.
- Guidelines for postexposure evaluation (scabies, chickenpox, herpes) should be followed. Prophylaxis and follow-up after exposure.

Surveillance

The surveillance process should:

- Define the population at risk.
- Surveillance data must be analyzed appropriately and used:
  - To monitor skin infections
  - To improve skin infections in future.

Employee Health

- At the time of employment, all facility personnel should be evaluated for conditions relating to communicable skin diseases (Leprosy, Scabies).
- The evaluation should include:
  - Medical history.
  - Immunization status.

Education and Training of Healthcare Workers

- Educational programs should meet the needs of dermatology.

- Resources should be provided for continuing professional education.

Threat of Emerging Infectious Diseases

- Many new contagious diseases have been identified, such as AIDS, Ebola, and hantavirus.
- Increased travel between continents makes the worldwide spread of disease a bigger concern than before.
- Additionally, many common skin/infectious diseases have become resistant to treatments.

Precautionary Measures

- Avoid areas with a lot of insects, (leishmania, pruritis, urticaria).
- Be cautious around with: Wild or unfamiliar animals, animals that are unusually aggressive. Do not purchase exotic animals as pets.
- Find out about infectious diseases when you make travel plans. Advisory on Schistosomiasis for Egypt. Leishmaniasis/leprosy for India, Pakistan. Fungal diseases in subtropical regions. Cutaneous larva migrans in south America and subtropical zones.
- Do not engage in unprotected sex and avoid intravenous drug use to protect from Syphilis, Gonorrhea, Genital herpes and AIDS for Far East and India especially.

Conclusion

- Personnel health and safety measures should be adopted.
- Clinicians should have the know how regarding various skin diseases thus enabling them to diagnose/manage and prevent the spread of such infections.
- Health education
  - In schools.
  - In higher educational institutions.
  - Information in print media.
  - Through electronic media radio/TV.
  - By organizing seminars/symposiums.
  - National and international conferences in the country.

  Infection control courses to be imparted as curriculum in medical education.
  - General practitioners.
  - Doctors, nursing staff and paramedics working in hospitals and primary health care centers.
- Special monitoring for:
  - Fungal/bacterial/viral infections, scabies and venereal diseases. In religious festivals and cultural festivals.
  - In institutions with large boarding facilities.
  - In army barracks, police quarters, prisons.

  Periodic, skin examination for various dermatological problems: Scabies, warts, tinea infections is important: In hospitals, schools/colleges, nursing homes, child care centers, orphanages.

DRESSING TECHNIQUES

Patients with wounds or ulcers should be treated as in general surgical wards, using sterile dressing (SSD pack) and no touch technique. It is preferable to have a special room for performing surgical techniques like biopsies. Dressing of patients with non-surgical patients is different, as it is not necessarily an aseptic procedure.

1. Dressing rooms should be adjacent to the bathroom.
2. Dressing room should have exhaust fans.
3. Dressing material used to cover broken skin should be sterilized.
4. Large bags should be provided for disposal of contaminated dressing.
5. Dressing should be done with sterile instruments or gloves as far as possible. Creams and ointments should be applied when possible with a gloved hand.

6. Staff should wash their hands thoroughly with soap or an antiseptic detergent preparation and water after handling each patient.
7. Staff should wear plastic disposable aprons, which should be discarded, at the end of each dressing.
8. Floors should be cleaned with vacuum cleaner that is capable of removing skin scales.
9. Special attention should be paid to the disinfection of baths and washbowls after each use.

In general, cleaning methods and techniques are similar to these recommended for containing infected patients.

ANTIBIOTIC TREATMENT

Resistance to antibiotics is common in patients with skin disease because of large populations of bacteria on the skin. Antibiotic treatment (especially topical treatment) should be avoided whenever possible, and other antimicrobial agents should be used if they are available or suitable (e.g. silver nitrate, chlorhexidine). Resistance emerges readily to erythromycin, lincomycin (or clindamycin) and fusidic acid, and their use should be controlled.

Neomycin and bacitracin are useful topical antibiotics, although resistance of *Staphylococcus aureus* and hypersensitivity to neomycin are common. Gentamycin is a useful systemic antibiotic and should not be used topically in hospital. The combination of neomycin and chlorhexidine in a topical preparation may reduce the likelihood of resistance emerging. Mupirocin is particularly effective in removing *Staphylococcus aureus* from carriage sites and eczematous lesions. However resistant strains are now emerging, and its use should preferably restricted to treatment of MRSA carriers. If applied to skin, its use (and often topical antibiotic agents) should be limited to a period of 7 days.

OINTMENTS AND OTHER MEDICAMENTS

Patients with widespread lesions of the skin are susceptible to infections, and since large amounts of topical medicaments are often applied, care must be taken that the applicant is free from pathogenic bacteria. Tubes should be used whenever possible for creams and ointments. In wards, ointments or creams should be supplied for individual patient. If jars are used, ointment should never be removed by fingers. Jars or bottles should be thoroughly cleaned (preferably disinfected) and dried before refilling.

NEUROSURGERY DEPARTMENT

INTRODUCTION

Infections occurring in the neurosurgery departments may occur in different ways and the meninges are particularly susceptible to infection. Postoperative central nervous system infections range from 5–7%.[12] These infections can manifest themselves as wound, meningitis, subdural empyema, bone-flap infection and or brain or epidural abscesses.

CAUSES OF INFECTION IN NEUROSURGERY

Infection may be caused by:[13,14]

- Contamination occurring at operation or during a lumbar or ventricular puncture, by gram-negative bacilli of low pathogenicity, as well as by the usual organisms (e.g. *Pseudomonas aeruginosa, Acinetobacter* species, *Serratia marcescens* and *Flavobacteria*).
- These opportunistic organisms have also caused infection because of inadequate sterilization or maintenance of sterility of instruments or water applied topically.
- Organisms normally present on the skin (e.g. coagulase-negative staphylococci),

which is usually of low pathogenicity may also cause low-grade infections with Spitz-Holter valves and other prosthesis.

- *Staphylococcus aureus* is the commonest pathogen isolated from wound infections. MRSA is an emerging multi-resistant pathogen.
- Infections may also be transmitted on the hands of staff from infected patients, or following the use of contaminated hand-creams, soaps or detergents.
- Inadequate cleaning of patient's skin preoperatively, or use of contaminated shaving equipment may also be followed by infection.
- As in case of other departments, infection may be caused by indwelling catheters, tracheostomy or endotracheal intubation.
- Patients of ear infection may be admitted to wards if infection spreads to mastoid or meninges.
- Unconscious patients may acquire chest infection or bedsores.
- Although cerebral abscesses are usually endogenous in origin, hospital strains of gram-negative bacilli and *Staphylococcus aureus* are likely to spread in the ward and may be acquired in the nasal or intestinal flora, becoming a potential source of endogenous infection, unless effective control measures are employed.

RISK FACTORS IN NEUROSURGERY[15,16]

Risk factors in neurosurgery are:

1. Multiple operations.
2. Prologed preoperative hospitalization.
3. Large size of incision.
4. CSF leak.
5. Duration of surgery.
6. Altered sensorium.
7. Age.
8. Use of corticosteroids.
9. Diabetes.

PREVENTION OF INFECTION[13,14]

The important measures of prevention of infection in the neurosurgical units are:

- Isolation and barrier nursing particularly in case of patients with pseudomonas or multi-resistant staphylococcal infection.
- Dressing of wounds exposing the meninges should be done in the operating theater, if not in a plenum ventilated room.
- Patient's own single-bedded room, if the facilities are adequate, may be suitable for many of the routine procedures.
- Special wards are required for intensive care treatment, including patients with tracheostomies.
- Procedures like lumbar puncture and catheterization may be performed in non-specialized wards.
- Preoperative shaving should be performed on the day of operation to avoid the possibility of small scratches or excoriations, which sometimes occur and may become heavily colonized.
- Shaving of either head or pubic hair for vertebral angiography should be completed before the disinfection of scalp or skin.
- Shaving brushes should not be used.
- Razors should be sterilized or disinfected and individual guaze swabs should be used to apply shaving cream.
- Shaving cream if used should contain an antiseptic cream to prevent the growth of organisms that might cause infection.
- A Povidone-iodine shampoo or chlorhexidine detergent may also be used before shaving.
- Subsequent procedure in the operation theater can be done by 0.5% alcoholic-chlorhexidine
- All equipments and instruments, etc. used for various procedures, e.g. lumbar puncture, catheterization, wound dressing and tracheostomy should be autoclaved.
- Particular care should be taken to avoid contamination of lotions.

- If aspiration of effusion from a craniotomy wound is required, insert the needle through intact skin and not through the suture line.
- Organisms may enter the blood stream from monitoring equipment, and set up infection at the operation site. The equipment should be regularly disinfected or sterilized preferably by heat.

Antibiotic prophylaxis reduces the infection rate in craniotomy operations. Cloxacillin, a cephalosporin or vancomycin with or without gentamicin, appear to be effective and are commonly given for 24 hours.

REFERENCES

1. Ayliffee GAJ, Fraise AP, Geddes AM, Mitchell K. Control of Hospital Infection—A Practical Handbook, 4th edition. Oxford University Press, New York; 2000.pp.309-12.
2. Das A, Dey AK, et al. Nosocomial ocular infection—a perspective study. Journal of Indian Medical Association (JIMA). 2003;101(8).
3. Outbreaks of Postoperative Bacterial Endophthalmitis caused by intrinsically contaminated ophthalmic solutions—Thailand, 1992, Canada, 1993 CDC. MMWR Weekly. 1996;45(23);491-4. From net.
4. The prophylactic use of vancomycin for intraocular surgery—a joint statement of the American Academy of Ophthalmology and the Centre for Disease Control and Prevent ionht tp://www.aao.org/aao/ education/library/ information/vancomycin. efm from net.
5. Control of Infection in Ophthalmic Practice. Community Eye Health. 2003;16(47):40-41. Accessed on 15th July 2015.
6. UTMB On-line Documentation Subject: Healthcare Epidemiology Policies and Procedures Topic: 02.12 - Ophthalmology. Accessed on 15th July 2015 from www.utmb.edu/policies_and_procedures/4229967.
7. Ayliffee GAJ, Fraise AP, Geddes AM, Mitchell K. Control of Hospital Infection—A Practical Handbook, 4th edition. Oxford University Press, New York; 2000.pp.312-3.
8. George R. Paediatric Departments, Chapter 16. In: Ayliffee GAJ, Fraise AP, Geddes AM, Mitchell K (Eds). Control of Hospital Infection. A Practical Handbook, 4th edition. Oxford University Press, New York; 2000.pp.314-6.
9. Elward AM, McGann KA. Steps to Reduce Nosocomial Infections in Children. Infect Med. 2002;19(9). Accessed on 18/7/2015 from: www.medscape.com/viewarticle/442779-9.
10. Ayliffee GAJ, Fraise AP, Geddes AM, Mitchell K. Control of Hospital Infection—A Practical Handbook, 4th edition. Oxford University Press, New York; 2000.pp.306-9.
11. Samdani AJ. Role of infection control in dermatology. Available at www.slideshare.net/icsp/role-of-infection-control-in - dermatology. Accessed on 25th July 2015.
12. Sturm LK. Neurosurgical surgical site infection: Rates and Prevention Strategies. Int J Infect Control. 2009;v5:i2. Accessed from www.ijic.info/article/download/3705/3162. Accessed on 21/7/2015.
13. Ayliffee GAJ, Fraise AP, Geddes AM, Mitchell K. Control of Hospital Infection—A Practical Handbook, 4th edition. Oxford University Press, New York; 2000.pp.308-9.
14. Gentz NM, Godofsky EW. Nosocomial central nervous system infections. In: Mayhall CG (Ed). Hospital Epidemiology and Infection Control, Baltimore, MD; Williams and Wilkins; 1996.p.246.
15. Buang SS, Haspani MS. Risk factors for neurosurgical site infections after a neurosurgical procedure: a prospective observational study at Hospital Kuala Lumpur. Med J Malaysia. 2012;67(4):393-8. Accessed from www.e-mjm.org/2012/v67m4/surgical-site-infection.pdf on 21/7/2015.
16. Bellusse GC, et al. Risk factors for surgical site infection in neurosurgery. Acta Paul Enferm. 2015;28(1):66-73. Accessed from www.scielo.br/pdf/ape/v28n1/en_1982-0194- ape-028-001.pdf on 21/7/2015.

Chapter 21

Infection Control in Ancillary Units

Chapter Outline

Microbiology and Pathology Laboratories
- Introduction
- Special Risks of Infection
- Prevention of Infection
- Transport of Specimens
- Procedures within the Laboratory
- Immunization of Laboratory Staff
- Training and Instructions for Staff
- Precautions Against Laboratory Infections
- Infections in Containment Category 3 Laboratories
- Fungi

Radiology and Radiotherapy
- Introduction and Principles of Control
- Care and Control of Infection in Radiotherapy

Postmortem Room and Mortuary
- Introduction and Causes of Infection
- Prevention of Infection

MICROBIOLOGY AND PATHOLOGY LABORATORIES

INTRODUCTION

The advisory committee on dangerous pathogens has classified organisms into four hazards and containment categories.[1]

Category 1 includes agents unlikely to cause human disease, and requires no special precautions. Category 2 includes most organisms isolated in clinical laboratories and requires good microbiological practice. Category 3 includes organisms of special risk to laboratory workers (e.g. *Salmonella typhi*, *Mycobacterium tuberculosis*) and requires special containment facilities. Category

4 includes organisms that are extremely hazardous to laboratory workers and which may cause serious epidemic disease (e.g. Lassa, Ebola, Marburg viruses) which require particularly stringent containment. It should be kept in mind that Category 3 organisms may be isolated in routine laboratories, and on identification, subsequent work on them must be carried out in the appropriate containment category. Requirements may be modified for handling samples from patients with hepatitis B or HIV antibody, but work in a cabinet may be preferred. These viruses are transferred by contact with blood and not by airborne route.

Extensive recommendations have been made regarding these codes and guidelines, which demand, a lot from the laboratory workers, as well as from those who design and direct the laboratory. It includes all the necessary precautions, which need to be taken in diagnostic (clinical) laboratories. In spite of this, no one can prevent infections due to negligence or poor technique of the laboratory worker. Everyone who works in a laboratory must develop habits of safe and careful technique.

However, precautions against laboratory-acquired infections should be reasonable. They should be based on scientific or clinical evidence. For example, ventilated rooms cannot be expected to influence the transmission of blood-borne infections such as HBV or HIV or organisms transferred by fecal-oral route such as *Salmonella typhi.*

SPECIAL RISKS OF INFECTION[2]

There are several ways by which infection can be spread in the laboratories. Infection may be carried to the patients from the laboratory by the laboratory staff collecting specimens from wards or outpatient departments, and may also be infected by procedures performed by the technician involving transfer of microbes from one patient to another.

Laboratory staff is at risk both from the patients and from the specimens of biological material and cultures examined in the laboratory. Risk to laboratory staff from biological specimens is more likely to have serious consequences. Many of the risks are known and precautions can be taken to prevent them, but infections can also arise from unsuspected sources (e.g. request form contaminated by feces and handled by clerical staff, or serum containing HBV examined in microbiology or pathology laboratories).

There are different routes by which infections are acquired in the laboratory. It may be due to infected aerosols or sprays generated while pipetting or pouring liquids in the laboratory, which may be inhaled by the workers or HBV or HIV may enter through skin abrasions. Tuberculosis has also been important in hospital and laboratory infections. Recently such infections have become less common as a result of better training in safe working. HIV, HBV and HCV may also be transferred to laboratory workers from clinical samples, but since it is a dangerous infection, a lot of care is essential.

In general, it is not usually a specimen which is already known to be infective that causes an infection, but one which is not suspected of being dangerous. Some areas such as animal houses, tuberculosis laboratories, and hospital mortuaries are especially hazardous and require special precautions.

PREVENTION OF INFECTION[2]

Risk of infection can be minimized in the following way:

1. All samples should be handled with care, as far as possible wearing disposable gloves.
2. They should be transported in sealed plastic bags.

   The above precautions are necessary, as the diagnosis may not be known until laboratory tests have been completed.
3. Specimens must be received in an area used exclusively for that purpose only.
4. Staff handling the specimens should be adequately trained.

5. A hand washbasin with pedal or elbow taps should be readily available.
6. Appropriate materials and disinfectants for disposal of spillage.
7. Laboratory staff visiting wards must be trained in barrier nursing techniques and must follow very carefully the instructions for handling infected patients.

TRANSPORT OF SPECIMENS[2]

Special attention has to be given to the containers used to transport specimens to the laboratories. The containers should be robust and leak-proof, and transported in trays or boxes which will hold the specimens upright. They may be sealed in plastic bags to keep the forms from contamination. If metal boxes are used for transporting specimens, they should be autoclaved weekly. Staff involved in transport of specimens should be trained to cope with spillage.

PROCEDURES WITHIN THE LABORATORY[2]

While handling specimens attention has to be given to many things, for example:

1. Attention should be given to centrifuge while using it, as it is a possible source of infective aerosols.
2. Infected material such as slides, pipettes should be discarded into jars containing phenolic or chlorine-releasing disinfectant, which is, replaced daily.
3. Plastic pipettes should be used rather than glass to reduce the hazards of trauma when handling. One of the most important measures of reducing risk of blood-borne infection is elimination of glassware.
4. Plastic petri dishes may involve problems of disposal, if possible they should be made safe before removal from the laboratory, and this is best achieved by autoclaving them in a suitable container or stainless steel buckets. The resultant lumps of polyethylene can be handled by the refuse collectors, but they should be kept in sealed plastic bags. The plates should not be discarded without treatment, as they will then be included in the general waste at local refuse sites. Incineration without autoclaving is acceptable provided the work is effectively contained during transport. Of course, there is one disadvantage of incineration of plastic plates that is if they are incinerated in bulk, it may lead to unacceptable level of smoke pollution.
5. Used glass petri dishes should be autoclaved by trained staff before being handled for washing, etc.
6. Other glass containers like bijou bottles containing infective material should be similarly autoclaved before leaving the laboratory, whether they are going to be reprocessed or disposed off.

IMMUNIZATION OF LABORATORY STAFF[2]

The laboratory staff should be immunized against tuberculosis, poliomyelitis and tetanus (female staff should also be offered rubella vaccination preferably after testing the immune status), especially in countries where this infection is common. None of these vaccinations are mandatory except BCG protection for staff members who are tuberculin—negative. They must be excluded from work with material that contains or is likely to contain tubercle bacilli until conversion has taken place.

Hepatitis B vaccine is offered to all laboratory staff handling clinical specimens, or those involved in invasive procedures.

TRAINING AND INSTRUCTIONS FOR STAFF[2]

Staff should be trained in aseptic procedures and methods of handling; this is a part of routine education in the microbiology departments. But in other department like biochemistry and pathology, some basic instructions should be given on methods of spread of infection; aseptic procedures and handling of potentially-infected biological or toxic materials. Relevant documents should be prepared which should be readily available for consultation.

PRECAUTIONS AGAINST LABORATORY INFECTIONS[2]

The following information should be given to the laboratory staff:

Any specimen entering the laboratory may be infectious. Some will certainly contain agents like HBV, HCV, and HIV infection, agents of typhoid, tuberculosis and other infections. So for your own safety, the safety of your family and safety of your colleagues, following instructions should be observed carefully.

General

1. There should be no eating, smoking or drinking in the laboratory.
2. The benches should be kept clean and tidy.
3. Wash your hands thoroughly on leaving the laboratory, before taking food, drink or handling any personal belongings.
4. Also wash hands after handling specimens, after changing tubing or dialyzers or diluters in autoanalyzers and if you think you have contaminated them, wash them thoroughly with soap and water.
5. If contamination with bacterial cultures has occurred, and also in high-risk laboratories, an antiseptic hand washing method should be used. For this a thorough application of 70% alcohol after washing is particularly effective.

Handwashing

This is a very important safeguard. Wear gloves when handling high-risk specimens (or when cleaning spillage). Wash hands after removing gloves.

Cuts and Abrasions[2]

1. If you have a cut or abrasion, immediately wash in running water. Cover it with waterproof protective dressing.
2. If you splash your eye with serum or a culture, wash it thoroughly with saline or tap water and report to the laboratory officer immediately and enter the incident in the accident book. Needlestick injuries must also be entered and immediately reported.

Spilt Specimens—Treatment of Contaminated Area, Floor or Other Surfaces[2]

If there is a spill on the floor, or other surfaces, immediately swab with 2% clear phenolic solution on the areas of contamination or with chlorine-releasing agents containing 10,000 ppm (1%) available chlorine when cleaning up blood or other organic materials that may contain viruses. 1000 ppm (0.1%) is adequate for small amounts of spillage or routine cleaning. Thoroughly covering the spillage with chlorine-releasing agent is also effective. However chlorine-releasing powder or granules should not be used for large amounts of spillage, as excessive amounts of chlorine may be released. Wear gloves when handling contaminated materials or disinfectants.

Pipettes[2]

Avoid mouth suction, use automatic pipettes or ones with rubber bulbs or teats. Discard all Pasteur pipettes and graduated pipettes into 2% phenol or a chlorine-releasing solution—0.25% (2,500 ppm of available chlorine) to cover them completely. It is preferable to use a jar with a screw lid.

Other Equipment[2]

Disposable plastics should be incinerated. Slides should be autoclaved in the discard jars in which they have been placed. Syringes and needles should be discarded into an approved container.

Centrifuging[2]

Only closed centrifuges should be used. They should preferably have sealed buckets, which should be opened only within protective exhaust cabinet if dangerous pathogens are involved.

The centrifuge bowl should be cleaned with a swab immersed in phenol, for viral infection it may be cleaned with 70% alcohol after washing. Wear disposable gloves.

If breakage occurs, autoclave the bucket and its contents and swab the bowl as described above.

White Coats[2]

Actually there should be a plentiful supply of white coats (though not feasible in India) coats must be changed immediately if they become contaminated, all coats should be treated as infected linen in the laundry. Coats known to be contaminated with particularly hazardous pathogens should be autoclaved in the laboratory autoclave. Fully protective coats should be worn when handling Category 3 pathogens.

1. Do not wear your laboratory coat to visit the wards.
2. Do not wear any white coat to visit the coffee room or toilet.

INFECTIONS IN CONTAINMENT CATEGORY 3 LABORATORIES[2]

This containment category is required for handling sputum specimens that may contain *Mycobacterium tuberculosis*; therefore most of the large laboratories will have this facility. This room should contain a cabinet with exhaust ventilators that are filtered before discharge usually to the outside. The cabinet and system should be disinfected with formalin both routinely and before maintenance, and airflows should be regularly checked. Gloves should be worn for all manipulations and staff must be adequately trained in order to avoid a false sense of security when using a cabinet.

In case you are working with HIV or HBV, it is safer to work on open bench very carefully, as they do not spread in air. So this can be carried out at a definite work place, which allows sufficient seclusion to avoid inoculation accidents.

A fully protective gown or plastic apron as well as disposable gloves should be worn for more dangerous manipulations. Staff must be adequately trained in the use of aseptic measures and provided with this protective clothing, otherwise a false sense of security may lead to simple errors which would not arise if gloves were not being worn.

FUNGI

Cultures of fungi that cause communicable systemic infection (e.g. histoplasma) should be processed in a ventilated cabinet, as recommended for tubercle bacilli.

RADIOLOGY AND RADIOTHERAPY

INTRODUCTION AND PRINCIPLES OF CONTROL

The principles of control are same as those, which apply in other areas of the hospital. Staff should be informed of any patients with communicable disease like tuberculosis, etc. Precautions are required for radiological procedures involving the gastrointestinal tract, particularly for *Clostridium difficile* infection or colonization, which can spread by contact to other patients in the radiography department as well as in the wards. Radiographers should also pay attention to the recommended barrier nursing routine, paying particular attention to hand washing and gowning techniques. X-ray equipment is not an important source of infection and, routine cleaning with detergent, then allowing drying, will usually suffice. Cleaning the equipment between patients is not necessary except if patient is known to be infected. Disinfection by wiping with 70% alcohol is quick and fairly effective and it may be necessary after X-raying an infected patient or if the equipment is taken into the operating theater.[3]

Nowaday, many procedures involving aseptic techniques are performed in the X-ray department, and therefore facilities should be adequate, with a handwashing basin, a room, which is well, ventilated, with no unnecessary equipment, with as few a people as possible in the room. Good surgical techniques are necessary for these procedures, as they are in operating theaters. Instruments, dressings, etc. should be supplied by SSD (Sterile supply department).[3]

Radiologic procedures in which health care workers have contact with any of the substances like blood, body fluids (Cerebrospinal fluid, peritoneal fluid, pleural fluid, pericardial fluid amniotic fluid, synovial fluid), vaginal secretions, semen, saliva in dental procedures, may pose a risk of exposure to blood-borne pathogens. Almost all angiographies and interventional procedure will fall into this category, as would some others which are not thought of as particularly risky. These include hysterosalpingography and related interventions, arthrography, myelography and fluoroscopically-guided lumbar puncture and amniocentesis, procedures such as urethrography, cystography, contrast studies of gastrointestinal tract, sialography and dacryocystography.[4]

Exposure to blood may occur in any procedure in which intravenous access is obtained or used such as for injection of a contrast agent or medications because there is a risk of needlestick injury in any such procedure. In addition although, a given procedure may not itself carry any risk of exposure (e.g. a diagnostic ultrasound study) radiology personnel may still be exposed to blood or body fluids in the course of transfer almost all angiographic and interventional procedures in the patient, emptying urine bags, changing linens, performing cardiopulmonary resuscitation (CPR) and so forth. This is particularly true in a setting of trauma because patients are often critically injured, may have visible bleeding, and may often require several radiological procedures.[4]

CARE AND CONTROL OF INFECTION IN RADIOTHERAPY

Since most of the patients in these wards are immunosuppressed and therefore susceptible to infection, these patients should be nursed in single-bed cubicles with protective, isolation precautions. Trained staff should be appointed, as special skills are required over here for nursing the patients. Other patients may be sources of infection. Isolation of these patients and techniques to prevent contact infection (e.g. handwashing and wearing of plastic gowns) is necessary. The equipment is often difficult to sterilize or disinfect. Whenever possible, it should be autoclaved and supplied in packs by SSD. If equipment is heat labile, ethylene oxide or low temperature steam and formaldehyde treatment in the SSD is preferable to chemical solutions.[3]

Immersion in 70% alcohol (with or without 0.5% chlorhexidine) for 5–10 minutes will be appropriate for most purposes, but great care is necessary when drying after immersion in alcohol, if equipment is likely to contact mucous membranes or the conjunctiva. For rapid disinfection of larger items of equipment, wiping with 70% alcohol is satisfactory and is preferable to the use of aqueous disinfectants.[3]

It is essential that the radiotherapy staff be trained in aseptic techniques and control of infection, so as to ensure that appropriate precautions are taken as these patients are at high risk of blood-borne infection.

POSTMORTEM ROOM AND MORTUARY

INTRODUCTION AND CAUSES OF INFECTION[5]

The dead body, whether it is infected or not, may be a source of infection for the staff in the mortuary and the postmortem staff. Bacteria may spread by air or by contact, but there are special hazards when a postmortem examination is being performed. Contaminated aerosols or splashes may be released by means of squeezing sponges, cutting tissues such as lung or incising abscesses, and the sawing of bones may also release small-contaminated chips in the air. A common mode of infection is by cutting or pricking a finger with a contaminated instrument or a ragged bone edge. Usually, most of the organisms in the dead body are not likely to infect healthy individuals with intact skin, but still there are some special hazards.

Tubercle bacilli may spread in large numbers in aerosols. *Salmonella, Shigella* and other intestinal pathogens may be transmitted from the intestinal tract. If there is a break in the skin of the operator, large numbers of *Staphylococcus aureus* or *Streptococcus pyogenes* may be introduced into the skin leading to severe local infection and sometimes to septicemias. HBV, HCV or HIV introduced by a cut or a needle prick is a major potential hazard. The conjunctiva may be infected by splashes or aerosols and a severe local infection may follow. Blood-borne viruses may also enter the body by this route.

PREVENTION OF INFECTION[5]

If adequate precautions are taken, the risk of infection is not much.

1. Keep the mortuary, the postmortem room and refrigerator clean.
2. Good personal hygiene of members of the staff is also essential.
3. The postmortem room should be mechanically ventilated and designed, so that cleaning can be readily achieved.
4. There should be efficient fly proofing arrangements in the mortuary and postmortem room.
5. A shower with soap and towels should be available for the postmortem room staff.
6. When performing postmortem, the staff should completely change their outer clothing, and wear a disposable plastic apron, disposable gloves and rubber boots.
7. Visitors to the postmortem room, who are not going to be in contact with the body, should wear a gown and overshoes.
8. There should be a washbasin with disposable paper towels, soap and an antiseptic hand washing preparations (povidone-iodine or chlorhexidine detergent or 70% ethanol).
9. The staff members should wash their hands thoroughly after handling any contaminated surface or material, irrespective of whether gloves are worn and always on leaving the postmortem room. If the hands are contaminated, they should also be washed before handling case-notes.
10. If the skin or eye is splashed, it should be thoroughly washed. An eyewash bottle containing sterile saline should be available.
11. In case you get a fingerprick or cut it should be immediately washed thoroughly under running water and an antiseptic applied (e.g. 0.5% alcoholic or aqueous chlorhexidine or 1% iodine in 70% alcohol). This should be reported to the pathologist or microbiologist.
12. All preexisting cuts or open lesions on the hands should be covered with a waterproof dressing. Any open injuries other than minor ones should be treated in the casualty department.
13. All the instruments should be routinely cleaned before disinfection. This is because the organic matter may protect the organisms from the disinfectant. The instruments should preferably be autoclaved, but if not possible then boiling in water or immersion in 2% phenol for 10 minutes though less sensitive are safe alternatives to autoclaving if properly carried out. After treatment with disinfectant, all instruments should be rinsed and

dried. Immersion in chlorine-releasing solution (1,000 ppm available chlorine) rather than a phenolic is advised after a postmortem in a patient with an HBV or HIV infection. Most preferable is a washer-disinfector as washing by hands is avoided.

14. The room and equipment should be thoroughly cleaned after use with a phenolic disinfectant (e.g. 2% stericol) or with a chlorine-releasing agent (1000 ppm available chlorine) if HBV, HCV, HIV infection or poliomyelitis was diagnosed in the patient before death. If chlorine-releasing agents are used on metal surfaces, they should be immediately rinsed in order to avoid corrosion.
15. Linen should be sent in a sealed bag and treated as infected by the laundry. Dressing, waste materials and body tissues should be sealed in plastic bags and treated as clinical waste.
16. Special precautions should be taken with certain infections. In postmortem examination of patients with untreated pulmonary tuberculosis, operators should wear filter type masks.
17. Postmortems on patients with known or suspected HBV, HCV or HIV infection should be avoided unless absolutely essential. Special care is necessary to avoid cuts and needle pricks.
18. Viruses which cause spongiform encephalopathies (e.g. Creutzfeldt-Jakob disease) and other slow virus infections are relatively resistant to heat and also to chemical disinfectants like aldehydes. The environment should be disinfected with a strong chlorine-releasing solution (containing 0.25% available chlorine and blood should be mopped up with a solution containing 1% (10,000 ppm) available chlorine. If the skin is contaminated, wash thoroughly with soap and water and apply 2 M sodium hydroxide for 10 minutes. Instruments should be autoclaved at 134°C for 18 minutes (e.g. six 3 minutes cycles) after thorough washing. Immersion in 2 M sodium hydroxide is a possible alternative if autoclaving is not possible.
19. Formaldehyde used for preservation of tissues is an effective antimicrobial agent. Thorough penetration should be ensured before handling, particularly if lesions are caused by potentially dangerous infections like tuberculosis, typhoid or hepatitis. It is ineffective against prions.
20. Lastly, it is important that the mortuary staff and undertakers should be informed about the bodies of patients who have died or were suffering from a communicable disease. These should be enclosed in a plastic bag, and it would be useful to attach a warning label to them in the ward. Training of mortuary staff in the prevention of infection is also necessary. Immunization should be offered as for the laboratory staff.

REFERENCES

1. Advisory Committee on dangerous pathogens. Categorisation of biological agents according to hazard and categories of containment, 4th edition. HMSO. London; 1995.
2. Ayliffee GAJ, Fraise AP, Geddes AM, Mitchell K. Control of Hospital Infection—A Practical Handbook, 4th edition. Oxford University Press, New York; 2000.pp.341-6.
3. Ayliffee GAJ, Fraise AP, Geddes AM, Mitchell K. Control of Hospital Infection—A Practical Handbook, 4th edition. Oxford University Press, New York; 2000.pp.328-30.
4. Hansen ME. Blood-borne pathogens: Occupational risk and infection control in radiology. Emergency Radiology. 1994;1(2):89-92. Accessed from www.link.springer.com/article/10.1000%2FBF02614909on 27.7.2015.
5. Ayliffee GAJ, Fraise AP, Geddes AM, Mitchell K. Control of Hospital Infection—A Practical Handbook, 4th edition. Oxford University Press, New York; 2000.pp.346-8.

Chapter 22

Laundry

Chapter Outline

- Types of Laundry
- Precautions for the Laundry Staff
- Decontamination and Washing of Blankets
- Decontamination and Washing of Mattresses
- Practical Aspects of Laundry

INTRODUCTION[1]

Bed linen, clothing used by the patients in the hospital can be a source of infection to the staff handling it. Therefore, adequate measures for collection, transportation, processing and storage of hospital linen are essential to prevent the transmission of infection to the hospital staff handling the linen.

Used linen is usually heavily contaminated with bacteria, but these are mainly gram-negative bacilli from the intestinal tract or coagulase-negative staphylococci from the skin. These organisms are usually found as common environmental contaminants and are unlikely to cause infection in staff handling linen. *Staphylococcus aureus* is usually present in small numbers (less than 1% of the total) and therefore does not pose much hazard if normal precautions are taken. Large numbers of *Bacillus cereus*, have been isolated from clean laundry (they are not usually killed by routine heating process) and have been responsible for outbreaks of infection (meningitis following neurosurgery and umbilical infections in neonatal units).[2,3]

Linen used by patients infected with specific pathogens (e.g. *Salmonella* and *Shigella* species) may be soiled with the excretions or secretions of these patients and be a source of infection.[4]

TYPES OF LAUNDRY

According to current UK recommendations, laundry is categorized into three types (1) used, (2) infected, and (3) heat labile.[5]

Used Linen (Soiled or Foul)

Includes all linen, irrespective of its state and which may on occasion be contaminated by body fluids or blood and often with excretion.

It excludes linen from patients in linen category 2 (infected).

Visibly fouled or soiled linen is usually contaminated with the same organisms as other used linen, but the numbers are usually higher. Fouled linen if handled with care is unlikely to infect laundry workers.

Infected Linen

This is linen from patients who are suffering with specific infections which have a potential to infect healthy staff, as well as other patients, e.g. patients suffering from enteric fever, other *Salmonella* infections, dysentery, cholera, pulmonary tuberculosis, hepatitis A, B or C, HIV infection and other notifiable diseases including infections in hazard groups 3 and 4,[6] or other infections specified by ICT. Although the risk of handling this linen is minimal, unless visibly soiled, even then handling by laundry workers should be avoided. Linen from patients with most notifiable diseases (e.g. measles, chickenpox) is not hazardous and could be treated as used linen. Whenever, there is any doubt about the safety of routine processing of linen, treatment should be discussed with the ICT. This linen should then be placed in an impermeable outer bag for storage or transport.

In USA linen is not segregated as described above.[7] As it is then unknown whether or not the linen is from an infected patient, sorting of used linen is carried out using universal precautions, and there is no evidence of acquired infection in laundry workers, provided that precautions are taken. In India, the same policy as in USA could be followed.

It has been recommended that all hospital linen should be heat disinfected during the washing process. This can be done at a temperature of 65°C for 10 minutes or 71°C for 3 minutes. Though these temperatures are effective, in practice higher temperatures or longer times have been used. These recommended times and temperatures were calculated from the killing of over 10^6 enterococci, which are more resistant to heat than most of the vegetative organisms and viruses. Usually, a temperature of 71°C for 3 minutes associated with thorough washing should be adequate, but if there is a problem with heat resistant strains in the hospital, temperatures and times of disinfection should be reviewed by ICT.

All washing machines should be fitted with accurate heat sensors to indicate the temperature reached during the disinfection cycle. The temperature of the coolest part of the load should be raised to the required temperature.

For testing the survival of heat resistant vegetative organisms (e.g. cultures of enterococci applied to patches of material or sealed in narrow bore planting tubing and attached to an item of linen in the load) are commonly used.[8]

Usually microbiological testing of linen after processing is not required, but it may occasionally be useful if there is an evidence or suspicion that this route has transmitted infection. Contact plates taken from processed linen awaiting distribution should not show more than one colony forming unit (cfu)/cm^2 and should not average more than 2 cfu/cm^2. The organisms should be predominantly gram-positive cocci and aerobic spore-bearing bacilli. Gram-negative bacilli should not be present. As some of the bacteria are destroyed during the heat drying and finishing process, counts taken from the load after washing, but before drying are likely to be higher. If substantial number of gram-negative bacilli or spore-bearing bacilli is present in samples taken after washing, it will be an evidence of recontamination from the surrounding environment or from contaminated water used to rinse after disinfection.

It should be remembered that organisms could grow in wet linen kept in the machine overnight. Machines should therefore be emptied at the end of the day and rinse sections should be heat disinfected before production starts each day.

Heat Labile Linen

The problem now a days is that heat disinfection is becoming more and more difficult, as there is an increasing use of fabrics (e.g. knitted polyester, etc.), which are likely to be damaged at the disinfecting temperatures. For these, thorough washing and rinsing at low temperature (e.g. 40–50°C) would remove most organisms.

Disinfection could also be done by chemical disinfection say using a chlorine-producing agent to give a final concentration of 150 ppm[9] available chlorine for a minimum exposure time of 5 minutes.[9] Heat labile linen should be enclosed in a white bag with an orange stripe. If sorting of infected linen has not been done, the bag could be labeled as 'Infected'.

Since most of the used linen is contaminated and contain sufficient moisture to allow microbes to multiply, it would immediately be enclosed in bags, which are impermeable to moisture. The linen should be handled with minimal disturbance to prevent dispersal of organisms. After enclosing the linen in a suitable bag, it could be transported through the wards and corridor. If the bag used is not a disposable one, it should be processed through a heat disinfection cycle before reuse. If this linen has to be stored temporarily, then select a properly designated area, which is secure from any tampering from pests.

PRECAUTIONS FOR THE LAUNDRY STAFF

The laundry staff while handling linen should wear aprons, gloves, and overalls, they should be provided with adequate facilities for washing and changing when starting and finishing the work at each shift. Staff handling the linen should be given training to ensure, that they understand the measures required to protect themselves and others. Staff should be offered immunization against poliomyelitis, tetanus, hepatitis B, and BCG if they are tuberculin negative. Staff with unhealed lesions or rashes or any exfoliative skin conditions should not handle clean laundry unless the lesions can be covered with an impermeable dressing.

Single vehicle should not be used for transfer of processed linen and used linen. This can be done only if the vehicle is divided into two compartments with separate loading doors for both and the partition between the two is impervious and complete. In places where use of 2 vehicles is not possible, a single vehicle may be used if it is adequately cleaned between loads.

Domestic type of washers can be used for small units if the patients are physically healthy.

Labeling of bags with the ward number will help to reduce hazardous practices.

Infection control staff to ensure that standards are acceptable should periodically visit the laundry.

In a country like India, most hospitals do not have washing machines, especially those that have a heat disinfection cycle facility, and washing of linen is done manually by dhobis (washer man). Special care is necessary when washer man does washing. The contaminated linen must be disinfected before giving to washer man for washing. This can be done by chemical disinfectant, or by boiling or autoclaving at low pressure of steam. These facilities for disinfection of contaminated soiled linen should be available in the hospital near the discarding of contaminated linen.

Then both the clean contaminated and contaminated linen should be packed separately in thick polythene bags of different colors and transported to the laundry. The clean contaminated linen can be transported in thick cotton bags also.

If the washing is done mechanically by washing machines, the decontamination of contaminated soiled linen can be done in the laundry itself with hot detergent in the washing machine.

Handling, separating and counting of clean and contaminated linen is hazardous and hence there should be minimum handling.

It is always good to have a suitable washing machine with built in cycle for decontamination.

Drying of linen in the sun after washing should be discouraged, as it is usually spread on roadside or other contaminated area.

DECONTAMINATION AND WASHING OF BLANKETS

Usually cotton and acrylic/synthetic blankets are preferred as they can be easily decontaminated when soiled. Washing them is also cheap and easy. They can be handled like linen.

If woolen blankets are used and they are soiled, they can be decontaminated either by exposing to formaldehyde vapors or autoclaving. Liquid disinfectants may damage woolen blankets.

DECONTAMINATION AND WASHING OF MATTRESSES

It is advisable to cover all mattresses with waterproof synthetic material like rexine or plastic. This makes disinfection of the mattresses easier. Big autoclaves are available for disinfection. Washing manually is not easy, though it can be done.

PRACTICAL ASPECTS OF LAUNDRY

We have already seen that laundry can be a source of microbial contamination. To prevent this, adequate precautions during collection, segregation, transportation processing and storage have to be taken.

To protect the staff working in the laundry, adequate instructions should be given to them. They are as follows:

1. Linen should be sorted out into clean contaminated (used) and contaminated (soiled).
2. They should be put in separate polythene bags (with different colors); this should be done at the location of use.
3. Linen should be removed from beds and handled with minimal agitation so as to avoid air-borne microbial contamination.
4. Soiled linen should not be sorted out in patient care unit.
5. Linen should be removed daily from patient care units and blankets should be laundered after each use by each patient.
6. Mattresses should be enclosed with covers of impervious plastic in order to prevent contamination and to permit easy cleaning.
7. Linen known to be contaminated with infected material should be clearly labeled and handled with special care.
8. Cloth bags used for soiled linen will also require the same laundering as their contents.
9. All soiled linen should be transported in well-covered clearly identified carts, used exclusively for that purpose. The linens of these carts (trolleys) should be cleaned and laundered frequently.
10. Rooms for sorting soiled linen in the hospital laundry should be separate from other processing rooms. The soiled linen area should be thoroughly cleaned and disinfected daily.
11. In addition to this, separate rooms should be available in the hospital laundry for processing, for clean storage, sewing and for an office. There should be facilities for hand washing and a toilet.
12. The flow of air (ventilation) in the laundry should be from the cleanest to the dirtiest area.
13. The floor and all equipments in the laundry should be cleaned at the end of each working day and a regular schedule should be established and maintained.
14. The conventional practice of washing linen with effective detergent at water temperature above 71°C (160°F) for 25 minutes is effective for hospital use.

15. It is recommended that all heavily soiled launderable linen should be handled as little as possible and be wrapped or covered before transportation.
16. Clean linen seldom needs to be sterilized except for use in operating and delivery rooms, for high-risk newborn infants and for patients of severe burns.
17. All laundry staff should be immunized, against poliomyelitis, hepatitis B, tetanus and BCG for tuberculin negative individuals.

REFERENCES

1. Barrie. Laundry hygiene and handling of contaminated linen—Chapter 12. In: Ayliffee GAJ, Fraise AP, Geddes AM, Mitchell K. Control of Hospital Infection—A Practical Handbook, 4th edition. Oxford University Press, New York; 2000.pp.239-43.
2. Birch BR, Perara BS, Hyde WA, et al. Bacillus cereus cross infection in a maternity unit. J Hosp Infect. 1981;2:349.
3. Barrie D, Wilson JA, Hoffman PN, Kramer JM. Bacillus cereus meningitis in two neurosurgical units: an investigation into the source of the organism. J Infect. 1992;25:291.
4. Standeert SM, Hutcheson RH, Schaffner W. Nosocomial transmission of Salmonella to laundry workers in a nursing home. Infection control and hospital epidemiology. 1994;15:22.
5. Department of Health NHS. Executive. Hospital laundry arrangements for used and infected linen Heywood: Health Publication Unit; 1995.
6. Advisory committee for dangerous pathogens. Categorisation of pathogens according to hazard and categories of containment. London, HMSO; 1990.
7. McDonald, Pugliese G. Laundry service. In: May Hall CG (Ed). Hospital epidemiology and infection. Baltimore MD, Williams and Wilkins; 1996.p.805.
8. Collins BJ, Cripps N, Spooner A. Controlling microbiological decontamination levels, Laundry and Cleaning News; 1987;30:31.
9. Laundry treatment at high and low temperatures. Health and Safety Executive (HSE). Accessed from www.hse.gov.uk/biosafety/ blood-borne-viruses/ laundrytreatments.htm. on 16th August 2016.

Chapter 23

Kitchen Hygiene

Chapter Outline

Infection Control in Hospital Kitchen

- Introduction
- Medical Examination of Staff
- Training
- Hazard Analysis Control Points
- Responsibility
- Pests—Eradication and Control
- Questionnaire for Catering Staff
- Catering Staff Agreement to Report Infection

Practical Aspects Regarding Kitchen

- Kitchen Architecture and Facilities
- Health Check-up for Food Handlers
- Personal Hygiene
- Washing of Crockery and Cutlery
- Disposal of Refuse
- Cleaning
- Education and Training of Food Handlers

INFECTION CONTROL IN HOSPITAL KITCHEN

INTRODUCTION

All the patients receive food from a single kitchen in the hospital, hence, if the hygiene of the kitchen is not maintained; it can lead to outbreaks of infection involving the whole hospital. Infection from contaminated food is particularly hazardous in debilitated or elderly people, and can cause severe illness or even death.[1]

It is also important to prevent food-borne infection among the staff, as subsequent transfer to patients would have similar unfortunate results.

Outbreaks of food poisoning are usually caused by *Salmonella* species, or the toxins of certain strains of *Staphylococcus aureus*,

Clostridium perfringens and *Bacillus cereus. Campylobacter* species is also now a common cause of food-borne infection, although outbreaks in hospital are infrequent. Outbreaks caused by *E. coli 0157:H7* have been frequently reported, but mainly occur in the community. Very small numbers of *E. coli O157:H7* is required to initiate an infection, and therefore, it becomes difficult to control an outbreak with this organism. These organisms especially *Salmonella* species, may be transferred to the patient directly from contaminated raw foods (e.g. meat, poultry if inadequately cooked) or indirectly from initially contaminated food by hands of staff or from inadequately cleaned surfaces or equipment. Staphylococcal and *Salmonella* carriers on the staff may also contaminate food if their personal hygiene is poor, but are infrequently responsible for outbreaks. Inadequately cooked food, which is left without refrigeration for several hours, and particularly if it is subsequently warmed, is an important source of infection. Any food that is capable of supporting bacterial growth should be stored either below 8° or above 63°C. It should not be allowed to remain between these temperatures for more than 2 hours and sufficient time must be allowed for complete thawing before cooking.

According to the UK Food Safety (Temperature control) Regulations 1995,[2] 8°C is satisfactory for cold storage, but 5°C is preferable if possible. Some bacterial species like *Listeria* can grow slowly at low temperatures, and therefore chilled food should be kept at a temperature of 0–3°C.

Good personal hygiene of the kitchen staff and effective methods of cleaning food preparation areas are very important in preventing the spread of infection. The kitchen structure, i.e. walls, floors and ceilings though not of much relevance should be kept clean and in a good condition.

Sources of Contamination

- Most viruses and bacteria that cause colds, flu and food-borne illnesses are spread by hand to hand or hand to food contact. People with hepatitis A, Norwalk -like virus (norovirus), or the bacteria *Staphylococcus* and *Streptococcus* can pass these illnesses on to others by handling food. Also a person who is ill from a food-borne illness, like hepatitis A, can pass that illness on to others by handling food.
- Raw meats, poultry, and fish carry a large variety of harmful bacteria. One of the most serious is *E. coli* O157:H7. This is the organism found most abundantly in undercooked hamburger. It is one of the most common causes of food-borne illness, according to CDC. This bacterium causes hemolytic uremic syndrome, an often-deadly disease that strikes mostly children. Older adults are also at high risk.
- Chicken, turkey and fowl are associated with *Shigella*, *Salmonella* and *Campylobacter*. These are bacteria that cause diarrhea, cramping and fever. Most meat can be contaminated with toxoplasmosis. This is a parasitic disease dangerous to both pregnant women and fetuses.
- Sea food particularly oysters, clams and other shell-fish, can be contaminated with *Vibrio* species of bacteria that causes diarrheoa, or with hepatitis A virus.
- Unpasteurized cheese and some meat can be contaminated with *Listeria monocytogenes*, a strain of bacteria that can cause disease in people and miscarriage or damage to the fetus in pregnant women. *Listeria* is often found in soft cheese. *Listeria* is one of the few bacteria that grow well at 4°C temperature of the refrigerator.
- Contaminated vegetables and fruits can carry a variety of organisms and parasites, depending on where they were grown and how they were processed.

Contaminated Kitchen Gadgets

Items in the kitchen become contaminated by contact with contaminated people, food, pets, or other environmental sources.

The first and foremost suspect "gadget" in the kitchen is the human hand. Too, often people do not wash their hands before preparing food. More often people do not wash their hands between handling contaminated foods like meat and other foods that are less likely to be contaminated like vegetables. The 'cross-contamination is the leading cause of food-borne disease according to CDC.

Kitchen items that often become contaminated include:

- Can openers
- Cutting boards
- Countertops: Most people use countertops not only for food preparation, but also for possibly contaminated items like grocery bags, mail, or household objects.
- Towels, sponges and scrubbers.
- Garbage disposals.
- Sink drains and P-trap: This is the J-shaped pipe under the sink that retains a quantity of water to block sewer gas from seeping back up through the sink.
- Refrigerators.
- Complex appliances like food processors, blender and egg beaters.

MEDICAL EXAMINATION OF STAFF

History and Physical Examination

A history and physical examination of the staff should be carried out.

A past history of typhoid, paratyphoid fever, dysentery, persistent diarrhea, or attacks of diarrhea and vomiting lasting for more than 2 days within the past 2 years, tuberculosis, boils, skin rashes, discharges from eye, ear, nose or other site, and also place and dates of all visits abroad should be noted.

A questionnaire on the above illnesses and all other relevant information should be filled by the medical officer-in-charge, and signed by the employee. Later, the medical officer should carry out a more detailed examination. Tuberculin test should be done, and if negative BCG should be offered. Examination of feces, blood, other laboratory tests and X-ray chest should be done only if indicated. The microbiologist or Infection Control Officer should be consulted if laboratory tests are considered necessary. If examination of feces is required, at least three samples taken in successive days should be examined.

Sickness

All incidents of vomiting and diarrhea in the catering staff should be noted. An assessment of fitness to return to food-handling duties should be made in the hospital only and not by the general practitioners, as they may regard the hospital staff fit to return to work when they are still excreting *Salmonella* or *Shigella*. So also all the catering staff that has been exposed to enteric infection requires counseling on hand washing techniques and other measures required to prevent possible spread.

Food handlers suffering from diarrhea or vomiting while at work should immediately be referred to an appropriate authority for assessment like the medical officer-in-charge. The incidence should be properly documented and appropriate specimens obtained. If they are decided to be unfit for duty, they should be reminded that they must report back before returning to normal duties. Skin rashes, boils and other lesions or rashes should be reported in a similar manner.

All food handlers should report to the staff medical officer or infection control nurse:

1. If they have been sick and taken off for any of the above said reasons.
2. If they have suffered from diarrhea or vomiting of more than 2 days duration while on leave.
3. If other members of the household are suffering from diarrhea or vomiting.

To encourage prompt reporting of such conditions, staff should be made aware that sending them off duty would not lead to loss of salary.

TRAINING

Introduction

All food handlers should be given training in personal and kitchen hygiene both at the time of employment and at intervals thereafter. Posters demonstrating different aspects of hygiene should be prominently displayed in catering food storage areas, and changed at frequent intervals.

Personal Hygiene

The main route of transfer of infection to food is via hands of staff. Hands therefore must be washed frequently, especially after using toilet. In addition to hands and fingernails, the face and other parts of the body should be kept clean, including the hair and scalp and forearms when short sleeves are worn. The nails should be kept short, and the nose, the hair and lips should not be touched while handling food. Even after washing hands, it cannot be assumed that the hands are free from pathogenic organisms and therefore food should be handled as little as possible. If possible non-sterile gloves should be worn, when handling food, which is to be eaten without further processing (e.g. Sandwiches).

Washing of Hands

Hands should be washed with hot water using a soap or detergent and must then be well rinsed, and thoroughly dried on a fresh paper towel. Nailbrushes should be used only if there is heavy soiling of fingers, for they damage the skin. So also nails brushes lying in soap dishes are likely to be heavily contaminated with gram-negative bacilli, so that using them will both damage the skin and inoculate it with bacteria. Nailbrushes if have to be used should be sterile or adequately decontaminated, and should be reprocessed after use.

Washbasins must be provided in the food preparation area, with a plain bar, a liquid soap or detergent. Bar soap should be kept in a dry state in between uses. If liquid dispensers are used, they should be thoroughly cleaned at regular intervals and must not be refilled without prior cleaning and disinfection.

Food handlers should keep their personal clothing clean, and should change their protective clothing daily. Protective clothing should be worn only for catering duties. Hospital authorities should arrange laundering. Staff should not smoke while handling food or while in a room where food is exposed. All cuts, etc. must be completely covered with a waterproof dressing.

Cleaning and Maintenance

Detailed schedules should be made and responsibilities fixed. Kitchen should be well maintained with floors, which can be easily cleaned. Walls and ceilings should have smooth impermeable surfaces. The cooking equipment should be placed at a site, the areas around which can be cleaned easily. All cleaning should be carried out with a freshly prepared and accurately diluted detergent solution. The cleaning equipment like scrubs and mops should remain in the kitchen, but not in the food preparation area, and should be examined at intervals and disinfected when necessary. If it is damaged, it should be repaired if possible or replaced.

Special attention should be paid to the food preparation area, especially the surfaces. Preparation surfaces should be impervious to water and should be maintained in a good condition. Stainless steel surfaces are advised. Preparation surfaces should always be cleaned with a recently prepared hot cleaning solution and a fresh disposable or laundered cloth. If there are separate areas for different types of food, the surfaces should be cleaned with different cloths, for if the same cloth is used for all surfaces, contamination will be transferred from one surface to the other. Each individual surface should be dried with a disposable or freshly laundered cloth, as most gram-negative bacilli die on drying if the surface is initially clean.

Usually, disinfectants are not necessary for cleaning, but they may be recommended if there is an outbreak of infection. Usually, chlorine-releasing agents releasing 250 ppm of available chlorine are often used. Cleaning removes grease, food residues and dirt as well as a large number of bacteria. Disinfecting kills organisms (bacteria, virus and parasites).

Transfer of contamination from one product to another is likely with meat mincers and slicers. Cooked and uncooked meat must never be processed with the same machine without thorough cleaning between operations.

The following are the ways to prevent infections from kitchen gadgets:

- *Can openers:* Whether hand or electric, clean after each use. After cleaning, wipe with bleach solution (or commercial disinfectant) and allow to air-dry.
- *Cutting boards:* If practical, keep two cutting boards, one for meat and one for vegetables and fruits. Clean after each use. The meat cutting board should be sprayed or wiped with the bleach solution and allowed to air-dry. Rinse the board in clear water before the next use to help remove residual bleach taste from the board.
- *Countertops:* Clean them thoroughly, then spray or wipe with bleach solution. Allow to air dry, If there is residual "frost" from bleach, it may be wiped off with a clean cloth.
- *Dishrags, towels, sponges and scrubbers:* These tend to be highly contaminated. You should not use a sponge in the kitchen. Use a clean dish-cloth daily. After use rinse thoroughly and dry. Scrubbers (metal or plastic) should be washed in the dish washer each time you run it. If you do not have a dish washer, rinse them thoroughly to remove any visible food residue and soak them in the bleach solution for 10 minutes.
- *Garbage disposals:* The film that builds up in the inside of the disposal, i.e. teeming with bacteria. Use a long-handled angled brush with a chlorinated cleansing powder to scrub the inside walls of the disposal and the underside of the rubber splash guard. Allow the cleanser to remain in place (do not rinse) until the next time the disposal is used. This gives the chlorinated disinfectant time to kill bacteria. This should be done at least once a month.
- *Sink drains and P-trap:* Before going to bed pour 1 cup of hot water into the drain. Wait a minute for the drain to soak up heat from the water, then pour in 1 cup of chlorine bleach (undiluted). Allow to stand overnight. This should be done every one to 2 weeks. Not only will this help sanitize the drain and keep odor down, but it will also help the drain running freely.
- *Refrigerators:* The fridge should be periodically cleaned thoroughly. After cleaning, it should be wiped with bleach solution and the food replaced. Spills should be cleaned up immediately. Food should not be allowed to mould or decay in the refrigerator.
- *Complex appliances such as food processors, blenders and eggbeaters:* The dish washer remains the best method for cleaning these items. Visible food materials must be removed from crevices, recesses, or tight areas and the washable parts of the appliances placed in the dish washer.
- Dish washers should be drained and flushed daily. Ensure that dishwashers reach the required wash temperature of 60°C and rinse cycle temperature of 80–82°C.[3,4]
- All serving carts must be sanitized. Ensure carts that collect soiled trays are sanitized as well.[4,5]

Crockery and Cutlery: Pots and Pans

In our country, crockery and cutlery is usually washed by hands. In such circumstances, two sinks should be used to ensure sufficient rinsing. Detergent solution and rinsing water should be changed frequently and should be as hot as possible. Nylon brushes could be used which should be washed and thoroughly dried after each use. However, it is most preferable to use a disposable material rather than non-disposable cloth or nylon brushes.

In developed countries, crockery and cutlery is machine washed at a minimum temperature of 60°C and a final rinse at 80°C for 1 minute, or another appropriate temperature and time. After washing, it is very important that all crockery, cutlery, pots and pans and kitchen equipment is dried thoroughly. The use of linen drying cloths (e.g. tea towels) should be discontinued and replaced by heat drying in air drain in racks. When drying by hand is necessary disposable or recently laundered towel is preferred.

Crockery, cutlery, pots, pans and other kitchen equipment must be regularly examined. If any of them are worn-out or chipped or stained or broken, they should be replaced. Whenever these items are not in use they should be stored under conditions in which recontamination is reduced to a minimum. If it is not possible to carry out heat disinfection, then disposable cutlery and crockery may be recommended by the Infection Control Team for certain infections (e.g. enteric fever and gastrointestinal infections).

Storage and Transportation of Food

Prepared food is transported to other areas in closed food carts or covered containers (use separate carts for serving clean trays and collecting dirty trays.

Food is served with clean tongs, scoops, forks, spoons, spatulas or gloves to avoid direct contact with food.

Contamination of food during storage and transportation is likely to occur. Especially food like raw meat, fish, and poultry is likely to be contaminated by harmful bacteria. Therefore, such type of food should be prepared and cooked in such a way that these organisms are destroyed before serving.

Periodic checking of temperature in the coldest part of the food is recommended. A temperature of at least 70°C for 2 minutes should be achieved. Poultry food may be contaminated with *Salmonella* species, and if adequate thawing of frozen poultry is not done before cooking, these organisms may survive the cooking process. The multiplication of bacteria should be prevented by careful storage of food at the correct temperature before and after cooking. *Clostridium perfringens* is a common cause of food poisoning, and its spores may survive the cooking process. These bacteria will multiply if the food is left unrefrigerated for more than 2 hours. Subsequent heating of food will further increase the number of bacteria, and when large numbers are eaten, toxins may be released into the intestine and cause food poisoning.

Food like raw meat, fish and uncooked vegetables (prepared or unprepared) must not be stored with food, which is to be served without further heat treatment, so that the two do not come into contact with other. These may be stored in separate refrigerators or closed compartments in the same refrigerator or cold room. Food must not be stored on the floor of the cold rooms, or below foods, which may leak or be spilt. The temperature of the cold rooms and refrigerators should be monitored routinely.

Food that requires cooling must not be left in the kitchen area, but should be transported to a cooling area and cooled rapidly to at least 8°C. Stored food should be protected from recontamination. Food, which is transported within the hospital (e.g. from stores to kitchen), or from the kitchen to the ward, should be transported under clean conditions and properly covered to prevent contamination. Transportation should be carried in a clean closed container, especially if the vehicle is used for other purposes. The vehicles used for this purpose should be appropriately designed and kept clean. Contaminated materials (e.g. refuse or soiled linen) must not be carried in these vehicles.

Refuse and food waste must not be allowed to accumulate in the kitchen and should be removed at frequent intervals.

Staff trained in food hygiene should serve food. Clean plastic aprons should be worn. Adequate serving equipment should be provided in order to prevent unnecessary handling. Leftover food in ward refrigerator should be discarded daily.

Good Catering Practice

The catering staff with advice from the Infection Control Team should prepare policy for safe handling and processing of food. The decisions should be made for each type of food with regard to the minimum internal temperature required, the maximum time allowed at room temperature after cooking, and how long it can be kept refrigerated before use or disposal. As far as possible meat should be cooked on the day that it is to be served. There should also be a strict policy on the maximum time for which uncooked food like sandwiches; salads, etc. are kept at room temperature or in chilled storage before they are discarded.

Bacteriological Standards for Food

Usually, routine microbiological testing is not necessary, but if the control of the different processes carried out is unreliable or if the services have been set up recently, then the following standard is suggested.

A sample of 100 g of each item of food from each batch to be tested should be taken immediately before reheating.

The following criteria are suggested:[6]

1. Total aerobic count—less than 100,000/g (agar plates incubated at 37°C for 48 hours).
2. *Salmonella* species and *Listeria monocytogenes* should not be detected in 25 g.
3. *E. coli*—less than 10/g, *E. coli 0155 H7* should not be detected.
4. *Staphylococcus aureus* and *Clostridium perfringens*—less than 100/g.

Listeria monocytogenes has emerged as a potential hazard, as it grows at lower temperatures than most other pathogens. It is found in the environment and as a contaminant of raw foods, but the number of food-borne infections is low. Although, the number of clinical infections reported in recent years has increased, the overall number is still relatively less. However susceptible groups like pregnant patients or immune compromised patients should not eat food that is likely to contain *Listeria*.

HAZARD ANALYSIS CONTROL POINTS (HACCP)

This is a system for identifying and assessing microbiological and other hazards in production, processing, preparation, storage and distribution of food. In this way, a periodical review of this system can be done.[2,7,8] Different points of operation can be checked to eliminate or minimize hazard like the temperature of food during cooking, time of the food left at room temperature and refrigerator temperatures. This review system should immediately detect any failure in procedures.

RESPONSIBILITY

Operational policies should be formed and kept in writing. It should be seen that the functioning of the whole system is proper. These should cover training of the staff, pest control, critical control systems, and cleaning and waste disposal. Ward staff that handle or serve food should be adequately trained and supervised. The catering manager or in-charge of kitchen is responsible for cleaning and hygiene. The responsibility for maintenance of structure and equipment should be clearly defined. One annual inspection should be done by the catering manager and the infection control team and a member of the engineering or building staff should examine the catering area with respects to the aspects of hygiene.

PESTS—ERADICATION AND CONTROL

The common pests in the kitchen, the laundry, the staff restaurants, etc. are cockroaches, mice and ants, and every effort should be made to eradicate them. The eradication or control will depend on the type of pest, the extent of infestation, the complexity of the buildings and other local factors.

The role of pests in transmission of hospital-acquired infection is uncertain, but some reports indicate the carriage of specific pathogens including *Salmonella* species. These pests not only transmit diseases, but they can spoil food, and damage fabrics and building structure. Ants have been responsible for penetration of sterile packs and patients dressings. To get rid of pests, not only is the use of insecticides and rodenticides necessary, but it is also essential to pay attention to good hygiene and structural maintenance. Pests usually require food, warmth moisture, harbourage and a means of entry. Therefore, it is essential that the staff should be encouraged to keep the food covered, to remove spillage and waste, and to avoid accumulations of stagnant water.

The structure of building should be well maintained, drains should be covered, if there are pipes leaking, they should be repaired, and damaged surfaces should be done. There should be no cracks in the plastic or the woodwork, no unsealed areas in the pipes, damaged tiles or badly fitting equipment and kitchen units, because these all can provide an excellent harbourage. Applying fly screens, close fitting doors and windows, bird nets will help to exclude pests from hospital buildings.

Most of the pests come in the nights, so surveys should be preferably conducted at night. You can either see the pests yourself or droppings, nests, rodent smears, fragments of insects, damage to the structure of the building, or damaged fabrics will all indicate infestation. Pyrethrum aerosols are useful for flushing cockroaches and other crawling pests.

Usually, the task of pest control is given to a commercial company, but the hospital should appoint a pest control officer to coordinate pest control activities.

The pesticides used should be approved by the Pesticides Regulations and should be considered by the Health Authority to be suitable for use within premises.

QUESTIONNAIRE FOR CATERING STAFF (TABLE 23.1)[1]

Table 23.1: Questionnaire for catering staff

	Yes	No	When (year)	How long off work	If yes name of doctor, etc. hospital
1. Have you even had any of the following? • Typhoid fever • Paratyphoid fever • Dysentery • Persistent diarrhea • Tuberculosis					
2. Have you suffered from any of the following within the past 2 years: • Diarrhea and/or vomiting for more than 2 days • Skin rash • Boils • Discharge from eye					

Contd...

Contd...

	Yes	No	When (year)	How long off work	If yes name of doctor, etc. hospital
• Discharge from ear • Discharge from nose • Other infections					
3. Have you ever been abroad: Yes/No If Yes : Where When I declare that all the foregoing statements are true and complete to the best of my knowledge and belief					
4. Investigations • Chest X-ray • Feces • Blood • Other Comments:					

CATERING STAFF AGREEMENT TO REPORT INFECTION[1]

I agree to report to the catering officer or his/her deputy.

1. If suffering from an illness involving:
   - Vomiting
   - Diarrhea
   - Skin rash
   - Septic skin disease (boils, infected cuts, etc.) discharge from ear, eye, nose.
2. After returning and commencing work following an illness involving vomiting and/or diarrhea or any of the above conditions.
3. After returning from a holiday during which an attack of vomiting and/or diarrhea lasted for more than 2 days.
4. If any other member of my household is suffering from diarrhea and/or vomiting.

I have read (or had explained to me) and understood the accompanying rules on personal hygiene

Signed Date:

PRACTICAL ASPECTS REGARDING KITCHEN

INTRODUCTION

Kitchen is a very important part of the hospital. Food-borne diseases are important particularly in the immunocompromised patients. The community incidence of enteric infection is also high in our country, which makes it more important to pay special attention in food preparation and handling.

It is also important to prevent food-borne infection among staff; they can subsequently transfer the infection to patients. Bacterial food poisoning is usually caused by *Salmonella, S. aureus* and *C. welchii.* These organisms particularly *Salmonella* may be transferred directly to patient from raw food (improperly cooked meat and poultry) or it may be transmitted indirectly by contamination of cooked food by raw food, hands of staff, inadequately cleaned surfaces or equipment. Staphylococcal and *Salmonella carriers* on the staff may also contaminate food if their personal hygiene is poor. Inadequately cooked food, left at room temperature for several hours without refrigeration and especially if subsequently warmed up is an important source of infection.

To prevent food-borne infection attention should be paid to (1) Kitchen architecture and facilities; (2) Food handlers; (3) Education and training of personnel in food preparation and distribution.

KITCHEN ARCHITECTURE AND FACILITIES

- Location—kitchen should never be close to any area where there is accumulation of refuse, filth, or open drain or laboratory block.
- Floors should be impervious, smooth, non-slippery and easy to clean.
- Doors and windows should be fly proof; rat proof and doors should be self-closing type. Window opening should be 25% of the floor area.
- Ventilation should be good (29% of floor area). There should be a proper exhaust and smoke pipe. Good circulation of air is necessary.
- Walls should be smooth with rounded corners, impervious and easily washable. It is better to have washable emulsion paint and not tiles.
- Lighting—should be adequate. There should be ample natural light aided by artificial lighting.
- Storage of cooked food—separate room to be provided. For long storage, refrigerator/deep freeze/cold room are necessary.
- Storage of raw food—should be separate from cooked food. Perishable and non-perishable articles of food to be kept separately, in rat proof and vermin proof space. For perishable articles temperature control is essential.
- Water supply should be adequate, continuous supply should be available. Water should be clean and safe/potable.
- All work surfaces and food storage areas must be kept clean.
- There should be no false ceiling.
- Proper rodent and pest control should be done.
- Preparation of food must be done taking all hygienic precautions.
- Food should be served as soon as possible after preparation.
- Food storage refrigerators and freezers should be properly maintained and the temperature checked daily by the provided thermometers.
- Leftover food should be discarded.
- Dishwashing equipment must be used if possible.

HEALTH CHECK-UP FOR FOOD HANDLERS

1. Complete check-up (medical examination) of all food handlers before employment. This includes history of past illness (enteric fever, diarrhea and jaundice) and resent illness, complete physical examination, culture of feces, urine and X-ray chest, and laboratory tests. Laboratory tests and X-ray chest are repeated yearly and whenever indicated.
2. Food handlers are instructed to immediately report to the incharge Medical Officer and I/c Kitchen regarding any evidence of intestinal disease, skin infection or superficial sepsis, or sore throat, during the course of employment. Food handlers, who are sick, should be excluded from food handling.
3. Any infectious illness in the family of the food handlers should also be notified immediately to the In-Charge Medical Officer and Infection Control Officer or Nurse.
4. Food handlers are required to report to the hospital Medical Officer on his return from sick leave for inquiry regarding intestinal infections and other illnesses.

Close monitoring of health of food handlers should be done.

PERSONAL HYGIENE

- *Hands:* Hands should be washed with soap and water immediately after a visit to the toilet, after handling raw food or refuse and before handling, cooking and distributing food. Fingernails should be kept clean and trim.
- *Hair:* Head should be covered to prevent loose hair entering the food.
- *Overall:* Clean overall (white) should be worn.
- *Habits:* Coughing and sneezing in the vicinity of the food, licking the fingers, touching nose or hair should not be done.

WASHING OF CROCKERY AND CUTLERY

- Utensils, crockery and cutlery should be cleaned with soap and hot water.
- All crockery should be scraped and wiped with a paper to remove food remnants.
- Crockery should be rinsed before washing. There should be two sinks, pre-rinsing and washing is done in one sink.
- Water, which is not too hot, is used for washing along with suitable detergent.
- After washing the utensils are put in a rack and lowered into hot rinsing sink in which the temperature of water is 77–82°C; one minute should be allowed for immersion. This wills disinfect/sanitize the crockery and cutlery. The dishes are stocked in a rack and they will dry spontaneously. Do not wipe to dry.

DISPOSAL OF REFUSE

Refuse should be collected in covered, impervious container and disposed of twice a day.

CLEANING

The food preparation area and equipment should be cleaned with soap and water after finishing work. It is better to use a disinfectant (hypochlorite) also.

EDUCATION AND TRAINING OF FOOD HANDLERS

- There should be written standards and work procedures for daily operation. Procedures for preparation and serving of food must be such as to minimize contamination by microorganisms and chemicals.
- Programs should be undertaken for the education and training of food handlers in food preparation procedures maintaining cleanliness and sanitation of work area and equipment and observing personal hygiene and cleanliness.
- Purchasing specification should be made. They should meet the requirement of safety and sanitation of food, equipment, service ware and cleaning material.
- Written manuals should be prepared for procedures for cleaning and sanitizing crockery, cutlery, utensils, trays and work surfaces after use.
- Services in isolation rooms should be planned in consultation with the ICN and nursing staff.
- Procedures for storage, handling and disposal should be decided upon and responsibilities fixed.
- During transportation of food to wards, the containers of food should be properly and tightly covered. The food trolley should be separate and not used for transporting patient or laundry.

REFERENCES

1. Hobbs and Roberts (1993). Kitchen Hygiene. Chapter 12. In: Ayliffe GAJ, Fraise AP, Geddes AM, Mitchell K (Eds). Control of Hospital Infection. A practical handbook. 4th edi. Oxford University Press. Inc. New York; 2000. pp. 243-52.
2. Department of Health NHS Executive (1996). Management of food hygiene and

food services in the National Health Service. London. Department of Health (Quoted by Ref. No. 1).
3. Ref: Infection Prevention and Control. Food Hygiene Guidelines. East Cheshire NHS Trust. Accessed from www. Eastcheshire.nhs.ur/../Fo1%20Disclosure%20589%20may%20 2010%20-%20 policies%20. On 28/8/2015.
4. Infection Control Assessment and Oversight of Food Services at Children's Hospital, Los Angeles. Accessed from www.apictrivalley.weekly.com/../infection-control-oversight-of-food-services-greater-la-epic-march 2012.pptx.
5. Ref: In the Kitchen: Prevent the spread of Infection—Online Medical encyclopedia. Accessed from www.urmc.rochester.edu/../content.aspx?...1. 0n 28/8/2015.
6. Sandys GH, Wilkinson P. Microbiological evaluation of a hospital-delivered meals service using precooked chilled foods. J Hosp Infect. 1988;11:209.
7. Richards J, Parr E, Risborough P. Hospital food hygiene: The application of hazard analysis critical points to conventional hospital catering. J Hosp Infect. 1993;24:273.
8. Barrie D. The provision of food and catering services in hospital. J Hosp Infect. 1996;33:13.

Chapter 24

Waste Disposal

Chapter Outline

- Classification of Biomedical Waste (Hospital Waste)
- General Waste
- Infectious Waste
- Communicable Disease Transmitted Through Biomedical Waste
- Injuries to Waste Handlers During Procedures
- Objectives of Biomedical Waste Management
- Biomedical Waste Categories and their Segregation, Collection, Treatment and Processing, and Disposal Options
- Biomedical Waste Categories, Color Coding, Type of Container and Treatment Options
- Waste Management Policy
- Hospital Waste Contract
- Landfills
- Occupational Hazards
- Safety Measures for the Medical and Paramedical Staff
- Safety Measures for Cleaning and Transportation Staff
- Training and Motivation
- Training Modules for Different Levels of Staff
- Training for Medical and Laboratory Personnel
- Administrative and Management Staff
- Incentives and Motivation
- Awareness
- Standard Operative Procedures for Waste Disposal

INTRODUCTION[1,2]

Hospital waste is extremely hazardous. If it is not managed properly it can lead to serious health and environmental problems. Hospital waste is different from domestic waste and must therefore be segregated, collected, stored, transported and disposed off properly. If it is not managed, according to the set guidelines, it can get mixed with general waste within the hospital and subsequently with the solid municipal waste outside. This can expose the entire community to highly infectious diseases like HIV, hepatitis B and C, tuberculosis and other skin and respiratory infections.

In most hospitals, it is a practice to burn off the waste, which is very unscientific. This can lead to emission of dangerous levels of dioxins and furans in the environment that can cause various types of cancers. The residual ash when not disposed off in secured landfills can also pollute the underground water and contaminate the soil.

Therefore, it is essential that all the hospital staff including the superintendent and its administrative officers should be trained and educated regarding the methods of waste disposal to be adopted and a policy should be set up for every hospital according to the resources and finances available to them.

Biomedical waste: It is defined as any waste solid/liquid, including its container and any intermediate product generated in the diagnosis, treatment and research or immunization of human beings or animals/testing of biologicals and waste from slaughter houses.

Medical waste or healthcare waste: Waste generated from healthcare facilities in the diagnosis, treatment, immunization and research activities.

Tons of waste is produced by hospitals, clinics and laboratories every day. This waste poses risk to those who generate the waste and come in contact with it, as well as the environment and the public.

Proper waste disposal has now become mandatory with the legislation being passed by Government of India for biomedical waste from 20th July 1998. Therefore, it became necessary that each health care facility should implement a framework for the management of biomedical waste, keeping in view the resources available to them and financial constraints. Proper training of staff is essential for this. Usually, the least educated staff that collects the waste is most neglected, so training should start from those people, and then the nurses, the technical staff, the doctors and administrators.

Nowadays, the healthcare industry has shifted to the use of disposable products rather than reusable ones (i.e. like glass syringes, hospital laundry, etc.). The unscrupulous recycling of all those disposables is largely responsible for the spread of infections like hepatitis B, C and HIV.

Waste can also be contaminated with pathogens of diseases notifiable under epidemic controlled regulations, such as cholera, gastroenteritis, plague, etc., which should not leave the premises unless suitably disinfected.

Hospital waste still finds its way to roadside heaps of rubbish, where it mixes with municipal waste rendering it hazardous for the environment and public. Even animals are not spared, for stray cattle near dumped waste may ingest polythene packets and sharps and die from internal hemorrhage. Incidence of bovine tuberculosis has also gone up, increasing the already existing threat of tuberculosis in the community.

The waste from hospitals is mostly non-biodegradable which will really destroy our environment if not disposed of properly.

Awareness regarding biomedical waste rules is very low even among qualified medical personnel, including superintendents of hospitals and hospital administrators. Knowledge regarding the various technological options available to treat biomedical waste also remains minimal.

Low-quality incinerators have been installed in many hospitals, which do more harm than good. They release toxic emissions like dioxins, furans, heavy metal vapors and other harmful particulates, polluting the environment besides causing a major public health hazard. The incinerators presently in use in the hospitals of the country only reduce the amount of garbage and give rise to harmful ash, which is disposed off with the municipal waste. These incinerators are mostly single chambered, and do not reach temperatures more than 300°C, thus the combustion is ineffective and does not reach the standard laid down in biomedical waste rules, the combustion efficiency must be at least 99% with zero emission standards.

CLASSIFICATION OF BIOMEDICAL WASTE (HOSPITAL WASTE)[1,2]

Biomedical waste—materials generated as a result of patient diagnosis, treatment or immunization of human beings or animals or in research activities or in production or testing of biologicals. Hospital waste can be broadly classified as:

- *Hospital household waste or general waste:* Waste generated at kitchen, store and offices.
- *Infectious waste:* That portion of medical waste that can transmit an infectious disease. This forms only 10–15% of the total waste.
- *Hazardous waste:* Waste that is not infectious but hazardous. This forms 5% of the total waste (e.g. chemicals, discarded disinfectants, etc.).

GENERAL WASTE

About 80–85% of the waste generated in the hospital is non-infectious or general. General waste includes items like paper, cardboard boxes, plastic packaging, metal boxes, etc. Kitchen waste (left over food, vegetable peals, meat, fish, tea-bags, etc.) is another kind of general waste.

General waste can be sold for recycling if possible or disposed of with municipal waste going ultimately to the sanitary landfill. The kitchen waste can be composted at a convenient site in the hospital and turned into manure that can be used in the gardens of the hospital.

All hospitals produce a substantial amount of general waste. This waste though easy to handle, needs to be managed with care. It must be segregated from the infected waste, for even if small quantity of infectious waste gets mixed with general waste, the entire waste can turn infectious, thus increasing the problems of waste handling and management.

INFECTOUS WASTE[10]

Human and Animal Anatomical Waste

Human or animal tissue, organs, body parts, fetus below viability period, experimental animal carcasses or waste generated from animals used in experiments or testing in veterinary hospitals or colleges or animal houses. These are segregated in **yellow**-colored nonchlorinated bags.

Such waste is treated by incineration, or plasma pyrolysis or deep burial.

Soiled Waste

- Items contaminated with blood, body fluids like dressings, plaster casts, cotton swabs and bags containing residual or discarded blood and blood components.
- Should be collected in **yellow** non-chlorinated bags.
- They can be incinerated, or undergo plasma pyrolysis or deep burial. In absence of these facilities, autoclaving or microwaving or hydroclaving followed by shredding or mutilation. Treated waste to be sent for energy recovery/(Energy recovery includes any process that converts non-recyclable materials into usable heat, electricity, or fuel through a variety of processes including combustion, pyrolization, anaerobic digestion and landfill gas recovery).[13]

Expired or Discarded Medicines (Including Cytotoxic Drugs)

Pharmaceutical wastes like antibiotics, cytotoxic drugs including all items contaminated with cytotoxic drugs along with glass or plastic ampoules, vials, etc. They are collected in **yellow**-colored nonchlorinated bags or containers.

Expired cytotoxic drugs and items contaminated with cytotoxic drugs should be returned back to manufacturer or supplier for incineration at temperature >1,200°C or to a common biomedical waste treatment facility or hazardous waste treatment storage and disposal facility for incineration at >1,200°C or encapsulation or plasma pyrolysis at >1200°C.

All other discarded medicines shall either be sent back to manufacturer or disposed by incineration.

Chemical Waste

Chemicals used in production of biological and used and discarded disinfectants, pesticides, or chemically contaminated containers. Such wastes also need to be managed and handled with proper care.

This waste is collected in **yellow**-colored containers or nonchlorinated plastic bags.

This is disposed by incineration or plasma pyrolysis or encapsulation in hazardous waste treatment and storage facility.

Chemical Liquid Waste

Liquid waste generated due to use of chemicals in production of biological and used or discarded disinfectants, silver X-ray film developing liquid, discarded formalin, infected secretions, aspirated body fluids, liquid from laboratories and floor washings, cleaning and house-keepimg and disinfecting activities. They should be collected via a separate collection system leading to effluent treatment system. After resource recovery, the liquid waste shall be pretreated/neutralized before mixing with waste water.

Discarded Linen

These include mattresses, beddings contaminated with blood or body fluid. They are collected in nonchlorinated **yellow** plastic bags or suitable packing material.

Nonchlorinated chemical disinfection followed by incineration or plasma pyrolysis or for energy recovery.

In absence of above facilities, shredding or mutilation or combination of sterilization with shredding should be used. Treated waste to be sent for energy recovery or incineration or plasma pyrolysis.

Microbiology, Biotechnology and Other Clinical Laboratory Waste

Blood bags, laboratory cultures, stocks or specimens of microorganisms, live or attenuated vaccines, human and animal cell cultures used in research, industrial laboratories, production of biological, residual toxins, dishes and devices used for cultures.

These should be autoclaved in autoclave safe plastic bags or containers. Or

Pretreat these with nonchlorinated chemicals on site as per NACO or WHO guidelines.

Infectious Plastics

Disposable items like syringes, tubing, intravenous tubes and sets, bottles, cannulas, ventilator tubings, gloves, catheters, urine bags, etc. are segregated in **red**-colored nonchlorinated plastic bags or containers and autoclaved/microwaved/ hydroclaved, then shredded and then sent for recycling. Such treatment prevents their reuse and renders them sterile and useless. It is essential that such waste be treated entirely at site to avoid any risk of infection and reuse.

Plastics should never be incinerated as their incineration can emit dioxins in the air and can cause cancer.

Plastic waste should not be sent to land fill sites.

Sharps

Most dangerous of the hospital waste. They can injure the healthcare workers, and all those coming in contact with hospital waste.

Sharps include needles, syringes with fixed needles, scalpels, needle tips from needle cutter or burner or any other contaminated items that can puncture or cut including metal sharps.

These are collected in **white** transluscent puncture proof containers.

Treatment of sharps can be done as follows:

- Sterilized by autoclaving or dry heat sterilization followed by shredding or mutilation or encapsulation in metal container and sent for final disposal to iron foundries or sanitary landfill or designated concrete waste sharp pit.
- Chemically disinfected, shredded and disposed, if above facility not available.

Discarded Glassware

Broken or discarded and contaminated glass including medicine vials and ampoules except those contaminated with cytotoxic waste. These should be collected in cardboard boxes with **blue**-colored marking.

They should be disinfected (by soaking the washed glass waste after cleaning with detergent and sodium hypochlorite treatment) or through autoclaving or microwaving or hydroclaving and then sent for recycling.

Metallic Body Implants

These should be put into cardboard boxes with **blue**-colored marking.

Radioactive Waste

Radioactive waste is generated at the site of diagnosis and treatment. In diagnosis, X-rays, chemical dyes and isotopes of various elements are frequently used for treatment.

Radioactive waste may be in solid or liquid form. Such waste must be stored in special lead containers until ten times their half-life period, before waste is transported. It is then disposed off according to Bhaba Atomic Research Center (BARC) regulations in India. Radioactive waste especially Cobalt needles used for Brachy must be returned to BARC. Liquid radioactive waste is discharged into drains only after its ten times half-life period is over.

COMMUNICABLE DISEASE TRANSMITTED THROUGH BIOMEDICAL WASTE

1. Hepatitis B and C
2. HIV
3. Other infections like tuberculosis, cholera, diphtheria, gastroenteritis, etc.
4. Other new viruses like transfusion associated viruses.

INJURIES TO WASTE HANDLERS DURING PROCEDURES

About 60% of all hospital staff may sustain injuries from sharps knowingly or unknowingly, during various procedures undertaken by them in the health care facilities. Hospital personnel working in operation theaters are especially prone to needle injuries while suturing. Cases are reported of surgeons developing positivity to hepatitis B significantly due to needle injuries.

OBJECTIVES OF BIOMEDICAL WASTE MANAGEMENT

General

1. To reduce the impact of waste on community.
2. To reduce the chance of infection and accidental injury to workers.
3. To reduce the cost of total treatment of waste.

Specific

1. Motivation and sensitization of healthcare personnel.
2. Training of healthcare personnel.
3. Segregation of waste, so that each type is treated in a suitable manner thus minimizing harms.
4. Using proper disinfection technology depending on type of waste.
5. Fixing responsibility in institution for biomedical waste disposal and treatment.

In general, the quantity of waste generated from hospital ranges from 1.5 to 2.5 kg per day per patient. It may be more in specialized health care facilities like dialysis centers.

BIOMEDICAL WASTE CATEGORIES AND THEIR SEGREGATION, COLLECTION, TREATMENT AND PROCESSING, AND DISPOSAL OPTIONS (TABLE 24.1)

Table 24.1: Biomedical waste categories and their segregation, collection, treatment and processing, and disposal options[3,10]

Category	Types of waste	Types of bag or container to be used	Treatment and disposal options
Yellow	• *Human anatomical waste:* Human tissues, organs, body parts and fetus below the viability period (as per the Medical Termination of Pregnancy Act, 1971 amended from time to time) • *Animal anatomical waste:* Experimental animal carcasses, body parts, organs, tissues, including the waste generated from animals used in experiments or testing in veterinary hospitals or colleges or animal houses	Yellow-colored non-chlorinated plastic bags	Incineration or plasma pyrolysis or deep burial*
	• *Solid waste:* Items contaminated with blood, body fluids such as dressings, plaster casts, cotton swabs and bags containing residual or discarded blood and blood components		Incineration or plasma pyrolysis or deep burial * In absence of above facilities, autoclaving or microwaving or hydroclaving followed shredding or mutilation or combination of sterilization and shredding. Treated waste to be sent for energy recovery.
	• *Expired or discarded medicines:* Pharmaceutical waste like antibiotics, cytotoxic drugs including all items contaminated with cytotoxic drugs along with glass or plastic ampoules, vials, etc.	Yellow-colored non-chlorinated plastic bags or containers	Expired cytotoxic drugs and items contaminated with cytotoxic drugs to be returned back to the manufacturer or supplier for incineration at temperature >1200°C or to common biomedical waste treatment facility or hazardous waste treatment, storage and disposal facility for incineration at >1200°C or encapsulation or plasma pyrolysis at >1200°C All other discarded medicines shall be either sent back to manufacturer or disposed by incineration
	• *Chemical waste:* Chemicals used in production of biologicals and used or discarded disinfectants	Yellow-colored containers or non-chlorinated plastic bags	Disposed of by incineration or plasma pyrolysis or encapsulation in hazardous waste treatment, storage and disposal facility
	• *Chemical liquid waste:* Liquid waste generated due to use of chemicals in production of biological and used or discarded disinfectants, silver X-ray film developing liquid, discarded formalin, infected secretions,	Separate collection system leading to effluent treatment system	After resource recovery, the chemical liquid waste shall be pretreated before mixing with other waste water. The combined discharge shall confirm to the discharge norms given in schedule

Contd...

Contd...

Category	Types of waste	Types of bag or container to be used	Treatment and disposal options
	aspirated body fluids, liquid from laboratories and floor washings, cleaning, housekeeping and disinfecting activities, etc.		
	• *Discarded linen:* Mattresses, beddings contaminated with blood or body fluid	Non-chlorinated yellow plastic bags or suitable packing material	Non-chlorinated chemical disinfection followed by incineration or plasma pyrolysis or for energy recovery. In absence of above facilities, shredding or mutilation or combination of sterilization and shredding. Treated waste to be sent for energy recovery or incineration or plasma pyrolysis
	• *Microbiology and biotechnology and other clinical laboratory waste:* Blood bags, laboratory cultures, stocks or specimens of microorganisms, live or attenuated vaccines, human and animal cell cultures used in research, industrial laboratories, production of biological, residual toxins, dishes and devices used for cultures	Autoclave safe plastic bags or containers	Pretreat to sterilize with non-chlorinated chemicals on-site as per National AIDS Control Organization or World Health Organization guidelines, thereafter for incineration
Red	*Contaminated waste (Recyclable):* Waste generated from disposable items such as tubings, bottles, intravenous tubes and sets, catheters, urine bags, syringes (without needles and fixed needle syringes) and vacutainers with their needles cut) and gloves	Red-colored non-chlorinated plastic bags or containers	Autoclaving or microwaving/hydroclaving followed by shredding or mutilation or combination of sterilization and shredding. Treated waste to be sent to registered or authorized recyclers or for energy recovery or plastics to diesel or fuel oil or for road making whichever is possible Plastic waste should not be sent to landfill sites
White	*Waste sharps including metals:* Needles, syringes with fixed needles, needles from needle tip cutter or burner, scalpels, blades or any other contaminated sharp object that may cause puncture and cuts. This includes both used, discarded and contaminated metal sharps	Puncture proof, leak proof, tamper proof containers	Autoclaving or dry heat sterilization followed by shredding or mutilation or encapsulation in metal container or cement concrete; combination of shredding cum autoclaving, and sent for final disposal to iron foundaries (having consent to operate from the state Pollution Control Board or Pollution Control Committee) or sanitary landfill or designated concrete waste sharp pit
Blue	• *Glassware:* Broken or discarded and contaminated glass including medicine vials and ampoules except those contaminated with cytotoxic wastes	Cardboard boxes with blue-colored marking	Disinfection (by soaking the washed glass waste after cleaning with detergent and sodium hypochlorite treatment) or through autoclaving or microwaving or hydroclaving and then sent for recycling
	• *Metallic body implants:*	Cardboard boxes with blue-colored marking	

*Disposal by deep burial is permitted only in rural or remote areas where there is no access to common biomedical waste treatment facility. This will be carried out with proper prior approval from the prescribed authority and as per the standards specified in schedule. The deep burial facility shall be located as per the provisions and guidelines issued by Central Pollution Control Board from time to time.

Some Important Rules

1. Chemical treatment using at least 1% hypochlorite solution having 30% residual chlorine for 20 minutes or any other equivalent chemical reagent, that should demonstrate $Log10^4$ reduction efficiency for microorganisms.
2. Mutilation/shredding must be done in a manner that can prevent the unauthorized use of biomedical waste.
3. There will be no chemical treatment before incineration, except for microbiological, laboratory and highly infectious waste.
4. Incineration ash shall be disposed through hazardous waste treatment and disposal facility, if toxic or hazardous constituents are present beyond the prescribed limits as given in the hazardous waste Rules 2008, or revised from time to time.
5. Syringes should be either mutilated or needles should be cut or stored in tamper proof, leak proof and puncture proof containers for sharps storage.

BIOMEDICAL WASTE CATEGORIES, COLOR CODING, TYPE OF CONTAINER AND TREATMENT OPTIONS (TABLE 24.2)

Table 24.2: Biomedical waste categories, color coding, type of container and treatment options[3,10]

Color coding	Types of container	Category	Treatment options
Yellow	Non-chlorinated plastic bag or container (Use autoclave safe bags or containers for microbiology, biotechnology waste)	• Human anatomical waste • Animal anatomical waste • Soiled waste • Expired or discarded medicines • Chemical waste • Discarded linen, mattresses, beddings contaminated with blood or body fluids • Microbiology, biotechnology and other laboratory waste	Incineration/deep burial/ plasma pyrolysis
Red	Non-chlorinated container/ plastic bag	Contaminated waste recyclable (plastic)	Autoclaving/microwaving/ hydroclaving followed by shredding or mutilation. Then sent to authorized recyclers
White	Puncture and leak- proof container	Waste sharps including metals	Autoclaving/dry heat sterilization and destruction/shredding or mutilation. Sent to iron foundaries or sanitary landfill or designated concrete waste sharp pit
Blue	Cardboard boxes with blue-colored marking	Glassware	Cleaning with detergent and disinfection with sodium hypochlorite/autoclaving/ microwaving/hydroclaving and then sent for recycling
Black bag	For general waste including kitchen waste, office waste, store waste, paper, orange peels, etc. thrown in ward by patient's relatives	All non-infectious waste or general waste	This will be picked up by the municipal corporation

WASTE MANAGEMENT POLICY[1,2]

A waste management policy has to be decided by the hospital authorities and documented. It should clearly describe all levels of responsibilities from the highest administrative authority to lowest staff (ayas, ward boys, etc). It should be written officially and approved by the regulatory authority and be available to all the employees in all the departments. The policy must clearly state the standard operative:

a. Identification, collection, and separation (segregation of waste)
b. Storage
c. Transport
d. Measurement
e. Treatment
f. Disposal
g. Worker training
h. Worker health and safety records.

Identification, Collection, and Segregation of Waste[1,2]

Segregation of waste is the most important step of biomedical waste management. By segregation, the quantities of waste needing special attention are considerably reduced and therefore more manageable. Different types of wastes need different treatment and therein lay the importance of segregation. Different types of containers should be available at each point.

1. General waste—black
2. Infected non-sharp waste (pathological waste/anatomical waste)—yellow
3. Infected soiled waste—yellow
4. Expired or discarded medicines including cytotoxic waste—yellow
5. Infected sharp waste—white puncture proof container
6. Infected plastic waste—red
7. Infected glassware—blue.

Internal Waste Segregation—Key to Success

This includes waste management process (Fig. 24.1):

- Make someone in-charge of waste management.
- Appropriately placed containers.
- Appropriately labeled containers.
- Appropriate bag liners and containers.
- Mandatory staff education about biomedical waste management program.
- Feedback system.
- Regular monitoring.
- Continuous process.

Transport and Storage[1,2]

Precautions during transport are essential to prevent the public as well as the operators from being exposed to hazardous waste. There are two types of transport of waste.

Internal Transport—Transport within the Hospital (Fig. 24.2)[11]

Refers to the transport of waste from the point of generation, collection and storage in the wards to the point outside the building premises, where it is kept pending till it is the transported to the actual site of disposal. A pushcart or a trolley designed to have bins or containers can be used to carry the waste from the wards to outside the building from where it is carried for final disposal. But if it is going for disposal in the hospital premises itself the same trolley can be used to carry it till there. This should be made of stainless steel, of robust construction and should be of good quality and durable.

Within the hospital waste routes must be designated to avoid the passages of waste through patient care areas.

Separate time should be fixed for transportation of biomedical waste to reduce chances of mixing with general waste.

Dedicated covered wheeled containers, trolleys or carts should be used to transport the waste bins/plastic bags to the site of storage/treatment.

Trolleys or carts should be thoroughly cleaned and disinfected in the event of any spillage.

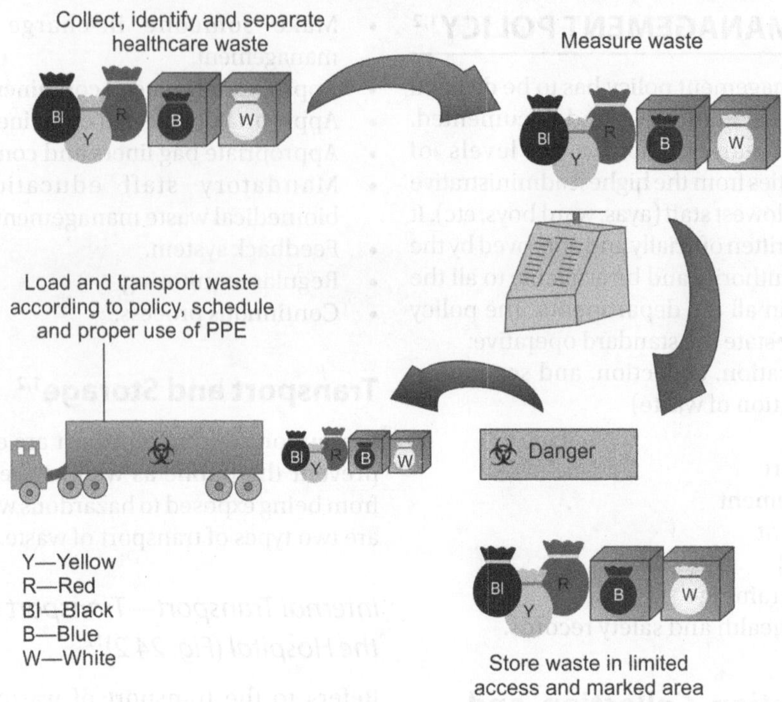

Fig. 24.1: Waste management process
(For color version, see Plate 1)

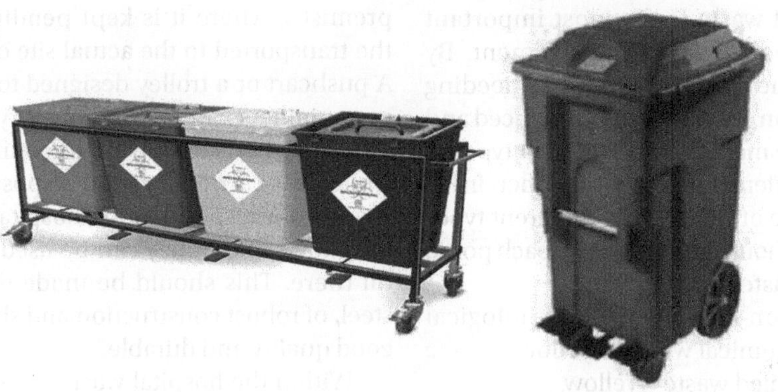

Fig. 24.2: Internal transport[11]
(For color version, see Plate 2)

The wheeled containers should be designed, so that the waste can be easily loaded, remains secured during transportation, does not have any sharp edges and is easy to clean and disinfect.

Waste Storage (Fig. 24.3)[1,2]

It is very necessary to arrange a certain place to store all kinds of wastes resulting from health care and treatment in the hospitals before appropriate disposal.

1. Technical specifications of waste store:
   - The store should be prevented from being used as a food source of pests or animals or breeding site of insects or germ carriers.
   - Water should be available for washing it.

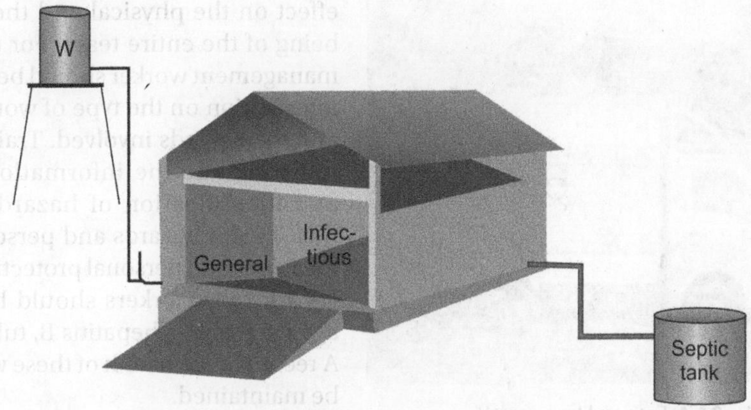

Fig. 24.3: Waste storehouse

- Drainage system should be available to receive polluted water from cleaning store floor.
- Capacity of store should be three times the daily accumulation of wastes.

2. Types of components of waste store:
   - Compartment for general waste.
   - Compartment for infectious waste.
3. Components of waste storehouse:
   - Should have a roof, and should be made up of durable building material.
   - Should be made of concrete, smooth walled and one meter high, the upper parts should be lined with wire net.
   - Should have a smoothened basement with slopes leading to septic tanks.
   - Should have wide doors for easy access that is bringing in and taking out wastes.
   - Water supply should be available near the waste store for convenient cleaning.
   - Septic tank should be available nearby.
   - In the compartment arranged for infectious waste, a steel grating or mesh stand arranged for punctured waste bags to allow to drain into the waste water system should be available.

Storage areas should be:

- Protected from water, wind, and rain;
- Protected from rodents, insects, and other animals;
- Located away from patients and the public;
- An enclosure that can be locked when not in use;
- Accessible only to authorized personnel;
- Kept clean, free at all times of debris and standing water;
- Disinfected weekly and whenever a spill occurs.
- Waste that can **decompose** and smell should not be stored longer than **1 day** (warm weather) to **2 days** (cool weather).

External Transport (Fig. 24.4)[12]

Refers to transport of waste from a central collection site outside the building premises to the site of final disposal. A lorry or van should be used for this. It should be labeled with" Biomedical waste" symbol on both sides and the rear part. It should be fully covered and lined internally with aluminum or stainless steel to give smooth impervious finish. It should have rounded corners without edges for effective cleaning and disinfection. The driver's cabin should be fully separated and the load compartment should be securely locked during transit. If the final waste disposal area is too far, then the load compartment should be refrigerated. Or it should have roof vents for ventilation.

Measurement of Waste[1,2]

This can be done in the wards or at the end when waste from all wards have been brought

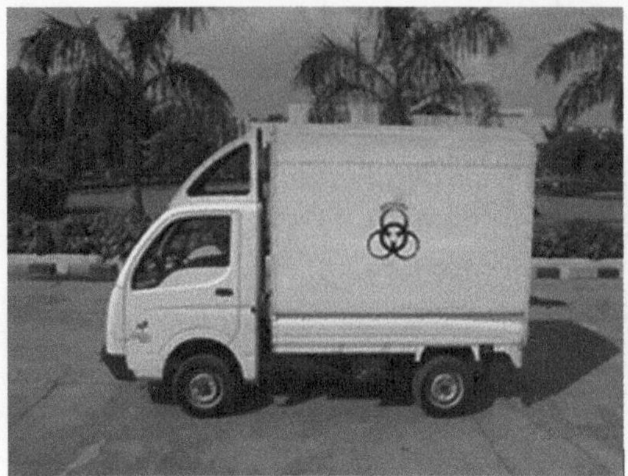

Fig. 24.4: External transport[12]

to a common site outside the building for storage before final treatment and disposal. Weighing is essential to know the exact amount of waste generated in the hospital and thus decides the method of treatment and disposal.

Worker Training[1]

Training is desirable in all health care institutions to sensitize the personnel regarding various aspects of waste management. Basic training should be given to all health care personnel especially those who are going to directly handle the waste. This should include:

- Information on hazards of health care waste.
- Methods of preventing nosocomial infection related to waste handling methods.
- Various safety procedures for dealing with chemical, pharmaceutical, radioactive waste and sharps. Proper waste segregation, handling, packaging, transport, treatment and disposal.
- Action and notification to supervisors in case of accidents.

The content of this program should be periodically reviewed and updated as necessary.

Workers Health and Safety[1]

Occupational safety and health issues related to biomedical waste treatment are important issues. They have a far reaching effect on the physical and the mental well-being of the entire team. For this, the waste management worker should be given detailed information on the type of work he has to do and the hazards involved. Training for safety must include the information on labeling and identification of hazardous material, their health hazards and personal protective measures and personal protective equipment. Health care workers should be immunized against tetanus, hepatitis B, tuberculosis, etc. A record of the health of these workers should be maintained.

Instructions for Personnel Handling Biomedical Waste[1,2]

Staffs who handle clinical waste bags and containers should be trained so as to be aware of the following to avoid injury and accidents.

While handling waste bags, the most likely danger is a needle prick injury, if needles have not been properly disposed off in sharp containers.

- When waste bags/containers are 3/4th full, they should be sealed.
- The bags and containers must confirm to the different color coding. Labeling can be done by writing the information on the bags and the outer container (date, ward no, name of person who has done this job, type of waste, etc.).
- Separation of the biomedical waste should be done at source (in different color coding bags).
- Check that the bags are properly sealed or tied.
- Bags should be picked up by the neck and placed, so that they can be picked up again by the neck for further handling.
- Manual handling of waste bags should be minimized to reduce the risk of needle prick injuries.
- Bags should not be held close against the body and too many bags should not be carried at one time.
- Yellow bags and blue bags or white bags should not be thrown or dropped.

- Sharp containers should preferably have a handle.
- Clinical waste should be kept in a specified storage area.
- Staff should know the appropriate cleaning and disinfection procedures in case of accidental spillage and how to report an incident.
- Plastic color coded bags before handling waste should be made available.
- Porter should wear protective clothing, gloves, overall, etc.
- If the bag is soiled, it should be placed in another clean bag of the same color.
- Under no circumstances should anyone insert their hands into any waste container.

Care of the HCW's Handling Waste[1,2]

Personal protective clothing (PPC) and personal protective equipment (PPE) must be available to the staff and its usage ensured (Fig. 24.5).

They must wear:

1. Heavy duty thick rubber gloves.
2. Aprons—a reusable heavy duty, autoclavable rubber apron may be worn.
3. Footwear—gumboots should be worn by waste handlers. The trousers must remain outside the gumboots.
4. Masks—simple, reusable masks must be worn.

Immunization of these workers especially with hepatitis B vaccine is essential.

In case, there are any potential problems or if additional training or education is required the housekeepers should notify the hospital infection control committee of the same. Mistakes in segregating are to be corrected by the house keeping/nursing staff by placing the incorrectly filled bag into another bag of correct color. Incorrectly segregated waste should never be taken out of a waste bag or container once deposited.

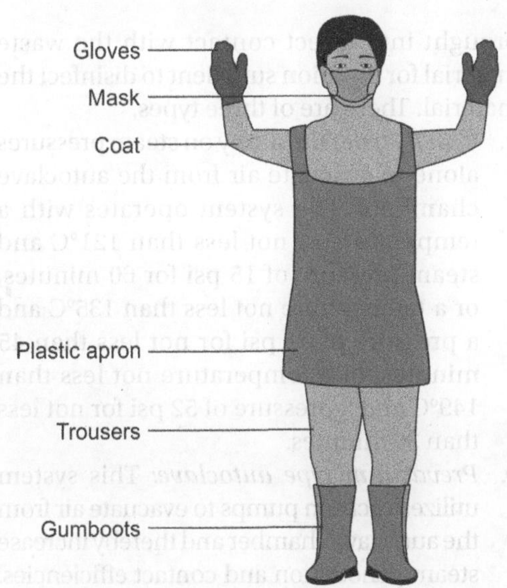

Fig. 24.5: Personal protective clothing

Technologies for Treatment of Biomedical Waste[1-3]

Various technologies have been developed for treatment of biomedical waste. The purpose of treatment of biomedical waste is to reduce or eliminate the number of pathogens thereby minimizing or eliminating the potential for disease transmission.

There are various categories of waste treatment process:

a. Mechanical processes
b. Thermal processes:
   - Autoclaving
   - Hydroclaving
   - Incineration
   - Pyrolysis
   - Plasma-plasma pyrolysis systems
c. Chemical process
d. Irradiation processes
e. Biological processes.

a. Mechanical Processes[1]

Mechanical processes are used to change the physical character of the waste to facilitate handling or to process the waste in conjunction with other treatment steps. The two primary mechanical processes are compaction and shredding. By compaction, the waste is compressed into containers, thus reducing the volume, shredding which also includes grinding, pulping, granulation, etc. used to break waste into smaller pieces.

But shredding and compaction are not considered to be good alternative techniques because aerosols or spills of microorganisms may be created which are dangerous and may infect the person working on a shredder. This happens especially if the untreated medical waste is shredded.

However, if waste is shredded after it has been decontaminated in order to make it unrecognizable, then there are no ill effects.

Shredding: According to BMW 1998 rules, plastics (IV bottles, IV sets, syringes, catheters, etc.), sharps (needles, blades, glass, etc.) should be shredded, but only after either chemical treatment/microwaving/autoclaving. Needle destroyers can be used for disposal of needles directly without chemical treatment.

b. Thermal Processes[1]

Most living organisms are killed at a temperature of 100°C.

There are two categories of thermal processes:

1. Low heat system
2. High heat systems.

Low heat systems use steam, hot water or electromagnetic radiation to heat and decontaminate the waste. They typically operate at temperature of less than 300°F, which is insufficient to combust or destroy the materials.

High heat system employs combustion, pyrolysis and high temperature plasmas to decontaminate and destroy waste. These systems operate at temperatures ranging from as low as 1,100°F to more than 10,000°F.

The basic thermal treatment processes are as follows:

Autoclave (Figs 24.6A and B)[1-4,10]

This is a process of steam sterilization under pressure. It is low heat in which steam is brought into direct contact with the waste material for duration sufficient to disinfect the material. These are of three types.

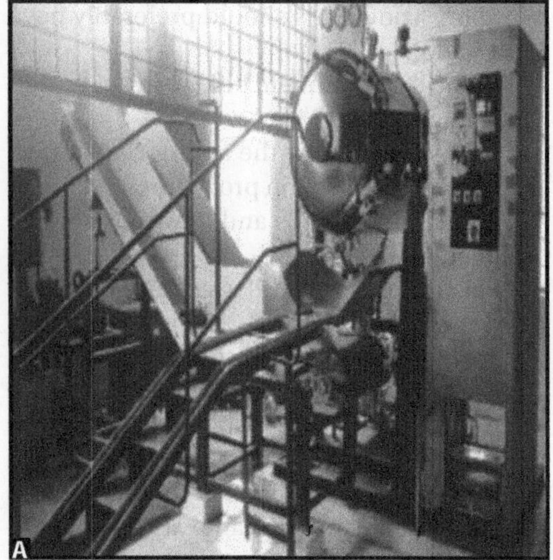

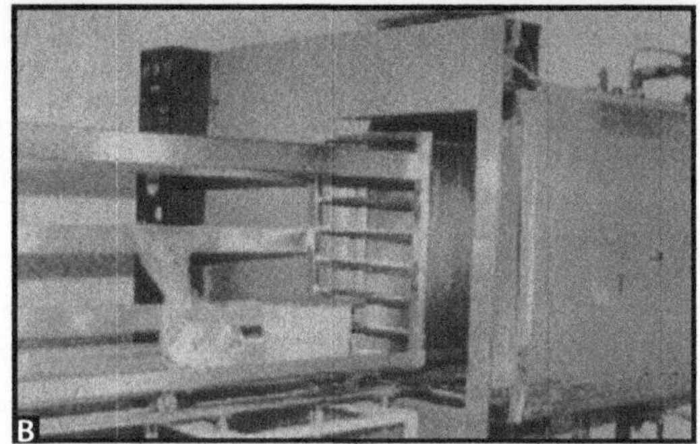

Figs 24.6A and B: (A) Autoclave with shredder; (B) Autoclave without shredder

a. *Gravity type:* These rely on steam pressures alone to evacuate air from the autoclave chambers. The system operates with a temperature of not less than 121°C and steam pressure of 15 psi for 60 minutes, or a temperature not less than 135°C and a pressure of 31 psi for not less than 45 minutes, or a temperature not less than 149°C and a pressure of 52 psi for not less than 30 minutes.
b. *Prevacuum type autoclave:* This system utilizes vacuum pumps to evacuate air from the autoclave chamber and thereby increase steam penetration and contact efficiencies. In this the medical waste will be subjected

to three prevacuum pulse to purge the autoclave of all air. The waste will be subject to a temperature not less than 121°C and pressure 15 psi for not less than 45 minutes or a temperature of not less than 135°C and pressure of 31 psi for not less than 30 minutes. The air removed during the prevacuum cycle should be decontaminated by means of HEPA and activated carbon filtration, steam treatment or any other method to prevent release of pathogen.

c. *Retort type autoclave:* These systems have large chambers designed to operate at higher temperatures and pressures than others. These autoclaves are designed to handle much larger volumes and operate at much high steam, temperature and pressure. They have been used on applications having capacities of up to 60 tons per day per unit. These systems are not as yet available in our country.

Until recently, conventional steam autoclaving was not used for treating large volumes of medical waste. This is primarily because autoclaving does not provide a post-shredding step, which is required to provide disfigurement.

Parameters, which influence effectiveness of steam autoclave treatment are:

- Temperature and pressure achieved by the autoclave.
- The size of waste load.
- The steam penetration of the waste.
- Packaging of the waste for treatment.
- The orientation of the waste load within the autoclave.

Steam autoclave operates most effectively when temperature, measured at the center of the waste load approaches 121°C (250°F) and there is adequate steam penetration of the load under pressure.

Autoclave with shredder: Autoclave treatment has been recommended for microbiology and biotechnology waste, waste sharps, soiled and solid wastes. This technology renders certain categories of biomedical waste as innocuous and unrecognizable (Fig. 24.6B).

Hydroclave (Figs 24.7A and B) [1-4]

It is also classified as a steam sterilization technology. It is an innovative form of autoclave. It is a double-walled container, in which steam is injected into the outer jacket to heat the inner chamber containing the waste. Moisture contained in the waste evaporates as steam builds up the requisite pressure (35–36 psi). There are paddles inside the chamber, which tumble the waste continuously against the hot wall mixing it as well as fragmenting the waste. In absence of enough moisture, additional steam is injected. The system operates at 132°C and 36 psi for 20 minutes. The total time for a cycle is about 50 minutes, which includes start-up, heat-up, sterilization, venting and depressurization and dehydration. The treated material can further be shredded before disposal. The expected volume and weight reductions are upto 85% and 70% respectively. The waste material is dehydrated and reduced in volume. The space required to install and operate the hydroclave is the size of an average room.

The hydroclave is horizontally mounted and has one or more top side loading doors and a smaller unloading door at its bottom.

The vessel is fitted with a motor driven shaft to which are attached powerful fragmenting/mixing arms, that slowly rotate inside the vessel.

When steam is introduced in the vessel jacket, it transmits heat rapidly to the wet fragmented waste, which in turn produces steam of its own.

The resultant dynamic interaction:

1. Sterilizes the waste by high temperature and pressure steam, similar to autoclave but with greater and more heat penetration.
2. Hydrolyses the organic components of waste.
3. Fragments and totally dehydrates the waste.
4. Reduces the volume by 85% and weight unto 60%.
5. Allows self-unloading after treatment cycle.

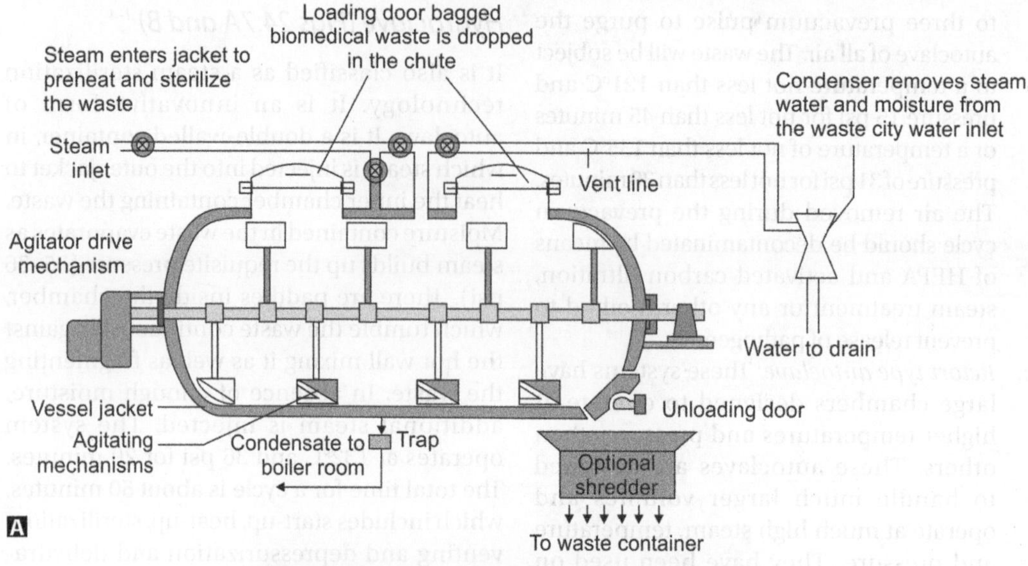

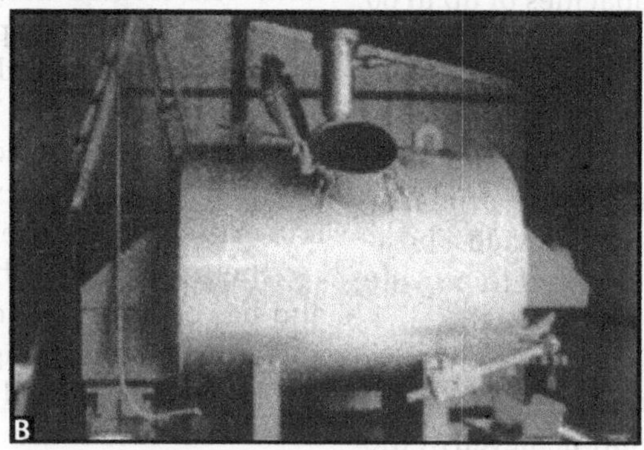

Figs 24.7A and B: Hydroclave

Advantages of hydroclave technology:

- No pretreatment of waste required.
- Complete waste dehydration.
- Disposal costs are greatly reduced
- Pathological waste treatment—sterilizes, dehydrates and renders unrecognizable.
- Environmentally friendly emissions.
- Treatment cost is low ₹1/kg—so economical
- Operation and maintenance—relatively simple, easy-to-operate and maintain.
- Operation is push button automatic.

The treatment cycle:

a. Loading.
b. Heat up and fragmentation.
c. Sterilization period—15 minutes at 132°C, or 30 minutes at 121°C (to achieve log level 6–8 sterilization).
d. Depressurization.
e. Dehydration.
f. Unloading.
g. Shredding.

Hydrolysis of organic waste in the hydroclave: The hydroclave can hydrolyse segregated, organic waste to a homogenous substance ready for use as soil supplement. The main advantage here is the speed at which the waste is converted as compared to the traditional method of composting.

The hydroclave can treat the same waste as the autoclave plus the waste sharps. The sharps are also fragmented. This technology has certain benefits, such as, absence of harmful air emissions, absence of liquid discharges, non-requirement of chemicals, reduced volume and weight of waste, etc.

Tata Memorial Hospital in Mumbai has installed the first hydroclave in India in September 1999.

Incineration (Fig. 24.8)[1-4]

Historical overview: Incineration comes from a Greek word meaning "burn to ashes". It signifies a combustion process. It was first introduced in the mid-fifties.

Initially, the incinerators were just uncontrolled single chamber fireboxes with smoke stacks. But the modern incineration systems are well engineered and designed, well controlled and well monitored. In our country, the norms laid down for incinerator by the Central Pollution Board regarding incinerators are still not followed. In fact because of environmental considerations the dropout rate of incinerators is constantly increasing and has reached up to a level of 60% or more.

Advantages and disadvantages of incineration:

Advantages:
- It reduces waste volume and weight.
- It renders the waste unrecognizable.
- Suitable for all types of waste.
- Heat recovery potential.
- Can treat chemotherapeutic waste.

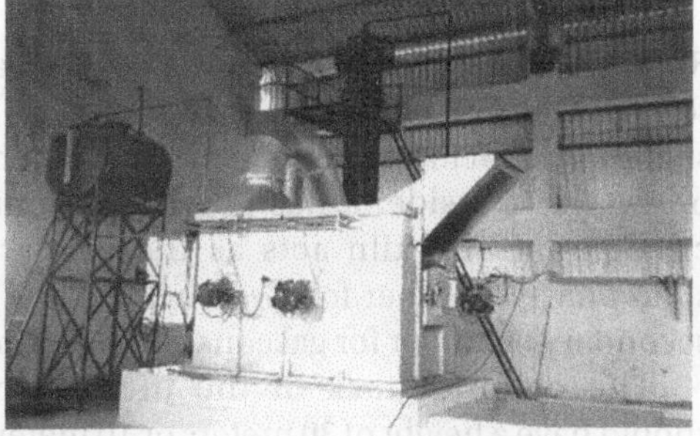

Fig. 24.8: Incinerator

Disadvantages:
- High capital costs.
- High maintenance and repair costs.
- Stack emission and concerns.
- High energy output and low efficiency.
- Siting difficulties.
- Permission difficulties.
- Public opposition.

Design, concepts and principles of incineration (Figs 24.9 and 24.10): Incineration is a high temperature thermal process employing combustion of the waste under controlled conditions for converting them into inert material and gases. They can be electrically operated or oil fired or a combination of both.

There are three types of incinerators used for hospital waste:
1. Multiple chamber type.
2. Rotary kiln.
3. Controlled air and rotary kiln types.

All types have primary and secondary combustion chambers to ensure optimal combustion.

In a nutshell, the primary chamber has pyrolytic conditions with a temperature range of about 800 (+/- 50°C). The secondary chamber operates under excess air conditions at about 1050 (+/- 50°C); the volatiles are liberated in the first chamber, whereas they are destroyed in the second chamber. Some models are filled with eductor mechanism, which maintains the system under negative pressure and helps control the flue gases more effectively. The chimney height should be minimum 30 meters above ground level. Installation of incinerators in congested area is not desirable.

In biomedical waste management, the incinerator has been recommended for human anatomical waste, animal waste, discarded medicines and soiled wastes.

Multiple chamber hearth incinerators: Solid phase combustion takes place in the primary chamber, whereas secondary chamber is for gas phase combustion. The tertiary chamber when present condenses the gases and air particulates.

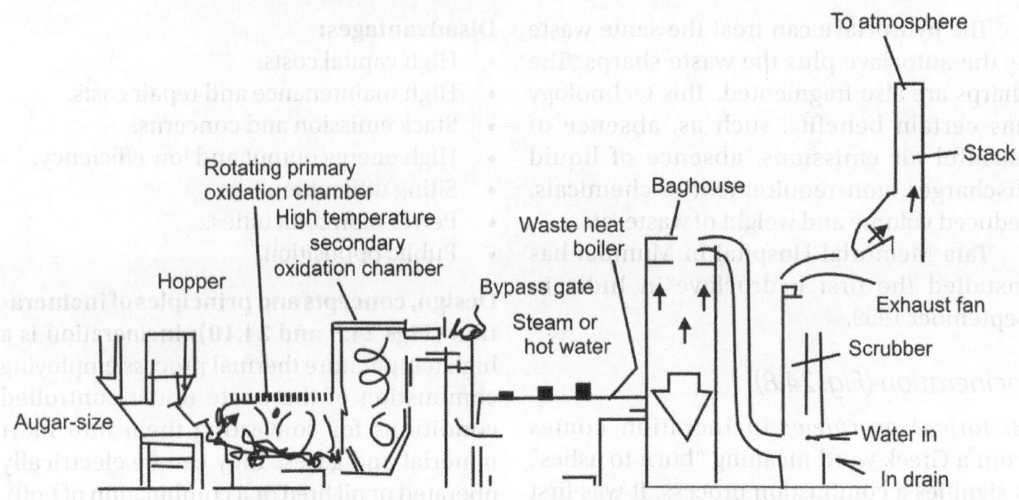

Fig. 24.9: Schematic diagram of three-stage incinerator

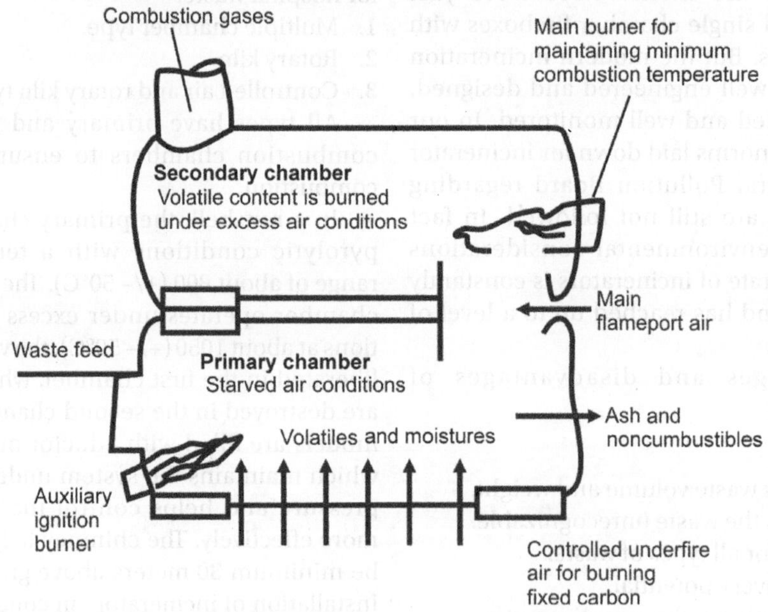

Fig. 24.10: Two chamber incinerator

These are also referred to as excess air incinerators, as excess air is present in both chambers.

Controlled air incinerator: In this type, its first chamber is operated at low air level, followed by an excess air chamber. Due to low oxygen levels in the primary chamber, there is better control of particulate matter in the flue gas.

Rotary kiln incinerator: This is a cylindrical refractory lined shell that is mounted at a slight tilt to facilitate mixing and movement of the waste inside. It has provision for air circulation. The kiln acts as the primary solid phase chamber followed by which is a secondary chamber for gaseous combustion.

The chimneystack of the incinerator should have a height of 30 meters or 10 meters higher than the nearest tallest building.

The main problem with incinerator is it poses an environmental threat. The system is complex and requires personnel trained in the technology of operation and maintenance of the equipment.

Regulation and standards for biomedical waste rules: Under EPA (Environmental Protection Act) Rule 1986, biomedical waste rules were framed in which emission standards for incineration were laid down. According to them, the incinerator should be a two-chamber incinerator with a combustion efficiency of 99%, temperature in the first chamber 800 (+/- 50°C) and second chamber 1050 (+/- 50°C) with 3% oxygen in stack gas.

The incinerator should be installed and made operational as per specifications under the BMW rules 1998 and March 2016 rules, and a certificate may be taken from CPCB/State Pollution Control Board.

Innovative and emerging technologies: Presently research programs are on all over the world and newer technologies are emerging, which aim at better combustion, better emission control and lower costs.

Microwave Treatment (Fig. 24.11) [1-4,10]

This is also a wet thermal disinfection technology, but unlike the other thermal treatment systems, which heat the waste externally, microwave heats the targeted material from inside out providing a high level of disinfection or sterilization.

Microwave treatment shall not be used for cytotoxic, hazardous or radioactive wastes, contaminated animal carcasses, body parts and large metal items.

Biological indicators (*Bacillus atrophaeus* spores) should be used for testing the microwave using vials or strips with at least 1 × 10^4 spores per strip. The biological indicator shall be placed with the waste and exposed to same conditions as the waste during a normal treatment cycle.

Method: The material is first put through a shredder. The shredded material is pushed into a treatment chamber, where it is moistened with high temperature steam. The material is then carried by a screw conveyor beneath a series (normally 4–6 numbers) of conventional microwave generators, which heat the material to 95–100°C and uniformly disinfect the material during a minimum residence time of 30 minutes. A second shredder fragments the material further into unrecognizable particles before it is automatically discharged into conventional or general waste container. This treated material can be land filled, provided adequate care is taken to complete the microwave treatment. In the modern versions, the process control is computerized for smooth and effective control.

Benefits (Advantages) of microwave technology:

1. Absence of harmful air emission (when adequate provision of containment and filters is made).

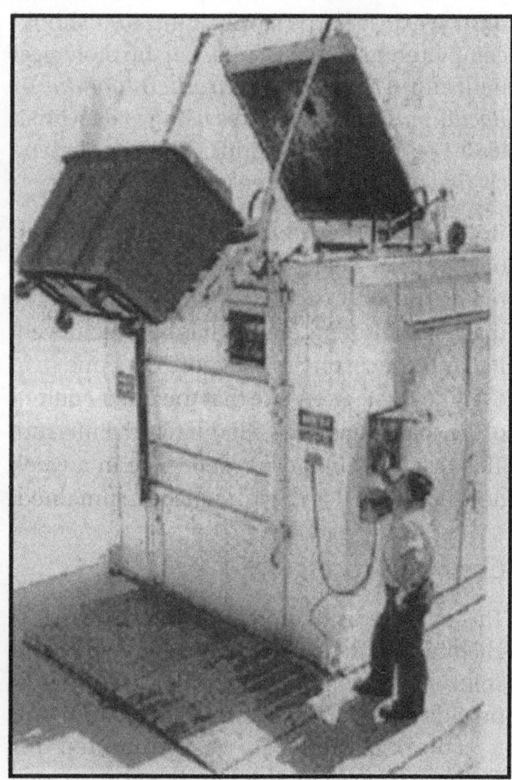

Fig. 24.11: Microwave

2. Absence of liquid discharges.
3. No chemicals required.
4. Reduced volume of waste (due to shredding and moisture loss).
5. Operator safety (due to automatic hoisting arrangements) for the waste bins into the hopper, so that manual contact with the waste bags is not necessary.
6. It is a cost-effective utility system.
7. It is worker friendly, operates quietly and is environment friendly.

Disadvantage: The investment costs are high at present.

Dry heat sterilization:[10] Waste sharps can be treated by dry heat sterilization at a temperature not less than 185°C for at least a residence period of 150 minutes in each cycle, of which sterilization period is of 90 minutes. There should be automatic recording system to monitor operating parameters.

Validation test for sharps sterilization unit: Wastes sharps sterilization unit should completely and consistently kill the biological indicator *Geobacillus stearothermophilus* or *Bacillus atropheaus* spores using vials with at least Log 10^6 spores per mL. The test shall be carried out once in three months.

Routine test: A chemical indicator strip or tape that changes color when a certain temperature is reached can be used to verify that a specific temperature has been achieved. It may be necessary to use more than one strip over the waste to ensure that the inner content of the sharps has been adequately disinfected. This test shall be performed once in a week and records in this regard shall be maintained.

Chemical Processes[1,2]

This is same as chemical disinfection. Most chemical waste treatment uses a disinfectant solution in combination with shredding to provide decontamination and disfigurement.

This treatment is recommended for waste sharps, solid and liquid waste, as well as chemical wastes. Chemical treatment involves use of 1% hypochlorite solution with a minimum contact period of 30 minutes. Other equivalent chemical reagents also can be used, such as phenolic compounds, iodine, hexachlorophane, iodine-alcohol, or formaldehyde-alcohol combination, etc. pre-shredding of the waste is desirable for better contact with waste material.

Standards for efficacy of chemical disinfection:[10] Microbial inactivation efficacy is equated to "Log 10 kill" which is defined as the difference between the logarithms of number of test microorganisms before and after chemical treatment. Chemical disinfection treatment methods shall demonstrate a 4 Log 10 reduction or greater for *Bacillus subtilis* (ATCC 19659) in chemical treatment systems.

Irradiation Processes[1,2]

In this electromagnetic or ionizing radiation is used. These systems require postirradiation shredding to render the waste unrecognizable.

Biological Processes[1,2]

In this method, biological enzymes are used for treating medical waste. Biological reactions are supposed to not only decontaminate the waste but also cause destruction of all the organic constituents so that only plastics, glass and other inerts remain in the residues.

A conveyor transports the waste to a shredder. The shredder residue is mixed with water and pumped slurry to a tank-containing enzyme where biological reactions take place. Treated residue is pumped from the tank through a screw press to separate solids, solid residues are compacted and collected in a bin for disposal.

Plasma Torch Technology[1,2]

The waste is pyrolyzed (heated without air) at temperature beyond 1150°C producing combustible gases and vitreous or glasslike rods substances by deploying plasma technology. The residue is suitable for concrete and asphalt construction and gases may serve as a source of energy.

Effluent Treatment Plant (Table 24.3)[14]

In hospitals that have ETP facility, the treatment is carried out using special scientific process and generally involves three stages, primary, secondary, and tertiary levels of treatment.

Primary treatment: It consists of temporarily holding the sewage in a basin where the settled and floating materials are removed and the remaining liquid subjected to secondary treatment. Primary treatment usually removes from 30% to 40% of the BOD. After this treatment the BOD and COD levels usually comes down to 25% of its initial levels.

Secondary treatment: It removes the dissolved and suspended biological matter and is typically performed by indigenous, water-borne microorganisms in a managed habitat. This treatment uses microbial degradation, aerobic or anaerobic, to reduce the concentration of the organic compounds. The combined use of primary and secondary treatment reduces approximately 80–90% of the BOD. In this stage, there is settling down of the suspended solid contents of the biological waste as thick slurry called sludge, while the treated fluid undergoes tertiary treatment. Through this process, 95% of the pollutants from the waste water are removed.

Table 24.3: Standards for liquid waste

Parameters	Permissible limits
pH	6.5–9.0
Suspended solids	100 mg/L
Oil and grease	10 mg/L
BOD	30 mg/L
COD	250 mg/L

Bioassay test 90% survival of fish after 96 hours in 100% effluent
These limits are applicable to those hospitals which are either connected with sewers without terminal Sewage Treatment Plant or not connected to public sewers:

- BOD—biochemical oxygen demand is the amount of dissolved oxygen needed by aerobic biological organisms in a body of water to break down organic material present in a given water sample at certain temperature over a specific time period
- COD—chemical oxygen demand is used to indirectly measure the amount of organic compounds in water. It is a useful measure of water quality

Tertiary treatment: It uses chemicals to remove inorganic compounds and pathogens. This is the final stage of treatment where the effluent after secondary treatment first is mixed with sodium hypochlorite and then the effluent is passed through dual media filter (DMF) and activated carbon filter (ACF) where sand, anthracite, and activated carbon are used as filtration media. Finally, the treated water is let into a small well to recharge the water table. This treated waste water now can be used for gardening, toilets, and laundry purposes.

Comparison of Various Technologies Used for Treatment of Biomedical Waste[1,2]

There are five different technologies, which can be used for treating biomedical waste.

1. Hydroclave
2. Autoclave
3. Microwave
4. Incinerator
5. Chemical.

Comparing the costs of all these methods, the:

1. Capital cost of hydroclave and autoclave is lowest, that of chemical is moderate and of incinerator and microwave high.
2. As far as sterilization efficacy is seen, sterilization efficacy of hydroclave is high. It is 6–8 logs, so also of incinerator (provided it is used properly), that of autoclave and microwave is lower about 4 logs. Efficacy of chemicals depends on strength of chlorine and disbursement through the waste.
3. Operating cost of hydroclave and autoclave is low:
   - Hydroclave—approximately ₹0.68–1.34/kg
   - Autoclave—approximately ₹1.26–1.50/kg
   - Microwave uses only electric energy, cost is ₹5–6/kg to ₹95/kg
   - Incineration—₹20–25/kg.

4. Operator maintenance skill: Low skill is required with hydroclave and autoclave, whereas high skill, and maintenance skill too is required in case of microwave and incinerator.
5. Air emissions

Hydroclave	Autoclave	Microwave	Incineration
Somewhat odorous but nontoxic	Highly odorous but nontoxic	Somewhat odorous but nontoxic	Can be highly toxic

6. Water emissions

Hydroclave	Autoclave	Microwave	Incineration
Odorous but sterile	Odorous, may contain live organisms at base	Negligible	None

7. Treated effluent acceptance

Hydroclave	Autoclave	Microwave	Incineration
High-dehydrated, shredded, mostly unrecognizable weight reduction and volume reduction	Low. Wet waste 10% heavier. All material recognizable	High, shredded but wet waste 10% heavier unless dried post-treatment	High-mostly ash and metals. May contain toxic substances

8. Description

Hydroclave	Autoclave	Microwave	Incineration	Chemical
Steam sterilization combined with dehydration, weight, volume reduction, steam recycled	Steam sterilization weight increased. No volume reduction, when door opens, all steam is lost	Heating of preshredded waste	High temperature waste incineration	Mixing preground waste with chemicals such as chlorine

Disposal[1-4]

In case disposal facility for sharps is not readily available in a town, healthcare establishments, especially hospitals having suitable land, can construct a concrete lined pit of about 1 m length, breadth and depth and cover the same with a heavy concrete slab having a 1-1.5 m high steel pipe of about 50 mm diameter. Disinfected sharps can be put through this pipe. When the pit is full, the pipe should be sawed off and the hole sealed with cement concrete. This site should not be water logged or near a borewell.

General Waste

The waste material generated from the office, kitchen, garden, store, chemicals counter, etc., which are nonhazardous and nontoxic, may be taken care of as follows:

- Composting of green waste—to be carried to a municipal facility or a private facility, if available. If suitable land is available, a hospital may consider composting its green waste within the campus itself taking all precautions regarding health and hygiene and safety to patients.
- Recycling of packaging material (caution—medical supplies such as unused or scantily used disposable items or those of uncertain history should never be allowed to be recycled).

Certificate indicating origin and of non-contamination, issued by the concerned medical authorities of the healthcare establishment before these wastes are handed over to the municipality/private operator is essential from the point of safety.

Site for sanitary landfill

- Must be authorized by a regulating authority, as clinical waste can cause significant risk to ground water.
- Should be securely fenced to prevent entry of animals/rag pickers.
- Should be far enough from public view.

Method to make a sanitary landfill for PHC: This is an effective option in waste disposal, if the community hospital has sufficient land plot and wishes to operate its own disposal (Fig. 24.12).

The functional steps are as follows:

- *Dig up a trench:* In case, it is a plateau and the ground water level is low, the trench should be dug up wide and long enough along the area. Several trenches can be made according to requirements. Each side of the trench should have 30 degrees slope. The recommended depth and width of trench are 1.20 × 1.20 m. Soil dug up should be piled up beside and along the trench for the convenience of covering wastes when required.
- *Dump:* The collected waste is collected in the trench and it is spread along the trench with an average thickness of about 50 cm. Press tractor or any kind of compacting machine should be applied to make the waste as compact as possible.
- *Cover:* To cover the surface of the compacted wastes, use the soil piled beside the trench and recompact the covering soil. Thickness generally recommended for each layer is 50 cm. This will prevent foul smell and will be protected from pests or animals.

Once the trench is filled up, a new trench can be dug up, and the same procedures followed. The wastes being buried in this manner for 2–3 years will reduce themselves by 10–30%. After they have been completely decomposed, the place can be converted into a garden or children's playground.

Standards for Deep Burial[3,10]

1. A pit or trench should be dug about 2 meters deep. It should be half filled with waste, then covered with lime within 50 cm of the surface, before filling the rest of the pit with soil.
2. It should be ensured that animals do not have access to burial sites. Covers of galvanized iron/meshes may be used.
3. On each occasion, when wastes are added to the pit, a layer of 10 cm of soil shall be added to cover the waste.
4. Burial must be performed under close and dedicated supervision.
5. The deep burial site should be relatively impermeable and no shallow well should be close to the site.
6. The pits should be distant from habitation, and sited so as to ensure that no contamination occurs of any surface water or ground water. The area should not be prone to flooding or erosion.
7. The location of the deep burial site will be authorized by the prescribed authority.
8. The institution shall maintain a record of all pits for deep burial.

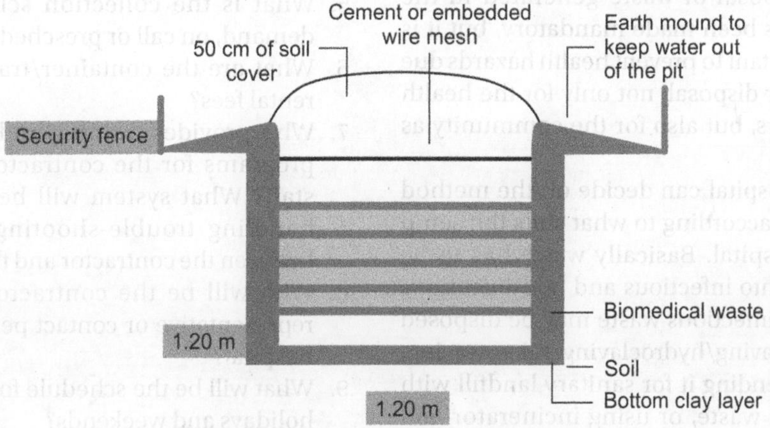

Fig. 24.12: Sanitary landfill at PHC

9. The ground water table level should be a minimum of six meters below the lower level of deep burial pit.

Certification of noncontamination and origin, by the concerned medical authorities of the health care establishment, before these wastes are handed over to the municipality/private operator is essential from the points of safety.

The recent legislation has fulfilled a long-standing necessity. However now, it is important that a clear policy regarding the acceptability of alternative technologies must be developed and issued by the central government. Such a policy can include an approval process for hospitals wishing to purchase an alternative technology, and also companies desiring to market a technology in the country.

Proper biomedical waste management system should be implemented by each hospital, nursing home, pathological laboratory etc. Each one can slightly modify the way, they are going to dispose the waste according to the availability at their institute and finances available.

There are significant comparative advantages and disadvantages, between each of the various alternatives, treatment technologies. But because of the rapid developments in this field, and because of the sparsity of data, at present it is difficult to select the best technology. To summarize proper disposal of waste generated in the hospital has been made mandatory, but it is more important to prevent health hazards due to improper disposal, not only for the health care workers, but also for the community as such.

Each hospital can decide on the method of disposal according to what suits the setup of their hospital. Basically waste has to be separated into infectious and non-infectious waste. The infectious waste may be disposed of by autoclaving/hydroclaving/microwaving, and then sending it for sanitary landfill with the general waste, or using incinerator and sending the ashes for disposal to sanitary landfill/secured landfill. If however such treatment facilities are not available, then till the time such facilities become available, the infected or biomedical waste should be sent to a secured landfill.

HOSPITAL WASTE CONTRACT

There are some things, which have to be kept in mind before planning waste disposal and giving the contract to a "hospital waste contractor". It has been seen that privatization of this service has proved to be economically and technically effective in most hospitals and this trend is on the increase throughout the country.

The checklist includes the following considerations:

1. What is the extent and range of services offered by the contractor?
2. Who provides the containers (leased, lease purchase, purchased)?
3. How many and what type of containers will be needed? How will new containers be obtained and in what time frame, if a program is expanded? Who provides container maintenance and on what schedule (explain what constitutes a clean container)?
4. Who provides service and maintenance for equipment like handcarts, tractor, trolley, broom, wet mop, soap and water?
5. What is the collection schedule—on demand, on call or prescheduled?
6. What are the container/tractor trolley rental fees?
7. Who provides training and awareness programs for the contractors working staff? What system will be set up for handling trouble-shooting problems between the contractor and the hospital?
8. Who will be the contractors account representative or contact person for the hospital?
9. What will be the schedule for service on holidays and weekends?

10. What documentation will be provided to identify the cleaning of the hospital area and lifting of hospital waste—weight slip, report from the wards and so on?

Is there a provision for cancellation or amendment of the contract within a time period if the services no longer meet the needs of the hospital? These standard operative procedures have been suggested as broad guidelines. Each health care facility should make alterations as per their requirements and needs, within the framework of biomedical waste management rules 1998 and 2016.

LANDFILLS[5,6]

The forerunner of a landfill was the dump. Webster's Dictionary refers to the verb "dump" as "to get rid of" and this is exactly what happened. Garbage was disposed of on any cheap and convenient piece of land; waste was dumped into the ground. Pest control, litter, soil, and water contamination were not of any real concern. People began to associate dumps with rats, seagulls, poor drinking water, and foul smells. Gradually, these problems were rectified, resulting in the creation of landfills. In the past, dumps took all wastes; industrial, commercial, and hazardous household materials. Landfills are now designed and regulated to hold specific materials. This has led to the creation of three general types of landfills: sanitary landfill, secure landfill, and monofill.

All landfills must have some level of engineering, both for the protection of the environment and for esthetic reasons. The specific protection required is determined on a case-by-case basis; each landfill is judged individually based on the waste it is to contain and the geographical properties of the area.

Gas and leachate are the two major problems landfills generate. Landfill gas is roughly 50% carbon dioxide and 50% methane. It is the methane that poses the greatest danger; the gas becomes explosive when mixed with oxygen. Without proper control, methane can seep into pipes and buildings. Homes built near old, improperly constructed landfills have exploded from methane leaks.

Leachate starts as rain or other precipitation. Upon falling on a landfill, or flowing past as surface water, the moisture passes down into the landfill. As water moves through the waste, metal, soluble chemicals, suspended particles and other contaminants are gathered by the liquid. Unless measures are taken, these pollutants end up in the groundwater and bodies of surface water (lakes, rivers). In general, the ministry prefers sites that have a high degree of natural protection against environmental damage.

Sanitary Landfill (Fig. 4.13)[6]

The sanitary landfill requires a layer of bedrock or compacted soil starting at the bottom. Preferably, this base would be a clay soil. Clays have physical properties which inhibit the movement of water. This is useful in a landfill, as the water percolating through the waste can carry contaminants into groundwater supplies.

Rolls of synthetic, *impermeable* membrane liner are placed on top of the soil/bedrock. When sealed together, the rolls form a large "bowl". Again, this protection is used to limit the flow of leachate out of the landfill. Immediately above the liner is a layer of sand or gravel and the leachate collection system. Liquids that cannot penetrate the liner accumulate in the sand/gravel. A network of pipes buried in this material allow leachate to be drawn up and out of the landfill. The liquid removed is treated as sewage, to allow for its safe disposal.

Lying on top of the leachate recovery layer is a bed of clay. As mentioned, the clay is helpful in controlling the downward movement of liquid. Another synthetic membrane bowl is placed over this clay later, then a second leachate collection system in a bed of sand/gravel. Groundwater monitoring wells and methane gas monitoring equipment are inserted into the landfill before waste is added. Water samples are taken, while the site is empty, as a benchmark of groundwater

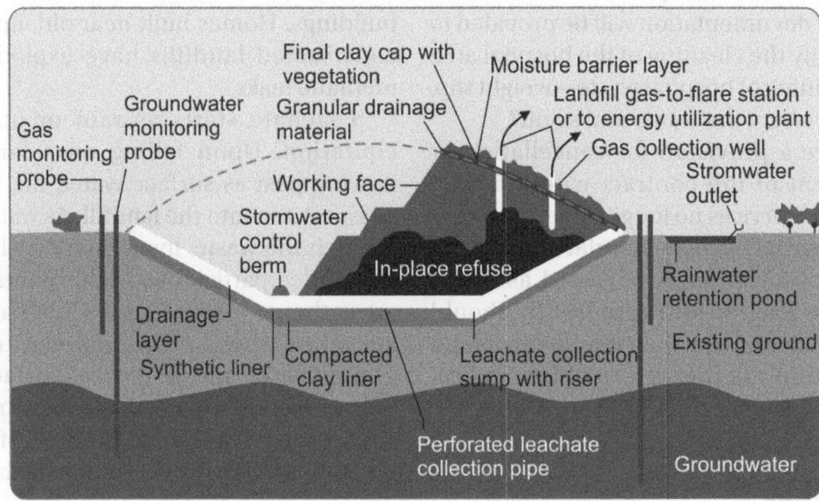

Fig. 24.13: Modern sanitary landfill cross-section *(For color version, see Plate 2)*

quality; future samples will be measured against the initial sample. Now the landfill is ready to accept waste.

Refuse is placed in a small working area called cells. Layers of garbage are compacted using heavy equipment, such as a packer tractor, in a cell before being covered with soil at the end of each day. Daily cover keeps odors, pests, contamination and litter to a minimum. When a sufficient number of cells have been completed a layer of soil called intermediate cover is added. This allows the landfill workers and their equipment to start on another series of working areas.

Once enough layers of cells have been filled, to complete the landfill's capacity, a top cover is placed above the last row of cells to seal the site. Grading of the cover and ditches controls surface water run-off. Beams and trees are used to make the perimeter of the landfill visually appealing. Fences and locked gates ensure illegal dumping or mishaps are avoided during nonoperating hours. Many landfills, today, refuse to accept material that can be recycled. Others do not take commercial/building/demolition waste. The materials accepted by the site depends upon what the MOE (Ministry of Environment) has licensed; the ministry establishes what each facility is allowed to receive. In the case of hazardous waste, a secured landfill is the only type of landfill legally allowed to take this material (Fig. 24.14).

An engineered or secured landfill: It is singly or doubly lined with some impervious material like cement that does not allow seepage of leachate into the ground (Leachate is liquid waste percolating through solid waste and dissolving suspended particles and gases from it). There is a pipe to collect this from the dump and is treated before disposal. With every layer of waste dumped in the landfill, it must be covered with a layer of earth and then finally, it must be covered with multiple layers of earth to facilitate plantation later. However, the best engineered landfills leak and is a potential threat to community's fish and wildlife, and to air quality.

India does not have a single engineered landfill. A low-lying area is selected and dumping begins there. Once a landfill gets over, a new low-lying area is designated. When the landfill is 'dead,' it is finally covered with a thick layer of soil and left unused for about twenty years, after which housing colonies too can be developed here. There is thus an increasing problem and danger of ground water pollution. Plus there is almost no segregation of waste, and toxic and hospital waste contributes to the leachate.

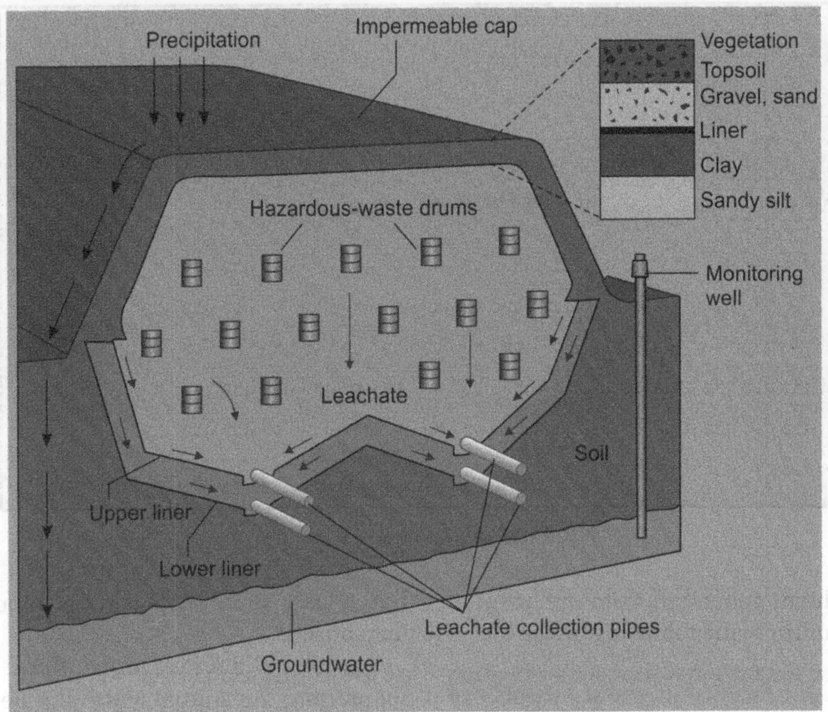

Fig. 24.14: Secure landfill[7,8]
Source: www.britannica.com/technology/hazardous-waste-management#ref593344.[8]
(For color version, see Plate 3)

Landfilling of hazardous solid or containerized waste is regulated more stringently than landfilling of municipal solid waste. Hazardous wastes must be deposited in so-called secure landfills, which provide at least 3 meters (10 feet) of separation between the bottom of the landfill and the underlying bedrock or groundwater table. A secure hazardous-waste landfill must have two impermeable liners and leachate collection systems. The double leachate collection system consists of a network of perforated pipes placed above each liner. The upper system prevents the accumulation of leachate trapped in the fill, and the lower serves as a backup. Collected leachate is pumped to a treatment plant. In order to reduce the amount of leachate in the fill and minimize the potential for environmental damage, an impermeable cap or cover is placed over a finished landfill (Fig. 24.15).

A groundwater monitoring system that includes a series of deep wells drilled in and around the site is also required. The wells allow a routine program of sampling and testing to detect any leaks or groundwater contamination. If a leak does occur, the wells can be pumped to intercept the polluted water and bring it to the surface for treatment.[8]

Disposal of Waste Water and Liquid Waste

Waste waters and liquid wastes from the kitchens, cafeteria and laundry should be drained into the municipal/civic drains. In case no sewer connections are available in the hospital, they should develop their own sewerage treatment plants. Generally, cytotoxic and hazardous wastes are not discharged into the sewers without treatment.

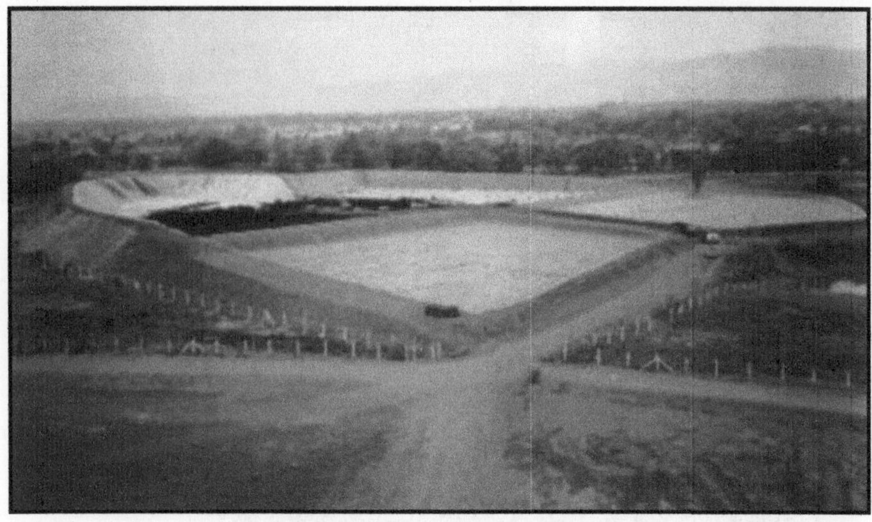

Fig. 24.15: Aerial view of a landfill

The effluent generated from the hospital should conform to the following limits:

Sl. No.	Parameters	Permissible limits
1.	pH	6.5–9.0
2.	Suspended solids	100 mg/L
3.	Oil and grease	10 mg/L
4.	BOD	30 mg/L
5.	COD	250 mg/L
6.	Bioassay test	90% survival of fish after 96 hours in 100% effluent

These limits are applicable to those hospitals which are either connected with sewers without terminal sewage treatment plant or not connected to public sewers.

For discharge into public sewers with terminal facility, the general standards as notified under the environment protection act 1986 will be applicable.

Disposal of Animal Waste[4]

Animal waste comprises animal tissue, organs, body parts, experimental animal carcasses (used for research), animal waste from veterinary hospitals, animal houses, etc.

According to rules, such waste has to be incinerated. In towns with population less than 5 lakh, such waste can be subjected to deep burial.

In towns having more than 5 lakh population, the animal waste can be sent to the common treatment facility meant for other type of biomedical waste and incinerated there. The animal waste must be put in leak-proof bags and should be transported safely taking precautionary measures.

OCCUPATIONAL HAZARDS[4]

The following types of occupational hazards occur/can occur in case of medical/paramedical personnel or staff involved with cleaning/collection or transportation of waste, etc.:

- Accidental cut or punctures from infected sharps such as, hypodermic needles, scalpels, knives, etc.
- Contact with infected material like pathological waste, used gloves, tubing, etc., especially from the operation theater.
- Bedding and dress material of the patient or from the doctors (used during check-up/ surgery, etc.).
- Contact with stool, urine, blood, pus, etc. of the patients during cleaning job.

SAFETY MEASURES FOR THE MEDICAL AND PARAMEDICAL STAFF[4]

The following instructions need to be notified and strictly adhered to:

- Clear directives in the form of a notice to be displayed in all concerned areas.
- Issuance of all protective clothes such as, gloves, aprons, masks, etc. without fail.
- Sterilization of all equipment and issue of only properly sterilized equipment and tool, such as, surgical tools to the medical personnel.
- Maintenance of registers for this purpose.
- Provision of disinfectant, soap, etc. of the right quality and clean towels/tissue paper.
- Regular medical check-up (half-early).

SAFETY MEASURES FOR CLEANING AND TRANSPORTATION STAFF [4]

- Display of illustrated notices with clear instructions for do's and don'ts in Hindi and the local language.
- Issuance of all protective gears such as, gloves, aprons, masks, gum boot, etc. without fail.
- Provision of disinfectant, soap, etc. of the right quality and clean towels.
- Provision of a wash area, where they can take bath, if needed/desired.
- Washing and disinfecting facility for the cleaning equipment and tools.
- Regular medical check-up (at least half-yearly).

TRAINING AND MOTIVATION[4]

The training program aims at sensitizing the management and equipping the medical, paramedical and auxiliary staff with necessary working knowledge and clear instructions about their respective roles. At the same time a core group of trainers should be organized for continued in-house training of the auxiliary and sanitation staff. For the success of the program, it is essential that training and orientation courses are planned for the following categories of functionaries and people according to their qualification and experience, their role and responsibility:

- Policy makers.
- Civic authorities.
- Hospital administration, medical superintendent, deans and head of the departments.
- Doctors, surgeons and specialists.
- Auxiliary and nursing staff.
- Ward boys and cleaning/sanitation staff.

The training program for the various categories need to be repeated, especially for the auxiliary staff. The interval between two programs has to be decided by the management, depending upon available staff strength, resources, etc.

TRAINING MODULES FOR DIFFERENT LEVELS OF STAFF[4]

Training modules should be developed for the following category of personnel:

- Medical and laboratory personnel.
- Paramedical personnel, e.g. nurses, ward boys, etc.
- Sweepers/cleaning staff, guards, etc.
- Administrative and management staff.

Each category has different duties and accordingly, they should (i) understand their specific role regarding waste management, (ii) comply with the policy decisions taken by the management of the establishment, and (iii) contribute to the success and betterment of the overall biomedical waste management plan in their own health care establishment as well as in their town.

TRAINING FOR MEDICAL AND LABORATORY PERSONNEL[4]

This training capsule should include:

- Detailed discussion regarding the existing rules and regulations, supply of copies of the rules to each individual.

- Review of the hazards and impact of improper management of biomedical waste, citing case studies if possible.
- Discussion regarding the policy of the specific health care establishment.
- Detailed description of each step involved, including use of equipment and tools (for example, needle cutter/melter, containers for used sharps, sterilizing equipment, etc.), use of forms, monitoring, etc.
- Discussion regarding their specific role.
- Measures for accidents, incidents and emergency situations (regarding hospital waste management).
- Comments and suggestions which subsequently be considered for the success and betterment of the system.

Paramedical Personnel[4]

This training capsule should include:

- Health hazards and impact of improper management of biomedical waste, implication of neglect and not following the instructions, examples.
- Brief outline regarding the existing rules in simple language which they can understand.
- Supply of relevant charts indicating the practical implications of the rules and the policy of the hospital management.
- Detailed description of each step involved from their point of view.
- Discussions and instructions regarding their specific role and activities in this respect.
- Do's and don'ts regarding biomedical waste management.
- Measures to be taken during accidents/incidents/emergency situations.
- Incentives and punishments.
- Comments and suggestions.

Sweepers, Cleaning Staff and Guards[4]

This training should preferably be carried out in the local language. The material for this category may contain the following:

- Awareness generation, highlighting the importance of proper management of infectious and hazardous biomedical waste and the health hazards and diseases caused by them.
- A brief introduction of the rules framed by the Ministry of Environment and Forests, Government of India and the advantages in following them.
- Providing them simple illustrated charts showing their responsibilities, the pit falls, how to be vigilant (especially for the guards).
- How to cope with accidents/incidents related to infectious, toxic and hazardous waste, how to help their colleagues in such situations.
- How to maintain personal hygiene in the environment of a health care establishment, the use and importance of protective gear such as, gloves, gum-boots, mask, apron, etc. as well as of disinfectant and soap.
- How to cooperate with the management in this matter and how to report in case of any problem.
- The incentives and punishments program of the management.

ADMINISTRATIVE AND MANAGEMENT STAFF[4]

The management of the healthcare establishment should make an action plan to implement the recommendations of the rules framed by the Government of India (Ministry of Environment and Forests). This would include the following:

- Formation of a Waste Management Committee as outlined above.
- Clear indication of the role of each member of the committee.
- Action plan for proper waste management in the particular health care establishment and its documentation. This plan should be reviewed once a year.
- Development of a format for reporting accidents and incidents relating to biomedical waste management and its meticulous following.

- Assessment of all the survey results and their utilization—once in every 6 months.
- Awareness generation, the responsibilities and accountabilities formulation of policy.
- Highlighting the social, ethical and legal responsibilities of the management, case studies.
- Discussion on the Biomedical Waste (Management and Handling) Rules, 1998 and March 2016, emphasizing the legal, financial and contractual issues.
- The steps required for formulating a policy for the specific health care establishment, keeping in view the government rules.
- Coordination with the civic and health authorities as well as with the prescribed authority of the state.
- Administrative and managerial support mechanism necessary for implementing and sustaining a proper biomedical waste management system.
- How to motivate and elicit cooperation from various staff members.
- The concept of common treatment facility—the legal, financial and contractual issues.

INCENTIVES AND MOTIVATION[4]

These are important components for the success of the program. Awards and punishments—both are required for this purpose. The following steps are recommended:

- The medical, surgical, laboratory and research staff should be encouraged to think on this problem and suggest innovative ideas/designs/systems, etc. which may be adopted for improvement in the waste management situation.
- Suitable awards may be instituted for this purpose.
- Similarly, the nursing and the auxiliary staff may also be encouraged to suggest practical ideas for improvement in their sphere of activities.
- Awards should be instituted on annual basis for the sanitation staff for the best work in each ward/suitable units.
- Awards may also be instituted for the most hygienic and clean department for which the award may be given to the respective team.
- Punishment for dereliction of duty and noncompliance or not obeying the orders/directives should be decided in advance and notified prominently.
- Prompt action should be taken for such lapses.

AWARENESS[4]

Sustained awareness generation is essential. The management of the hospital should organize awareness programs, especially for the auxiliary staff.

Debates, drama, essay competition, etc. may be considered for this purpose.

STANDARD OPERATIVE PROCEDURES FOR WASTE DISPOSAL[1]

This includes:

1. Standard operative procedures (SOP) for clinical specimens.
2. SOP for disposal of sharps.
3. SOP for anatomical waste and soiled waste.
4. SOP for expired/discarded medicines/cytotoxic drugs.
5. SOP for chemical waste.
6. SOP for liquid waste.
7. SOP for radioactive wastes or radioactively contaminated items.
8. SOP for dealing with mercury spills.

SOP for Clinical Specimens

All clinical samples come under the category of infectious waste and therefore transportation of these samples from the wards to the laboratory require special care, because there are chances of accidental spillage. All the clinical specimens must be transported in spill-proof screw-caped bottles. Special precautions are also required for samples taken from patients suffering from AIDS or hepatitis B and C. In these cases leak proof, screw capped bottles should be covered by polythene bags. Any accidental contamination or spill on the way from the ward to the laboratory must be informed to the authorities immediately and immediate disinfection should be carried out.

Blood specimens and other specimens contaminated with blood and tissues must not spill on tabletop, floor, papers or any surface. In case of spillage, the surface must be disinfected immediately under no circumstances should mouth pipetting be permitted.

After carrying out the tests, all the specimens must be discarded in a container with disinfectant. These containers must be autoclaved and disposed off. All reusable material like culture plates, should be chemically disinfected or autoclaved and then washed thoroughly and cleaned with soap and water, and reused.

SOP for Disposal of Sharps

Correct disposal of sharps is important because they form a major threat of risk of blood-borne diseases from biomedical waste.

- Needles, syringes and sharp instruments must be placed in a puncture resistant plastic/metal container at the place of work (White).
- These should be autoclaved or dry heat sterilizer, mutilated or shredded and then disposed and sent to iron foundries or sanitary landfill or designated concrete waste pits.
- Reuse the containers if at all, only after cleaning and disinfecting.
- About 40% needle prick injuries are due to recapping, so do not recap.
- For reusable glass syringes and needles:
  - Aspirate hypochlorite solution
  - Immerse in flat tray containing hypochlorite for 20 minutes.
  - Rinse with water several times.
  - Autoclave (or boil for 20 minutes).

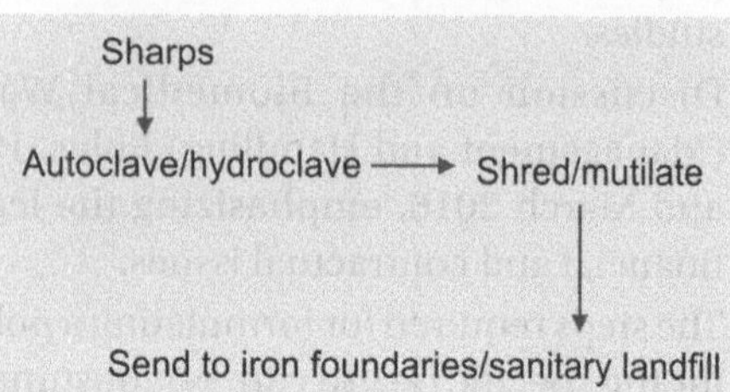

In many hospitals autoclave and shredders may not be available, so we can chemically disinfect the sharps using sodium hypochlorite solution and then send for disposal in sanitary landfill or can be sent directly for incineration.

Important Don'ts

- Do not chemically treat incinerable waste.
- Blood coated instruments reduce potency of chemical, therefore, the solution must be changed daily.

SOP for Anatomical Waste and Soiled Waste

Human or animal anatomical waste, soiled waste

↓

Sent in yellow bag for incineration or plasma pyrolysis or deep burial

SOP for Expired/Discarded Medicines/Cytotoxic Drugs

Expired/discarded medicines/cytotoxic drugs

↓

Returned back to manufacturer or to common biomedical waste treatment facility for incineration at temperature >1200°C

SOP for Chemical Waste

Chemicals found in medical and public health services come in both solid and liquid forms.

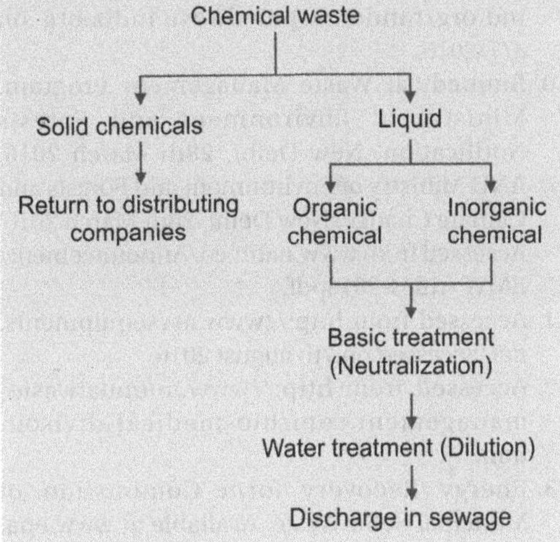

SOP for Liquid Waste

These include secretions, aspirated body fluids, liquid from laboratories, housekeeping or urine, should be disposed through the following procedure.

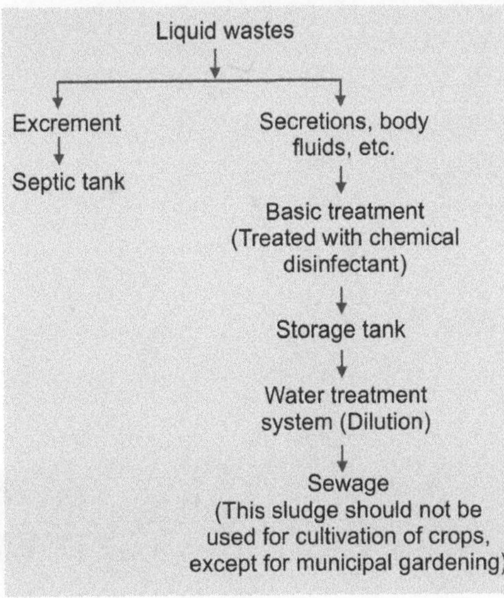

SOP for Radioactive Wastes or Radioactively Contaminated Items

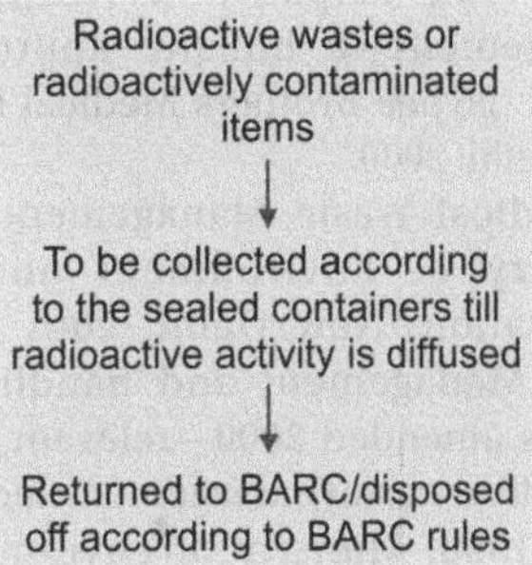

SOP for Dealing with Mercury Spills

1. Do not touch mercury with bare hands as mercury gets absorbed quickly through the skin.
2. Clean the area around the spill.
3. Wear heavy-duty protective gloves or two layers of latex gloves.
4. A regular syringe can be used to suck all the mercury. Small spills can be managed by using stiff paper to scoop and gather the mercury. Large droplets of mercury may be sucked by a syringe.
5. The collected mercury should be poured into a plastic container with 5 to 10 ml of water.
6. Seal the container that contains the mercury by using scotch tape.
7. Put the used syringe in a separate plastic container for further use.
8. Dispose off the used gloves carefully after disinfection.

What materials can be recycled?[9]

- Glass after cleaning and disinfection/sterilization.
- Paper.
- Corrugated cardboard.
- Aluminum.
- X-ray film.
- Reclaimed silver from X-ray film.
- Plastics—noninfectious component only.

REFERENCES

1. Acharya DB. The textbook of hospital waste management. Minerva Press; 2003.
2. Anand RC, Satpathy S. Hospital waste management—a holistic approach. 2nd edition. Jaypee Brothers Medical Publishers, New Delhi; 2000.
3. Biomedical Waste Management Program. Ministry of Environment and Forests Notification. New Delhi; 20th July 1998. AND (Management and handling) rules, 1998 as amended 2000—relevant provisions biomedical waste (management and handling) rules, 1998. Ministry of environment and forests notification, New Delhi; 20th July, 1998.
4. Biomedical waste. Chapter 7. Accessed from www.localbodies.up.nic.in/swm/chap7.pdf on 4/7/2015.
5. Topic 3 collection, segregation, transport, treatment and disposal methods (Sadat International, Inc. Engineering and Environmental Services). Accessed from www.worlbank.org/INTUSWM/Resources/463617.
6. Landfills. Blue water recycling association. 2004;1-5. Accessed from www.bra.org/landfills.html. Accessed on 8/11/04.
7. Secured landfill in Globar time magazine—centre for science and environment. Page 2&3a. Available at www.gobartimes.org/gt20030415/gt_askme.htm.
8. Nathanson JA. Hazardous waste management. Secure landfills. Available at www.britannica.com/topic/hazardous-waste-management #ref 593344.
9. ISHWM. Indian society of waste management. June 27, 2015. Acessed from www.medwaste.ind.org/randomaspmedwasteindia.org on 4/7/2015.
10. Biomedical Waste Management Program. Ministry of Environment and Forests Notification. New Delhi, 28th March 2016. AND Ministry of Environment and Forests and Climate Change. New Delhi, 28th March 2016. Accessed from www.nabh.co/Announcement/BMW -rules-2016pdf.
11. Accessed from http://www.arvsequipments.net/accessed on 7th august 2016.
12. Accessed from http://www.mumbaiwaste-management.com/bio-medical-divison.htm.
13. Energy Recovery form Combustion of Muncipal Solid Waste. Available at www.epa.gov>smm>energy-rec.
14. Liquid biomedical waste management: An emerging concern for physicians. Review article. Muller Journal of Medical Sciences and Research. 2013;4(2). Accessed from www.mjmsr.net.on Friday August 2016 IP 117.223.98.238. Available at http://aksharqhse.in/Blog/bio-medical-waste-management-rules-2016/on 7th August 2016.

Chapter 25

Use of Antibiotics and Chemotherapeutic Agents

Chapter Outline

INTRODUCTION

The era of chemotherapeutic agents started long back. Since then there has been a continuous development and introduction of antibiotics. Newer and newer antibiotics are being introduced but the problem of drug resistance has also emerged. This is increasing the necessity to find more new drugs.[1]

CHANGES IN CHARACTER OF NOSOCOMIAL INFECTIONS[1]

Since 1950's, there also has been a change in the character of nosocomial infections. In the 1940's and 1950's, B hemolytic *Streptococcus* and *Staphylococcus aureus* were common, in 1950's and later, only *Staphylococcus* especially the one resistant to penicillin, tetracycline, erythromycin, chloramphenicol and streptomycin emerged to cause epidemics in hospitals. In 1960's, *Staphylococcus* was replaced with gram-negative bacilli, enterococci and fungi.

Today once again infections due to staphylococci, especially methicillin resistant staphylococci and infections due to gram-negative bacilli are common in hospitals. At present almost all staphylococci are resistant to penicillin and so also there is a widespread dissemination of methicillin-resistant *Staphylococcus aureus* and methicillin resistant coagulase negative staphylococci. So also there is emergence of penicillin resistant streptococci[2,3] and penicillin resistant clostridial strains which was once very uncommon. *Treponema pallidum* still remains sensitive to penicillin. There is also an increasing prevalence of ampicillin resistant *Haemophilus influenzae* and beta-lactamase producing gonococci.

The increased and indiscriminate use of antimicrobial drugs and development of newer medical technologies all have a profound effect in shaping the characteristic of nosocomial infections.

INDISCRIMINATE USE OF ANTIBIOTICS

There has been a steady increase of use of antibiotics both for therapeutic as well as for prophylactic purposes. Most of the times, it is given for prophylaxis. Many times it was noticed that drugs were being used inappropriately that is either the wrong drug was given, or the dose was inappropriate, or the administration of antimicrobial therapy or prophylaxis was considered unjustified. Such massive use of antibacterial drugs in hospitals whether appropriate or inappropriate, has effects on both the hosts who receive the drugs and the bacteria exposed to them.

AIM OF CHEMOTHERAPY AND PROPER CHOICE

If a patient is known or suspected to be suffering from an infection, the clinician must decide as to which organism is likely to be responsible and the antibiotic to which it will probably be sensitive. He also must take into consideration, the purpose for which he is choosing the antibiotic, the range of activity of the antibiotic and the possible side effects of the antibiotic.

The aim of chemotherapy is to help the natural defenses of the body to eliminate the microbes from tissues by preventing their multiplication. In order to have this effect, the blood and infected tissues must contain a concentration of the antibiotic, which is ideally 2-5 times higher than the minimal inhibitory (i.e. bacteriostatic) concentration (MIC) of the antibiotic for the infecting organism. There are a limited number of circumstances where chemotherapy must aim to kill the infecting organisms (i.e. tissue fluids must contain more than the minimal bactericidal, i.e. killing) concentration (MBC) of the antibiotic. Such situations include endocarditis and infections in patients who are immunosuppressed.

DEVELOPMENT OF RESISTANCE TO ANTIBIOTICS

Antibiotic-resistant strains of certain organisms are becoming common in hospital. *Staphylococcus aureus* and gram-negative bacilli that may cause hospital infection have become increasingly resistant to the commonly used antibiotics. These resistant strains may have appeared as a result of selection of intrinsically resistant strains by extensive and indiscriminate use of antibiotics, or by mutation of the previously sensitive bacteria, and selection following exposure to the antibiotics. Some of these resistant bacteria especially gram-negative bacilli can transfer antibiotic resistance to other bacteria. These antibiotic resistance genes can reside on plasmids or segments of DNA which are capable of moving between organisms (transposons).

Though majority of the hospital staphylococci and also most strains of the community are now resistant to penicillin, all hemolytic streptococci of group *A (Streptococcus pyogenes)*, *Clostridia* and the *Treponema* of syphilis remain sensitive to the antibiotic—an example of extreme variability, of bacterial resistance.

There is also an increasing prevalence of ampicillin resistant. *Haemophilus influenzae*, the increasing frequency of b-lactamase producing gonococci, the wide spread dissemination of methicillin-resistant *Staphylococcus* and emergence of penicillin resistant pneumococci.

VIRULENCE OF ANTIBIOTIC-RESISTANT BACTERIA

Studies regarding virulence of antibiotic-resistant bacteria have been carried out. It was found that infection of patient with drug-resistant strain of a bacterium will increase the rate of hospitalization, the hospital stay and the mortality rate by two fold as compared to an infection with a drug-sensitive organism. However, it could not be determined, whether the poorer prognosis is due to the shortcomings of the antibiotic therapy or to correlate bacterial properties that enhanced virulence.

FACTORS INDICATING A LINK BETWEEN HOSPITAL USE OF ANTIMICROBIALS AND DEVELOPMENT OF ANTIMICROBIAL DRUG RESISTANCE

There are few factors which link the antimicrobial use in the hospital with the antimicrobial resistance in hospital bacteria[4] (1) Antimicrobial resistance is more prevalent among bacteria causing infection in the hospital setting than in the community, (2) In outbreak situations, patients infected with resistant bacteria are more likely to be those who have received prior antibiotic therapy than are patients colonized or infected with susceptible strains of the same species, (3) Antibiotic resistant strains are more prevalent in areas of the hospital, where there is intense use of antibiotic (e.g. ICU, Burns unit etc), these are also generally the areas where mostly highly susceptible patients are encountered, (4) Increased duration of exposure to antibiotics in hospital, also generally increases the colonization with resistant organism, and (5) Finally, antibiotic therapy produces marked effects on the host's endogenous flora and exerts selective pressure in favor of resistant organisms.

Drug resistant organisms (mutants, transductants, containing plasmids or conjugate containing 'R' factors) selected by the pressure of antibiotics are at a disadvantage, however slight, in the absence of selective pressure. 'R' determinants represent energy "load" for the bacteria. If it were not so, wild bacteria in the community would have been drug-resistant, or at least a mixture of sensitive and resistant strains. Although 'R' factor containing bacteria persist for some time in the community, free of the selective pressure of antibiotics, but they decay in the absence of selective pressure.

CLASSIFICATIONS OF ANTIBIOTICS

The easiest way to classify the antibiotics is to classify them according to which microorganism they are likely to affect (Table 25.1). The table is summary of the classification used in Parker and Collier, 1990.[5]

Though we talk about antibiotics as being either bactericidal or bacteriostatic, and the importance of bactericidal activity as compared to bacteriostatic activity the

Table 25.1: Classification of antimicrobial agents according to activity

Active against gram-positive bacteria and gram-negative cocci	Mainly active against gram-negative bacteria	Broad spectrum antibiotics	Specific antibacterial agents	Antifungal and antiviral agents
• Benzyl penicillin • Phenoxymethyl penicillin • Flucloxacillin • Erythromycin • Clindamycin • Rifampin • Vancomycin • Teicoplanin	• Ampicillin[a] • Mezlocillin[a] • Piperacillin • Ciprofloxacin • Ofloxacin • Temocillin • Aztreonam • Gentamicin • Amikacin • Nitrofurantoin[b] • Nalidixic acid[b]	• Sulfonamides • Co-trimoxazole • Cephalosporins • Imipenem • Tetracyclines • Chloramphenicol • Meropenem	*Anaerobes* • Clindamycin • Metranidazole *Tuberculosis* • Isoniazid • Rifampicin • Ethionamide • Pyrazinamide, etc *Chlamydia*[c] • Erythromycin • Tetracycline • Chloramphenicol *Campylobacter species* • Erythromycin • Ciprofloxacin *Legionella species* • Erythromycin • Rifampicin	*Antifungals* • Nystatin • Amphotericin B • 5-Fluorocytosine • Imidazoles • Griseofulvin *Antivirals* • Acyclovir • Ganciclovir • Zidovudine

[a]Some activity vs Gram-positive bacteria
[b]Urinary tract infection only
[c]Also mycoplasma, *Rickettsia*

clinical significance of this distinction is questionable. Many agents, which are bacteriostatic, become bactericidal at higher doses, and the clinical situation in which bactericidal activity is required is limited.

USE OF BROAD-SPECTRUM ANTIBIOTICS

It is very tempting to use broad-spectrum antibiotics for the treatment of many infections as they cover a large range of less common pathogens; this has the advantage of selecting out resistant strains. Broad-spectrum antibiotics can in particular increase the risk of antibiotic-associated diarrheas and other infections caused by *Clostridium difficile.* Therefore, broad-spectrum antibiotics should not be used to treat specific pathogens that are sensitive to narrow range agent (e.g. *Streptococcus pyogenes*).

For guidance on complex treatment and its control, the clinician should consult a clinical microbiologist or a physician experienced in chemotherapy.

ANTIBIOTIC COMBINATIONS

Most of the infections respond to a single antibiotic, but in some cases a combined therapy may be valuable, for example:

1. For prevention of development of drug resistance—as in case of tuberculosis.

2. Infections caused by more than one organism (polymicrobial sepsis), for example—case of intra-abdominal sepsis—infection is caused by both aerobes and anaerobes.
3. Septicemia and endocarditis: Combinations of antibiotics are required for treatment of septicemia and certain forms of endocarditis.

WHEN IS A COMBINATION THERAPY SUPERIOR TO SINGLE AGENT?

Combination therapy is useful in serious sepsis such as endocarditis or septicemia because the mixture of the two agents has greater activity than the sum of the individual activities of the agents. This phenomenon is called as synergy, and laboratory methods are available for testing of chemotherapeutic agents for this interaction.

SELECTION OF AN ANTIBIOTIC

Selection of antibiotic should not be haphazard. It should be based on careful consideration of certain factors. They are:

Sensitivity (or Probable Sensitivity) of the Infecting Organisms

Normally, antibiotic sensitivity testing is done and after the culture report and report of antibiotic sensitivity testing, the appropriate antibiotic is chosen.

But in some severe infections, it may take time to get the culture and sensitivity of the organism immediately, so it is necessary that a presumptive clinical diagnosis is made, the probable organism causing it is considered and the treatment is started with a potentially appropriate antibiotic (e.g. in infective endocarditis, where the commonest organisms is *Streptococcus viridans* or in purulent meningitis, organisms like meningococci or pneumococci are common, in our country, *Haemophilus* too is common (but in foreign countries *H. influenzae* is now a rare cause of meningitis since the introduction of childhood vaccine against type b strain). Some severe infections like endocarditis require detailed sensitivity testing including determination of MIC and MBC of the organism.

Clinical Pharmacology of the Various Antibiotics

The important factors of the antibiotics are absorption, excretion and distribution. Some antibiotics like ampicillin are excreted in bile and urine, while some like chloramphenicol and penicillin penetrate the inflamed blood brain barrier. There are drugs which are excreted predominantly by the renal route and it is important to be aware that renal failure will delay its excretion. It is also important to know how different antibiotics are cleared by hemodialysis and hemofiltration, so that dosages can be adjusted appropriately.

Route of Administration

Usually, oral therapy is satisfactory, but in severe infections, intravenous injections may be required. In order to achieve high blood levels, intravenous antibiotics may be administered by 'bolus' IV infusion. In some cases, topical applications may be needed as in eye, ear and superficial skin infections.

Toxicity of Antibiotics

All antibiotics have side effects, and therefore toxic drugs should not be used when safer drugs are available. For example, chloramphenicol may cause fatal aplastic anemia, and is thus rarely indicated systemically.

Aminoglycoside antibiotics cause eight nerve damage if blood concentrations are allowed to exceed accepted safe levels. In the presence of renal failure, longer intervals between doses are required to prevent toxic blood levels.

Prophylaxis

There are well-defined indications for prophylactic antibiotics discussed below.

Cost of Antibiotics

The least expensive antibiotic should be chosen, when all other factors are satisfied.

INDICATIONS FOR PROPHYLAXIS WITH ANTIBIOTICS

Systemic Chemoprophylaxis

Chemoprophylaxis should be given only when indicated. Routine prophylactic use of antibiotics leads to an increase in the proportion of resistant organisms and may cause the replacement of sensitive strains by resistant ones in the patient's flora, increasing the hazards of infection. Whenever prophylaxis is indicated it is important that the most appropriate antibiotic or antibiotics are given, and that the dosage, duration of course and route of administration should be optimized. Prophylaxis in case of post-operative infection should involve a very short perioperative administration, which is most unlikely to cause selection of resistant strains.

In open heart surgery, there is a very low incidence of infection, but the risk of mortality is high if infection (e.g. with coagulase-negative staphylococci) occurs. Antibiotic prophylaxis can prevent the lodgment of microorganism in the heart and some clinical trials suggest that this is beneficial.

Medical Indications for Systemic Prophylaxis

These include the following:

- Prevention of endocarditis in patients with heart valve lesions, septal defect, patent ductus or prosthetic valve.
- For non-immune diphtheria contacts.
- For contacts of meningococcal infection.
- Following acute rheumatic fever for at least 5 years or until the child leaves school.
- Following splenectomy, especially in children.

Indications, for Systemic Prophylaxis in Clean Surgery (Table 25.2)

These include the following:

- Arterial grafts.
- Cardiac surgery.
- Neurological operations involving foreign materials.
- Joint prosthesis.
- Severe injuries and burns (e.g. *Clostridium tetani* and *Clostridium perfringens*).
- High amputation of ischemic legs (*Clostridium perfringens*).

Prophylaxis Against Surgical Sepsis (Table 25.2)

Prophylaxis against surgical sepsis is advisable, whenever an internal organ, the contents of which contain high concentrations of bacteria is opened. The type and extent of bacterial colonization within the gastrointestinal tract are related to the site and nature of an underlying disease. Prophylaxis should be used for the following groups of operations:

Group 1: Operations on the stomach or esophagus in patients with carcinoma or bile reflux gastritis.

Group 2: Cholecystectomy in selected patients who may have infected bile. Patients at risk for sepsis can be selected on the basis of a history of jaundice, rigors, recent acute cholecystitis, age over 70 years, or a previous biliary operation.

Group 3: All intestinal operations in patients with inflammatory bowel disease.

Group 4: All colorectal operations involving resection and/or anastomosis.

Group 5: Patients with a perforated gangrenous appendix should be given a therapeutic course of antibiotic. The need for prophylaxis in non-perforated, non-gangrenous appendicitis is not yet established.

Group 6: Pelvic operations.

There are also other indications for prophylaxis for which there is often no general agreement.

- Recurrent cystitis in women of child-bearing age with a normal urinary tract.
- Infants of mothers with sputum-positive tuberculosis (if the child cannot be separated from the mother).
- Siblings of patients with whooping cough
- All instrumentations in the presence of bacteriuria.
- Transrectal prostatic biopsy.
- Urethral dilatation.

Choice of Chemotherapeutic Agent

This should be based on the nature of the organisms that are likely to contaminate the operative field. For patient's in-group 1 and 2, the organisms most likely to cause sepsis are streptococci, *E. coli* and other aerobic gram-negative bacilli.

Operations in group 3, 4, and 5 require antibiotics active against anaerobic bacteria, *E. coli* and other aerobic gram-negative bacilli. Anaerobic and microaerophilic bacteria are mainly responsible for pelvic sepsis in group 6 patients.

Suitable prophylactic regimens for the above groups are as follows:

Group 1: A single preoperative dose of gentamicin or a cephalosporin by IM or IV injection.

Group 2: A single preoperative injection of gentamicin or cephalosporin IM or IV.

Groups 3 and 4: A single preoperative injection of gentamicin IM or IV and metronidazole is recommended. Preoperative oral, bowel preparations with antibiotics is often effective, but is not recommended because of the risk of emergence of resistant gram-negative bacilli.

Group 5: Metronidazole given as a suppository or IV is the most rational prophylactic for appendicectomy.

Group 6: Metronidazole combined with cefuroxime is effective prophylaxis against pelvic sepsis.

Timing and Route of Prophylaxis in Surgery (Tables 25.2 and 25.3)

Prophylaxis is only effective if high blood and tissue levels of an appropriate antibiotic are present at the time of bacterial contamination of the surgical wound. Effective antibiotic concentrations are therefore required from the time of incision to 8 hours after surgery. Up to three doses can be given during this period. Usually single dose is enough, but if surgery is prolonged beyond 4 hours, then an additional dose is required. Prophylaxis should not continue after completion of the operation.

Table 25.2: Recommendations for surgical antimicrobial prophylaxis[6]

Sl. No.	Type of surgical procedure	Predominant infecting organism(s)	Recommended agents[a,b]	Alternative agents in patients with β-lactam allergy	Strength of evidence
1. Cardiac	Coronary artery by pass	**Common**: *Staphylococcus aureus, coagulase-negative Staphylococcus* **Less common:** *Enterobacter* species, *Pseudomonas aeruginosa, Escherichia coli, Klebsiella pneumoniae, Proteus mirabilis, Acinetobacter* species, Rarely *Propionibacterium acnes*	Cefazolin or Cefuroxime or Vancomycin (only if high incidence of MRSA)	Clindamycin[d], Vancomycin[d] for gram-positive coverage Gram-negative: An aminoglycoside aztreonam or a fluoroquinolone	A
	Cardiac device insertion procedures (e.g. pacemaker implantation)	As above	Cefazolin, cefuroxime	Clindamycin, vancomycin	A
	Ventricular assist devices	As above	Cefazolin, cefuroxime	Clindamycin, vancomycin	C
2. Thoracic	Noncardiac procedures including lobectomy, pneumonectomy, lung resection, and thoracotomy	*S. aureus, S. epidermidis, Streptococcus* species, gram-negative bacilli like *Haemophilus influenzae, Enterobacter cloacae, Klebsiella pneumonia, Acinetobacter* species, *Pseudomonas aeruginosa, Moraxella catarrhalis,* and fungal (*Candida* species)	Cefazolin, Ampicillin-sulbactam	Clindamycin[d] , vancomycin[d]	A
	Video-assisted thoracoscopic surgery	As above	Cefazolin, ampicillin-sulbactam	Clindamycin[d], vancomycin[d]	C
3. Gastroduodenal[e]	Procedures involving entry into lumen of GIT (pancre-aticoduodenectomy)	Most common organisms are coliforms (*E. coli, Proteus* species, *Klebsiella* species), staphylococci, streptococci, enterococci, and occasionally *Bacteroides* species	Cefazolin	Clindamycin or vancomycin + aminoglycoside[g] or aztreonam or fluoroquinolones[h-j]	A
	Procedures without entry into GIT (antireflux, highly selective vagotomy) for high-risk patients)	As above	Cefazolin	Clindamycin or vancomycin + aminoglycoside[g] or aztreonam or fluoroquinolone[h-j]	A

Contd...

Contd...

Sl. No.	Type of surgical procedure	Predominant infecting organism(s)	Recommended agents[a,b]	Alternative agents in patients with β-lactam allergy	Strength of evidence
4. Biliary tract	Open procedure	*E. coli, Klebsiella* species, and enterococci; less frequently, other gram-negative organisms, streptococci, and staphylococci are isolated. Anaerobes are occasionally reported, most commonly *Clostridium* species	Cefazolin, cefoxitin, cefotetan ceftriaxone[k] ampicillin-sulbactam[h]	Clindamycin or vancomycin + aminoglycoside[g] or aztreonam or fluoroquinolone[h-j] Metronidazole + aminoglycoside[g] or fluoroquinolone[h-j]	A
	Laparoscopic procedure Elective, low risk[1] Elective, high risk[1], e.g. >70 years, Acute cholecystitis, acute cholangitis, Common duct stone	As above	 None Cefazolin, cefoxitin, cefotetan ceftriaxone[k], ampicillin-sulbactam[h]	 None Clindamycin or vancomycin + aminoglycoside[g] or aztreonam or fluoroquinolone[h-j] Metronidazole + aminoglycoside[g] or fluoroquinolone[h-j]	A A
5. Appendicectomy for uncomplicated appendicitis		Most common are anaerobic and aerobic gram-negative enteric organisms. *Bacteroides fragilis* is the most commonly cultured anaerobe, and *E. coli* is the most frequent aerobe, aerobic and anaerobic streptococci, *Staphylococcus* species, and *Enterococcus* species occasionally. *P. aeruginosa* has been reported infrequently	Cefoxitin, cefotetan cefazolin + metronidazole	Clindamycin + aminoglycoside [g] or aztreonam or fluoroquinolone [h-j] Metronidazole + aminoglycoside[g] or fluoroquinolone[h-j]	A
6. Small intestine	Nonobstructed	The most frequent microorganisms in lower abdominal surgery *E. coli*, followed by *Enterococcus* species, *Streptococcus* species , *P. aeruginosa*, and *S. aureus*; (resistant to methicillin). Upper abdominal tract surgery did not show any significant differences compared with SSIs of the lower	Cefazolin	Clindamycin + aminoglycoside[g] or aztreonam or fluoroquinolone[h-j]	C

Contd...

Contd...

Sl. No.	Type of surgical procedure	Predominant infecting organism(s)	Recommended agents[a,b]	Alternative agents in patients with β-lactam allergy	Strength of evidence
		tract, though there are relatively more staphylococci, *K. pneumoniae*, *Enterobacter* species, *Acinetobacter* species, and *Candida albicans* isolates and fewer *E. coli*, *B. fragilis*, and *Clostridium* species in the upper abdominal surgery group			
	Obstructed	As above	Cefazolin + metronidazole, cefoxitin, cefotetan	Metronidazole + aminoglycoside[g] or fluoroquinolones[h-j]	C
7. Hernia repair	(Hernioplasty and herniorrhaphy)	Aerobic streptococci, *Staphylococcus* species, and *Enterococcus* species are common, and MRSA is commonly found in prosthetic mesh infections	Cefazolin	Clindamycin, vancomycin	A
8. Colorectal[m]		*B. fragilis* and other obligate anaerobes are the most frequently isolated organisms from the bowel 1000 to 10, 000 times higher than aerobes *E. coli* is the most common aerobe. *B. fragilis* and *E. coli* comprise approximately 20–30% of the fecal mass	Cefazolin + metronidazole, cefoxitin, cefotetan, ampicillin-sulbactam[h], ceftriaxone + metronidazole[n], ertapenem	Clindamycin + aminoglycoside[g] or aztreonam or fluoroquinolones[h-j], metronidazole + aminoglycoside[g] or fluoroquinolones[h-j]	A
9. Head and neck					
	Clean		None	None	B
	Clean with placement of prosthesis (excludes tympanostomy tubes)		Cefazolin, cefuroxime	Clindamycin[d]	C
	Clean-contaminated cancer surgery	Postoperative SSIs are usually polymicrobial due to the flora from oropharynx. The predominant oropharyngeal organisms include	Cefazolin + metronidazole, cefuroxime + metronidazole, ampicillin-sulbactam	Clindamycin[d]	A

Contd...

Contd...

Sl. No.	Type of surgical procedure	Predominant infecting organism(s)	Recommended agents[a,b]	Alternative agents in patients with β-lactam allergy	Strength of evidence
		various streptococci (aerobic and anaerobic species), other oral anaerobes including *Bacteroides* species (but not *B. fragilis*), *Peptostreptococcus* species, *Prevotella* species, *Fusobacterium* species, *Veillonella* species, Enterobacteriaceae, and staphylococci. Nasal flora includes *Staphylococcus* species and *Streptococcus* species.			
	Other clean-contaminated procedures with the exception of tonsillectomy and functional endoscopic sinus procedures	Same as above	Cefazolin + metronidazole, cefuroxime + metronidazole, ampicillin-sulbactam	Clindamycin[d]	B
10. Neurosurgery					
	Elective craniotomy and cerebrospinal fluid shunting procedures	SSIs are primarily associated with gram-positive bacteria, *S. aureus*, and coagulase-negative staphylococci (75–80% have been shown to be MRSA) Other skin organisms such as *P. acnes* may be seen after CSF shunt placement, craniotomy and other procedures Gram-negative bacteria have also been associated, many of them in polymicrobial infections	Cefazolin	Clindamycin [d], vancomycin [d]	A
	Implantation of intrathecal pumps		Cefazolin	Clindamycin[d], vancomycin[d]	C
11. Cesarean delivery		Group B β-hemolytic streptococci, enterococci, *E. coli*, anaerobic streptococci (*Peptococcus* species and *Peptostreptococcus* species),	Cefazolin	Clindamycin + aminoglycoside[g]	A

Contd...

Contd...

Sl. No.	Type of surgical procedure	Predominant infecting organism(s)	Recommended agents[a,b]	Alternative agents in patients with β-lactam allergy	Strength of evidence
		Bacteroides species (e.g. *Bacteroides bivius, B. fragilis*), *Ureaplasma urealyticum* and *Staphylococcus* species			
12. Hysterectomy (vaginal or abdominal)		Postoperative infections associated with vaginal hysterectomy are frequently polymicrobial, with enterococci, aerobic gram-negative bacilli, and *Bacteroides* species isolated most frequently Postoperative SSIs after abdominal and radical hysterectomies are also polymicrobial; gram-positive cocci and enteric gram-negative bacilli predominate, and anaerobes are frequently isolated	Cefazolin, cefotetan, cefoxitin, ampicillin-sulbactam[h]	Clindamycin or vancomycin + aminoglycoside[g] or aztreonam or fluoroquinolone[h-j] Metronidazole + aminoglycoside[g] or fluoroquinolone[h-j]	A
13. Ophthalmic		Coagulase-negative *Staphylococcus* species, primarily *S. epidermidis. Other gram-positive organisms include* *S. aureus, Streptococcus* species, *Enterococcus* species, *P. acnes*, and *Corynebacterium* species. Gram-negative organisms like *Serratia* species, *Klebsiella* species, *P. mirabilis* and *P. aeruginosa.*	Topical neomycin-polymixin B-gramicidin or fourth-generation fluoroquinolones (gatifloxacin or moxifloxacin) given as 1 drop every 5–15 minutes for 5 doses.[o] Addition of cefazolin 100 mg by subconjunctival injection or intracameral cefazolin 1–2.5 mg or cefuroxime 1 mg at the end of procedure is optional	None	B
14. Orthopedic		Skin flora are the most frequent organisms The most common pathogens in orthopedic procedures are			

Contd...

Sl. No.	Type of surgical procedure	Predominant infecting organism(s)	Recommended agents[a,b]	Alternative agents in patients with β-lactam allergy	Strength of evidence
		S. aureus, gram-negative bacilli, coagulase negative staphylococci (including *S. epidermidis*), and β-hemolytic streptococci. polymicrobial infection that includes gram-negative bacilli A contributing factor to SSIs in arthroplasty is the formation of bacterial biofilm, particularly with *S. aureus* and *S. epidermidis*, on inert surfaces of orthopedic devices. Increasing concern about MRSA and VRE			
	Clean operations involving hand, knee or foot and not involving implantation of foreign materials		None	None	C
	Spinal procedures with and without instrumentation		Cefazolin	Clindamycin[d], vancomycin[d]	A
	Hip fracture repair		Cefazolin	Clindamycin[d], vancomycin[d]	A
	Implantation of internal fixation devices, e.g. nails, screws, plates, wires		Cefazolin	Clindamycin[d], vancomycin[d]	C
	Total joint replacement		Cefazolin	Clindamycin[d], vancomycin[d]	A
15. Urologic		*E. coli* is the commonest and other gram-negative bacilli can cause infection *Enterococcus* may also cause infection Organisms such as *S. aureus*, coagulase-negative *Staphylococcus* species, and group A *Streptococcus* species			

Contd...

Contd...

Sl. No.	Type of surgical procedure	Predominant infecting organism(s)	Recommended agents[a,b]	Alternative agents in patients with β-lactam allergy	Strength of evidence
		biofilm-forming bacteria (*S. epidermidis* and *P. aeruginosa*) in patients with prosthesis implantation			
	Lower tract instrumentation with risk factors for infection (includes transrectal prostate biopsy)		Fluoroquinolone[h-j,] trimethoprim-sulfamethoxazole, cefazolin	Aminoglycoside[g] with or without clindamycin	A
	Clean without entry into urinary tract		Cefazolin (the addition of a single dose of an aminoglycoside may be recommended for placement of prosthetic material, e.g. penile prosthesis)	Clindamycin[d], vancomycin[d]	A
	Involving implanted prosthesis		Cefazolin + /– aminoglycoside, cefazolin + /– aztreonam, ampicillin-sulbactam	Clindamycin + /– aminoglycoside or aztreonam, vancomycin + /– aminoglycoside or aztreonam	A
	Clean with entry into urinary tract		Cefazolin (the addition of a single dose of an aminoglycoside may be recommended for placement of prosthetic material, e.g. penile prosthesis)	Fluoroquinolone[h-j,] aminoglycoside[g] with or without clindamycin	A
	Clean-contaminated		Cefazolin + metronidazole, cefoxitin	Fluoroquinolone[h-j,] Aminoglycoside[g] + metronidazole or clindamycin	A
16. Vascular[p]		The predominant organisms involved are *S. aureus, S. epidermidis,* and enteric gram-negative bacilli. MRSA is an emerging organism of concern	Cefazolin	Clindamycin[d], vancomycin[d]	A

Contd...

Contd...

Sl. No.	Type of surgical procedure	Predominant infecting organism(s)	Recommended agents[a,b]	Alternative agents in patients with β-lactam allergy	Strength of evidence
17. Heart, lung, heart-lung transplantation[q], heart transplantation[f]		*Staphylococcus* species, are the primary pathogens , MRSA and Vancomycin-resistant *Enterococcus faecalis* have also been reported. Other gram-positive pathogens (e.g. coagulase-negative staphylococci, *Enterococcus* species) and gram-negative organisms (e.g. Enterobacteriaceae, *P. aeruginosa, Stenotrophomonas maltophilia*), *Candida* species	Cefazolin	Clindamycin[d], vancomycin[d]	A (based on cardiac procedures)
Lung and heart-lung transplantation[r,s18.]		*P. aeruginosa, S. aureus* (including MRSA), *B. cepacia, Enterobacter* species, *S. maltophilia, Klebsiella* species, *S. epidermidis, E. coli, Aspergillus* species and VRE. Similarly, organisms frequently seen in pediatric lung infections are nonfermenting gram-negative bacteria, such as *Pseudomonas* species, *Stenotrophomonas* species, *Alcaligenes* species, and fungi, including *Aspergillus* species	Cefazolin	Clindamycin[d], vancomycin[d]	A (based on cardiac procedures)
18. Liver transplantation[q,t]		*E. coli, Klebsiella* species, *Enterobacter* species, *Acinetobacter baumannii*, and *Citrobacter* infections due to *P. aeruginosa* may also occur but are much less common in the early postoperative period Enterococci are particularly common, *S. aureus* (frequently MRSA) and coagulase negative staphylococci, *Candida* species commonly cause both early and late postoperative infections	Piperacillin-tazobactam, cefotaxime + ampicillin	Clindamycin or vancomycin + aminoglycoside[g] or aztreonam or Fluoroquinolone[h-j]	B

Contd...

Contd...

Sl. No.	Type of surgical procedure	Predominant infecting organism(s)	Recommended agents[a,b]	Alternative agents in patients with β-lactam allergy	Strength of evidence
19. Pancreas and pancreas-kidney transplantation[f]		Majority of superficial SSIs after pancreas or transplantation are caused by *Staphylococcus* species (both coagulase positive and coagulase-negative) and gram-negative bacilli (particularly *E. coli* and *Klebsiella* species) Deep SSIs also are frequently associated with gram-positive (*Enterococcus* species, *Streptococcus* species, and *Peptostreptococcus* species) and gram-negative organisms (*Enterobacter* species, *Morganella* species, and *B. fragilis*), as well as *Candida* species. Although anaerobes are occasionally isolated, the necessity for specific treatment of anaerobes in SSIs after pancreas transplantation remains unclear	Cefazolin, flucanazole (for patients at high risk of fungal infection (e.g. those with enteric drainage of the pancreas) Cefazolin	Clindamycin or vancomycin + aminoglycoside[g] or aztreonam or fluoroquinolone[h-j] Clindamycin or vancomycin + aminoglycoside[g] or aztreonam or fluoroquinolone[h-j]	A A
20. Plastic surgery	Clean with risk factors or clean contaminated	The most common organisms after plastic surgery procedures are *S. aureus* other staphylococci, and streptococci Procedures involving macerated, moist environments (e.g. under a pannus or axilla of an obese individual), below the waist, or in patients with diabetes are associated with a higher rate of infection with gram-negative organisms such as *P. aeruginosa, Serratia marcescens*, or Enterobacteriaceae, including *E. coli, Klebsiella* species and *P. mirabilis*	Cefazolin, ampicillin-sulbactam	Clindamycin[d] vancomycin[d]	C

Contd...

Contd...

[a]The optimal time for administration of preoperative doses is within 60 minutes before surgical incision.

Some agents, such as fluoroquinolones and vancomycin, require administration over one to two hours; therefore, the administration of these agents should begin within120 minutes before surgical incision.

Single dose prophylaxis is usually sufficient; the duration of prophylaxis for all procedures should be less than 24 hours. If an agent with a short half-life (e.g. cefazolin, cefoxitin) is used, it should be readministered if the procedure duration exceeds the recommended redosing interval (from the time of initiation of the preoperative dose (see table). Readministration may also be warranted if there is prolonged or excessive bleeding or if there are any other factors that may shorten the half-life of the prophylactic agent, e.g. extensive burns. Readministration may not be warranted in patients in whom the half-life of the agent may be prolonged (e.g. in patients with renal insufficiency or failure.

[b]For patients known to be colonized with methicillin-resistant *Staphylococcus aureus*, it is reasonable to add a single dose of vancomycin to the recommended agents.

[c]Strength of evidence that supports the use or non-use of prophylaxis is classified as A (levels I–III), B (levels IV–VI) or C (level VII). Level I evidence is from large well conducted, randomized controlled clinical trials. Level II is from small well-conducted randomized controlled clinical trials. Level III evidence is from well-conducted cohort studies. Level IV evidence is from well-conducted case-control studies. Level V evidence is from uncontrolled studies that were not well conducted. Level VI evidence is from conflicting evidence that tends to favor the recommendation. Level VII evidence is expert opinion.

[d]For procedures in which organisms other than staphylococci or streptococci are likely then additional agents with activity against that particular pathogen may be considered. For example, if there are surveillance data showing that gram-negative organisms are a cause of surgical site infections (SSIs) for the procedure, practitioners may consider combining clindamycin or vancomycin with another agent (cefazolin if the patient is not beta-lactam allergic, aztreonam, gentamicin or single dose fluoroquinolones if patient is allergic to beta-lactam antibiotics).

[e]Prophylaxis should be considered for patients at highest risk for postoperative gastroduodenal infections such as those with increased gastric pH (e.g. those receiving histamine H_2- receptor antagonist s or proton-pump inhibitors), gastroduodenal perforation, decreased gastric motility, gastric outlet obstruction, gastric bleeding, morbid obesity, or cancer. Antibiotic prophylaxis may not be needed when the lumen of the intestinal tract is not entered.

[f]Consider additional antibiotic coverage with infected biliary tract.

[g]Gentamycin or tobramycin.

[h]Due to increasing resistance of *Escherichia coli* to fluoroquinolones and ampicillin-sulbactam, local population susceptibility profiles should be reviewed prior to use.

[i]Ciprofloxacin or levofloxacin.

[j]Fluoroquinolones are associated with an increased risk of tendonitis and tendon rupture in all ages. However, this risk would be expected to be quite small with single-dose antibiotic prophylaxis. Although the use of fluoroquinolones may be necessary for surgical antibiotic prophylaxis in some children, they are not drugs of first choice in pediatric population due to an increased incidence of adverse events as compared with controls in some clinical trials.

[k]Ceftriaxone use should be limited to patients requiring antimicrobial treatment for acute cholecystitis or acute biliary tract infections which may not be determined prior to incision, not patients undergoing cholecystectomy for noninfected biliary conditions, including biliary colic or dyskinesia without infection.

[l]Factors that indicate a high risk of infectious complications in laparoscopic cholecystectomy include emergency procedures, diabetes, long procedure duration, intraoperative gallbladder rupture, age of >70 years, conversion from laparoscopic to open cholecystectomy. American Society of Anesthesiologists classification of 3 or greater, episode of colic within 30 days before the procedure, reintervention in less than one month for non-infectious complication, acute cholecytitis, bile spillage, jaundice, pregnancy, non-functioning gallbladder, immunosuppression, and insertion of prosthetic device. Because a number of these risk factors are not possible to determine before surgical intervention, it may be reasonable to give a single dose of antimicrobial prophylaxis to all patients undergoing laparoscopic cholecystectomy.

[m]For most patients a mechanical bowel preparation combined with oral neomycin sulfate plus oral erythromycin base or with oral neomycin sulfate plus oral metronidazole should be given in addition to IV prophylaxis.

[n]When there is increasing resistance to first and second generation cephalosporins among gram-negative isolates from SSIs, a single dose of ceftriaxone plus metronidazole may be preferred over the routine use of carbapenems.

[o]The necessity of continuing topical antimicrobials postoperatively has not been established.

[p]Prophylaxis is not routinely indicated for brachiocephalic procedures. Although, there are no data in support, patients undergoing brachiocephalic procedures involving vascular prosthesis or patch implantation (e.g. carotid endarterectomy) may benefit from prophylaxis.

[q]These guidelines reflect recommendations for perioperative antibiotic prophylaxis to prevent SSIs and do not provide recommendation for prevention of opportunistic infections in immunocompromised transplantation patients (e.g. antifungal or antiviral medications).

[r]Patients who have left-ventricular assist devices as a bridge and who are chronically infected might also benefit from coverage of the infecting microorganism.

[s]Prophylactic regime may need to be modified to provide coverage against any potential pathogens, including gram-negative (e.g. *Pseudomonas aeruginosa*) or fungal organisms, isolated from the donor lung or the recipient before transplantation. Patients undergoing lung transplantation with negative pretransplantation cultures should receive antimicrobial prophylaxis as appropriate for other types of cardiothoracic surgeries. Patients undergoing lung transplantation for cystic fibrosis should receive 7–14 days of treatment with antimicrobials selected according to pretransplantation culture and susceptibility results. This treatment may include additional antbacterial or antifungal agents.

[t]The prophylactic regimen may need to be modified to provide coverage against any potential pathogens, including vancomycin-resistant enterococci isolated from recipient before transplantation.

Table 25.3: Recommended doses and redosing intervals for commonly used antimicrobials for surgical prophylaxis[6]

Sl. No.	Antimicrobial	Recommended dose		Half-life in adults with normal renal function, hour	Recommended redosing interval (from initiation of preoperative dose), hour[c]
		Adults[a]	***Pediatrics***[b]		
1.	Ampicillin - sulbactam	3 g (ampicillin 2 g/sulbactam 1 g)	50 mg/kg of the ampicillin component	0.8–1.3	2
2.	Ampicillin	2 g	50 mg/kg	1–1.9	2
3.	Aztreonam	2 g	30 mg/kg	1.3–2.4	4
4.	Cefazolin	2 g, 3 g for patients weighing ≥120 kg	30 mg/kg	1.2–2.2	4
5.	Cefuroxime	1.5 g	50 mg/kg	1–2	4
6.	Cefotaxime	1 g[d]	50 mg/kg	0.9–1.7	3
7.	Cefoxitin	2 g	40 mg/kg	0.7–1.1	2
8.	Cefotetan	2 g	40 mg/kg	2.8–4.6	6
9.	Ceftriaxone	2 g[e]	50–75 mg/kg	5.4–10.9	NA
10.	Ciprofloxacin	400 mg	10 mg/kg	3–7	NA
11.	Clindamycin	900 mg	10 mg/kg	2–4	6
12.	Ertapenem	1 g	15 mg/kg	3–5	NA
13.	Fluconazole	400 mg	6 mg/kg	30	NA
14.	Gentamicin[g]	5 mg/kg based on dosing weight (single dose)	2.5 mg/kg based on dosing weight	2–3	NA

Contd...

Contd...

Sl. No.	Antimicrobial	Recommended dose		Half-life in adults with normal renal function, hour	Recommended redosing interval (from initiation of preoperative dose), hour[c]
15.	Levofloxacin[f]	500 mg	10 mg/kg	6–8	NA
16.	Metranidazole	500 mg	15 mg/kg Neonates weighing <1200 g should receive a single 7.5 mg/kg dose	6–8	NA
17.	Moxifloxacin[f]	400 mg	10 mg/kg	8–15	NA
18.	Piperacillin-tazobactam	3.375 g	Infants 2–9 months: 80 mg/kg of the piperacillin component. Children >9 months and ≤40 kg: 100 mg/kg of the piperacillin component	0.7–1.2	2
19.	Vancomycin	15 mg/kg	15 mg/kg	4–8	NA
Oral antibiotics for colorectal surgery prophylaxis (used in conjunction with a mechanical bowel preparation)					
20.	Erythromycin base	1 g	20 mg/kg	0.8–3	NA
21.	Metronidazole	1 g	15 mg/kg	6–10	NA
22.	Neomycin	1 g	15 mg/kg	2–3 (3% absorbed under normal gastrointestinal conditions	NA

[a]Adult doses are obtained from studies cited in each section of the article. When doses differed between studies, expert opinion used the most-often recommended dose.

[b]The maximum pediatric dose should not exceed the usual adult dose.

[c]For antimicrobials with a short half-life (e.g. cefazolin, cefoxitin) used before long procedures, redosing in the operating room is recommended at an interval of approximately two times the half-life of the agent in patients with normal renal function. Recommended redosing intervals marked as "Not Applicable" (NA) are based on typical case length; for unusually long procedures redosing may be needed.

[d]Although FDA-approved package insert labeling indicates 1 g, experts recommend 2 g for obese patients.

[e]When used as a single dose in combination with metronidazole for colorectal procedures.

[f]When fluoroquinolones have been associated with an increased risk of tendinitis/tendon rupture in all ages, use of these agents for single-dose prophylaxis is generally safe.

[g]In general, gentamicin for surgical antibiotic prophylaxis should be limited to a single dose given preoperatively. Dosing is based on the patient's actual body weight. If the patient's actual weight is more than 20% above ideal body weight (IBW), the dosing weight (DW) can be determined as follows: DW = IBW + 0.4 (actual weight – IBW).

FORMULATION OF ANTIBIOTIC POLICY

Necessity of Formulation of Antibiotic Policy

Formulation of an antibiotic policy is essential for every hospital. The reasons are:

1. It is a way of ensuring that patients receive appropriate therapy.
2. When the use of antibiotics is restricted, the appearance of resistant strains will be delayed and thus incidence in the hospital kept low. MRSA and gram-negative bacilli like *Klebsiella* species and *Pseudomonas aeruginosa* have caused cross infections problems in urological, intensive care and burns units. In these organisms, resistance is transferred from one organism to the other even when the organisms are unrelated. Transferable resistance to one antibiotic is often linked to resistance to other antibiotics, so that excessive use of one antibiotic may be the cause of high incidence of resistance to several others.
3. Up-to-date information should be provided for the prescriber, and the incidence of adverse reactions should be reduced by restricting the use of certain potentially toxic agents.
4. Costs are reduced by controlling the use of expensive drugs.

The type of policy must be adapted to the needs of the staff, the type of patients and organisms prevalent in the hospital or unit. It must therefore be flexible, and where necessary adapted to the needs of individual units (e.g. burns and intensive care).

Components of Antibiotic Policy

The policy could have the following components:

1. *Personal advice discussion:* There should be daily discussion between the senior and junior doctors on prescribing habits. Effective use of antibiotics requires experience and this is not readily available. So all hospitals must have a doctor (usually a medical microbiologist or infectious disease consultant) with a special interest in and knowledge of antibiotics, which should be available to other members of the staff.
2. *General advice and education:* If possible every hospital must have booklets on antibiotics prescription, which could be made available in wards. It is particularly important that advice is available on the use of topical agents on prophylaxis and on expensive preparations. Postgraduate lectures on chemotherapy are also helpful, but are less important than personal advice and discussion.
3. *Provision of surgery data:* The antibiotic policy depends to a considerable extent on the sensitivity patterns of currently isolated bacteria. This information should be made available from the laboratory regarding the current resistance patterns. This gives the clinician a valuable guide to the therapy that is most likely to be of use. Some type of information can be made available to the general practitioners. This information can be given only once a year in general practice because of the small changes in resistance of bacteria among general community compared to those found in hospitals.
4. *Reservations of antibiotics:* Some hospitals group antibiotics into different categories in order to hold some in reserve for particular organisms or specific types of patients. Restricting the use of specific compounds can preserve the useful life of an antimicrobial agent. In large hospitals, where there is a resident population of organisms 'waiting to acquire resistance', and large amounts of antibiotics may be used, it is essential to keep some in reserve.

Examples of the ways in which antibiotics can be classified for the purpose are shown in Tables 25.4 and 25.5, which summarize the policy adopted in a general hospital (Table 25.4) and in a hospital with many specialized services and departments (Table 25.5).

Table 25.4: Example of antibiotic policy used in a general hospital

Unrestricted use	Restricted use (On advice of infectious disease physician or microbiologist)	Not recommended (and not in stock in the hospital)*
• Penicillin • Ampicillin and derivatives • Flucloxacillin • Tetracyclines • Erythromycin • Metronidazole • Gentamicin • Cefuroxime • Co-trimoxazole (or trimethoprim)	• Azlocillin • Ceftazidime • Netilmicin • Clindamycin • Vancomycin • Chloramphenicol • Ciprofloxacin	• All other cephalosporins • Amikacin • Tobramycin • Ureidopenicillins

* Some of these agents (e.g. amikacin) may be on the restricted list in some hospitals.

Table 25.5: Antibiotic policy employed by a complex teaching district hospital with many specialist units:

a. The antibiotics are divided into five categories with different degrees of accessibility. (A) Oral and parenteral compounds which are available for prescription by all doctors. (B) Compounds, which are restricted to certain units or indications. (C) Compounds, which can only be started by senior doctors, usually consultants. (D) Drugs, which are undergoing trial in the hospital and only available to trialists. (E) All other antibiotics available in the UK. These are not in stock and can only be ordered via consultants
b. (O+P) Oral and parenteral prescriptions of these compounds are available to all doctors

Category A	Category B	Category C	Category D	Category E
• Amoxycillin (O+P) • Phenoxymethyl penicillin • Cephalexin • Erythromycin stearate • Flucloxacillin (O+P) • Fusidic acid • Metronidazole (O+P) • Nalidixic acid • Nitrofurantoin • Ciprofloxacin • Trimethoprim • Chloramphenicol • Cefixime • Co-amoxiclav • Benzylpenicillin • Cefuroxime • Erythromycin lactobionate • Gentamicin • Piperacillin • Teicoplanin • Nystatin	• Ampicillin/sulbactam (surgical prophylaxis) • Cefotaxime (STD; pediatrics) • Ceftazidime (ITU) • Dapsone (dermatology) • Doxycycline (STD; dermatology) • Minocycline (dermatology) • Netilmicin (renal unit) • Vancomycin (hematology, renal unit) • Piperacillin (hematology) • Anti-TB drugs (chest unit)	a. Amikacin • Aztreonam • Ciprofloxacin (Injection) • Clindamycin • Imipenem • Rifampicin (Injection) b. Category B compounds used for non-listed indications c. Antivirals • Acyclovir • Ganciclovir • Ribavirin • Zidovudine d. Antifungals • Fluconazole • Amphotericin	Variable list	Variable list

New agents should be carefully considered by a drug and therapeutics committee. They should be purchased only if they are superior in one or more respects to the existing drugs. By this means the clinician can be guided in the use of the numerous antibitotic preparations now available.

Changes in Antibiotic Policies

Stopping the use of antibiotic in question (i.e. if resistance to that particular antibiotic has developed) will lead to a large reduction or elimination of the resistant organisms. This happened more often in the early years of antibiotic era, before multiple and genetically linked resistance became common in hospital bacteria. When multiple resistances are present, all of the antibiotics involved in the resistance pattern may need to be withdrawn and not be used again until these strains have been eliminated. In some outbreaks, withdrawal of antibiotics has not been effective. Transfer of all patients carrying or infected with strains, which show the resistance pattern should be shifted to one ward, which is kept closed to new admissions until all carriers of the resistant strain have been discharged. This proves effective in eliminating the resistant strains.

The antibiotic resistant pattern is constantly changing and it is necessary to change a policy in response to alterations in resistance. Often one unit in the hospital may require a policy which is different from that used by other units. For example, methicillin resistant *Staphylococcus aureus* or cephalosporin-resistant *Enterobacteria* may appear in one unit and not in others. A change could then be made to a reserve antibiotic in the ward with the newly acquired resistant strains.

Antibiotics and Laboratory

The hospital clinician can use the antibiotics rationally only if adequate laboratory services are available. There are several ways in which the laboratory can provide assistance:

- Most important is provision of accurate sensitivity tests on the relevant isolates from individual patients to the most appropriate antibiotics.
- The choice of agents and susceptibility guidelines employed should be kept under regular summary data on the prevalence of resistant bacteria, and facilities for monitoring of certain antibiotic levels (particularly aminoglycosides) should be available.
- Laboratories should report sensitivities to appropriate antimicrobial agents to the clinicians in order to restrict the range of antibiotics used (e.g. the sensitivity of *Staphylococcus aureus* could be reported to flucloxacillin and erythromycin only).

IDENTIFICATION OF IDENTICAL STRAINS DISSEMINATED IN THE HOSPITAL

Whenever strain dissemination is suspected, various techniques can be applied to determine the probable identical nature of the strain. The earliest and the most available are those used in routine evaluation of the isolates in the clinical laboratory, species identification, biotype and antimicrobial susceptibility patterns all provide useful clue to strain identity. More information is often necessary, however, because many common nosocomial pathogens provide little variability in biotype or susceptibility pattern. This makes accurate determination of the sameness of isolates difficult using the readily available data, additional laboratory study of the strains becomes necessary.

Additional information is obtained from referral centers by (1) Serotyping, (2) Phage typing, and (3) Bacteriocin production or bacteriocin susceptibility can be useful, depending on the organism.

Nowadays, additional procedures that have provided useful information are analysis of total plasmid content by agarose gel electrophoresis (AGE), or analysis of total

DNA by field inversion gel electrophoresis (FIGE). The electrophoretic analysis of total plasmid DNA is extended to whole cell DNA and used for typing as well. Whole cell DNA is digested by restriction endonucleases and electrophoresed using pulsed-field electrophoresis. Similar to plasmid analysis a fingerprint of the strain is created by the resulting digest.

REFERENCES

1. Ayliffe GAJ, Fraise AP, Geddes AM, Mitchell K. Control of Hospital Infection: A Practical Handbook. 4th edition. Oxford University Press, New York; 2000.pp.263-80.
2. Kunin CM, Twpasi T, Craig WA. Use of antibiotics: A brief exposition of the problem and some tentative solutions. Quoted in antibiotics and nosocomial infections. In: Bennet JV, Brachman PS (Eds). Chapter 12 by Theodore (Eickloff M). Hospital Infections. 3rd edition, Ann Intern Med. 1973;79:555.
3. Stevens GP, Jacobson JA, Burke JP. Changing patterns of hospital infections and antibiotic use: Prevalence surveys in a community hospital. Arch Intern Med. 1981;141:587.
4. McGowan JE Jr. The antimicrobial resistance in hospital organisms and its relation to antibiotic use. Rev Infect Dis. 1983;5:1033.
5. Parker MJ, Collier LH. Topley and Wilson's principles of bacteriology, virology and immunity, 8th edition. London: Edward Arnold; 1990.
6. Bratzler DW, Dellinger EP, Olsen KM, Peri TM, et al. Clinical practice guidelines for antimicrobial prophylaxis in surgery. Am J Health-Syst Pharm. 2013;70:195-283.

Chapter 26

Hospital Antibiotic Policy and Standard Treatment Guidelines

Chapter Outline

- Antibiotic Policy
- Surveillance of Antimicrobial Resistance
- Cumulative Antibiogram
- Development of Standard Treatment Guidelines
- Strategies for Promoting Rational Antibiotic Prescription
- A Model Standard Treatment Guideline for Community-acquired Pneumonia at the Hospital Level
- Antimicrobial Stewardship
- Summary of Antibiotic Policy and Standard Treatment Guidelines

INTRODUCTION[1]

Antimicrobial resistance (AMR) has emerged as a major public health problem all over the world. Infections caused by resistant microbes fail to respond to treatment resulting in prolonged illness and greater risk of death. Choice of antibiotic becomes difficult as there are very few new drugs available and there is scarcity of the old drugs. Prevalance of multidrug resistant bacteria lead to prescription of limited number of active antibiotics, especially the broad spectrum antibiotics which affects the bacterial ecology leading to appearance of more and more drug resistant strains. Treatment failures lead to longer periods of infectivity and increase numbers of infected people moving in the community. This exposes the general population to the risk of contracting a resistant strain. When these strains become resistant to the first-line antimicrobials, the prohibitive high cost of the second line drugs may lead to failure to treat these diseases in many individuals. Most alarming are the multidrug resistant microbes which are virtually non-treatable and thereby create a postantibiotic era scenario.

Antimicrobial Resistance in Healthcare-associated Infections[1]

Antimicrobial resistance has assumed great importance in Healthcare settings. This is due to the presence of compromised individuals in an environment of variety of infectious agents which are continuously under heavy antibiotic pressure which results in emergence and spread of resistant organisms to other patients in the form of cross-infections. There is also an increased number of ageing population living with immunocompromised states. Such people spend more time in hospitals or long-term care facilities, where they are exposed to these drug-resistant organisms. Therefore, strategies to prevent the emergence and spread of healthcare-associated antimicrobial resistant population are essential.

Hospital epidemiologists are still trying to solve the problem associated with preventing the spread of the multidrug resistant aerobic gram-negative bacilli and multidrug-resistant *Staphylococcus aureus* (MRSA) in healthcare settings. Developing simple effective strategies to ensure adherence to hand hygiene is also still a problem. An effective strategy to limit this problem of multidrug resistance must be multifaceted and must include the education of patients and physicians about the appropriate drug, dose and duration, use of effective infection-control practices to prevent transmission from infected to uninfected patients, surveillance of antimicrobial resistance and antimicrobial use and improved use of immunization. Campaigns must be taken to educate the public about the dangers of antimicrobial resistance and what may be done to control it.

Availability of New Antimicrobial Agents[1]

There are hardly any new antimicrobial agents in the pipeline especially for treatment of some common multidrug-resistant nosocomial organisms grouped under the acronym of **ESKAPE**:

- *Enterococcus faecium* (Vancomycin-resistant enterococci—VRE)
- *Staphylococcus aureus* (Methicillin-resistant *Staphylococcus aureus*).
- *Klebsiella* and *Escherichia coli* that produce extended spectrum beta-lactamases (ESBL) and carbapenemases.
- *Acinetobacter baumanni.*
- *Pseudomonas aeruginosa.*
- *Enterobacter* species.

Strategies Against Antimicrobial-resistant Microorganisms in Hospitals[1]

Strategic Objectives

- To develop a system to recognize and report trends in antimicrobial resistance within the institution.
- To rapidly detect and report resistant microorganisms in individual patients and ensure prompt treatment.
- To assure increased adherence to basic infection control policies and procedures.
- To incorporate the detection, prevention and control of antimicrobial resistance into institutional strategic goals and provide the required resources.
- To develop a plan for identifying, transferring, discharging and readmitting patients colonized with specific antimicrobial resistant pathogens.
- To establish a policy and practices for the rational use of antimicrobials.

Strategic Approaches

- Optimizing the duration of choice and dose of empiric therapy-antimicrobial stewardship.
- Optimizing antimicrobial prophylaxis for operative procedures.
- Developing and implementing an antibiotic policy and standard treatment guidelines (STG).
- Monitoring and providing a feedback regarding antibiotic resistance.
- Improving antimicrobial prescribing by educational and administrative means.

To achieve these, a comprehensive approach through a hospital policy on the rational use of antibiotics is essential (Fig. 26.1).

ANTIBIOTIC POLICY[1]

Aim

1. To minimize morbidity and mortality due to antimicrobial-resistant infection.

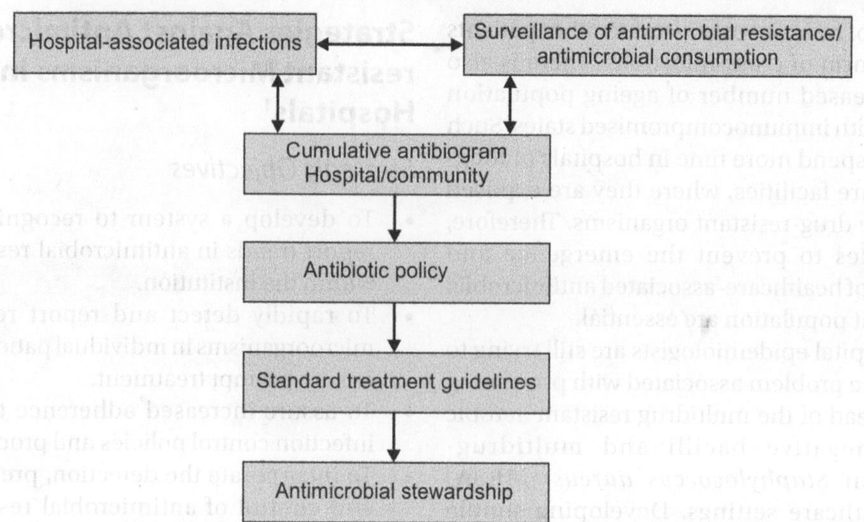

Fig. 26.1: Process for development of hospital antibiotic policy

2. To preserve the effectiveness of antimicrobial agents in the treatment and prevention of communicable diseases.

Scope

The antibiotic policy is essentially for prophylaxis, empirical and definitive therapy. The policy shall incorporate specific recommendations for the treatment of different high risk/special groups such as immunocompromised hosts; hospital-associated infections and community acquired infections.

The hospital antibiotic policy will be based upon:

- Spectrum of antibiotic activity.
- Pharmacokinetics and pharmacodynamics of these medicines.
- Adverse effects.
- Potential to select resistance.
- Cost.
- Special needs of individual patient groups.

The hospital antibiotic policy will also set *levels for prescribing antibiotics*, e.g.

- First choice antibiotics can be prescribed by all doctors.
- Restricted choice antibiotics can only be prescribed after consulting the head of the department or the antimicrobial team (AMT).
- Reserve antibiotics will be prescribed only by designated experts.

Development of Antibiotic Policy

For the development of antibiotic policy following steps to be taken:

Establishing a Multidisciplinary Antibiotic Management Team to Draft Policy

- For an efficient antibiotic policy to be developed, full commitment of the top management as well as their total support is essential.
- To develop an antibiotic policy each hospital should establish a multidisciplinary antibiotic management team (AMT). Functions of this team should include.
  a. Developing an antibiotic policy.
  b. Monitoring the implementation of the antibiotic policy.
  c. Receiving feedback.
  d. Assessing outcome and discussing with clinicians.

e. Conducting a revision of the policy every year based on the experience of the prescribers and the antimicrobial susceptibility profile.

f. Setting audit targets.

The AMT team should be a multi-disciplinary group consisting of 8–10 members. These should be from different disciplines usually infectious diseases, internal medicine, surgery, pediatrics, clinical microbiology, pharmacology and hospital pharmacy. At least one member should have the skills to conduct literature and systematic reviews. There should be inputs from all concerned including trainees in order to ensure "ownership" of guidelines.

The other functions of the AMT team include:

- Antimicrobial dose and regimen alteration.
- Streamlining and sequential therapy.
- Discontinuation of antimicrobials.
- Advice on and as a result of therapeutic drug monitoring.
- Automatic stop orders for antimicrobial prophylaxis.
- Restricted antimicrobials.
- Approval of restricted antimicrobials.
- Assistance in interpretation of laboratory results.
- Indication for use of specific anti-microbials.
- Suggestion for ordering additional laboratory testing and formal educational events.

Review Available for Antibiotic Policies and Evidences

To set up antibiotic policy the available evidence-based antibiotic policy from other institute or the national policy if formulated may be reviewed. If it is appropriate, it may be adapted for local circumstances. The advantage of adapting from national policy is that clinical, managerial and technical skills as well as time and financial resources needed for the task are available. But the knowledge at the local level is unlikely to be sufficiently broad, hence opinion of the local personnel may introduce bias into the decision making process. However, the advantage with local guidelines is that it requires fewer resources for effective dissemination and implementation.

Draft Antibiotic Policy Based Upon Available Evidence

The policy should be based on a systematic review of scientific evidence which would minimize the risk of bias. Literature should be identified according to explicit search strategy and defined inclusion criteria assessed against consistent methodological standards. In addition, the search terms and the period of search should be mentioned.

When enough evidence is not available then a combination of varying degree of evidence and expert opinion may be used to develop the antibiotic policy. However, the recommendation should be done and graded according to the strength of evidence supporting them and it should be validated based on the study design and quality of consistency and clinical relevance.

Attributes of Antibiotic Policy

The policy should be simple, clear, clinically relevant, flexible, and applicable to day-to-day practice and should be available in a user friendly format such as pocket guide, web based form, etc.

The recommended antibiotic should be effective against pathogens seen in that locality.

- Recommendations should be provided regarding optimal selection, dosage, route of administration, duration, and alternatives for allergy to first-line agents and for adjusted dosage for patients with impaired liver disease or renal function.
- Recommendations for prophylaxis should specify procedures for which antibiotic are needed, optimal agents, dosage timing, route and duration of administration, so that adequate antibiotic concentrations are available at the time

of bacterial contamination. Prophylaxis recommendations should mainly focus on clean as well as contaminated procedures. The prophylactic dose is recommended for a short duration, free of side effects and should be relatively cheap. Also the antibiotics used for prophylaxis should not be used therapeutically, as this may lead to the emergence of antimicrobial resistance.

Identification of Gaps and Research Priorities

The Policy Group must identify evidence that is lacking and areas for further research. For example, if empiric therapy results in clinical failure, then review of cumulative antibiogram may be needed to change the policy accordingly. For example, an elderly male patient with cystitis seen in the emergency room does not respond to empiric ciprofloxacin treatment though previously the same was successful. Culture is performed and result shows *E. coli* resistant to ciprofloxacin. Then the research question would be—what percentage of urine isolates from emergency room patients are susceptible to ciprofloxacin?

Monitoring and Review of Policy

The policy group should identify sample outcome measures that would form the basis for both the process and outcome of the policy, for example, ciprofloxacin is recommended for the treatment of typhoid fever, only if MIC of ciprofloxacin is $\leq$25 µg/mL. Auditing should include whether this recommendation is followed? Has ciprofloxacin MIC been determined for every *Salmonella typhi* identified? Furthermore, the audit should also monitor and evaluate the quality of antimicrobial prescriptions for right duration and dosage.

Policy should be reviewed by experienced peers who are not the members of the policy development group, but are experts in the relevant field.

Policy is not static. It is a living document. It should be reviewed at periodic intervals, updated according to current medical knowledge, clinical practice and local circumstances.

Hospital versus National Antibiotic Policy

Generally, the hospital policy should be more or less similar to the national antibiotic policy except for a few changes as warranted by the local antimicrobial resistance profiles. If there is a wide variation from national to hospital and hospital to hospital then the desired purpose is defeated i.e. to minimize the morbidity and mortality due to antimicrobial-resistant infections; to preserve the effectiveness of the antimicrobial agents in the treatment and to prevent microbial infections.

Important Issues that may be Addressed in the National Antibiotic Policy

A national antibiotic policy should include all issues for antibiotic use, both in the community and the hospital, as well as veterinary and agricultural use. The important issues that need to be included in the policy are as follows:

- Existing laws should be enforced to prevent antibiotics without prescription and over the counter sale of antibiotics.
- Guidelines for antibiotic treatment and prophylaxis should be prepared and adapted institutionally at a local level.
- Consumption of antibiotics should be monitored to estimate the national consumption of antibiotics.
- A national antimicrobial resistance surveillance system should be established and coordinated with international systems.
- A national infection control program should be implemented.
- A national institute of excellence with mandate to make recommendations

on various microbiological culture and susceptibility tests and disk diffusion and minimum inhibitory concentration breakpoint interpretive criteria should be established.

- External quality assessment scheme (EQUAS) to ascertain the quality of laboratory results should be launched and sustained.
- Educational programs should be taken for both health care workers and the public.
- Collaboration should be established with international organizations.
- Appropriate funding should be made available by the government or any other organization.

Limitation of the National Antimicrobial Policy

The limitations of the national antimicrobial policy are

- Local resistance problems.
- Different prescribing practices within a defined geographical region.
- Huge economic and social differences between the different regions which will demand different approaches at different levels.

SURVEILLANCE OF ANTIMICROBIAL RESISTANCE[1]

The antibiotic policy will depend upon the surveillance of antibiotic resistance and the antibiotic consumption in any setting. Hence, it is mandatory to have an efficient surveillance system.

Introduction to Surveillance of Antimicrobial Resistance

Antimicrobial surveillance data will help to formulate, monitor and identify the prevailing and emerging problem, which can be contained by effective strategy. Currently, majority of the surveillance programs are laboratory based. Very few clinical data are collected and the data collected by most surveillance programs are not useful to implement control and/or prevention measures. One strategy to improve the collection, collation and dissemination for effective use in the hospital/community is to integrate this function of antimicrobial surveillance activities into the existing disease surveillance activities.

A comprehensive laboratory-based antimicrobial surveillance programme has been addressed in other WHO documents. However, the following four features must be considered while establishing a surveillance mechanism:

Use of Standards

Laboratories should use standards for reporting quantitative resistance data (e.g. minimal inhibitory concentration or zone diameters) that will detect decreased susceptibility. This is because numerical test results reported qualitatively (e.g. susceptible, intermediate or resistant) may hide an emerging resistance character in a microorganism with a small decrease in susceptibility that may still be classified as susceptible.

Generate Reliable Numerator

It is crucial to avoid duplicating results since a patient may have either consecutive cultures obtained from the same body site or cultures from different body sites yielding the same organism (e.g. urine and blood culture). Therefore, only the first positive culture from the patient for each disease episode should be reported for surveillance purposes. This will be the reliable numerator for the antimicrobial resistance surveillance.

Express Resistance as an Incidence Rate

It is important to express antimicrobial resistance rates as incidence rates within a defined human population instead of using the number of isolates as the denominators. This is imperative because the submission of microbiology specimens to the laboratory is inconsistent and varies broadly in hospital settings. It is recommended to use the number of admissions and the number of days of hospitalization, which are particularly useful for inter- or intra-healthcare facility comparison. It should be recognized that this process captures data only from patients admitted to health facility and excludes those who attend as outdoor patients.

Participate in External Quality Assessment Schemes

The validity and reliability of surveillance data is deemed acceptable only when the clinical laboratories providing data for the surveillance program should have routinely participated in pertinent training and proficiency testing (external quality assessment) programs with good performance.

Other considerations for effective antimicrobial resistance surveillance include:

- Clinical microbiologists should be trained in health care epidemiology.
- The choice of microorganisms and antimicrobials to survey should be based on their relative public health importance, using criteria such as expected number of cases, severity of the infectious diseases as measured by its mortality rate and case fatality ratio, medical costs of such infections, and preventability.
- Microbiologists should collect not only laboratory data, but also the clinical data that is often missing from surveillance reports.

A well-structured computer system with WHO (WHONET) open source software can be used for data entry and analysis (*http://www.who.int/drugresistance/whonetsoftware/en/*). The analysis should be done at regular intervals and the results/observations should be shared within the institution, with community and collaborative study groups.

Attributes of Good Surveillance Systems

The attributes of a "good" surveillance system are:

- Simplicity
- Flexibility
- Representativeness
- Timeliness
- Usefulness.

A surveillance system should accurately describe the occurrence of antimicrobial resistance during a particular period at a particular place and its distribution in the population. This is a difficult task as the spectrum of microorganisms under surveillance includes uneven distribution of pathogens and opportunistic pathogens.

The surveillance system should be flexible, so that any change in information can be incorporated easily, and any new diseases can be included. An example is the capacity of an *S. aureus* surveillance system to conduct special surveillance for glycopeptides—intermediate or resistant *S. aureus*

The timeliness of surveillance program is also important since antimicrobial resistance is rapidly evolving and delay does not fit in an efficient policy. The published data does not reflect the current state of antimicrobial resistance.

Evaluation of a Surveillance System

The evaluation of surveillance can be measured by investigating the following aspects:

- Does the system detect trends that signal changes in the occurrence of diseases?
- Does the system provide estimates of the magnitude of morbidity and mortality related to the health problem under surveillance?
- Does the system stimulate epidemiologic research and action likely to lead to control and prevention?
- Does the system identify risk factors associated with disease occurrence?

- Does the system permit assessment of the effects of control measures?
- Does the system lead to improved clinical practice by the health care providers who are the constituents of the surveillance system?

Prediction of Evolution of Antimicrobial Resistance

To predict the short-term evolution of resistance, the behavior of antimicrobial use, and its dynamic relationship, time series analysis on antibiotic resistance and consumption data help to estimate the probability of susceptibility of the microorganism to every available antibiotic. This information facilitates to make recommendations about the empiric therapy, relevant to the local environment that would minimize the error in the therapeutic choice.

Surveillance of Antimicrobial Consumption[1]

It is essential to have a surveillance data on antibiotic use/consumption in the hospital/ community. This is an indispensible tool in the strategy to contain antimicrobial resistance. Hence, it is a must that all the hospital/community should generate a valid data on antibiotic prescriptions and sales. The same should be made publicly available to formulate antibiotic policy and Standard Treatment Guidelines.

To evaluate if antibiotic prescribing is rational, data on the number of prescriptions, indications, dose and duration of treatment, as well as different age groups are essential. Such data is essential in order to evaluate the impact of antibiotic prescribing on resistance, morbidity, complications and mortality.

However, drug consumption data with varying data collection system, time periods, and units of measurement makes it difficult to compare trends in antibacterial usage between geographical regions. Further in many developing countries, the lack of access to essential pharmaceuticals, over the counter sales, and suboptimal dosage are major problems in collecting reliable data.

Measurement of Antimicrobial Consumption

WHO collaborating center for Drug Statistics Methodology (1999) describes unit called as defined daily dose (DDD) according to the Anatomic Therapeutic Chemical (ATC) classification system. This defined daily dose is a unit based on the average adult dose used for the main indication of the drug. To make comparisons between geographical areas possible, the number of DDDs per 1000 inhabitants and day (DID) may be calculated. This measure will be influenced by several factors, for example, the dosage and duration of treatment, which may vary between hospitals even for the same indication.

The other measure of antibiotic use is the number of antibiotic prescriptions per 1000 inhabitants per year. This measure is probably more appropriate when evaluating antibiotic use in children.

It has been observed that instead of individual antibiotic pattern, better guidance is obtained using cumulative antibiogram. The cumulative antibiogram (CA) represents a report which summarizes the susceptibility of commonly isolated microorganisms to usual antibiotics in a defined period of time.

CUMULATIVE ANTIBIOGRAM[1]

The surveillance for antimicrobial resistance/ antibiotic consumption and preparation of a "Cumulative antibiogram" at the local level helps in clinical decision making, helps to design infection control measures, and antimicrobial containment strategies.

Attributes of Cumulative Antibiogram

The major attributes of a reliable cumulative antibiogram include:

- Analysis/presentation of data regularly, at least annually.
- Inclusion of only final verified results.
- Inclusion of only species with at least ≥30 isolates tested (under certain circumstances when you do not have >30 isolates, then combine two consecutive years' isolates into calculation.
- Inclusion of diagnostic isolates.
- Information only on drugs routinely tested.
- Inclusion of the first isolate per patient in the period analyzed, irrespective of body site from which the specimen was obtained or the antimicrobial susceptibility pattern.
- Calculation of the percentage susceptibility because clinicians generally avoid prescribing antimicrobials if a test result indicates intermediate susceptibility. Isolates with intermediate susceptibility should not be included in the calculation of percentage of isolates that are susceptible.
- Avoid the presentation of potentially misleading or confusing data, especially when presenting a table and ensure that all the details are provided in the accompanying footnotes.
- Providing confidence intervals and statistical significance of changes in the percentage of susceptible isolates.
- Utilizing statistical tools to analyze data.
- Undertaking data stratification to encourage optimal antimicrobial therapy. It is often useful to stratify results by specimens type or infection site, by nursing unit or site of care, by organism's resistance characteristics, by clinical service or patient population.
- Reviewing the cumulative antibiogram data if clinical failure occurs after empiric therapy, if changed the trend has to be followed.
- Ensuring the quality of cumulative antibiograms.
- Comparing the cumulative antibiogram with national data. However, care must be taken to make sure that there is no variation in drug panels of comparing antibiogram.

Antibiogram-derived Radical Decision Trees

This type of dissemination in the hospital helps to recognize the resistance to first-line drugs indicate susceptibility to second-line drugs and as well understand the probability of encountering such organisms.

Challenges in Cumulative Antibiogram

Variability in culture and susceptibility ordering practices is inevitable. Usually, a significant number of laboratory requests for the culture susceptibility from outpatients or inpatients are due to suspected infection with resistant organisms. Consequently, the number of requests received for susceptible infections are less as when compared with those for resistant cases. As a result, overcall of resistant rates are always introduced into most of the cumulative antibiograms.

Community-wide Antibiograms

Establishment of local surveillance systems improves appropriate antimicrobial use and curtailing antimicrobial resistance. To ensure that reliable data are presented, consistent mechanism to generate, collect and collate data at the local level is required that represents community prevalence of organisms.

Cumulative Hospital Antibiograms as a Quality Indicator

- Laboratories are often surveyed about their testing practices, but analysis of antibiograms may be a useful tool to measure whether laboratories are incorporating changes and updates in their testing methods.

- Analysis of antibiograms may provide useful information when deciding where to focus educational efforts.
- Increase compliance with standards and guidelines, particularly those with regard to daily verification of unusual or unlikely results, should result in decreased errors on antibiograms, and thus provide more reliable data to clinicians to guide antibiotic choice.
- Programs that provide and explain the antimicrobial susceptibility testing standards and guidelines may encourage compliance.

DEVELOPMENT OF STANDARD TREATMENT GUIDELINES[1]

Effective standard treatment guidelines (STG) improve patient care as well as enhance cost savings. The STG also reflects data on resistance, recognizing that local patterns of resistance often differ across geographical regions. The use of STG can be an effective means of changing behavior; hence the STG should be readily adaptable for local implementation.

Prerequisites of Effective STG

- Standard treatment guidelines should be based upon the findings of the cumulative antibiogram, antimicrobial policy, surveillance data on antimicrobial resistance and antibiotic consumption data and hospital-associated infection profile of the particular hospital or community.
- If a large number of STG documents are available from different sources on the same subject these can be compared for strengths and weaknesses in each guideline. Then a suitable guideline among the existing ones can be adapted with modifications for a desired local hospital, community/region.
- The STG should clearly specify for which disease/condition(s) they are stipulated, and also state who the intended users and the target population are, and what are the interventions and practices—such as evaluation, diagnostic studies, treatment and prevention-considered.
- The guideline developers should describe methods used to collect/select the evidence such as search of electronic databases and the number of documents sourced.
- All the major recommendations should be accompanied with levels of evidence (I-III) available and grades of recommendation (strong, moderate and weak). The quality and strength of evidence can be based on a rating scheme generally followed as listed below:
  - *Level 1 (High):* Evidence from well-conducted, randomized control trials.
  - *Level II (Moderate):* Evidence from well-designed controlled trials without randomization (including cohort, patient series and case control studies) Level II studies also include any large case series in which systematic analysis of disease patterns and/or microbial etiology was conducted as well as reports of data on new therapies that were not collected in a randomized fashion.
  - *Level III (low):* Evidence from case studies and expert opinions, in some instances, therapy recommendations come from antibiotic susceptibility data without clinical observations.

Summary of Prerequisites of STG

- Should be based on local antibiograms.
- Should be syndrome/disease based.
- Should specify type of clinical setting.
- Should specify rationale of guidelines.
- Should specify evidence-based strength of recommendations.
- Should involve treating physicians to bring ownership to the guidelines.

Development of STG

Recommendations are made and the methods used to formulate the recommendations are also declared. The strength of each recommendation is graded as "strong", "moderate" or "weak". Usually, the guideline committee independently grades each recommendation on the basis of the evidence and also includes their expert interpretation and clinical applicability. The final grading of each recommendation will be a composite of the individual STG developer group members' grades. For the final document, a strong recommendation requires that majority of the committee members to consider it to be strong. The moderate or weak management recommendations are usually not followed by the majority of the clinicians.

The description of the method used to analyze the evidence should be stated. This could either be a review or review of published meta-analysis. Also evidence supporting the recommendations, references and type of evidence supporting the recommendations must be mentioned, and a formal cost analysis should be performed and included.

Recommendations in STG

- Minor criteria and major criteria for the diagnosis are formulated and recommended for the clinical syndrome/ disease concerned.
- Recommendations are made for pathogen directed therapy. Once the etiology of the infection has been identified on the basis of reliable microbiological methods, antimicrobial therapy is directed at that pathogen.
- Decision of admission to hospital is advised on the basis of the severity of illness scores, or prognostic models. This can identify the level of care as outpatient, in-patient non-ICU admission or direct in-patient ICU admission.
- Recommendations on the empirical antimicrobial therapy are specified separately for outpatient treatment, inpatient treatment, on-ICU treatment and in-patient ICU treatment on considering the clinical condition and presence of co-morbidities.
- In addition to the constellation of suggestive clinical features, the STG should include suggestion for diagnostic testing of the disease condition such as chest radiograph, or other imaging technique, microbiological/pathological, hematological and biochemistry data/ values. The recommendations should focus on the investigation for specific pathogens that would significantly alter standard (empirical) management decisions.
- Recommendations are generally made for a class of antibiotics rather than a specific drug, unless outcome data clearly favors a specific drug. Since overall efficacy remains good for many classes of agents, the more potent drugs are given preference because of their benefit in decreasing the risk of selection for antibiotic resistance. Other factors for consideration of specific antimicrobials include pharmacokinetics/ pharmacodynamics, compliance, safety and cost.
- Early treatment (within 48 hours of the onset of symptoms) with appropriate antimicrobials is recommended, whereas for patients admitted through the emergency department, the first antibiotic dose should be administered while still in the department.
- Recommendation on the duration of therapy for patients with infection should lay emphasis that therapy should continue for minimum of 48–72 hours after the patient becomes afebrile and should have no more than one or two syndrome-associated signs of clinical instability before discontinuation of therapy.
- Recommendation on the criteria for clinical stability should be in place. Usually, this can be the minimum expected temperature, heart rate, respiratory rate, systolic blood pressure and arterial oxygen saturation.

- Recommendation on switch from intravenous to oral therapy can be made when the patient is hemodynamically stable and improving clinically, is fully conscious, and able to ingest oral medications.
- Recommendations on the use of antimicrobials should take into account, the use of antimicrobials within the previous three months (in which case an alternative from a different class should be selected). In case the individual is from a geographical region that has a high rate (>25%) of resistant organisms reported or where high-level minimal inhibitory concentration (MIC) is observed, then the use of alternate agent is mandatory.
- Recommendation on patient discharge can be suggested as soon as they are clinically stable, and have no other active medical problem.
- The locally adapted guideline should offer suggestion about the epidemiology and/or risk factors for alternative or specific additional antibiotics for the treatment.
- Suggestion for the management of "non-responding infections" can be outlined. Non-responding infection is defined as an inadequate clinical response despite adequate treatment.

Monitoring the Quality of Antimicrobial Prescriptions

Even with the use of STGs, one needs to monitor their application. Monitoring should be done to ascertain the following:

- Is the clinical picture compatible with an infection/Is there an indication for treatment with antibiotics?
- Is the choice of the antimicrobial drug adequate?
  - Efficacy: Is the (suspected) agent active?
  - Toxicity/allergy: Is there a less toxic alternative?
  - Cost: Is there a less costly alternative at equal efficacy and toxicity?
  - Broadness of spectrum: Is the spectrum unnecessarily broad?
- Is the duration of treatment appropriate?
  - Too long/too short?
- Is the dosage correct?
  - Dose/interval/mode of administration
- Is the timing appropriate?
  - Too early/too late?

Validation of STG

Guideline validation should be done by the internal peer review process. The STG is submitted to selected reviewers and changes recommended by the individual reviewer should be discussed by the STG developing group and incorporated into the final document. The STG is then reviewed by an eminent peer who was not part of the STG panel, but who is an expert in that particular specialty.

STRATEGIES FOR PROMOTING RATIONAL ANTIBIOTIC PRESCRIPTION[1]

Apart from conventional methods of communication, the effective strategies found to be aimed at appropriate practices for prescribing antibiotics by changing physician behavior are education outreach (academic detailing with interactive sessions) and the use of computer information systems and computer checks that can facilitate changes. Reminders to healthcare workers have to be used sparingly; otherwise too frequent reminders will be ignored, Computer checks can be programmed into hospital information system (HIS) to provide reminders and other suggestions to facilitate appropriate ordering of therapeutic and preventive treatments. Educational outreach is another effective strategy. For example, in academic detailing, there is one-on-one dialog and the exchange tends to be interactive rather than didactic. In the interaction, the provider being detailed can discuss the matter with the academic detailer until the provider understands the issue.

Barrier-oriented Interventions

Barrier-oriented interventions are critical and must be tended to specific local barriers. These possible local barriers would be disagreement among experts, availability of alternative practices, and inapplicability of guidelines to certain patient subgroups, patient refusal to comply, institutional inertia, vested interests, ineffective continuing medical education, and uncertainty of when and how to apply evidence-based medicine measures. The other barriers identified by Cabana et al.[2] in 1999 are listed in Table 26.1.

Using Checklist to an Effective Tool

A checklist should be used to assure that the right thing is done at the right time in the right place. This checklist is warranted because medical care has become complicated enough that one physician cannot remember everything that has to be done for a particular problem. A checklist for important interventions including use of antibiotics therefore should be helpful.

Finally, the most generally effective strategy to consider is multifaceted interventions. Multiple strategies are likely to be more successful than one.

Prescription Auditing

Prescription auditing is an indispensible and effective tool to monitor antimicrobial prescription practices. If properly done it can help treating physicians to improve their antimicrobial prescription skills and help an organization to adhere to, monitor and improve compliance to antibiotic policy.

Prescription auditing can be done by a team of physician, infectious disease specialists, clinical microbiologists and pharmacologists depending on their availability in an organization. The healthcare settings that lack hospital information management system (HIMS) or other form of computerization can also do the auditing by formulation of clear policy and procedures. An example of the prescription auditing method is described in Figure 26.2.

A MODEL STANDARD TREATMENT GUIDELINE FOR COMMUNITY-ACQUIRED PNEUMONIA AT THE HOSPITAL LEVEL[1]

Purpose

This document is developed for diagnosis, management and treatment of community-acquired pneumonia (CAP).

Table 26.1: Barrier-oriented interventions

Barrier	Explanation
Lack of awareness	Clinician unaware that guidelines exist
Lack of familiarity	Clinician aware of guidelines, but unfamiliar with specifics
Lack of agreement	Clinician does not agree with a specific recommendation made in guidelines or is averse to the concept of guidelines in general
Lack of self-efficacy	Clinician doubts whether he or she can perform the behavior
Lack of outcome expectancy	Clinician believes that the recommendations will be unsuccessful
Lack of motivation	Clinician is unable/unmotivated to change previous practices
Guideline-related barriers	Guidelines are not easy or convenient to use
Patient-related barriers	Clinician may be unable to reconcile guidelines with patient preferences
Environment-related barriers	Clinician may not have control over some changes (e.g. time resources, organizational constraints)

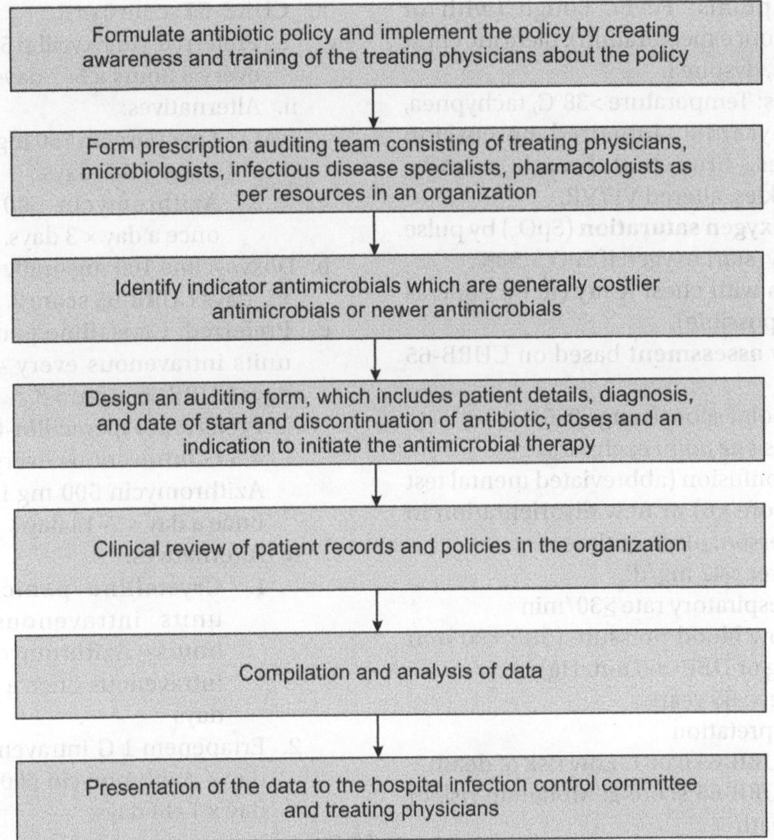

Fig. 26.2: Example of prescription auditing structure and process

Intended Use

This STG is intended for use in critical care, emergency medicine, family practice, infectious diseases, internal medicine and pulmonary medicine. However, these guidelines should be modified as per the need in CAP occurring in immuno-compromised patients, transplant patients, high-dose corticosteroid recipients and human immunodeficiency virus/acquired immunodeficiency syndrome (HIV/AIDS) patients.

The suggested reading references are considered along with the microbiology culture susceptibility data (antibiogram) for the previous five years for developing the hospital-based STG for CAP. The quality and strength of the evidence should be followed as stated in the adult CAP guidelines.

Among the recommended antibiotics (empirical or pathogen-specific therapy) included are crystalline penicillin, macrolides, doxycycline, fluoroquinolones, beta-lactam plus beta-lactam and carbapenems based on the severity of illness and the causative microorganisms often seen in this region.

Note: This STG is suggestive and health facilities need to modify it to suit their needs, match with local data and antibiotic usage policy.

Standard Treatment Guidelines for Community-acquired Pneumonia

1. **Suspect** if patient (not been hospitalized in the previous two weeks; not immuno-compromised) has any combination of the following:

a. Symptoms: Fever, cough (with or without expectoration), pleuritic chest pain, dyspnea.
b. Signs: Temperature >38°C, tachypnea, tachycardia, impaired percussion notes, bronchial breath sounds, crackles, altered VF/VR.

2. **Check oxygen saturation** (SpO_2) by pulse oximetry; start oxygen if SpO_2 <90%.
3. **Confirm** with chest X-ray (to be done as soon as possible).
4. **Severity assessment** based on CURB-65 score
   a. Six point score (range 0–5)
   b. Gives *one point* each for:
      i. Confusion (abbreviated mental test score ≤8) or new disorientation in person, place or time.
      ii. Urea >42 mg/dL
      iii. Respiratory rate ≥30/min
      iv. Low blood pressure (SBP <90 mm Hg or DBP <60 mm Hg)
      v. Age ≥65 years.
   c. Interpretation
      i. CURB-65 0 or 1: Low risk of death
      ii. CURB-65 score 2: Moderate risk of death
      iii. CURB score ≥3: High risk of death.
5. **Laboratory tests**
   a. Complete blood counts
   b. Urea, creatinine
   c. Antibiogram (only if CURB 65 score ≥2).
   d. Blood culture × 2 (only if CURB 65 score ≥2)
   e. Sputum Gram stain and culture (optional)
      i. *Only if* CURB 65 score ≥2 and patient can expectorate
      ii. Specimen (expectorated sputum) should be transported *promptly* to the laboratory
6. **Setting of care**
   a. CURB-65 score 0 or 1:Ooutpatient
   b. CURB-65 score 2: Inpatient (ward)
   c. CURB-65 score ≥3: Inpatient (M-ICU)
7. **Antibiotic management:** All patients should receive the first dose of antibiotics as soon as the diagnosis of CAP is confirmed.
   a. CURB-65 score 0 or 1
      i. Preferred: Amoxycillin 500 mg orally every 8 hours × 5–7 days
      ii. Alternatives:
         1. Levofloxacin 750 mg orally once a day × 5–7 days.
         2. Azithromycin 500 mg orally once a day × 3 days.
   b. Doxycycline 100 mg orally twice a day × 7 days CURB-65 score 2.
   c. Preferred: Crystalline penicillin 20 L units intravenous every 4 hours × 7 days CURB 65 score ≥ 3.
      i. Preferred: Piperacillin-tazobactam 4.5 G intravenous every 8 hours + Azithromycin 500 mg intravenous once a day × 7–14 days.
      ii. Alternatives:
         1. Crystalline penicillin 20 L units intravenous every 4 hours+ Azithromycin 500 mg intravenous once a day × 7–14 days
         2. Ertapenem 1 G intravenous once a day + Azithromycin 500 mg once a day × 7–14 days.

Note:

- Change to an oral regimen as soon as clinical improvement occurs and the temperature has been normal for more than 24 hours, and there is no contraindication to the oral route.
- Modify antibiotic regimen based on results of culture and susceptibility reports.

Other recommendations included in the hospital STG for CAP are:

- If patient is critical with signs of infection admitted through the emergency department, the first antibiotic of choice should be recommended for administration while still in the emergency room.
- Once the etiology of CAP has been identified and susceptibility reports are available the antimicrobial therapy should be either continued or altered according to the susceptibility report.
- Patients with CAP should be treated for a minimum of five days. Patient should be

afebrile for at least 48–72 hours and should have no more than 1 CAP associated sign of clinical instability before discontinuation of therapy.

- When patient is hemodynamically stable and improving clinically (temperature <37.8°C, heart rate 100 beats/min, respiratory rate <24 breaths/min, systolic blood pressure > 90 mm Hg, arterial oxygen saturation >90% or pO_2 >60 mm Hg and full conscious, able to take oral medications, then a switch from intravenous to oral therapy is recommended.
- Patients should be discharged as soon as they are clinically stable. At discharge, patient should have no other active medical problems, and have a safe environment for continued care.
- Failure to respond to initial therapy should raise questions of diagnosis, treatment adherence, and antimicrobial resistance.
- Polysaccharide pneumococcal vaccine (23-valent) may be given either at hospital discharge or during outpatient treatment.
- Smoking cessation and alcohol abstaining should be advised for patients to whom such habits contributed to the illness.
- Educating the patient regarding the hygiene measures, including the use of hand hygiene and masks or tissues for patients with cough, should be used to reduce the spread of respiratory infections.

STG Performance Measures to Improve/Track Outcome in the Hospital[1]

- Antibiotics should be administered within four hours of admission to the healthcare facility.
- Only the recommended antibiotics should be used and not others. Blood cultures if drawn, should be drawn before antibiotics are given.
- The patients should receive advice or administered pneumococcal vaccine before discharge.

ANTIMICROBIAL STEWARDSHIP[1]

Good antimicrobial stewardship involves selecting an appropriate drug and optimizing its dose and duration to cure an infection while minimizing toxicity and conditions for selection of resistant bacterial strains.

Benefits of Prescribing Against Non-prescribing of Antibiotics

The clinical syndromes should be carefully assessed based on the benefits of prescribing against non-prescribing of antibiotics as outlined below:

- Patient cure/improvement against failure/mortality.
- Development of resistance in pathogens infecting the patient.
- Risk for spread of resistance.
- Suppression of normal flora.
- Development of resistance in normal flora.

The other relevant issues to be considered are:

- In vitro susceptibility
- Antibiotic activity: Bactericidal/bacteriostatic.
- Site of infection and achievable antibiotic concentration.
- Dosage and pharmacodynamic principles
- Dosing and host factors like weight, immunosuppression, hepatic/renal failure.
- Cost-effective ratio.
- Drug interactions and poor absorptions.

Further, this can be effectively assisted by instituting various regulations such as formula restrictions, automatic stop-order, prior approval programs, therapeutic substitution, streamlining and antibiotic cycling, etc.

Maximizing Clinical Outcomes and Minimizing Selection of Resistant Organisms

What Should be Done

- Appropriate empirical antimicrobial therapy, with right dose, for right duration and at right time.

- Delayed therapy or modifying the initial antimicrobial therapy does not improve the outcome.
- Multidrug-resistance organism predisposes for inappropriate therapy.

- Early and accurate identification of the pathogen and susceptibility.
- Combination or monotherapy chosen on the basis of the pathogen identified.
- Deescalation of initial broad spectrum therapy after definitive diagnosis (generally based on microbiology reports).

What Should not be Done

- Treat non-infectious or nonbacterial syndrome.
- Treat colonization or contamination.
- Treat longer than necessary.
- Fail to make adjustment in a timely manner.
- Prescribe antibiotic with spectrum of activity not indicated.

Antimicrobial Stewardship, Hand Hygiene and STG

Hand hygiene compliance rates of 10–40% have been observed even in best of the units in the developed countries. Acceptability of such compliance rates and justifications of intense antimicrobial usage under the umbrella of "empirical therapy" has underscored the importance of increasing hand hygiene compliance efforts. In recent years, adoption by WHO of hand hygiene as the first global challenge and the availability of robust hand hygiene compliance monitoring tools has lead to an increase in hand hygiene compliance. Uniformity in monitoring hand hygiene compliance through these tools has also provided compatibility and credibility to the hand hygiene compliance figures. Improved hand hygiene compliance has also led to decline in "empirical antimicrobial therapy" in such units.

MRSA can be contained by active surveillance culture, admission culture, isolation, decolonization and decontamination. Scandinavian countries and The Netherlands effectively practices the "admission screening" for MRSA, but nowhere outside these countries is this implemented routinely. Although the importance of such activities is well known it is yet to be appreciated fully.

Antibiotic Use as a Cause of Hospital Infection

Third-generation cephalosporins and quinolones are implicated as a risk factor for increase MRSA/gram-negative bacilli colonization and infection. There is also ample evidence that MRSA incidence rates declined following the implementation and monitoring of antibiotic policies that reduced use of cephalosporins and quinolones. Similarly reports of VRE incidence rates declined following implementation of antibiotic policies that reduce use of vancomycin and *Clostridium difficile* following reduced use of clindamycin.

Studies had demonstrated the concept of 'squeezing the balloon' whereby reduction in use of one drug is reflected by increasing use of another.

Pitfalls of Practicing According to the Guidelines

The antibiotic stewardship achieves only "uniformity of prescribing "with adherence to policies, guidelines and formularies. Paradoxically, this may actually at times be harmful, as the best defense against resistance is probably "diversity of prescribing".

The other important issue is difficulty in reducing overall antibiotic use, as modern medical developments seem to have no end to the immunosuppression of the patient.

The earlier guidelines from the British and American Thoracic Societies for treatment of community-acquired pneumonia (CAP) resulted in over-use of cephalosporins, quinolones and macrolides triggering MRSA outbreaks. Though the guidelines are evidence based, the antibiotic recommendations are definitely not and leaning heavily to combination therapy in trying to cover all etiological agents.

SUMMARY OF ANTIBIOTIC POLICY AND STANDARD TREATMENT GUIDELINES

Introduction

Antimicrobial resistance has become a major public health problem. Infections caused by resistant microbes lead to treatment failure, resulting in prolonged illness and mortality. Choice of antibiotics is difficult as there are no effective antibiotics. There are very few new drugs available and there is scarcity of old drugs. Prevalence of multidrug resistant bacteria leads to prescription of number of active drugs especially the broad-spectrum antibiotics. This affects bacterial ecology and appearance of more and more drug-resistant bacteria. It is now essential to (1) Delay the emergence of such resistant strains, and (2) Prevent their spread. This can be done by proper use of antibiotics and proper antibiotic strategy.

Availability of New Antimicrobial Agents

The situation on the development of new antimicrobial agents is not very encouraging. There are hardly any new antimicrobial agents in the pipeline especially for treatment of some common multidrug resistant nosocomial organisms grouped under the acronym of **ESKAPE**:

- *Enterococcus faecium* (Vancomycin-resistant enterococci—VRE).
- *Staphylococcus aureus* (Methicillin-resistant *Staphylococcus aureus*).
- *Klebsiella* and *Escherichia coli* that produce extended spectrum beta-lactamases (ESBL) and carbapenemases.
- *Acinetobacter baumanni*
- *Pseudomonas aeruginosa*
- *Enterobacter* species.

Strategies Against Antimicrobial-resistant Microorganisms in Hospitals

Strategic Objectives

- To recognize and report trends in antimicrobial resistance within the institution.
- To rapidly detect and report resistant microorganisms in individual patients and ensure prompt treatment.
- To assure increased adherence to basic infection control policies and procedures.
- To incorporate the detection, prevention and control of antimicrobial resistance into institutional strategic goals and provide the required resources.
- To establish a policy and practices for the rational use of antimicrobials.

Strategic Approaches

- Optimizing the duration of drug of choice and dose of empiric therapy—antimicrobial stewardship.
- Optimizing antimicrobial prophylaxis for operative procedures.
- Developing and implementing an antibiotic policy and standard treatment guidelines (STG).
- Monitoring and providing a feedback regarding antibiotic resistance.
- Improving antimicrobial prescribing by educational and administrative means.

To achieve these, a comprehensive approach through a hospital policy on the rational use of antibiotics is essential.

Antibiotic Policy

Aim

- To minimize morbidity and mortality due to antimicrobial-resistant infection.
- To preserve the effectiveness of antimicrobial agents in the treatment and prevention of communicable diseases.

Scope

The antibiotic policy is essentially for prophylaxis, empirical and definitive therapy. The policy shall incorporate specific recommendations for the treatment of different high-risk/special groups such as immunocompromised hosts; hospital-associated infections and community acquired infections.

The hospital antibiotic policy will be based upon:

- Spectrum of antibiotic activity.
- Pharmacokinetics and pharmacodynamic of these medicines.
- Adverse effects.
- Potential to select resistance.
- Cost.
- Special needs of individual patient groups.

The hospital antibiotic policy will also set levels for prescribing antibiotics, for example:

- First choice antibiotics can be prescribed by all doctors.
- Restricted choice antibiotics can only be prescribed after consulting the head of the department or the antimicrobial team (AMT).
- Reserve antibiotics will be prescribed only by designated experts.

Development of Antibiotic Policy

- A multidisciplinary antibiotic management team (AMT) shall be developed, which will have full commitment and support from the top management. This team will consist of 6-10 members with expertise and experience in different subjects like infectious disease, internal medicine, surgery, pediatrics, clinical microbiology, and pharmacology and hospital pharmacy. This team will be responsible for developing, implementing, and revising the policy every year.
- Their main functions will be to decide the antimicrobial dose, duration of antimicrobial, decide about antimicrobial prophylaxis, empirical antimicrobials, restricted antimicrobials and their approval and indication for use of specific antimicrobials.
- The policy will be drafted based on scientific evidence and if enough evidence is not available a combination of expert opinion should be used.

Attributes of Antibiotic Policy

- Should be clear, flexible, applicable in day-day practice in the form of a pocket guide.
- The recommended antibiotic should be effective against pathogens seen in that locality.
- Details regarding dose, duration, route of administration, alternatives in case of allergy, in patients with liver or renal disease should be provided.
- Antibiotic used for prophylaxis should be free of side-effects, cheap and given for short duration. It should not be used for therapeutic purposes as it will lead to development of antimicrobial resistance.

Surveillance of Antimicrobial Resistance

- For surveillance of antimicrobial resistance, laboratory data as well as clinical data is essential (laboratory surveillance and disease surveillance). Quantitative resistance data is more useful (i.e. minimal inhibitory concentration or zone diameters) since this can detect an emerging resistance character in an organism.
- Duplicate results should be avoided since a patient may have consecutive cultures obtained from the same body site or cultures from different body sites yielding the same organism. Only the first positive culture from the patient for each disease episode should be reported for surveillance purposes.
- It is important to express resistance as incidence rates within a defined human population instead of using number of isolates as denominator. It

is recommended to use the number of admissions and the number of days of hospitalization. Of course, this process captures data only from patients admitted to the hospital and excludes those who attend as outdoor patients.

- The validity and reliability of this data is acceptable only when the clinical laboratories providing the data for surveillance have routinely participated in external quality assessment programs with good performance A well-structured computer system with WHO (WHONET) open source software can be used for data entry and analysis. The analysis should be done at regular intervals and the results/observations shared within the institution.
- It is also essential to have surveillance data on antibiotic use/consumption in the hospital/community. Hence, it is a must that all hospital/community should generate a data on antibiotic prescriptions and sales. The same should be made publicly available to formulate antibiotic policy and standard treatment guidelines (STG).
- It has been observed that instead of individual antibiotic pattern, better guidance is obtained using cumulative antibiogram. The cumulative anti-biogram (CA) represents a report which summarizes the susceptibility of commonly isolated microorganisms to usual antibiotics in a defined period of time.

Development of Standard Treatment Guidelines

Standard treatment guidelines should be developed based on:

- The findings of cumulative antibiogram.
- Antimicrobial policy.
- Surveillance data on antimicrobial resistance.
- Antibiotic consumption data and.
- Hospital-associated infection profile of the particular hospital.

These guidelines should be:

- Syndrome/disease based.
- Should specify clinical setting-outpatient clinics, inpatient clinics, ICU setting.
- Should provide evidence-based strength of recommendations.
- Should involve treating physicians.

Strategies for Promoting Rational Antibiotic Prescribing

Effective strategies are found to be aimed at appropriate practices for prescribing antibiotics:

- By changing physician behavior such as education outreach (academic detailing with interactive sessions)
- Use of computer information systems and computer checks that can facilitate changes.
- Prescription auditing is also an effective tool which can monitor antimicrobial prescription practices. If properly done, it can help physicians to improve their antimicrobial prescription skills and help an organization to adhere to and monitor compliance to antibiotic policy.

REFERENCES

1. Step-by-step approach for development and implementation of Hospital Antibiotic Policy and Standard Treatment Guidelines, WHO 2011. Accesses from www.apps.who.int/medicinedocs/documents/s19184en/19184en.pdf on 13th August 2015.
2. Cabana MD, Rand CS, Powe NR, et al. Why don't physicians follow clinical practice guidelines? A framework for improvement. JAMA. 1999;282:1458-65.

Chapter 27

Infection Control in Cardiac Catheterization Laboratory

Chapter Outline

Patient Preparation and Protection
- Hair Removal
- Skin Cleaning
- Drapes
- Antibiotics
- Catheterization Technique
- Sheath Removal and Vascular Closure Devices
- Wound Dressings

Laboratory Personnel—the Primary Operator and Staff
- Hand Scrub and Gloves
- Gowns and Shoe Covers
- Caps, Masks, and Eye Protection
- Ancillary Personnel
- High-risk Patients (For Staff Exposure)
- Skin Puncture or Laceration
- Vaccination

Laboratory Environment
- Cleaning
- Air Vents
- Maintenance of Environment
- Fixed and Disposable Laboratory Equipment
- Disposal of Waste

INTRODUCTION[1]

Till the 1970's sterile techniques, typical of those in the operating suite were followed in the cardiac catheterization laboratory, but by 1990s, these sterile techniques became less prevalent in the early years of diagnostic cardiac catheterization. Strict sterile precautions were required for cutdown procedures. Thirteen years ago, when the original guidelines were written, the brachial arteriotomy was still frequently utilized, femoral closure devices were uncommon, "implantables," such as intracoronary stents and patent foramen ovale (PFO)/atrial septal defect (ASD) closure devices, were in their infancy, and percutaneous valve replacement was not a consideration.

Since 2005, the cardiac catheterization laboratory became a complex interventional suite with percutaneous access routine and device implantation standard.

Despite frequent device implantation, strict sterile precautions are often not observed. Reasons for this include a decline in brachial artery cutdown, limited post-procedure follow-up with few reported infections, limited use of caps and masks in televised cases, and lack of current guidelines.

Proper sterile technique has the potential to decrease the patient infection rate. Hand washing remains the most important procedure for preventing infections. Caps, masks, gowns, and gloves help to protect the patient by maintaining a sterile field. Protection of personnel may be accomplished by proper gowning, gloving, and eye wear, disposal of contaminated equipment, and prevention and care of puncture wounds and lacerations. With the potential for acquired disease from blood-borne pathogens, the need for protective measures is as essential in the cardiac catheterization laboratory as is the standard Universal Precautions, which are applied throughout the hospital. All personnel should strongly consider vaccination for hepatitis B.

Maintenance of the cardiac catheterization laboratory environment includes appropriate cleaning, limitation of traffic, and adequate ventilation. In an Society for Cardiovascular Angiography and Interventions (SCAI) survey, members recommended an update on guidelines for infection control in the cardiac catheterization laboratory. The following revision of the original 1992 guidelines is written specifically to address the increased utilization of the catheterization laboratory as an interventional suite with device implantation. In this update, infection protection is divided into sections on the patient, the laboratory personnel, and the laboratory environment. Additionally, specific CDC recommendation sections highlight recommendations from other published guidelines.

In the cardiac catheterization laboratory, many other guidelines will thus have to be followed such as (1) the Centers for Disease Control (CDC) guidelines for prevention of intravascular catheter-related infections (2002), which are now considered the best clinical practice guidelines,[2] (2) guidelines on the prevention of surgical site infection[3] hand hygiene in healthcare settings[4] and (3) environmental infection control in healthcare facilities[5] which contain recommendations relevant to the cardiac catheterization laboratory.

PATIENT PREPARATION AND PROTECTION[1]

HAIR REMOVAL

Consideration should be made to avoid hair removal unless it directly interferes with the procedure. If it is necessary to remove hair at the access site, use a clipper or depilatory on the day of the procedure, and not before. Shaving with a razor should be avoided because it can injure the skin and increase the risk of infection.[6-8] Clipping the day before the procedure should be avoided, because it can be associated with dermal abrasions that could be a nidus for local infection.[9] Depilatories sometimes will produce hypersensitivity reactions, so the cardiac catheterization laboratory staff should be observant for these types of complications.

CDC Recommendations

Do not remove hair preoperatively unless the hair at or around the incision site will interfere with the operation.[3]

If hair is removed at an access site immediately before a procedure, it is preferable to use electric clippers or a depilatory cream.[3]

SKIN CLEANING

The skin at the cutdown or puncture site should be thoroughly cleaned. Immediately before the procedure, a broad-spectrum antimicrobial agent should be generously applied, in accordance with manufacturer's recommendations.[10]

CDC Recommendations

A 2% chlorhexidine-based preparation for skin antisepsis is preferred during central line insertion, but tincture of iodine (an iodophor) or 70% alcohol may be substituted.[2]

Allow the antiseptic to remain on the insertion site (do not swab excess) and air-dry before catheter insertion when possible. Povidone iodine is most effective when allowed to remain on the skin for at least 2 min or longer if it is not yet dry.[2]

For patient skin preparation in the operating room, iodophors, alcohol-containing products, and chlorhexidine gluconate (CHG) are most commonly used. CHG achieved both a greater reduction in skin microflora and had a greater residual activity after a single application when compared with povidone-iodine. Further, CHG is not inactivated by blood or serum protein, whereas iodophors may be.[3] CHG is bacteriostatic and effective as long as it is present on the skin.

DRAPES

Nonporous drapes should be used to cover the area surrounding the wound.[7] Maximum sterile barrier precautions should be utilized during catheter insertion.

The sterile sheet should be large enough to cover the entire patient and any other hardware attached to the table that could come in contact with long catheter or wires. Any adhesive material attached to the skin around the wound and to the drapes should isolate the wound site from the surrounding unprepared skin.

CDC Recommendations

Use surgical drapes that remain effective barriers when wet (i.e. materials that resist liquid penetration).[3]

Use aseptic technique, including the use of a cap, mask, sterile gown, sterile gloves, and a large sterile sheet, for the insertion of central venous catheters [including peripherally inserted central catheter (PICCs)] or guidewire exchange.[2]

ANTIBIOTICS

Antimicrobial drug prophylaxis is not routinely recommended for procedures performed in the cardiac catheterization laboratory. In fact, prophylaxis is generally not indicated for "clean" surgery unless it involves implantation of certain prosthetic material.[11]

Antibiotic prophylaxis should be considered for the immunocompromised patients and for any patient with probable or definite wound contamination during the procedure.[12]

If an antibiotic is used prophylactically, the activity should be against common skin organisms. A cephalosporin with a moderately long serum half-life, such as cefazolin, is a common drug of choice before the catheterization procedure.[11] A single dose of parenteral antimicrobial given within 30 minutes of device insertion usually provides adequate tissue concentration for several hours. This is common practice for device insertions, such as in patent foramen ovale closures.

A patient with an active bacterial infection at a site remote from a surgical wound has a greater risk of wound infection than an uninfected patient. This risk may be reduced by treating the remote infection before an invasive procedure is performed.[7] While this applies to bacterial infections, the approach for local fungal infections is less well defined. In these instances, avoidance of the infected site when possible or aggressive local skin cleaning is standard practice.

CDC Recommendations

Antibiotic prophylaxis is not routinely indicated for a sterile procedure, such as cardiac catheterization. In the rare circumstance when it is indicated, selection of the antibiotic agent should be based on its efficacy against most common skin pathogens.[3]

In most instances, when a prophylactic antibiotic is used, it should be given 30–60 minutes before the procedure.[3]

Whenever possible, identify and treat all infections remote to the surgical site before an elective-operation; postpone elective procedures until the infection has resolved.[3] If a fluoroquinolone or vancomycin is chosen, it should be given 120 minutes before the procedure.[12a]

CATHETERIZATION TECHNIQUE

Prolonged procedures and lapses in aseptic technique are important causes of wound infections.[7] Care should be taken to prevent large hematomas, which serve as a nidus for infection.[7] Although no data exist on the performance of cardiac catheterizations or coronary interventions in a febrile patient, those with ongoing infections should be appropriately treated before an elective cardiac catheterization. Fever is a relative contraindication for an elective cardiac catheterization. The risks versus benefits of performing urgent invasive procedures on a febrile patient must be weighed individually.

The choice of the access site is an issue if a second percutaneous procedure is performed shortly after the first. Local infection at the puncture site is more likely to occur after early repuncture of the ipsilateral femoral artery.[13] If a percutaneous intervention (PCI) procedure is performed after a 6 hour delay following a diagnostic catheterization, the operator should consider contralateral access for the PCI.

With advances in femoral and radial percutaneous access, brachial artery cutdown is now an infrequent method for artery access in patients undergoing cardiac catheterization. One study demonstrated a 10-fold increase in infectious complication with this approach.[14] If used, infection control precautions for cutdown procedures should be more rigorous than percutaneous procedures and should be similar to those used for any minor surgical procedure.

SHEATH REMOVAL AND VASCULAR CLOSURE DEVICES

Vascular access sheaths are routinely removed following diagnostic procedures but not infrequently left in place following femoral interventional procedures.

When this is necessary, a standard wound-dressing protocol should be followed, similar to that for other indwelling vascular catheters. For in-dwelling venous catheters, the duration of the catheter placement is the most important predictor for an infection.[15] Therefore, it is prudent to remove any in-dwelling sheath or catheter as early as clinically appropriate. When clinically indicated, a catheter and rarely even a sheath may be maintained for a period of days following the procedure. In this circumstance, appropriate wound dressings and daily wound inspections are critical.

Multiple vascular closure devices (VCDs) are available for establishing hemostasis following femoral artery access. While these devices are designed to eliminate the need for manual compression and allow for earlier ambulation post-procedure, they have not been shown to decrease vascular complications.[14,16-18] Vascular closure devices are used in many diagnostic catheterization laboratories. Occasionally, the complication with VCD is more severe than with manual compression.[19] One of the most significant of these is infection of the suture or collagen anchor leading to arteritis.[20] These complications occur in 0.5% of VCD procedures and can be limb and life-threatening.[14]

Special precautions may be warranted in patients receiving a VCD. Antibiotic coverage for common skin flora is recommended for the diabetic patient undergoing VCD placement.[14]

These devices should be avoided when arterial puncture is into a preexisting synthetic vascular graft, if local or systemic infection is a possibility, or if the sheath has been in-dwelling for an extended period of time.[17] Following prolonged procedures; consideration should be given to site recleaning as well as new sterile gloves for the operator before VCD placement. The presence of a hematoma before placement of a VCD may increase the incidence of infection. When sutures are involved, these should be cut so the ends retract well below the skin and a topical triple antibiotic cream applied to the puncture site. The patient should be instructed to avoid tub baths until the skin puncture site is healed and to report early any groin complications or signs of infection. A pseudoaneurysm following a closure device should be considered a possible early sign of infection and thus treatment by local injection of prothrombotic agents used with caution.[18]

WOUND DRESSINGS

Although more applicable for prolonged use, occlusive nonpermeable plastic dressings should be avoided because they increase the infection risk two- to four-fold compared with traditional gauze dressings.[21]

CDC recommendations. Use either a sterile gauze or sterile and transparent semipermeable dressing to cover the catheter site. Do not use nonpermeable (plastic) dressings.[2]

If the patient is diaphoretic, or if the site is bleeding or oozing, gauze dressing is preferable to a transparent semipermeable dressing.[2]

Topical antibiotic ointments or creams promote fungal infections and antibiotic resistance. They should therefore be avoided except with dialysis catheters.[2]

LABORATORY PERSONNEL—THE PRIMARY OPERATOR AND STAFF[1]

HAND SCRUB AND GLOVES

Handwashing is the single most important procedure for preventing nosocomial infections.[4] An operator should start the day in the laboratory with a hand scrub of at least 2 or 3 minutes, utilizing a sterile surgical scrub brush impregnated with detergents and a topical antiseptic agent that has a persistent chemical effect. For subsequent cases, it is best to avoid repeated scrubbing, which may irritate the skin and increase the likelihood of dermal abrasions. It is preferable to use an antiseptic solution or foam before subsequent procedures. All rings and bracelets should be removed before scrubbing. Ideally, fingernails should not extend past the fingertips and should be kept free of fingernail polish and artificial coverings.

Two types of agents are commonly used for hand washing: detergents (plain soap) and antiseptics. The primary action of plain soap and water is to remove viable noncolonizing organisms physically from the skin surface.[22] Antiseptic agents have additional important properties. No definitive clinical trial has yet conclusively demonstrated the effects of hand washing with an antiseptic agent on nosocomial infection rates.

The use of antiseptic hand scrubs is nearly universal in the operating room environment.[3,4] All agents have a bactericidal effect, killing and/or inhibiting growth of both "normal flora" of the skin as well as more virulent bacteria. Some antiseptics bind to the skin, resulting in persistent chemical activity that inhibits proliferation of organisms within the moist environment of rubber or plastic gloves.[22] Brushless, waterless scrubs containing alcohol are often preferred because of less hand irritation, increased efficacy, and immediate bactericidal activity.

Gloves should be applied in a sterile manner. They should be changed if a puncture occurs or blood is detected under the gloves during the procedure. As noted previously, surgical hand antisepsis using either an antimicrobial soap or an alcohol-based hand rub, with persistent activity, is recommended before donning sterile gloves. Damage to physician gloves was evaluated in one study during cardiac catheterization.[23] No punctures were detected in 25 pairs of unused control gloves, but 19% of 200 gloves worn during procedures had small punctures. The thumb and index finger were the sites of 81% of the punctures; this was attributed to glove trauma from manipulation of stopcocks. Therefore, consideration should be given to the use of double gloves when an operator has hand abrasions.

CDC Recommendations

Observe proper hand hygiene procedures either by washing hands with conventional antiseptic-containing soap or with waterless alcohol gels or foams. Observe hand hygiene before and after palpating catheter insertion sites, as well as before and after inserting, replacing, accessing, repairing, or dressing an intravascular catheter.[2]

When performing surgical hand antisepsis using an antimicrobial soap, scrub hands and forearms for the length of time recommended by the manufacturer, usually (2–5) minutes. Long scrub times (e.g. 10 minutes) are not necessary.[3,4]

Scrub hands with brushes only once per day; subsequent procedures require only repeated antiseptic foam/gel hand washing.[4]

When using an alcohol-based surgical hand scrub product with persistent activity, follow the manufacturer's instructions. Before applying the alcohol solution, prewash hands and forearms with a nonantimicrobial soap and dry completely. After application of the alcohol-based product as recommended, allow hands to dry thoroughly, approximately 15–25 seconds, before donning sterile gloves.[4]

Remove debris from underneath fingernails using a nail cleaner under running water before scrubbing the hands with either a brush or antiseptic gel or foam.[4]

GOWNS AND SHOE COVERS

The operator should wear a nonporous gown to prevent the contamination that occurs when porous cloth gowns become wet with blood or other fluids. The operator should wear a scrub suit or other clean hospital uniforms, and not street clothes, in the cardiac catheterization laboratory. There are no scientific data to support the role of shoe covers in preventing surgical wound infections. However, they may provide protection to laboratory personnel and are commonly used to prevent tracking contaminated fluids throughout the facility by soiled footwear.

CDC Recommendations

No recommendations exist on how or where to launder scrub suits, restricting the use of scrub suits to the operating suite, or for covering scrubs when out of the operating suite.[3] Change scrub suits that are visibly soiled, contaminated, and/or penetrated by blood or other potentially infectious materials.[3] Shoe covers are not required solely to prevent a surgical site infection, but are required by Occupational Safety and Health Administration (OSHA) if soiling of shoes is likely, in order to reduce contamination of other areas of the healthcare facility (i.e. room-to room transmission).[24]

CAPS, MASKS, AND EYE PROTECTION

Although masks protect the operator's mucous membranes from contamination by a patient's body fluids, the effect of caps and masks on the incidence of infection in the cardiac catheterization laboratory is unclear. Caps and mask are standard attire in a surgical suite, but there are diverse opinions and only limited data regarding their benefit in the cardiac catheterization laboratory.[25,26]

Because of the risk associated with exposure to blood-borne pathogens, the use of Universal Precautions, as applied throughout the hospital, are relevant to healthcare providers in the cardiac catheterization laboratory.[24] The operator is provided personal protection by following these precautions that include the wearing of a mask, eye protection, gloves, and nonporous gown. Therefore, it is recommended that all personnel exposed to bodily fluids in the cardiac catheterization laboratory use Universal Precautions.

Since the incidence of infections related to procedures in the cardiac catheterization laboratories is low, it is unlikely an adequately powered randomized study of caps and masks will ever be performed. However, the consequences from such infections are significant while the risk of using these precautions is nonexistent.[14]

Therefore, it is the recommendation of these guidelines that the use by the operator(s) of a cap, mask, and eye protection be strongly considered, if not mandatory, for all procedures performed in the cardiac catheterization laboratory for the protection of the operator. If an operator does not use a cap and mask routinely, they should at least be used for procedures in patients who are at increased risk for both an infection as well as for a serious complication, should one develop. Such patients include those with native valve disease or intracardiac prostheses, arterial access performed through a femoral arterial graft, prolonged catheter or procedure times, prolonged use of an indwelling sheath following the procedure, intra-aortic balloon pump insertion, percutaneous valvular procedures, and the use of implantable devices such as stents, septal closure devices, and/or VCDs. It may not always be known at the start of the procedure if one of these higher-risk situations will occur. Accordingly, each facility should consider the best policy for their laboratory, with patient safety given the highest priority.

CDC Recommendations

Use aseptic technique, including the use of a cap, mask, eye protection, sterile gown, and sterile gloves, for the insertion of catheters or for guidewire exchange. Maximum sterile barrier precaution is required during catheter insertion. The operator should ensure that assistants also use maximal barriers.[2]

ANCILLARY PERSONNEL

Technicians, nurses, and any other personnel in the catheterization laboratory should wear scrub suits, cap, mask, and gloves when they assist within the sterile field of the procedure. All should wear eye protection with proper splash protection.[14] Circulators should wear scrub suites and, as all should, observe Universal Precautions. Visitors in the laboratory should wear either a scrub suit or other appropriate available attire over their street clothes and should remain at an acceptable distance from the table as to avoid potential contamination of either the patient or the equipment.

HIGH-RISK PATIENTS (FOR STAFF EXPOSURE)

As discussed earlier, the potential for acquired diseases from blood-borne pathogens exists for all invasive procedures. Since screening for blood-borne pathogens is not routinely performed before referral to the cardiac catheterization laboratory, it should be assumed that every patient has the potential to transmit an infectious agent. This reinforces the need to apply. Universal precautions, used throughout the hospital, in the cardiac catheterization laboratory.[14] However, some patients referred for cardiac catheterization laboratory will be known to carry HIV or the hepatitis virus. If Universal Precautions are followed, there is no reason such patients should be managed differently.

Since the hands of the operator are most likely to come in contact with blood, some operators choose to wear two pairs of gloves when it is known that a patient has a blood-borne infection. Little is known about the adequacy of available sterile gloves, but some operators claim that 2% of gloves leak even before they are used. More is known regarding the integrity of gloves during surgical procedures. In a study by Gerberding et al.[27] about 17.5% of gloves developed a perforation during surgery. Wearing two pairs of gloves reduced the chances of a puncture hole in the inner glove by 60%. Though this practice has not been proven to prevent transmission of hepatitis or HIV, it seems prudent to use this technique when the operator is working with high-risk patients.

The active disposal of contaminated fluids into an open container, such as emptying a syringe or flushing a catheter, increases the risk of accidental spilling or splashing. This is prevented by discarding fluid through the manifold via an extra port that contains a one-way valve to a disposal bag. This constitutes a closed system within the manifold.

SKIN PUNCTURE OR LACERATION

Any person who suffers a puncture or laceration with a contaminated needle or blade in the catheterization laboratory should report this incident immediately to their supervisor. Each laboratory should have a protocol for the management of such events, which includes evaluation by a physician, baseline HIV, hepatitis B, and hepatitis C testing of both the patient and the person who received the puncture, along with follow-up HIV and hepatitis testing at regular intervals following the exposure. Tetanus vaccination should be updated if greater than 10 years since the last vaccination. The Centers for Disease Control has published guidelines for the management of occupational exposure to blood-borne pathogens.[28]

VACCINATION

Vaccination for hepatitis B virus should be strongly considered, if not mandatory, for all operators and other personnel who work in the cardiac catheterization laboratory.[29]

LABORATORY ENVIRONMENT[1]

CLEANING

The laboratory should be completely cleaned once a day and spot-cleaned between each case. The floor should be wet-mopped or wiped if gross spillage is evident. Trash should be removed between each case.

CDC Recommendations

After the last catheterization procedure of the day or night, wet-vacuum or mop the cardiac laboratory room floors with a single mop and an EPA-registered hospital disinfectant.[2]

No conclusive recommendations are available regarding the disinfecting of surfaces or equipment between cases in the absence of visible soiling.[3]

AIR VENTS

The air vents should be cleaned at least monthly. The ventilation system should ideally provide at least 15 air exchanges per hour of which at least three should be fresh air.[3,5]

MAINTENANCE OF ENVIRONMENT

The doors to the catheterization laboratory should be kept closed, except as necessary for passage of equipment, personnel, and the patient. After a catheterization procedure has started, the number of personnel allowed to leave or enter should be kept to a minimum.

FIXED AND DISPOSABLE LABORATORY EQUIPMENT

Single-use disposable catheters are the current standard for the majority of equipment utilized in the catheterization laboratory. Standard techniques should be employed to ensure proper sterilization of equipment that is reused. Reuse of equipment should be limited to only that currently permitted by regulations.[30] Equipment near the catheter entry site, which has the potential for blood contamination, such as foot switches, should be covered.

Suture material should be fine and monofilament, rather than thick or braided, and a minimal amount of sutures should be used.[7] Multidose vials should be avoided because of the potential for contamination. All containers of contrast material and flush solutions that are used for one procedure should be changed for the following patient, unless an approved device that is protected against backflow is used with an aim toward contrast conservation.

DISPOSAL OF WASTE

Blood-contaminated drapes, gowns, gloves, and sponges should be discarded in special containers and labeled as healthcare waste. Needles and blades should be placed in puncture-proof containers.[14]

REFERENCES

1. Chambers CE. Writing Committee Members: Chambers CE, Eisenhauer MD, McNicol LB, Block PC, Phillips WP, Dehmer GJ, Heupler FA, Blankenship JC, and the Members of the Catheterization Lab Performance Standards Committee for the Society for Cardiovascular Angiography and Interventions. Infection Control Guidelines for the Cardiac Catheterization Laboratory: Society Guidelines Revisited. Catheterization and Cardiovascular Interventions 67:78-86 (2006). Accessed from www.scai.org/asset.axd?id=4186da84-6b4e-45bd-ba16-t in 18 June 26, 2015.
2. O'Grady NP, Alexander M, Dellinger EP, et al. Guidelines for the prevention of intravascular catheter-related infections. Centers for Disease Control and Prevention. MMWR Recomm Rep. 2002;51(RR-10):1-29. Accessed from www.shea-online.org/images/guidelines/hicpac_catheter.pdf. in Oct 2016.
3. Mangram AJ, Horan TC, Pearson ML, et al. Guideline for the prevention of surgical site infection. Infect Control Hosp Epidemiol. 1999;20:247-80. Accessed from www.cdc.gov/hicpac/pdf/guidelines/ssi_1999.pdf in Oct 2016.
4. Boyce JM, Pittet D, et al. Guideline for hand hygiene in health-care settings. Recommendations of the Healthcare Infection Control Practices Advisory Committee and the HICPAC/SHEA/APIC/IDSA Hand Hygiene Task Force. Society for Healthcare Epidemiology of America/Association for Professionals in Infection Control/Infectious Diseases Society of America. MMWR Recomm Rep. 2002;51(RR-16):1-45. Accessed from www.cdc.gov/mmwr/pdf/rr/rr5116.pdf in Oct 2016.
5. Sehulster L, Chinn RY. CDC; HICPAC. Guidelines for environmental infection control in healthcare facilities. Recommendations of CDC and the Healthcare Infection Control Practices Advisory Committee (HICPAC). MMWR Recomm Rep. 2003;52(RR-10):1-42. Accessed from www.cdc.gov/mmwr/preview/mmwrhtml/rr5210a1.htm in Oct 2016.
6. Alexander JW, Fischer JE, Boyajian M, et al. The influence of hair removal methods on

wound infections. Arch Surg. 1983;118:347-52. Accessed from www.researchgate.net.publication/16375455_The_influence_0f_hair_removal_methods_on_wound_infections in Oct 2016.

7. Center for Infectious Diseases, Centers for Disease Control, Public Health Service, US Department of Health and Human Services. Guideline for prevention of surgical wound infections,1985, revised by Garner JS. Atlanta, GA: US. Department of Health and Human Services. Accessed from www.wonder.cdc.gov/wonder/PrevGuid/p0000420/p0000420.asp in Oct 2016.
8. Lazenby KW, Zelano JA, Isom OW, et al. Effects of shaving methods and intraoperative irrigation on suppurative mediastinitis after bypass operation. Ann Thorac Surg. 1991;53:301-5. Abstract available at www.ncbi.nim.nih.gov/pubmed/1731672 in Oct 2016.
9. Olson MM, MacCallum J, McQuarrie DG. Preoperative hair removal with clippers does not increase infection rate in clean surgical wounds. Surg Gynecol Obstet. 1986;162: 181-2. Abstract available at www.ncbi.nim.nih.gov/pubmed/3945897 in Oct 2016.
10. Rutala WA. APIC guidelines for infection control practice: APIC guideline for selection and use of disinfectants. Am J Infect Control. 1996;24:313-42. Accessed from www.salvatbiotech.com/Content/Media/80e61906544641ac992fd6de8423b819/Guideline_selection_disinf.pdf in Oct 2016.
11. Medical Letter on Drugs and Therapeutics. Antimicrobial prophylaxis in surgery. Med Lett. 1989;12:105-8. Abstract available at www.secure.medicalletter.org/article-share?a=1012a&p=tml&title=Antimicrobial%20prophylaxis%20in%20Surgery&cannotaccesstitle=1.in Oct 2016.
12. Dellinger EP, Gross PA, Barrett TL, et al. Quality standard for antimicrobial prophylaxis in surgical procedures. Clin Infect Dis. 1994;18:422-7. Accessed from www.ncbi.nlm.nih.gov/pubmed/8011827.

12a. Bratzler DW, Houck PM. Antimicrobial prophylaxis for surgery: an advisory statement from the National Surgical Infection Prevention Project. Clin Infect Dis. 2004;38:1706-15. Accessed from www.cid.oxfordjournals.org/content/38/12/1706.full.pdf+html OR www.ncbi.nim.nih.gov/pubmed/15227616 in Oct 2016.

13. Wiener RS, Ong LS. Local infection after percutaneous transluminal coronary angioplasty: relation to early repuncture of ipsilateral femoral artery. Cathet Cardiovasc Diagn. 1989:16:180-1. Quoted in Ref No. 1. Abstract available at www.ncbi.nim.nih.gov/pubmed/2522020. Accessed in Oct 2016.
14. Baddour LM, Bettmann MA, Bolger AF, et al. Nonvalvular cardiovascular device-related infections. Circulation. 2003;108:2015-31. Accessed from www.circ.ahajournals.org/content/circulationaha/108/16/2015.full.pdf in Oct 2016.
15. Polanczyk CA, Rohde LE, Goldman L. Right heart catheterization and cardiac complications in patients undergoing noncardiac surgery: an observational study. JAMA. 2001;286:309-14. Accessed from www.pmmp.cnki.net/Resources/CDDPdf/evd%5c200801%5cJAMA%5cjama20.
16. Bouchart F, Dubar A, Bessou JP, et al. Pseudomonas aeruginosa coronary stent infection. Ann Thorac Surg. 1997;64:1810-3. Accessed from www.annalsthoracicsurgery.org/article/S0003-4975(97)01151-x/pdf in Oct 2016.
17. Carey D, Martin JR, Moore CA, et al. Complications of femoral artery closure devices. Catheter Cardiovasc Interv. 2001;52:3-8. Quoted in Ref No. 1. Abstract available at www.ncbi.nlm.nih.gov/pubmed/11146512 accessed in Oct 2016.
18. Toursarkissian B, Mejia A, Smilanich RP, Shireman PK, Sykes MT. Changing patterns of access site complications with the use of percutaneous closure devices. Vasc Surg. 2001;35:203-6. Quoted in Ref. No. 1. Abstract available at www.ncbi.nim.nih.gov/pubmed/11452346 accessed in Oct 2016. Or www.ves.sagepub.com/content/35/3/203.fullpdf+html accessed in Oct 2016.
19. Samal AK, White CJ. Percutaneous management of access site complications. Catheter Cardiovasc Interv. 2002;57:12-23. Quoted in Ref No. 1. Abstract available at www.ncbi.nlm.nih.gov/pubmed/12203921 accessed in Oct 2016.
20. Cooper CL, Miller A. Infectious complications related to the use of the angio-seal hemostatic puncture closure device. Catheter Cardiovasc Interv. 1999;48:301-3. Quoted in Ref No. 1. Abstract available at www.ncbi.nim.nih.gov/pubmed/10525234 Accessed in Oct 2016.

21. Corona ML, Peters SG, Narr BJ, et al. Subspecialty clinics: critical-care medicine. Mayo Clin Proc. 1990;65:979-86. Available at www.researchgate.net/publication/7437277_Infection_Control_Guidelines_for_the_Cardiac_Catheterization_Laboratory_Society_guid .Accessed in Oct 2016.
22. Larson E. APIC guidelines for infection control practice: guideline for use of topical antimicrobial agents. Mundelein, IL: APIC National Office. Quoted in Ref No.1. Abstract available at www.ajicjournal.org/article/S0196-6553(88)80005-1/pdf. Accessed in Oct 2016. Or at www.ncbi.nim.nih.gov/pubmed/2849888 accessed in Oct 2016.
23. Palmisano JM, Meliones JN. Damage to physicians' gloves during "routine" cardiac catheterization: an underappreciated occurrence. J Am Coll Cardiol. 1989;14:1527-9. Accessed from www.ncbi.nlm.nih.gov/pubmed/2809014 in Oct 2016.
24. Department of Labor, Occupational Safety and Health Administration. Occupational exposure to blood borne pathogens: final rule. Fed Reg. 1991;56:64004-182. Accessed fro www.osha.gov/OshDoc/Directive_pdf/CPL_2-2_69.pdf.inOct 2016.
25. Laslett LJ, Sabin A. Wearing of caps and masks not necessary during cardiac catheterization. Cathet Cardiovasc Diagn. 1989;17:158-69. Accessed from www.ncbi.nlm.nih.gov/pubmed/2766345 in Oct 2016.
26. Banai S, Selitser V, Keren A, et al. Prospective study of bacteremia after cardiac catheterization. Am J Cardiol. 2003;92:1004-7. Abstract available at www.ncbi.nlm.nih.gov/pubmed/14556886 in Oct 2016.
27. Gerberding J, Littell C, Tarkington A, et al. Risk of exposure of surgical personnel to patients' blood during surgery at San Francisco General Hospital. N Engl J Med. 1990;322:1788-93. Accessed from http://www.nejm.org/doi/pdf/10.1056/NEJM199006213222506 in Oct 2016.
28. US Public Health Service. Updated US. Public Health Service Guidelines for the Management of Occupational Exposuresto HBV, HCV, and HIV and Recommendations for Postexposure Prophylaxis. MMWR Recomm Rep. 2001;50(RR-11):1-52. Accessed from http://www.cdc.gov/MMWR/preview/mmwrhtml/rr5011a1.htm in Oct 2016.
29. Protection against viral hepatitis. Recommendations of the Immunization Practices Advisory Committee (ACIP). MMWR Recomm Rep. 1990;39(RR-2):1-26. Accessed from http://www.cdc.gov/mmwr/preview/mmwrhtml/00041917.htm in Oct 2016.
30. Feigal DW. Reprocessing of single-use devices: letter in attachment on reprocessing of single use medical devices by hospitals, from Center for Devices and Radiologic Health, US Food and Drug Administration. Infect Control Hosp Epidemiol. 2000;21:801-4. Accessed from www.fda.gov/MedicalDevices/DeviceRegulationandGuidance/Reprocessingofsingle-useDevices/ucon121968.htm in Oct 2016.

Chapter 28

Central Sterile Supply Department

Chapter Outline

- Decontamination, Cleaning, Drying and Transportation
- Inspection and Tray Assembly
- Packaging and Packaging Material
- Storage
- Sterile Linen for Use on Operation Theaters
- High-temperature Sterilization
- Low-temperature Sterilization
- Quality Assurance and Monitoring of Sterilization
- Documentation
- Sterile Area—Maintenance and Handling of Sterile Supply
- Shelf Life
- Expiry Date
- Checks Before Issue
- Housekeeping Practices
- Transportation
- Handling
- Training of Staff and Standard Operating Protocols

INTRODUCTION[1]

CSSD is the abbreviation of Central Sterile Supply Department. The objective of establishing a CSSD is to make reliably sterilized articles available to the hospital at required time and place as economically as possible.

People come to health facilities to be cured from disease and injuries. Many of their diseases are caused by microorganisms. Therefore, health facilities are places with a high incidence of disease-causing microorganisms which are easily spread from patient-to-patient by the staff and equipment and other materials used for patient care. Moreover many people visiting hospitals are weak and therefore are extra susceptible for acquiring a disease. It is the task of the health facilities not only to cure diseases of its patients, but also to prevent transmission of diseases from one patient to the other.

An important measure against spreading of diseases is the requirement that all medical supplies, such as instruments, swabs, drapes, etc. which are used on open wounds or will be in touch with the inner fluids of the body, are free of any viable microorganisms. They have to be sterile. Some of these materials are sterilized at the factory and are designed for single use. However, many instruments and materials used for medical interventions are very expensive and are designed such that they can be re-used. A high-quality reprocessing cycle is necessary in which the used materials are treated such, that they can be used safely again. This reprocessing should be centralized in a single CSSD serving the whole facility.

CSSD is the key to control hospital-associated infections. It is the backbone of hospital and ensures infection free surgical instruments, linen, etc. Initially, it started only as an autoclave sterilization unit, but it is a now a full-fledged department with facilities to receive, clean, pack, disinfect, sterilize, store and distribute instruments.

An alarming rate of hospital-acquired infections (HAI) in Indian hospitals has highlighted the importance of CSSD.

Major Responsibilities and Objectives of CSSD[1]

- To provide sterilized material from a central department where sterilizing practice is conducted under conditions, which are controlled, thereby contributing to a reduction in the incidence of hospital infection.
- Monitoring sterilizing practices.
- To maintain record of effectiveness of cleaning, disinfection and sterilization process.
- To monitor and enforce controls necessary to prevent cross infection according to infection control policy.
- To maintain an inventory of supplies and equipment.
- To reduce the load of nursing staff, so that they can devote more time to patients.
- To provide a safe environment for the patients and staff.

To stay updated regarding developments in the field in the interest of efficiency, economy, accuracy and provision of better patient care.

Benefits of CSSD[2]

- Centralized management.
- Uniform standards of practice.
- Maximum utilization of human and material resources.
- Eliminates costly duplication of work and equipments.
- Efficiency due to good supervision of cleaning, maintenance and sterilization practices.
- Maintains consistently high standards for sterilization techniques and product quality throughout the healthcare facility.

Location of CSSD[2]

- Should be centrally located with proximity to the major departments to which it supplies materials, preferably in the same building.
- Should have easy access to the stores from where it gets its raw material and also to the laundry for a clean supply of linen.

A good layout and work flow is very important for CSSD.

Layout[2]

There are four zones in the CSSD:

1. *Dirty area (washing area):* Reusable equipment, instruments and supplies are cleaned and decontaminated by means of manual or mechanical cleaning process and disinfection.
2. *Assembly area or packing area:* Clean items are received here are then inspected and

packed for storage or further pro-cessing as for sterilization.

3. *Sterile area:* Sterilization is carried out and sent for storage to the sterile storage area.
4. *Sterile goods storing area:* Equipment and instruments are stored here till it is time for them to be issued.

Proper coordination is required between these for good work flow.

CSSD receives stores, sterilizes and distributes to all departments including the wards, outpatient department (OPD) and other special units such as operating theater (OT).

Workflow[2]

- There should be unidirectional flow of material from dirty to clean to sterile area, never in the opposite direction.
- Used dirty goods should be received in the dirty area packed in the clean area and clean packaged sterile goods issued from sterile area.
- Entry beyond receipt and delivery counters should be limited to staff only.

Central Sterile Supply Department Staff[1,2]

It consists of:

- A responsible officer (CSSD manager) who is responsible for technical supervision during the day time.
- He will liaise with the infection control team, OT manager and clinical departments.
- The CSSD manager is administratively responsible to the head of the health care facility (Dean).
- Under the CSSD manager are shift supervisors (usually a theater sister, laboratory technician or a male nurse).
- Under the shift supervisor are the other CSSD personnel.
- The number of staff and category will depend on the extent of automation and the type of facilities the hospital is catering to.
- The thumb rule is one staff for every bed.

Qualifications[2]

- CSSD personnel are an integral part of the hospital services and contribute greatly to patient care.
- They must therefore know to operate all the automated as well as other equipment in the CSSD.
- An entry level trainee must be able to effectively speak, read write and follow instructions in English. A science graduate is preferred.
- A 6 months to one year on job training must be given which can be reduced if he has an approved certificate or formal academic training in Central Service Technology.

Functional Flow of Activities in CSSD (Fig. 28.1)[1]

The functional flow of activities in CSSD may be generally specified as follows:

- *Rinsing:* Rinsing of articles after use should not be permitted in patient care areas unless carried out by a trained member of the staff.
- *Cleaning:* All reusable medical devices should be thoroughly cleaned prior to disinfection or sterilization.
- *Drying:* all articles should be dried appropriately.
- *Inspection and assembly:* Each item should be inspected for functionality, defects, breakage and then appropriately assembled.
- *Packaging:* Articles should preferably be packed in porous material.
- *Labeling:* Each pack should be marked with nomenclature of the article, contents of the pack, initials of the person who packed it, date and initials of the person who carried out the sterilization.
- *Sterilization:* To be entrusted to a responsible and fully-trained person. Instrument for sterilization should be kept in a state of good maintenance and repair.
- *Storage:* Should be properly managed separately for sterile and non-sterile

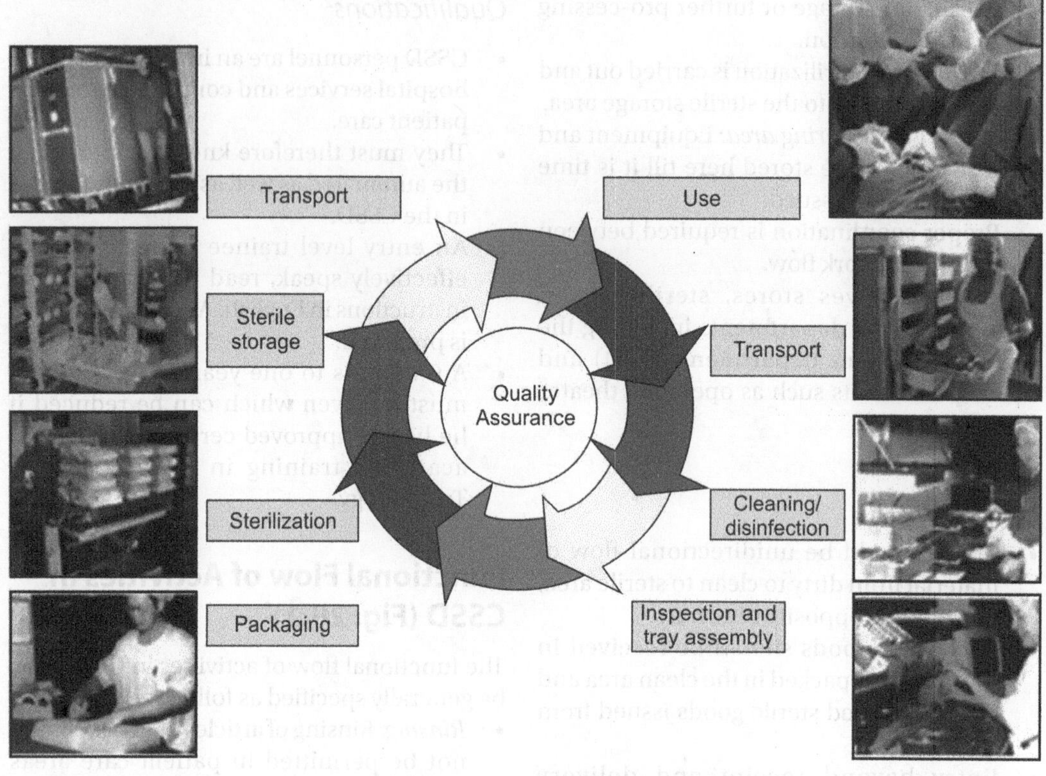

Fig. 28.1: Functional flow of activities in CSSD
Source: http://wfhss.deconidi.ie/html/educ/sbasics/sbasics01_en.htm[3]

stores. For sterile goods, clean room conditions should be followed.

- *Distribution:* Refers to clean and dirty articles exchange system. A program should be established for the collection of used items from patient care areas and distribution of sterilized goods.

DECONTAMINATION, CLEANING, DRYING AND TRANSPORTATION[4]

Definition

Decontamination is the use of physical or chemical means to remove, inactivate, or destroy blood-borne pathogens on a surface or an item, to the point where they are no longer capable of transmitting infectious particles and the surface or item is rendered safe for handling, use or disposal.

Introduction

- The decontamination process assumes that all items are contaminated and potentially infectious because microorganisms cannot be seen with the naked eye and the source is not always known or screened.
- Standard precautions must be used while handling such items to protect both patients and employees.
- It is a critical step in breaking the chain of cross infection between patient and patient and patient and worker.

Disinfection

- Disinfection kills or eliminates nearly all pathogenic microorganisms on inanimate surfaces but not necessarily bacterial spores.

- Chemicals are often used as disinfectants for devices, which cannot withstand high temperatures.
- The best disinfection procedure is the use of heat either in the form of steam or hot water between 70 and 90°C.
- It is further classified as high level, intermediate level and low level disinfection.
- A number of factors can affect the overall effectiveness of chemical germicides, like smoothness of the surface to be decontaminated, presence of organic soil, temperatures, contact time, concentration of disinfectant and hardness of water.

Cleaning

The used instruments and materials are taken to the cleaning section of the sterilization department, i.e. the 'dirty area' of the sterilization department. Cleaning implies the removal all (visible) debris and dirt. The large majority of microorganisms including any disease-causing agents are removed here. Adequate cleaning is considered the most essential step in the reprocessing cycle of sterile goods.

Objectives of Cleaning (Figs 28.2 to 28.4)

- It is the first and most important step in the sterilization process.
- One can clean without sterilizing but cannot sterilize without cleaning.
- Cleaning is a prerequisite to sterilization.

Cleaning involves:

- Removal of dirt, dust, soil, blood, remains of tissue, chemicals, fluids-especially from lumen—as they will enter sterile areas of body and may cause infection.
- Reduces bioburden (invisible soil, pathogens and microorganisms), so that the sterilization process is more effective,
- Dead organisms which may release pyrogens (endotoxin) are also removed.
- Immediate cleaning is essential, so that protein material does not stick to the instruments.

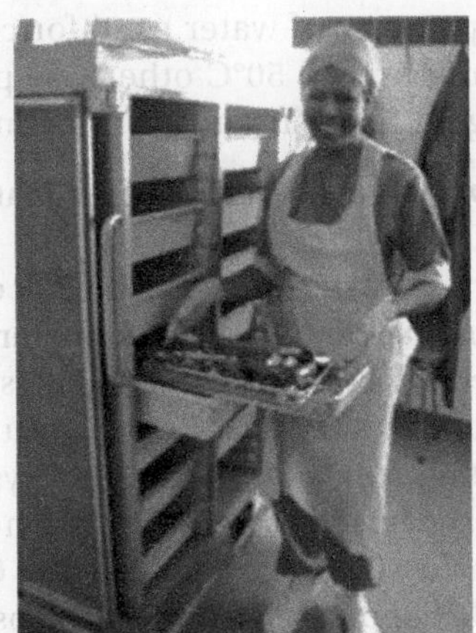

Fig. 28.2: Transportation of soiled instruments to the CSSD

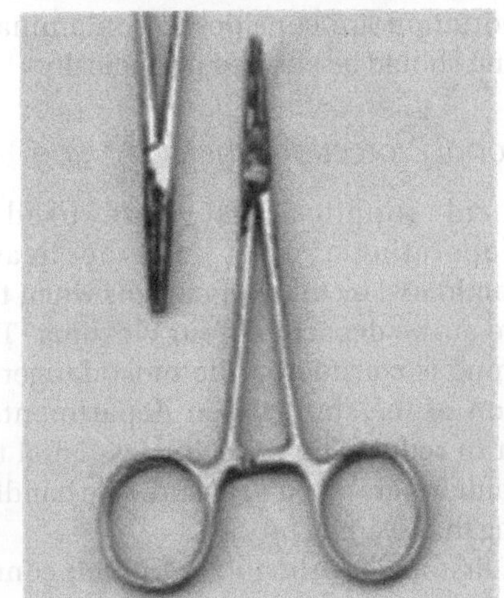

Fig. 28.3: Soiled instrument

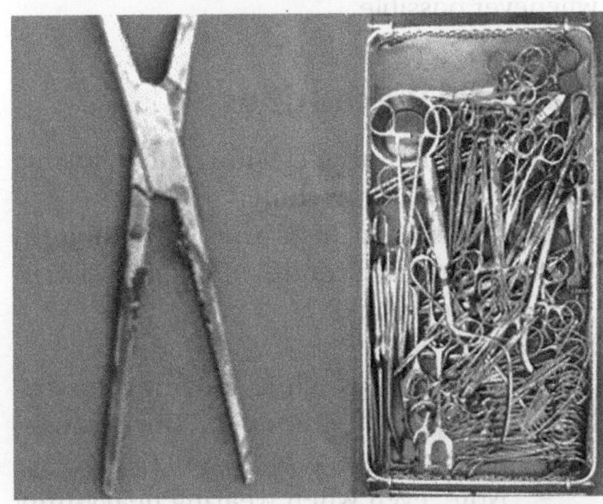

Fig. 28.4: Instruments encrusted with blood and tissues

Temperature of water used for cleaning should not exceed 50°C otherwise proteins will coagulate and stick to the instruments.

Transportation of used infected material to the CSSD:

- After use, in the operating theater or other treatment room, the soiled materials are collected and transported in suitable containers (leak-proof, puncture resistant, non-porous) and trolleys which have covers to the location where the reprocessing takes place: the Central Sterile Supply Department. In most of the standard hospitals, there is a separate lift to carry the soiled material to the CSSD.
- Containers and carts used for transportation are considered contaminated and should be cleaned periodically.

Personal Protection when Cleaning

Medical supplies that were used in the operating theater may be heavily contaminated by microorganisms when they arrive at the department for cleaning. Thus cleaning is considered the most dangerous section of the sterilization department. In order to reduce the risks, it is essential that precautions are taken to ensure safe handling during the cleaning process.

A first major principle is to limit contact with the materials as much as possible. That is why machine-cleaning is recommended whenever possible.

Standard Precautions

For protection during cleaning the following standard precautions should be used:

1. **Handwashing:** This is a basic technique in prevention and control of transmission of microorganisms.
2. **Gloves:**
   - Wear gloves while cleaning instruments and equipment. Thick household gloves may work well (Fig. 28.5).
   - Note: even when wearing heavy-duty utility gloves, care should be taken to prevent needlestick injuries or cuts when washing sharps.
   - When scrubbing ensure that any splashing moves away from you. Also you can do the scrubbing under water.
   - Gloves should be impervious to moisture and long enough to cover the sleeves of the apron or gown worn.
3. **Plastic apron:** The apron will prevent moisture reaching clothes. Should be made of water repellant material
4. **Masks and goggles or face shield:** If required to prevent exposure from splashes, sprays and aerosols.
5. **Shoe covers:** To prevent shoes from getting wet and contaminated especially if large quantities of fluids are involved example washing of trolleys, etc.
6. **Sharps:** It should be handled carefully to prevent accidental injuries.

Requirements of Washing Area

- Requirement of clean cold and warm water.
- If water is hard it needs to be softened or preferably demineralized to protect the instruments form hard ion deposits.
- Stainless steel sinks sufficiently deep at least 12 inches or more.

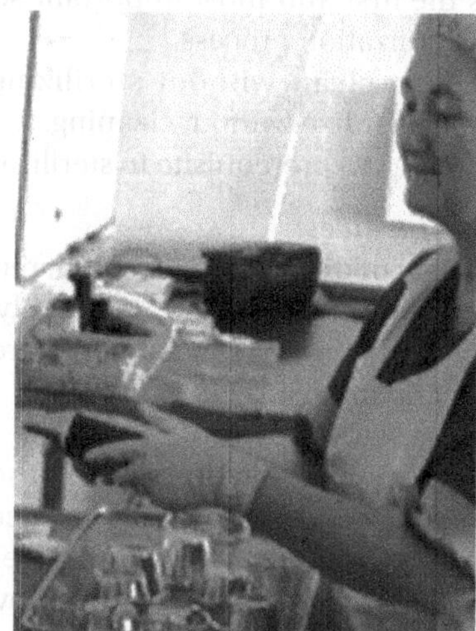

Fig. 28.5: During cleaning always wear gloves and apron

- Water, air pressure gun, sand water spray or shower.
- Perforated or preferably wire mesh trays.
- Cleansing agents—chemical/enzymatic.
- Disinfecting agents.
- Soft bristle brushes.
- Ultrasonic cleaners.
- Washer—disinfector.

Receiving of Used Items

- The personnel involved in cleaning must be properly attired in a protective gown or plastic apron, cap, mask, and should wear gloves.
- At CSSD, the instruments must be checked for proper count and examined for any obvious damage and sorted for manual and machine cleaning.

Cleaning Procedure

- Manufacturer's recommendations for operation of cleaning equipment as well as supplies like detergents and disinfectants, etc. should be strictly followed.
- Before cleaning is carried out, instruments that are made of more than one part must be dissembled. These parts must be tied together to avoid confusion while packing the instruments.
- Segregate the instruments, depending on the condition of surfaces to be cleaned (glass, steal, rubber, plastic, etc.).
- Pass water under pressure through cannulated items such as catheters.
- Take special care of areas which are readily exposed such as grooves in Atraugrip forceps, teeth in dissecting forceps, box locks of instruments, ratchets of handles, other instruments which are made up of more than one part.
- If certain devices cannot be submerged under water, they may be wiped with a detergent wetted cloth, followed by a clean cloth.
- If there is any dried blood on instruments, hydrogen peroxide can be used as a solvent. Do not leave the instruments in it as it could be corrosive.

Manual Cleaning

- Manual cleaning is done when machine cleaning is not possible, usually for delicate instruments and utensils.
- Manual cleaning involves placing the items to be cleaned in a sink or basin containing water and cleaning solution.
- Each item must be cleaned with a soft bristle brush.
- Drill bits and blades must be soaked and cleaned with toothbrush.
- Avoid using hard brushes or abrasive powder to clean, as the same will damage the instrument.
- Motorized hand pieces should be cleaned with sprays recommended by manufacturers, with the help of gauze pieces.

Principles of Ultrasonic Cleaning

- Ultra means 'beyond' and sonic means 'sound' hence these cleaners make use of vibrations with frequency greater than those of sound.
- When an ultrasonic wave passes through a liquid it makes the liquid vibrate very fast. Due to this small gas bubbles develop, becoming larger and implode.
- This draws out tiny particles of dirt from crevices such as the hinges and serrations on instruments resulting in thorough cleaning of especially hard to clean areas where manual scrubbing would not be possible.
- It has a brushing effect, more efficient than manual cleaning.

Ultrasonic Cleaning Method

- To prevent spillage, noise and aerosol formation the unit should have a lid.
- Recommended concentration of cleaning agent and a temperature between 35 and 50°C should be used.

- Use wire mesh trays and do not overload. The instrument tray is to be kept in a detergent bath for 5–10 minutes or as recommended by the manufacturer.
- Use warm water above 40°C to stimulate de-gassing in the bath, but not more than 60°C to avoid protein coagulation.
- Change the cleaning solution whenever it is dirty, at the start of every shift or as recommended by the manufacturer.

Washer-Disinfector Cleaning Method

- This equipment is programmable with respect to the concentration of the cleaning agent, number of rinse cycles, any other treatment post-washing like the use of lubricant/neutralizer. Thus depending on the items to be cleaned, appropriate program needs to be selected.
- Here, disinfection is achieved by hot water usually approximately 90°C for 1 minute; 80°C for 10 minutes or 70°C for 100 minutes.
- Temperature of water for pre-rinse wash, post-rinse and disinfection is controlled in the machine.
- Detailed operating protocol should be obtained from the manufacturer.

Cleaning Agents

- Water alone is not suitable for removing hydrophobic substances such as oils, fats and protein, etc.
- Cleaning agents like detergents or enzymatic cleaners should be used.
- Earlier soaps were used made from animal fats combined with alkalis like sodium or potassium hydroxide. These are very harsh and never used for cleaning instruments.
- Detergents lower surface tension and dislodge, disperse and hence remove soils from surface being cleaned by suspending them in a liquid medium.
- Detergents should be compatible with the equipment with which they are used, e.g. foaming detergents may not be suitable for mechanical washing.
- They should also be compatible with the material being cleaned and the quality of water (soft/hard).
- Enzymatic cleaners are biological catalyst molecules which help break down or digest large organic molecules like protein, fats and starch into smaller ones. Preferably, rinsing is done with high quality water, e.g. water prepared by deionization or reverse osmosis.

Rinsing

- After cleaning, residual loosened dirt and cleaning agent residues may be left on the instruments and if not rinsed properly, they will hamper sterilization or left over chemicals will cause erosion. That is why, it is essential that after cleaning, the load is rinsed thoroughly.
- The instruments must then be washed by spraying or washing under running water.
- Last rinse is preferably done with demineralized or deionized water to prevent stains, rust or corrosion.
- If possible, wash instruments in their racks/holders to protect from damage as long as all the parts are exposed.

Inspection

- It is essential to verify that the cleaning process has been effective in removing all the visible soil from every surface (external and internal) of the instrument/device, by visual inspection.
- When items are clean and free from dirt, soil and oil, water will run off in sheets. If the item is dirty, droplets or beads will form on the object.
- To carry out the visual inspection, it is mandatory to have sufficient illumination in the work place and if possible a magnifying lens/device.
- Reusable instruments/devices should be purchased only when assurance has been

provided by the manufacturer that they can be safely and effectively cleaned and further reprocessed.

Instrument Lubrication

- Water soluble lubricants (instrument milk) could be used after the cleaning process.
- Lubricants which inhibit the passage of steam, e.g. oil, paraffin should not be used. Steam penetrable lubricants and sprays should be used.

Drying

- After washing instruments need to be dried as water droplets would interfere with most of the sterilization processes, e.g. in case of steam sterilization, excess water would not be revaporized after the process, causing wet packs.
- The only exception is water droplets left in the lumen of articles which facilitates steam formation inside the lumens.
- EO reacts with the water molecules and the concentration of gas is reduced.
- In case of gas plasma, the cycle is aborted if any moisture is present in the load.
- In case of chemical sterilization/ disinfection residual water may dilute the agent. In this case, remove as much water as you can, since complete drying may not be possible.

Drying is achieved by (Fig. 28.6)

- Items can be wiped with a clean, non-fiber shedding cloth manually, usually followed for bigger items like basins, mayo trays, etc.
- Moisture, dust and oil free compressed air can be forced over the instruments and through lumens to remove water droplets.
- Items can be dried in a hot air oven with a thermostat and air circulation facility to maintain a fixed uniform temperature. This is the best method as it does not involve manual handling of the device after cleaning ,as well as saves labor.

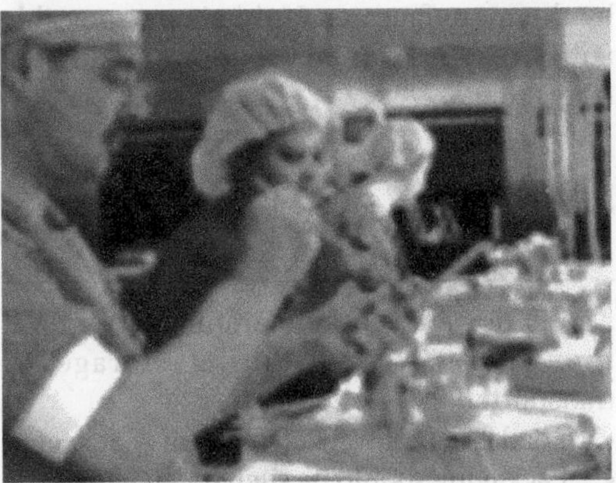

Fig. 28.6: Inspection

INSPECTION AND TRAY ASSEMBLY

- Instrument trays for all procedures are prepared.
- Vigorous inspection of each tray should be done.
- They should be double-checked for completeness.
- Instruments which are not working should be removed and replaced.
- The contents of the pack should be as per the user's requirements. For the same procedure/surgery, the set should be standardized.

Instrument Damage from Solutions and Chemicals

Instruments must not be left for long periods in solutions or chemicals. They can cause staining, rusting and harmful effects on surgical instruments. Chemicals that can be harmful are saline, bleach, iodine based preparations, abrasive powders used for cleaning, hand scrub, soap, laundry detergent, steam impermeable oils.

Instrument Marking

Instrument marking should be done to allow identification by department, specialty set, and surgeon, etc. Acid based and laser etching can be done by the instrument manufacturer or the hospital. Color coding also can be done by the manufacturer. If this is not possible adhesive tapes can be used for marking the instruments.

PACKAGING AND PACKAGING MATERIAL[5]

Aim to prevent contamination after removal from autoclave, or during storage or transportation (Fig. 28.7).

- Load is to be sterilized inside its packaging
- Packaging should be such that it allows the sterilizing agent to reach the actual load.
- It should act as a microbial barrier.
- Packaging should guarantee sterility up to the moment a product is used.
- Poor or damaged packaging makes all the work of cleaning, packaging and sterilization useless.

Packaging consists of:

a. **Primary packaging:** For wrapping of textile packs and instrument sets in trays.
b. **Secondary packaging**: For additional mechanical protection during storage and transport.

Primary Packaging

Aim is to prevent recontamination after removal from autoclave, or during storage or transportation (Fig. 28.8):

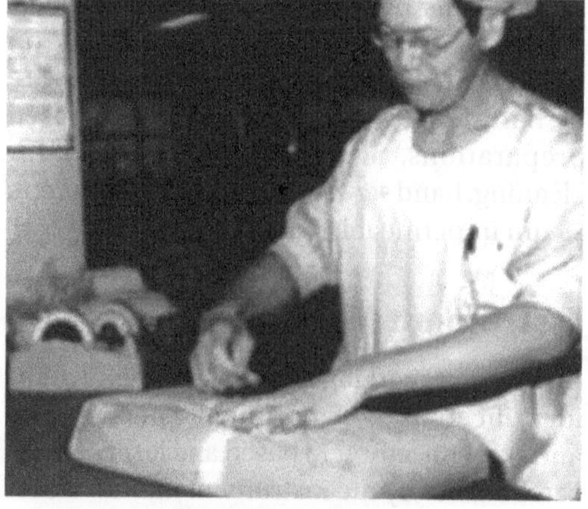

Fig. 28.7: Packaging

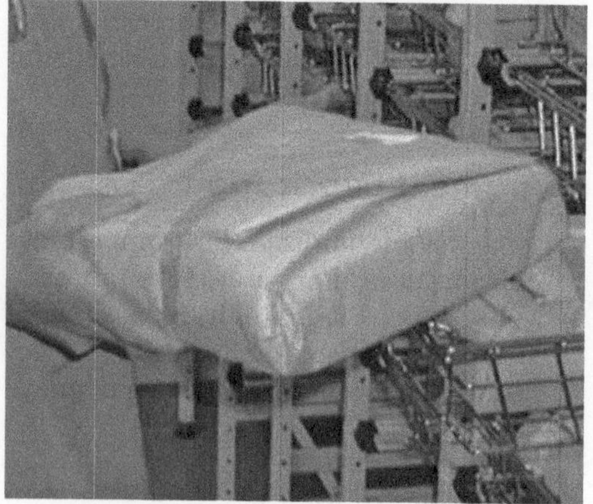

Fig. 28.8: An instrument set in its primary packaging

- Should be a good microbial barrier, allow penetration of steam and air.
- Package-consists of 2 layers of paper or 2 layers of non-woven sheets or single or double laminated film pouch, paper bag or container with adequate filter(s).

Secondary Packaging (Fig. 28.9)

- Used to facilitate proper storage and internal transport to user.
- An additional primary packaging, e.g. an extra, plastic wrapper, bag, cardboard box or container.
- It may offer extra-protection against dust and gives extra-mechanical protection, making handling easier.
- Commonly used for disposable sterile supplies.

Transport Packaging

A transport package is used for external transporting of sterile goods in their primary and secondary packaging. Usually, it is a strong cardboard box, cradle, closed trolley or other type of container (Fig. 28.10).

When the goods enter the clean area, e.g. operating theater, the transport packaging should be removed.

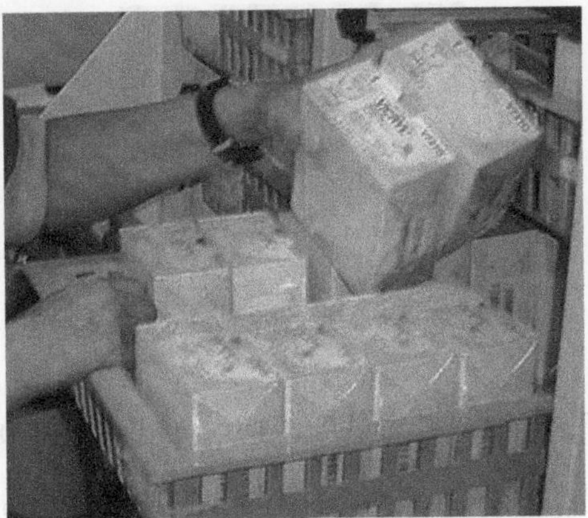

Fig. 28.9: Disposable sterile items in secondary packaging

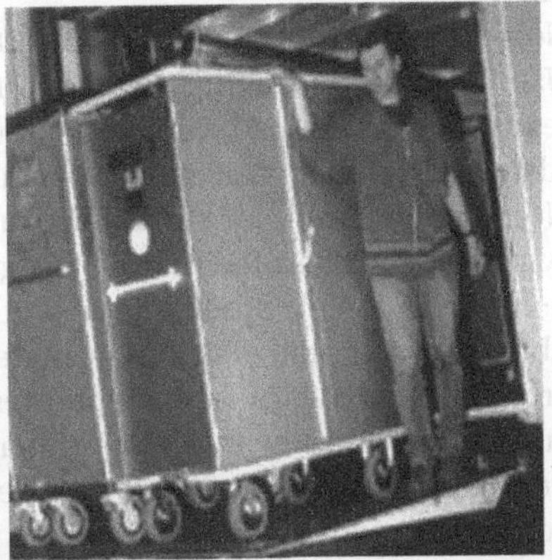

Fig. 28.10: Transport packaging (closed tralleys for external transport)

Packaging Materials

A wide range of materials used for packaging of sterile supplies are available.

Traditionally, packaging materials for sterile supplies were reusable, such as sterilizing drums and cotton ware. Due to their inadequate microbial barrier, most of these, traditional materials do not meet the requirements for primary sterile packaging anymore. They may still play a role as mechanical protection or additional dust protection layer. At the moment non-wovens, laminated film pouches, paper bags and containers are used as primary packaging materials.

The following is an overview of packaging materials in use in sterile supply:

Soft/Flexible Packaging Materials

a. **Textile sheets—cotton or linen (Fig. 28.11)**
Use: Inner wrapping of instrument sets or outer dust protection.
Textile alone is not suitable as primary packaging.
Cotton sheets have long been the standard packaging material for sterile goods. It has some major advantages:
   - Textile always has been a very common and well known hospital commodity.
   - Strong.
   - Well drapable and convenient in use
   - Can be reused.

The openings between the threads however are larger than most micro-organisms and thus the fabric does not provide an adequate microbial barrier. It therefore does not meet the requirements anymore as primary packaging for sterile goods. They however are still often used as an inner wrapping for protection or as an outer dust cover.
Linen wrappers can be used for steam and low temperature steam-formalin (LTSF). It is not recommended for EO, dry heat or plasma.

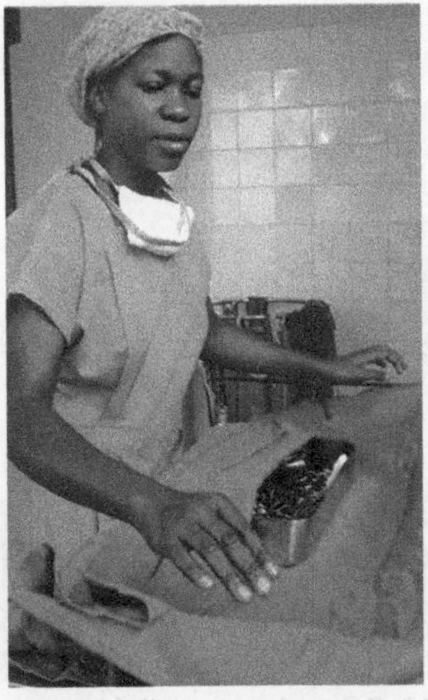

Fig. 28.11: Packaging in cotton still being used in health facilities with limited resources

b. **Paper sheets (Fig. 28.12)**
Use: Primary packaging for wrapping of textile packs and instrument sets in trays. Also used as inner packaging in containers
Paper was the first alternative that replaced textile. It has a smaller pore size than textile and thus can be used as primary packaging. Smooth papers are used for inner packaging. Crepe paper is stronger and is rough. Crepe paper can be used for inner and outer packaging.
During sterilization, steam penetrates through the packaging. When paper is wet, it loses much of its original strength. Therefore, stress in paper should be prevented. Wrapping should not be too tight, but also not too loose. It is essential that drying is adequate.
Paper sheets are for single use only. They can be used for steam, EO LTSF and dry heat, but not for gas plasma.

c. **Paper sterilization bags (Fig. 28.13)**
Use: For packaging of individual instruments or small sets used in nursing stations and wards.
Closing is usually done in a sealing device.
Disadvantages:
- They are not very strong.
- Opening is not convenient: tearing or cutting.

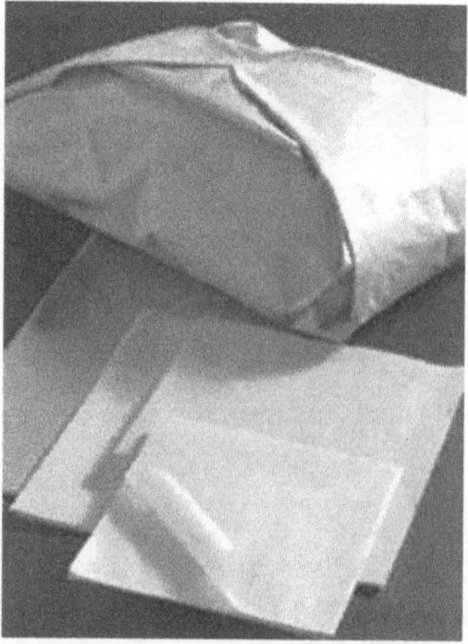

Fig. 28.12: Paper sheets available in many sizes and strengths

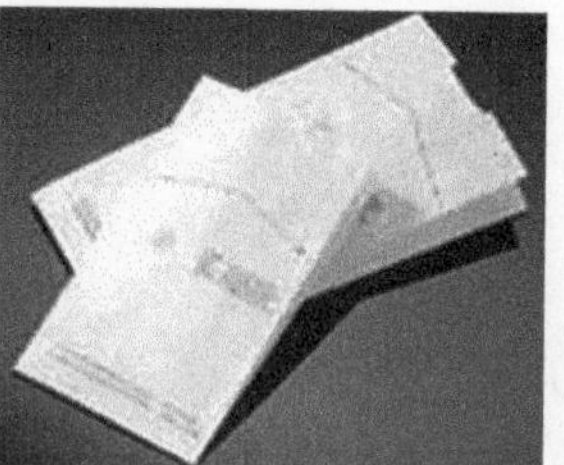

Fig. 28.13: Paper sterilization bags

- They do not facilitate aseptic opening.
- You cannot see what is inside.

Its use has decreased with the introduction of laminated film pouches.
Paper sterilization bags are for single use only.

d. **Non-woven sheets (Figs 28.14 and 28.15)**
Use: Primary packaging for wrapping of textile packs and instrument sets in trays. Also used as inner packaging in containers
Non-woven contain a certain amount of synthetic fibers. Added may be inorganic, textile, cellulose or other kind of synthetic fibers. These fibers of different materials are joined together, by for example pressing and heating. This means that the fibers are not woven together, but sealed together. For sterilization, special non-wovens have been developed to meet the requirements for the primary packaging of sterile goods. They combine the good characteristics of other packaging materials:
- Very strong
- Well drapable
- Allow air removal and penetration of the sterilizing agent.
- Very small pores, thus efficient microbial barrier.
- Virtually lint-free; free of particles and loose fibers.
- They repel liquids (hydrophobic) Fluids are not absorbed into the fabric.
- Various non-woven materials are available for a range of applications in the sterilization department: extra softness, extra strong, etc.

Non-woven sheets are for single-use only non-woven fabrics can be used for steam,

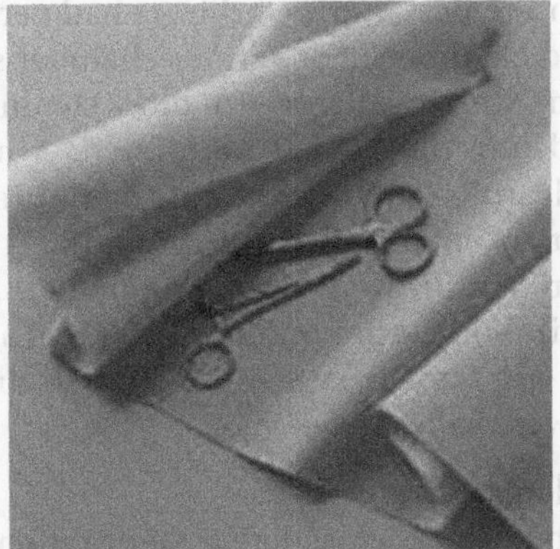

Fig. 28.14: Non-woven wrapper

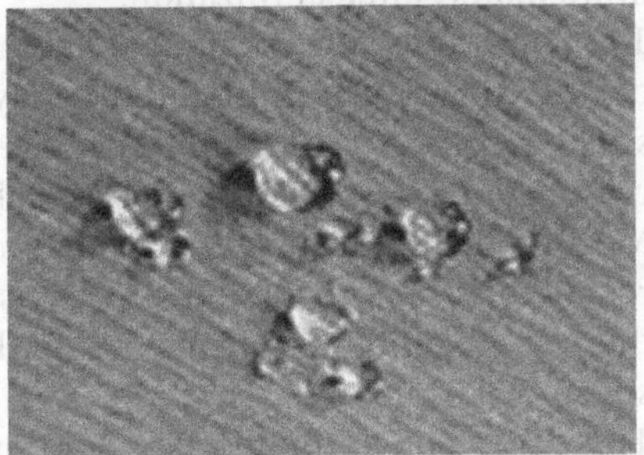

Fig. 28.15: Non-wovens are water-repellent

low temperature steam formaldehyde (LTSF), EO and in case of gas plasma, non-cellulosic only (Fig. 28.16).

e. Laminated film pouches (Figs 28.17 to 28.19)

Use: Primary packaging for individual instruments or small instrument sets.

They were the follow-up of paper sterilization bags. The pouches consist of a sheet of paper or non-woven and a sheet of laminated transparent plastic, which are sealed together. The film cannot be penetrated by steam or air. Removal of air and penetration of steam is through the paper/non-woven. The pouch is opened by peeling back the laminated sheet from the paper sheets, like opening a banana. Pouches are available in many sizes. The open end of the pouch is closed with a sealing device. It is essential that the sealing temperature and pressure are adjusted well in order to get an adequate seal.

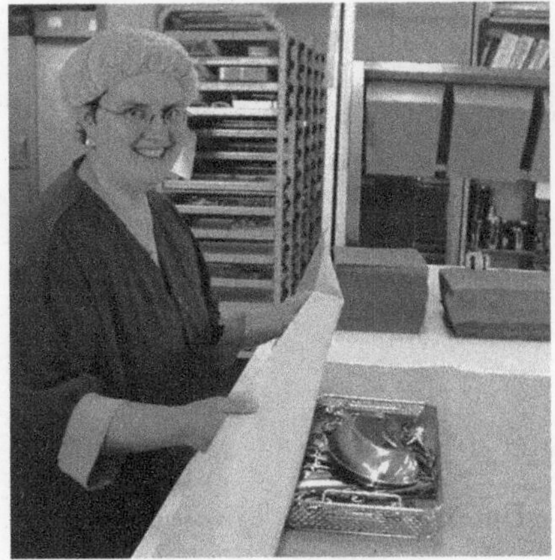

Fig. 28.16: Packaging an instrument set in a non-woven sheet using the parcel fold

Fig. 28.17: Typical laminated film pouch

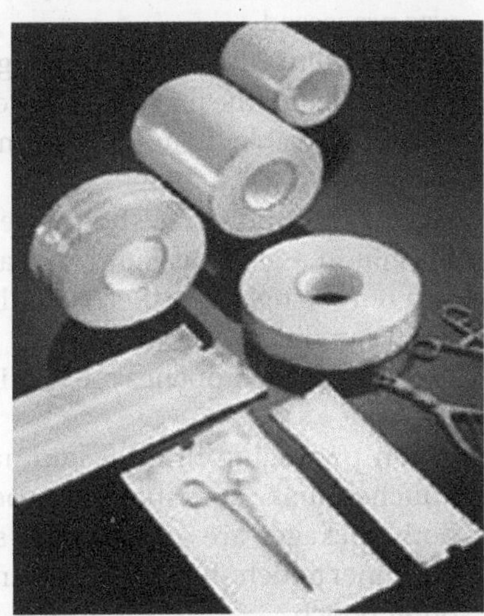

Fig. 28.18: Laminated film pouches in various sizes and on roll

Also laminated film packaging is available on roll. The user can cut pouches to any size needed. In that case both sides need to be sealed by the user.

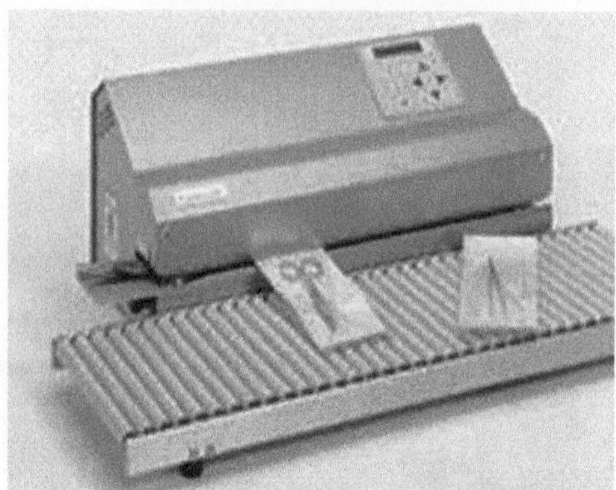

Fig. 28.19: Sealing device for pouches

- The peel-open system assures dust-free aseptic opening on presentation.
- The pouch should be such that when peeling it open, neither the paper nor the laminate will tear. It should open neatly along the seals.
- It should not release fibers or fluffs.
- The content is clearly visible.
- It should not be possible to reseal the pouch, when opening by mistake.
- A sterilizer indicator should be on the pouch indicating whether a product was processed.
- The content should not be tightly surrounded by the packaging material; it should be able to move freely inside the pouch.
- Sterilization pouches should be put upright in a grid basket or container and not too tight together, such that a hand can slide in between them.
- Laminated film pouches are for single use only.
- When packaging in dual laminated pouches, make sure that the paper of both packages are on the same side. The inner pouch should fit freely in the outer pouch.

Rigid Packaging Systems

Sterilizing drums (Fig. 28.20)

Use: As secondary packaging layer—mechanical protection of its content.

Not suitable as primary packaging.

In the past, most sterilizers had vertical, round chambers. For various chamber sizes, drums were available. To allow steam into the drum, the wall is perforated. A metal band around the drum can be shifted in order to open and close the perforations. Before sterilization they are opened. After sterilization the perforations are closed again. They are known as Schimmelbusch drums and were widespread.

Problems:

- The band is closed after sterilization and thus the content may be recontaminated immediately after sterilization.
- The band does not provide an adequate closure, thus contaminated air may be sucked inside the drum. Also the lid closure does not provide a proper seal.
- Most modern autoclaves have horizontal, rectangular chambers. Round drums are then very inefficient in using the sterilizer space.
- The drums have hinged lids, hindering aseptic opening.

Therefore, they are not suitable as primary packaging. They may only be used as an extra mechanical protection.

Drums with filters in top and bottom

Drums are available with filters in the lid and bottom. They can be considered as sterilizing containers for round, vertical autoclaves.

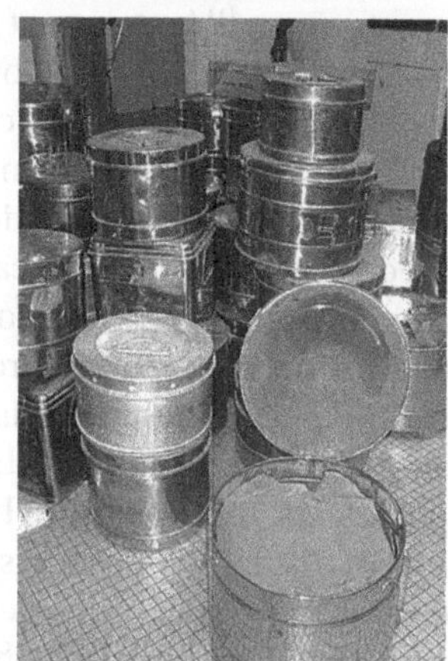

Fig. 28.20: Sterilizing drums are only suitable as additional mechanical protection (secondary packaging)

Sterilizing containers (Figs 28.21 to 28.23)

Use: Primary packaging of textile packs and instrument sets in trays.

Well-designed sterilizing containers offer the following features:

- Air removal and steam access through filters or valves. They ensure maintenance of sterility during storage.
- For autoclaves with downward displacement processes containers are available with filters in the lid and bottom.
- The sizing of most container systems is based on the Sterilizing Unit (1 StU = 30 cm × 30 cm × 60 cm). Thus, they fit in sterilizers, instrument washer disinfectors, and are compatible with packaging materials, that are also based on this unit.
- The lid is removed completely from the bottom part thus facilitating aseptic opening.
- They provide an effective mechanical protection during handling and transport.
- They can be stacked. However stacking should not hinder steam penetration, nor cause entering of condensate dripping down from higher containers. Proper drying is to be confirmed.
- Grid baskets can be stacked inside containers.
- Labeling system offers clear identification of the content, production data, etc.
- A tamper protection device shall give clear indication whether a container was opened.

Depending on the sterilizer process, containers shall be used with filters in top and bottom (for downward displacement process) or containers with filters only in the top (fractionated prevacuum process).

STORAGE

- All sterilized items should be stored in separate area.
- This area should be regularly cleaned.
- It should be free from dust, insects and vermins.
- It should be cool dry away from sunlight.
- It should have storage shelves which are non-porous and easy-to-clean.

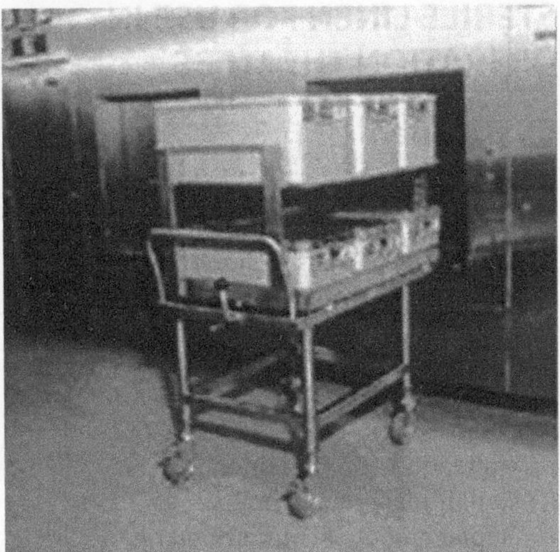

Fig. 28.21: Loading a sterilizer with containers

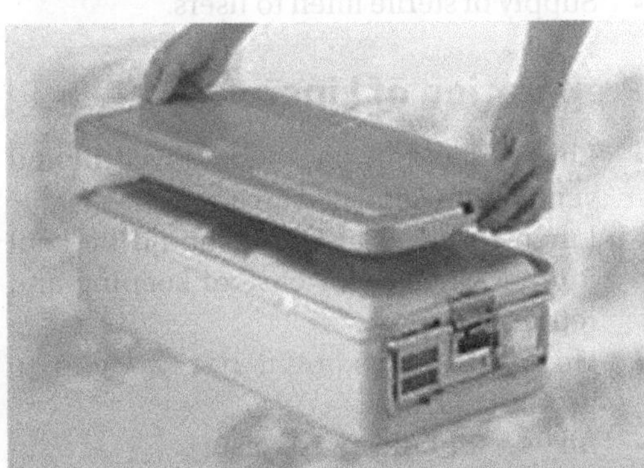

Fig. 28.22: Sterilizing container

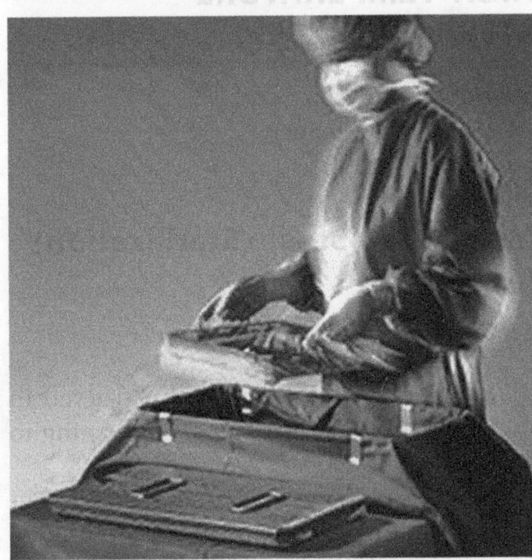

Fig. 28.23: Taking out a tray from container

STERILE LINEN FOR USE IN OPERATION THEATERS

CSSD Linen

- Green and blue are commonly used colors.
- A minimum of 4 sets of linen are desirable (1 in use, 1 in CSSD, 1 in laundry, 1 as buffer).

Written Procedures

In coordination with laundry and users, procedures should be laid down for:

- Collection of soiled linen.
- Repair of damaged linen.
- Replacement of condemned linen
- Supply of clean linen to CSSD
- Inventory management
- Supply of sterile linen to users.

Preparation of Linen

- Linen should be packed in a well-lit and ventilated segregated area.
- Linen received in CSSD should be kept in open shelves for ease of keeping and retrieval.
- Hospital linen should have a logo to prevent pilferage.
- All users should avoid misuse.

HIGH-TEMPERATURE STERILIZATION[2]

Methods used are:

- Moist heat (Steam) .
- Dry heat.

Moist Heat (Steam Sterilization) (Autoclave)

Equipment

- It consists of a chamber constructed to withstand high pressures, confirming to strict safety codes.
- Steam is either generated in the chamber in the non-jacketed or from an outside source in the jacketed sterilizers.
- The sterilizer may be horizontal or vertical and either gravity displacement or dynamic air removal type.
- Jacketed, horizontal, air removal type are preferred.

Types of Steam Sterilization

- Gravity displacement
- Dynamic air removal or high speed pre – vacuum (HPHV).
- Flash sterilization.

Gravity Displacement

- Here air being heavier is displaced by gravity when steam enters the chamber.
- In tabletop sterilizers water in the bottom of the sterilizer is heated to form steam.
- In larger sterilizers, steam is supplied from an outside source.
- In both cases, air is pushed out by the entry of steam.

Dynamic Air Removal

- Here, air is actively removed from the chamber and load
- Two types of sterilizers are available, the prevacuum sterilizer and the pulsing gravity sterilizer
- In the first type, a series of pulses is created where a vacuum is drawn by means of a vacuum pump followed by a pressure pulse.
- In the second type, a series of steam pressure pulses force the air out in a manner similar to the gravity displacement system.

Flash Sterilizers

- It is used for instruments which are accidentally dropped or not anticipated before the procedure began but not for instruments in short supply.
- Instruments should be processed near the point of use and used immediately, not stored.
- Open instruments without a wrapper have no shelf-life and hence should be used

immediately. If wrapped instruments are used a regular cycle with drying time included is required.

- The exposure time depends upon content of load.
- A minimum exposure time of 3 minutes is required for open instruments without lumens.
- Process should be monitored with the help of chemical indicator/Biological indicator specially designed for flash sterilizers. Daily or minimum weekly monitoring with BI may be done routinely.

Note: Implants should not be flash sterilized, but if it is unavoidable, then it becomes compulsory to monitor the patient closely for any signs of postoperative infection.

Common 121°C Gravity Displacement Steam Cycles (Table 28.1)

Table 28.1: Common 121°C gravity displacement steam cycles

Load contents	Temperature	Sterilization time (minutes)
Wrapped metal items without porous items	121°C/134°C	≥ 20/≥7
Packs containing fabric	121°C/134°C	≥30/≥10
Containers	121°C/134°C	≥30/≥10

Common 132–134°C Vacuum-assisted Steam Cycles (Table 28.2)

Table 28.2: Common 132–134°C vaccum-assisted steam cycles

Load contents	Temperature	Sterilization time (minutes)
Unwrapped metal instruments	121°C/134°C	≥7/≥3
Unwrapped metal instruments combined with porous items	121°C/134°C	≥20/≥4
Wrapped metal items, packs containing fabric containers, etc.	121°C/134°C	≥20/≥7

Dry Heat Sterilization (Hot Air Oven)

This is used for items that cannot be sterilized by steam or gas due to sterilant permeability constraint, thus killing of microorganisms is achieved by using heat transfer through conduction and convection. For example, anhydrous powders, vaseline, oils and other items where direct contact with steam or gas is not possible like assembled syringes. It cannot be used for fabric or rubber.

Parameters

Time and Temperature

The following time-temperature ratios are adequate (Table 28.3).

An important point to be noted is that the exposure period mentioned should be measured after the temperature is attained, e.g. the time required to heat a 4 ounce jar of petroleum jelly from room temperature to 160°C is 165 minutes. Hence, total time of sterilization is 165 + 120 = 285 minutes.

Equipment

- It consists of a hot air oven which can be a gravity convection oven or mechanical convection oven.
- The latter is preferable as it contains a blower that distributes heated air throughout the chamber uniformly.
- A temperature controller with thermostat and timer should be added for maintaining required temperature and cutting off supply after specified time.

Table 28.3: Time-temperature ratio

Temperature	Time
180°C	30 minutes
170°C	1 hour
160°C	2 hours
150°C	2 and ½ hours
140°C	3 hours
121°C	6 hours

Precaution

- Containers should withstand high temperature.
- During exposure period, temperature and circulation of hot air should be maintained by not disturbing the oven.
- Allow the sterile material to cool down gradually before exposing to room temperature.

LOW-TEMPERATURE STERILIZATION[2]

Many of the articles to be reprocessed by the CSSD are sensitive to heat and or moisture, hence cannot be sterilized by steam or any other high temperature method. Thus low temperature methods are used. They are:

- EtO sterilization.
- Gas plasma.
- Peracetic acid sterilization.
- Ionizing radiation (Gamma rays).
- Formaldehyde steam.
- Ultraviolet light (Only used for room sterilization).
- Filtration (Used only for pharmaceutical solutions and incoming air).
- Chlorine dioxide (No commercial product).
- Ozone (No commercial product).

Ethylene Oxide Sterilization

Ethylene oxide sterilization (EtO) gas is highly diffusible and has excellent penetration characteristics. Hence, products may be sterilized prepacked in sealed plastic bags, cellophane and cartons.

EO is used in combination with hydrofluorocarbon or CO_2 (available in cylinders) or as 100% EtO.

EtO is an effective alkylating agent, i.e. it replaces hydrogen atom within the cell with an alkyl group, thus making the microorganisms unable to metabolize and reproduce. Normally, it is an irreversible process, ultimately leading to killing of these microorganisms.

Commonly used gas concentration is 450 to 750 mg/liter of chamber volume. Relative humidity levels are generally kept between 40 to 80% in order to achieve a minimum of 35% at the site of microbial inactivation.

Moisture is required for microbial inactivation and also facilitates the transfer of EO through films like nylon and cellophane.

Temperature is usually kept between 37°C and 60°C. Increase in temperature increases the rate of microbial inactivation for every 10 degrees rise and may also facilitate transfer of EO through product and packaging by increasing permeability. Exposure time ranges from 1 to 5 hours for hospital cycles. There is a direct relationship between the above three parameters (temperature, humidity and gas concentration) and time required for sterilization.

Advantages of EtO

- Items can be prepackaged in plastic/polypropylene pouches giving them a long shelf life.
- It is non-corrosive to plastic, metal and rubber materials.
- It penetrates and sterilizes irregularly, shaped items and lumens efficiently.

Precaution

- Water droplets left in material to be sterilized lead to ethylene glycol formation, making it unsafe, therefore items must be thoroughly dried before packing.
- Paper and linen cannot be used for packaging, items need to be packed in non-woven polypropylene material.
- Lumen with inside diameters less than 6 mm and lengths greater than 31 cm need boosters to help penetration of gas.

Limitations

- It is more complex than steam or dry heat.
- Aeration is required to remove adsorbed gas from sterile articles, due to toxic nature of sterilant.

- Total turnover time is 12–16 hours.
- It is toxic, flammable, carcinogenic, mutagenic and a reproductive hazard.

Aeration

- Sterile items adsorb EO and aeration is a process that removes residual EO from sterilized material.
- Mechanical aeration is recommended at 55°C for 12 hours and at 37°C for 24 hours. In absence of a mechanical aerator, sterile material will have to be kept in a dedicated, enclosed area with minimum traffic and good ventilation for at least 7 days before use.

EtO monitoring for employee safety:

- Due its carcinogenic property and its potential as a reproductive hazard healthcare facilities must conform to stringent requirements when using EO.
- By OSHA standards 1 ppm exposure limits are over an 8 hour time weighted average period and 0.5 ppm at any given time.
- Monitoring systems are available for gas leakage, personnel and environment exposure.

Hydrogen Peroxide Gas Plasma Sterilization

- Gas plasma is a highly ionized or highly charged fourth state of matter, created by deep vacuum and electromagnetic energy.
- Plasma is a state of matter in which negatively charged particles or electrons exist in an unstable and excited state.
- Generally, hydrogen peroxide in the gaseous phase is used to create this plasma.
- Microbicidal activity is due to highly reactive electrons and ions.

Penetration

Gas plasma is not adsorbed through surfaces and thus has limitations for penetration.

Advantages

- Ninety five percent of medical devices are compatible with H_2O_2 plasma.
- It has short cycle time of 60-75 minutes.
- No aeration is required.
- No personnel monitoring is required.
- Easy installation.
- No toxic chemical residues, byproducts of sterilization being oxygen and water.

Liquid Peracetic Acid Sterilization

- Peracetic acid is a most commonly used liquid sterilant.
- It is highly microbicidal at a concentration of less than 1%.
- It maintains its efficacy in the presence of organic soils.
- Used for sterilization of reusable immersible devices like flexible and rigid endoscopes.
- Total processing time is 30 minutes at 50 to 56°C.
- This should preferably be carried out at the point of use to maintain sterility after sterilization.

Advantages

- Short cycle—30 minutes.
- Tabletop unit—Easy installation-water source, drainage and electrical line.
- Single use sterilant container.
- No personnel monitoring.
- No disposal precautions.

Limitations

- It is a strong oxidizing agent and concentrated solutions are irritating to the skin, mucus membranes and eyes.
- It has no shelf life.
- A large number of medical devices have been found to be compatible with this process. However, untreated metals could be subjected to oxidation.

- Since this is a liquid process and does not use any packing material, there is no shelf life of items sterilized.

Ionizing Radiation Sterilization

- They are high energy radiation emitted from radioactive isotopes.
- Gamma rays emitted from Cobalt 60 are used for continuous processing at BARC.

Formaldehyde Steam Sterilization

- In this method, articles are sterilized by placing them in a chamber and subjecting them to pulses of steam and formaldehyde vapor at subatmospheric pressure and relatively low temperatures like 60 to 80° C
- This method is also used for heat sensitive items.

QUALITY ASSURANCE AND MONITORING OF THE STERILIZATION[2]

Quality assurance is a comprehensive plan to maintain and improve quality. Quality is the consistent delivery of products and services according to established standards. For this, a quality control program has to be laid down.

Quality control program consists of:

- Written policies and procedures
- Orientation and training
- Monitoring
- Documentation

Policy: Is what must be done? A policy gives you an outcome of a product. For achieving good quality goods, a standard policy should be desired.

Procedure: Is How to do it? All procedures must be standardized and the written down in detail.

Regulations, guidelines and standards: It should be made to maintain compliance. Follow literature and regulations. Maintain professional standards.

Sterilization process monitoring: It is essential as proper sterilization of instruments and material is a critical aspect of infection control. Since microorganisms cannot be seen by naked eye there must be some way of determining that the item sterilized is really sterile.

Validation of sterilization process: The purpose of sterilization is to provide the end user with a sterile product. The only way of ensuring sterility is to test every pack. Since this is not feasible, it is necessary to employ monitors to assure that the parameters of sterilization have been met. For this, Technical quality control indicators in the form of mechanical, chemical and biological indicators have to be incorporated into the sterility assurance program.

Indicators

Mechanical

Pressure gauges: In jacketed sterilizers, there are two main pressure gauges to determine pressure in jacket and chamber.

Temperature and pressure graphs, recording charts and computer printouts: These describe temperature and pressure inside the sterilizer and various phases of sterilization can be known from the pattern.

Computer printouts: They describe accurately the sterilizer cycle giving heat up time, holding time, exhaust creation time, etc.

Leak rate test: It is performed in prevacuum sterilizers to check if the leakage in the sterilizer is within permissible range (i.e. below 13 millibars), otherwise sterility can be affected. Checks may be carried out preferably weekly or at least monthly.

Chemical Indicators

These may be substances which melt at high temperatures and are put in the load in sealed ampoules or strips impregnated with certain dyes that change color when the required temperature is reached.

There are different classes of chemical indicators depending on the information, they provide regarding the sterilization .They range from telling us whether the pack has been through the process (not necessarily sterile) upto the adherence of all parameters of the sterilization process (resulting in a sterile pack).

Class 1

- They are internal and external process indicators.
- External process indicators inform the user that the pack has been through the sterilization process and are often used as sealers for packages.
- Internal indicators show the penetration of steam to the inside of the pack (examples are sterilization tapes, indicators printed on peel pouches, etc.).
- They show that the item has been through the sterilization process NOT THAT THE ITEM IS STERILE.

Class 2

- It is used in the Bowie-Dick test for pre-vaccum sterilizers.
- It is used in other specific test procedures like process challenge device.

Bowie-dick test

- It is used only for Prevacuum sterilizers to monitor vacuum level, detect air leaks and steam quality.
- The test needs to be performed for 3.5–4 minutes at 132–134°C and 7 minutes at 121°C.
- Should be done in the first cycle each day, after warm up.
- A satisfactory result is indicated by a uniform color change of indicator on test sheet.
- This test should also be carried out during installation and relocation of the sterilizer, sterilizer malfunction, sterilization process failure and major repairs.

Class 3

- They are single-parameter indicators, i.e. they respond to only one parameter of sterilization (Usually temperature).
- They are usually used in steam or dry heat sterilizers.
- They indicate only the temperature reached and do not specify the exposure time at that temperature.

Class 4

- They are multiparameter indicators.
- They respond to two or more parameters of sterilization.
- They respond to a specific value of the chosen parameter usually printed on the indicator.
- They contain an ink that changes color when exposed to the correct combination of sterilization parameters.
- They have a plastic lamination which regulates their sensitivity and response time.

Class 5

- They also function as integrators.
- They respond to all parameters of sterilization over a specified range of temperatures.
- Their performance is compared to the inactivation of a test organism.
- They can be used in both steam and EtO cycles.

Class 6

- They are also known as emulators.
- They respond to all parameters of sterilization over a specified range of sterilization cycle.
- They will react only after 95% of the cycle is complete.
- Their performance is compared to the settings of the selected cycle.

Biological Indicators (BI)

- Standardized and certified biological indicators are used to monitor sterilization.

- They ensure proper packing, loading, sterilant quality and functioning of equipment.
- They contain a certain number of spores (about 1 million) of a microorganism most resistant to the sterilization process.

Types of BI

- They may be in the form of paper strips impregnated with spores contained in envelopes. This is the traditional form. They need to be placed aseptically into a growth medium after sterilization is complete. This step may however be responsible for contamination giving wrong results.
- Nowadays, the spore strip or disk is placed in a vial with a sealed ampoule of growth medium. These are activated by crushing the ampoule, allowing the microorganisms to come in contact with the growth medium. When incubated the spore grow and cause color change in medium within 24 to 48 hours.
- In the third method-biological indicators employ a fluorescent light to determine an enzymatic reaction that indicates that cell division is occurring. This type is 'Rapid readout" and results can be obtained as quickly as one hour.
- Steam sterilizers use *Geobacillus stearothermophilus* as the test organism.
- EtO, dry heat and hydrogen peroxide use *Bacillus atrophaeus*.

Method of Testing

- Two indicators are to be used per test, the experimental indicator and the control indicator.
- The experimental indicator is placed into the sterilizer at the place most difficult to reach (e.g above drain in steam sterilizer and diagonally to cartridge/inlet in EtO).
- The control indicator is not put in the sterilizer, but incubated along with the one that underwent sterilization.
- The control indicator is expected to grow but not the experimental indicator.

Frequency of Testing

- For steam sterilization, the BI should be used daily or at least weekly.
- For EtO, it should be in every cycle.
- For dry heat sterilization, it should be used weekly.

Note: In addition for any type of sterilizer, one should follow any major change/maintenance/shutdown. For pre-vacuum steam sterilizers, leak rate and B-D test are also essential.

DOCUMENTATION[2]

- Document all the sterilization records, for if your facility was sued for malpractice concerning a nosocomial infection, sterilization records can shift the burden of proof to the plaintiff.
- Remember not documented is considered as NOT DONE.
- If department wise records are maintained, it helps in 'recall" in case of sterilization failure.

Record Keeping

- Lot control numbers should be affixed on the product.
- At the beginning of the cycle, the date, time, the sterilizer operator and cycle identification should be marked on the chart.
- At the end of the cycle, the response of chemical indicators should be recorded.
- Results of BI should be recorded when obtained.
- The sterilization record should be examined and attested.
- Local record log should be maintained.

STERILE AREA—MAINTENANCE AND HANDLING OF STERILE SUPPLY STORAGE[2]

Introduction, Storage and Unloading

- All sterilized items—stored in separate area—the sterile area.

- This area should be regularly cleaned.
- Should be free from dust, insects and vermins, fluid and debris.
- Should be cool, dry away from sunlight.
- Storage shelves should be nonporous and easy-to-clean.
- Sterile goods should be stored in order of their date of expiry (fist in, first out FIFO method should be followed.
- Only items that are visibly dry must be removed wait till packages are cool before they are unloaded
- Store on wire mesh racks to allow for air circulation. Shelves should be 8 to 10 inches from the floor, at least 18 inches from the ceiling and at least 2 inches from the walls.
- Access to sterile storage area should be limited and separated from high-traffic areas.

Environment and Ventilation

- The air supply should be filtered by means of Hepa filters of 0.3 μ after filtering through a series of prefilters, free of dust and the rooms should be under positive pressure of minimum 0.1 mm of mercury level. There should be 10 or more air changes per hour.
- The temperature of the area should be controlled between 18 and 22°C.
- Relative humidity should be maintained between 35 and 50%.

Hygiene

- Personnel working in CSSD must follow good hand hygiene, wear appropriate attire like clean, fresh laundered clothes with cap. He must maintain a high level of hygiene including clean hair, body, nails and clothing. Hands should be washed with sanitizers frequently. Dedicated pair of shoes and shoe covers must be used. Finger nails should be short and no jewelery to be worn.
- It is important to maintain the sterility. Microbial contamination can take place due to improper handling, transport or storage. By controlling the environment and events that a sterile package is exposed to the probability of contamination can be minimized.
- Use wrapping material with better bacterial barrier properties.

SHELF LIFE[2]

- Depends on the quality of the wrapper.
- Also depends on storage conditions.
- Conditions during transport
  - Through dedicated lifts
  - Clean corridors.
- Amount of handling
  - Minimum handling.

EXPIRY DATE[2]

- Arrangement of sterile packs should be in sequence of their expiry date.
- Normally shelf life is given as follows:
  - Linen packed trays or sets 7 days.
  - Medical grade paper packing 1 month.
  - Non-woven packing material 3 months.
  - PVC peel pouch packing 1-2 years.

The above is a guideline and should be validated at site before implementation.

CHECKS BEFORE ISSUE[2]

Before issue packs must be observed for expiry date, dirt, puncture, evidence of moisture and compromised seals.

HOUSEKEEPING PRACTICES[2]

- Flooring should be cleaned at least once a day with mild detergents.
- Fogging should be done once a week.
- Air sampling should be done weekly to ensure that contamination is kept under check.
- Sterilizer panels, unloading trolleys, pass boxes should be part of the cleaning schedule.

- Shelves and racks should be cleaned with a disinfectant cum detergent weekly.
- A checklist can be prepared to facilitate total coverage.

TRANSPORTATION[2]

Transportation to and from sterile area must be done in covered or enclosed carts with solid bottom to prevent dirt from entering. The cart should be washed periodically and should be in good condition.

HANDLING[2]

- Minimum handling of sterile packs to be done.
- Any sterile items that fall on the floor or are wet must be considered contaminated and must be sent for reprocessing.

TRAINING OF STAFF AND STANDARD OPERATING PROTOCOLS[2]

- Staff must be trained not only theoretically, but also practically. They must be trained in the procedures of cleaning, disinfection and sterilization of equipment and surgical instrumentation. They must know to operate automated as well as mechanical equipment in processing areas.
- Approximate six months to one year of on job training experience with theoretical training by managers is necessary for an technician or a formal certificate in an approved CSSD course.
- Every department must have a manual, documented Standard Operating Procedures (SOP's) in the form of written policies.
- Also training ofaAdministrative aspects like inventory management, software applications, making check lists and making use of them at workplace, record keeping of process monitoring indicators are all important aspects which the CSSD personnel must be trained for.
- Lastly, human relation skills are mandatory for an CSSD employee.

REFERENCES

1. Central Sterile Supply Department (Amrita Institute of medical Sciences). Accessed from www.aimshospital.org/get-help/doctors/support-services/central-sterile-supply-department/ on Feb 2016.
2. Recommended guidelines for CSSD. Hospital Sterile Services Association (India). Executive Committee. PD Hinduja Hospital, Mumbai. Email:CSSD@hindujahospital.com. Setting Standards for Health Care, AIMS (Amrita Institute of Medical Sciences). Available at wwwcssd.mht accessed on 18/2/09.
3. Huys J. The Sterile Supply Cycle. http://wfhss.deconidi.ie/html/educ/sbasics/sbasics01_en.htm.Accessed in 2009 and 19th Feb 2016.
4. Huys J. Cleaning of equipment and materials to be sterilized. WFHSS. Accessed from http:// www.deconidi.ie/html/educ/sbasics/sbasics0102_en.htm. in 2009 and 19th Feb 2016.
5. Huys J. Packaging of Sterile Products. The Sterile Supply Cycle: Packaging http://www.deconidi.ie/html/educ/sbasics/sbasics0104_en.htm.Accessed in 2009 and 19th feb 2016.

Index

Page numbers followed by *f* refer to figure and *t* refer to table